VOID

Library of
Davidson College

Health and Health Care
Policies in Perspective

Preparation of this book was assisted by a
grant from The Robert Wood Johnson Foundation,
Princeton, New Jersey. The opinions, conclusions,
and proposals are those of the authors and
do not necessarily represent the views
of the Foundation.

Health and Health Care

Policies in Perspective

Anne R. Somers
Herman M. Somers

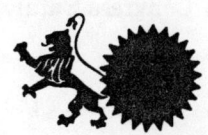

Aspen Systems Corporation
Germantown, Maryland
1977

Library of Congress Cataloging in Publication Data

Main entry under title:

Health and health care.

Includes index.
1. Medical policy—United States—Addresses, essays, lectures. 2. Medical care—United States—Addresses, essays, lectures. I. Somers, Anne Ramsay. II. Somers, Herman Miles, 1911—   [DNLM: 1. Community health services—United States—Collected works. 2. Delivery of health care—United States—Collected works. 3. Insurance, Health—United States—Collected works. W84 AA1 S65h]
RA395.A3H388   362.1'0973   77-76921
ISBN 0-912862-45-9

Copyright © 1977 by Aspen Systems Corporation

All rights reserved. This book, or parts thereof, may not be reproduced in any form or by any means, electronic or mechanical, including photocopy, recording, or any information storage and retrieval system now known or to be invented, without written permission from the publisher, except in the case of brief quotations embodied in critical articles or reviews. For information, address Aspen Systems Corporation, 20010 Century Boulevard, Germantown, Maryland 20767.

Library of Congress Catalog Card Number: 77-76921
ISBN 0-912862-45-9

Printed in the United States of America

To
Ward Darley
And
Franz J. Ingelfinger
Physicians, Scholars, Humanitarians, Exemplars
of Courage And Responsibility

Table of Contents

List of Tables xi

Preface xiii

Acknowledgments xvii

PROLOGUE—Medical Science: The Sorcerer's Apprentice? 1

    Selection 1—The Emergence of Scientific Medicine 3
    Selection 2—Grantsmanship and Stewardship: Federal Grants
                   Management in Biomedical Research 7

PART I—The Principal Actors and Some of Their Problems 17
    Selection 3—Who's in Charge Here?—Alice Searches for a King
                   in Mediland 17

Chapter One—The Physician and Other Health Professionals 21
    Selection 4—Dr. Smith and Dr. Jones: Two Portraits 21
    Selection 5—Professional Licensure: Is It Effective? 26
    Selection 6—The Development of Professional Performance
                   Standards 33
    Selection 7—Medical Education and The Community 38

Chapter Two—The Consumer-Patient 51
    Selection 8—Death and Disability Among American Workers 51
    Selection 9—The Fragmented Patient 56
    Selection 10—The Changing Doctor-Patient Relationship 60
    Selection 11—The Future of Demand: Some Influential Factors 76

Chapter Three—The Modern Hospital 85
    Selection 12—Bigger, Better, and Beleaguered 85
    Selection 13—The Rise in Hospital Use 92
    Selection 14—Those Who Ignore History 97
    Selection 15—Democratizing the Hospital 99
    Selection 16—The Rising Costs of Medical Care 100

**PART II—Assuring Access: Central Aim of Public Policy During the
               1950s and 1960s** 107

Chapter Four—Private Health Insurance 109
    Selection 17—A Mid-1950s Perspective: Some Definitions and
                   Problems 111

Selection 18—What Consumers Expect from the Blues 115
Selection 19—Comprehensive Prepayment Plans: The Original HMOs... 118
Selection 20—Self-Regulation: Can Voluntary Controls Work?..... 125
Selection 21—A Successful Past and Uncertain Future 130
Selection 22—Blue Shield: Special Problems, Special Remedies 136

Chapter Five—Public Programs..................................... 143
Selection 23—Workmen's Compensation: Medical Administration.. 145
Selection 24—Rehabilitation: The Trauma of Administrative and Professional Adjustment........................... 153
Selection 25—Medicare: Legislation and Administration—The Seamless Web 158
Selection 26—"Reasonable Costs" and "Reasonable Charges": Early Warning; Trouble Ahead 170
Selection 27—Medicaid: The Big Sleeper......................... 177
Selection 28—National Health Insurance: Story with a Past, Present, and Future 179
Selection 29—National Health Insurance: Criteria for an Effective Program and a Proposal........................... 192

Chapter Six—Rationalizing the Delivery System: Approaches to Comprehensive Care 205
Selection 30—The Hospital as Center of Community Health Services: A Proposed Model 206
Selection 31—The Franchised Hospital........................... 216
Selection 32—Alternative Models................................. 217
Selection 33—The Hospital Model in Action: A Lonely Experiment. 225
Selection 34—Redesigning the Delivery System: Unresolved Controversy 229

PART III—Inflation, Frustration, and the Search for New Policies .. 235

Chapter Seven—Regulation of Facilities: Moving Reluctantly Toward the Inevitable..................................... 239
Selection 35—Development of State Regulation.................... 241
Selection 36—The Philadelphia Medical Commons: The Choices Ahead.. 244
Selection 37—"Certificate-of-Need" versus the "Market" as Regulator... 255
Selection 38—The New Jersey Certificate-of-Need Experience.. .. 260

Chapter Eight—PSRO and Malpractice: Two Aspects of the Quality Quandry.. 277
Selection 39—PSRO: Friend or Foe?............................. 278

Selection 40—Public Accountability and Quality Protection in Ambulatory Care 281
Selection 41—The Malpractice Controversy and the Quality of Patient Care 288

Chapter Nine—Consumer Health Education: Revitalizing an Old Idea 307
Selection 42—A National Program of Consumer Health Education.. 309
Selection 43—Death Rates, Life Style, and National Morale: Two Proposals... 315
Selection 44—Health Education at Monmouth Medical Center: A Case Study 322
Selection 45—Consumer Health Education: Some Critical Questions 330

Chapter Ten—Some Special Problem Areas: Prevention, Violence, The Elderly 333
Selection 46—The Lifetime Health Monitoring Program 335
Selection 47—Violence, Television, and the Health of American Youth... 346
Selection 48—Homemaker Services: An Essential Option for the Elderly... 354

Chapter Eleven—Some Relevant Foreign Experience 363
Selection 49—The Rationalization of Health Services in Britain and Sweden 364
Selection 50—Geriatric Care in the United Kingdom: An American Perspective 377
Selection 51—Recharting National Health Priorities: A Canadian Perspective 391

PART IV—A Proposed Framework for Health and Health Care Policies 395

Chapter Twelve—Knowledge Development 401

Chapter Thirteen—The Environment 411

Chapter Fourteen—Individual Behavior and Life Style 419

Chapter Fifteen—Personal Health Services 427

EPILOGUE—Health Care, Technology, and the Political System: The Sorcerer's Apprentice Revisited 479

Appendix—Tables and Figure 491

Index 517

List of Tables and Figures

Table I — U.S. Death Rates: Crude; Age-Adjusted, by Sex and Race; and By Age. Selected Years, 1920-1975.................. 492

Table II — Life Expectancy at Birth: Selected Countries, Latest Available Period....................................... 493

Table III — U.S. Death Rates: Crude, Selected Causes, and Years, 1950-1975 494

Table IV — Health Manpower: Selected Occupations, Estimates, 1974   495

Table V — Doctor of Medicine: Total, Total Active, Primary Care - Potential, and Ratios to Population, Selected Years 1949-1975 496

Table VI — Community (Nonfederal Short Term) Hospitals, Selected Data and Years, 1950-1975............................. 498

Table VII — Nursing Homes: Selected Characteristics, 1964, 1969, and 1973-74... 500

Table VIII — Private Health Insurance: Estimated Percent of Population Covered, by Age and Specified Type of Care, Selected Years 1962-1974 502

Table IX — Private Health Insurance: Financial Experience, by Type of Carrier, Selected Years 1966-1974................... 504

Table X — Personal Health Expenditures[a]:Amount and Percentage Distribution, by Source of Funds, Selected FYs 1929-1976.   506

Table XI — National Health Expenditures: Aggregate and Per Capita Amounts and Percent of Gross National Product, Selected Fiscal Years 1929-1976................................ 507

Table XII — National Health Expenditures: Aggregate Amount and Percentage Distribution, by Type of Expenditure, Selected FYs 1929-1976 508

Table XIII — Public Programs: Expenditures for Health Services and Supplies, by Program, Type of Expenditure, and Source of Funds... 510

Table XIV — Consumer Prices and Medical Care Components, Average Annual Percentage Change, Selected Periods, 1950-1976, and Total Percentage Increases, 1965-1976.............. 515

Figure I — Proportion of Gross National Product Spent on Health Services, International Comparisons, 1960, 1969, and 1973 516

Preface

The spectacular development of health care during the past quarter century into one of the nation's largest and most pervasive industries has made it a major arena of public policy controversy. Its immense growth forced the rapid recruitment of tens of thousands of new personnel—not only physicians and others engaged in direct patient care, but also administrators, planners, educators, researchers, and regulators. The pressures of accelerating expansion soon immersed them in the day-to-day demands of decision making and action. Their impact on the lives of the public was large and direct.

Everywhere, educational institutions devised new, or augmented existing, curricula to train additional personnel to suit the occupational categories and the increasing number of jobs being created. The need for development and dissemination of expanded and better knowledge was quickly recognized. Great quantities of good research on specialized aspects of health care have been produced. Vast amounts of data now pour regularly from the presses. Indeed, the available information is far beyond the capacity of anyone to assimilate. Moreover, all these instructive bits and pieces do not necessarily add up to a whole picture. Even if they did, it would be a prodigious task to sort out the pieces and fit them together.

The resulting widely felt need for some convenient comprehensive view of the field as a whole, presented with historical perspective appropriate to its long traditions and special culture, has been strongly impressed upon us. We have had a steady flow of requests that we update *Doctors, Patients, and Health Insurance,* which made its appearance in 1961. This, a different type of book, has been written and assembled with the aim of partially meeting that need.

PLAN AND PURPOSE OF THE BOOK

The volume is divided into four parts with 13 chapters, in each of which are included several essays to which we refer as "selections." About one-third of the selections were written especially for this volume, although many of these have also been published in journals. For the balance, we turned to our own writings over the past 23 years. Through these "historical" selections, we hope to give the reader a sense of the evolutionary developments of the past quarter-century, not in hindsight but as viewed contemporaneously.

We believe it is important to view old and persistent problems not only as we see them today, but also as they appeared in earlier periods. This should contribute to a better appreciation of how we arrived where we are. The design of the book, therefore, requires the reader to note carefully the date of the original publication of each of the selections, which is recorded on each opening page. Each must be seen in contemporary perspective.

A straight chronological presentation would not yield the picture we were seeking of the interrelationships among this multifaceted set of problems and policies. Consequently, the book is organized along two overlapping lines—a cross-cutting mixture of the chronological and the thematic. The reader might find this dual approach confusing at times, but we hope not irritating. We have no desire to make the subject more complicated than it inherently is. But one of the fascinations and the aggravations of this field is its diversity, its disjunctions, and its complexity. To some degree, the organization of such a book must be affected by such phenomena. So must the reader's awareness. To paraphrase E.B. White, we predict a bright future for complexity!

Part I introduces the major private sector actors in the vast drama—the physician, the modern hospital, the consumer-patient—delineating their characteristics, roles, problems, and relationships. Most of these descriptions and appraisals were published before 1970. The reader will note that their essential elements remain valid today.

Part II moves into the historical development and controversies of health care programs in the 1950s and 1960s, as the nation moved to implement its then primary goal of assuring greater access to medical care. The role of private health insurance, the growth and variety of public programs, actual and proposed, and some prominent innovative approaches to improve delivery systems are all examined, including the continuing debate over national health insurance.

Part III deals with the disappointments and frustrations that followed the marred hope that opening wide the door of access would alone solve the problems of health care and health. The resulting burst of regulatory activity is described, and several chapters explore leads to potential new policies. A look at relevant foreign experience follows.

Part IV presents a framework for redesigning the nation's health policies and practices in recognition of the important changes that have taken place in health care, in society, and in our perceptions. Present policies are neither consonant with these changes nor in keeping with the increased sophistication the nation has acquired about the range and complexity of the problems that challenge us.

Several major themes run through most of the book, even when not explicitly identified. Among these are: the role of health care in the spectrum of forces determining health outcomes; its value and significance as symbol, surrogate, or vehicle for jobs and other human needs and aspirations; private and public sector relationships; the alleged "quality versus economy" conflict; the pervasive influence of science and new technologies versus rediscovery of the importance of individual responsibility for personal health.

The last is perhaps the overriding theme: Can we learn to enjoy the multitude of advantages from advancing technology without becoming passive captives of its powers and dictates? The metaphor of the Sorcerer's Apprentice has been part of the authors' lexicon, with mounting disquiet, since the early 1960s. The Prologue and Epilogue emphasize this concern.

Most of the selections have been published elsewhere; 21 before 1970. None has been rewritten or updated to take advantage of hindsight or more recent knowledge. We reiterate that this is deliberate because our purpose is to offer a view of "how it looked and felt at the time." Therefore, the reader must not only take note of the original date of publication but also understand that the data, analysis, and any recommendations were related to that period. It does not follow that differing positions taken over time are necessarily inconsistent. Where it seemed helpful, we have written explanatory introductions.

The original essays have, of necessity, been severely pruned. For the most part, references and footnotes that appeared in the originals are also omitted. However, the location of the original publication is identified for each selection, and the reader seeking specific documentation or amplification is referred to those sources.

* * *

The book has two authors who assume equal accountability for the product. Our views were not always identical; in fact, differences were sometimes substantial. But we believe these differences turned out to be an asset rather than a liability. They forced debate, further exploration, and reconciliation. In the complex field of health, dogmatism will not resolve many problems. Divergent views must be accommodated and resolution found. The process can be painful, but we commend it.

As many of our readers know, we have frequently been personally engaged in this living history as advocates and activists. But throughout we have always maintained a primary academic role. We trust this book reflects the honest objectivity that calling should imply.

Princeton, New Jersey A.R.S.
September 1977 H.M.S.

Acknowledgments

Since we have, in a sense, been writing this book for nearly 25 years, we have obviously accumulated a vast debt of gratitude, starting with the institutions with which we have been affiliated and their officers, who enabled us to devote the time and energy to this work: the College of Medicine and Dentistry of New Jersey, Princeton University, Haverford College, and The Brookings Institution; also The Robert Wood Johnson Foundation, which helped to finance the book.

We are also indebted to a large number of individuals—colleagues, friends, and strangers—who have provided the inspiration, insights, and technical assistance without which this ambitious project could not have been consummated. Many of their names appear in our previous works; we wish we could repeat them all again. Two, named in our dedication, must stand as surrogates for the others.

Finally, there would be no book had it not been for the sustained efforts and patience of a number of dedicated editorial assistants, secretaries, and students: Philippa Chapman, William Frist, Mary Hayden, Janet McElligott, Lorna Neuhaus, Thelma Shays, Laura Stabler, and Lois Walker.

We also wish to express appreciation to the journals and publishers identified at the opening of each selection for generous granting of permission to use material originally published by them.

Prologue

Medical Science: The Sorcerer's Apprentice?

Prologue

Medical Science: The Sorcerer's Apprentice?

Human beings have within reach the capacity to control or prevent human disease. Although this may seem an overly optimistic forecast, it is, in fact, a realistic, practical appraisal of the long-term future. The historical record of accomplishment to date, having plainly established that some of the most lethal, complex, and previously baffling human diseases can be eliminated (or at least held in check), seems to us a warrant for optimism.... There do not appear to be any impenetrable, incomprehensible diseases....

Report of the President's Biomedical Research Panel (1976)

Craving for Ambrosia [the divine potion which gave the gods unending life] has now spread to the common mortal. Scientific and political euphoria have combined to propagate the addiction. To sustain it a priesthood of Tantalus has organized itself, offering unlimited medical improvement in human health. The members of this guild pass themselves off as disciples of healing Aesculapius, while in fact they are pedlars of Ambrosia. The result of dependence on Ambrosia is Medical Nemesis.

Ivan Illich, *Medical Nemesis: The Expropriation of Health (1975)*

As America entered the last quarter of the twentieth century, following three decades of unprecedented expansion in medical care services—in volume and technical quality of care—many of the premises underlying national health policies were falling under increasing challenge. The major ongoing controversies of past and present—regarding methods of financing, strengthening delivery systems, quality protection, the appropriate role of government, etc.—were rooted in a context of commonly accepted assumptions as to the overriding importance of maximum access to ever-rising levels of scientific medicine and the central place of medical care in individual and national health.

By 1975 the consensus was breaking up. Views were segmenting in various gradations of rejection and defense of traditional assumptions. The conviction was growing that the Western societies' reliance on medical care had become excessive; that it was not, in fact, a primary determinant of health status, and that diversion of resources to more exotic high-technology procedures was socially wasteful.

Many members of the scientific community grew fearful that the growing revolt against medical care expansionism might carry over to a rejection of biomedical research, which had been a primary pillar of the traditional faith. Increasingly, the point was being emphasized that biomedical research served not only to improve the effectiveness of medical care, but also to eliminate previously baffling diseases and become a major source of prevention. The case for biomedical research was veering away from sole identification with medical care toward standing on its own.

While Ivan Illich's exaggerated polemics were generally discounted, the widespread attention paid to his thesis reflected real nagging questions disturbing an increasing number of scholars and policy makers: Had the obvious achievements of science and technology during the past century undermined the individual's responsibility for, and autonomy over, his own life and death? Did the relatively small improvement in health status attributable to medical care during the 1960s and early 1970s, despite tremendous increases in expenditures for medical care and, to a lesser degree, biomedical research, portend the approaching practical limits of scientific medicine? Have medical technology and biomedical research become ends in themselves, less concerned with human health and happiness than with elegant theories, challenging procedures, and jobs? Do the growing controversies over the ethics of medicated vegetative survival, as indicated in the notorious Karen Quinlan case, symbolize society's inability to control the technical processes which the scientists have let loose?

In short, has Western man become the Sorcerer's Apprentice, committing himself to medical policies that are no longer central to health, and may even be health-threatening? Or, do such questions represent merely the most recent examples of the skepticism and harrassment that have accompanied the advancement of science throughout history?

These are not idle academic questions. Assumptions as to the relevance of biomedical research, the prompt translation of research findings into higher medical care technologies, and the assurance of universal access to such care have constituted the underlying premises of health policies and activities not only in the United States but also in all the advanced industrial nations. The much publicized, but rapidly disappearing, distinctions in methods of financing between the United States and other Western nations tend to obscure the basic similarity in their health policies as opposed, for example, to that of China, which has consciously opted against high technology medicine and concentrated on the development of lower level health practitioners, broad public health measures, and individual responsibility.

These are questions that will have to be addressed with increasing rigor in the future as larger shares of our national resources are devoted to the official pursuit of health. They will surface from time to time throughout this volume, especially in Part III, where the frustrations and disappointments associated with existing programs and commitments become clearer. During the 1950s and early 1960s, however, where our story begins, such questions were almost totally absent.

The first selection, published in 1961, summarizes the long historic struggle for acceptance of scientific methodology as a basis for the understanding and treatment of disease. The second (1965) does not queston any of the basic assumptions underlying the need for extensive biomedical research but does note, with some concern, a number of disquieting effects.

Selection 1

The Emergence of Scientific Medicine*

When Galileo destroyed Aristotelian physics by his experiments at Pisa and Aristotelian astronomy by his discovery of a new star in a region of the heavens previously believed unchangeable, the scientific revolution had begun. In giving the world the first telescope and microscope, Galileo also made possible the indispensable techniques of scientific measurement.

A renewed interest in medicine and anatomy was part and parcel of this great intellectual and cultural revival. The artists Michelangelo, Raphael, and Dürer were among the first anatomists, and Leonardo da Vinci produced an anatomical notebook, based on extensive dissection, which flatly contradicted Galen. At the universities of Padua, Basle, and Bologna a few brave medical professors and students began to challenge ecclesiastical and scholastic authority and to revive the free inquiring spirit of Hippocrates.

The great names of the medical Renaissance—Vesalius, father of modern anatomy; Ambroise Paré, father of modern surgery; Paracelsus, whom Osler called "the Luther of Medicine, the very incarnation of revolt;" William Harvey, chief of staff at old St. Bartholomew's in London, who discovered the circulation of the blood; Malpighi of Bologna, who followed Harvey's lead by discovering the capillary blood vessels; van Leeuwenhoek, the Dutch draper and lens grinder, who constructed the first short-focal microscope and became the first man to penetrate the unknown world of microorganisms—these men launched modern medicine by shattering obsolete authority, by laying the foundation for an accurate knowledge of the structure of the human body, and by demonstrating how physiological functions could be studied intelligently.

---

*Excerpt from H.M. and A.R. Somers, *Doctors, Patients, and Health Insurance: The Organization and Financing of Medical Care* (Washington, D.C.: The Brookings Institution, 1961), pp.18-24.

From that time on, slowly and often painfully, the extension of knowledge in physics, mathematics, astronomy, chemistry, and biology and the development of scientific methodology and instruments capable of precise identification and measurement—even of unseen microorganisms and cells inside the living body—became part of the essential progress in medical science. Anatomy, physiology, pathology, histology, bacteriology, pharmacology, and anesthesiology (the first major American contribution to medical research) were developed before or during the nineteenth century, followed by biochemistry, biophysics, and even more specialized medical disciplines in the twentieth. The dependence of medicine on the basic sciences can hardly be exaggerated. . . .

SCIENTIFIC ADVANCE AND INSTITUTIONAL RESISTANCE

It would not have been possible for medical science to progress or even be meaningful apart from the total environment. Higher standards of living and of mass education, the acceleration of communication and transportation, industrialization, social organization, and the spread of humanism and democracy were all contributing forces. In one of Henry Sigerist's memorable phrases: "Nicotinic acid cures pellagra but a beefsteak prevents it." The causes of the "scientific revolution in medicine" are complex and interdependent. So are the results. Sooner or later, the new medical science had to be translated into medical practice.

This was no simple matter. At all stages, science and rationality have had to batter walls of resistance due to ignorance, inertia, and vested interests of mind and purse. The phenomenon is not peculiar to medicine. Socioeconomic institutions have been at odds with advancing science and technology in most human affairs throughout history. Science is inherently expansive. It spells disturbance to social arrangements attuned to an earlier technical setting. Science is a disinterested force, amoral, impersonal. It cuts across and violates traditional disciplines, respects no occupational and professional jurisdictions, and unsettles tradition. Resistance from, and conflict with, the custodians of the habitual and familiar often result in long periods of maladjustment.

Institutional resistance to change has long been characteristic of medical practice. Medical history is replete with persistent and costly obstruction to scientific innovation—on the part of doctors, patients, and society at large. The long standing public opposition to dissection, led originally by the medieval church with its inhibiting effect on medical research, is too well known to need recounting. Harvey correctly anticipated both professional and lay hostility to his theory of the circulation of the blood when he prefaced his account of it with these words:

> I not only fear injury to myself from the envy of a few, but I tremble lest I should have mankind at large for my enemies, so much doth wont and custom, that become as another nature, and doctrine once sown and that hath struck deep root, and respect for antiquity influence all men.

Later, he claimed that no man over 40 accepted his new theory. Moliere's picture of the foppish and pedantic court physician, immortalized in his *Malade Imaginaire,* while probably colored by his own tuberculosis (which no doctor of the time could cure) was one widely held by educated men of his day and contrasted all too obviously with the brilliant scientists of the seventeenth century. Blood-letting, purging, cupping, prescribing of all sorts of noisome and usually irrelevant medications, and a tremendous amount of quackery, within the medical profession as well as outside it, continued to dominate medical practice throughout the eighteenth and well into the nineteenth centuries.

Generations were required to overcome both the inertia and the active opposition to the germ theory of disease and the principle of antisepsis. Galen's second century assertion that pus in wounds was a natural condition, leading to healing, was challenged as early as the thirteenth.[1] The hostility of profession and populace alike to the necessity for surgical cleanliness, however, led to a 600-year delay before it was accepted. In the 1840s the same treatment was accorded Drs. Oliver Wendell Holmes in the Untied States and Ignaz Semmelweis in Vienna when, at about the same time but independently, they charged that obstetricians were unwitting vehicles for the transmission of puerperal fever in lying-in hospitals.

Louis Pasteur, father of modern germ theory, and Joseph Lister, developer of antiseptic surgery, were similarly mocked and opposed by the majority of their colleagues.[2] The controversy over germs and antisepsis shook the medical world of the 1860s and 1870s to its very foundations. One of Lister's German supporters felt so strongly on the subject that he advocated, in 1880, that any surgeon who ignored antiseptics and lost a patient through pyemia should be held guilty of malpractice. He, in turn, was vehemently reproached as a fanatic. One of his critics, a distinguished medical jurist, replied that "no medical jurist alive would reproach a practical surgeon who acted faithfully according to the teaching of the text books, recommended at the University, because a practical surgeon could neither buy all new books, nor ought he to allow his principles to be shaken by every new discovery."[3]

Within another generation the radical theory had become accepted doctrine. But the history of resistance repeated itself. Many who had been in the forefront of the fight for antisepsis were now resistant to the next improvement—asepsis. The new opposition stemmed not only from outmoded learning and wounded vanity but from resistance to the cost of establishing and maintaining an aseptic operating room, and a prescient foreboding of the enlarged role of the hospital vis-a-vis the individual surgeon.

Scientific advance is often long delayed but rarely is it permanently frustrated. Antisepsis and asepsis, as well as compulsory vaccination and most other public health measures, are modern medicine's tribute to the radical fighters for the once unpopular germ theory. Still the struggle for acceptance of new scientific findings goes on, albeit in changing context. The heirs of the Pasteurian rebels became the orthodox defenders of a mechanistic concept of disease, now widely challenged by a new school of medical thought growing out of psychiatry, endocrinology, and other comparatively recent specialties. With its emphasis on "the whole man" and "comprehensive care," this latest approach has in some ways more in common with the old Hippocratic ideal of physical, mental, and emotional balance, so well summarized in the Roman aphorism *"mens sana incorpore sano,"* than with the exclusive concentration on physiology characteristic of medical science in the sixteenth to nineteenth centuries.

Science has grown in power, and medical progress proceeds apace. From Pasteur's day to the present obscurantism has been declining, and science is being translated into practice at an accelerating rate. In contrast to the lonely isolation of earlier medical scientists and the widespread apathy or resistance to their findings, virtually the whole nation was leaning over the shoulder of Dr. Jonas Salk as he completed his research on polio vaccine. It is estimated that 90 percent of the drugs prescribed in 1960 were introduced in the previous two decades; 40 percent could not have been prescribed in 1954.

Because knowledge and skill are cumulative, their expansive force tends to grow geometrically. The accelerating pace of scientific developments, especially in recent decades, and their increasingly rapid translation into medical technology have taken on the character of a revolution. The results are writ large in the vital statistics of every land where the revolution has penetrated.

The triumph of the rational and naturalistic approach is still far from complete and may never be completed. The broadening of knowledge has opened up even vaster expanses of the unknown and the unexplained. The human psyche may also contain enduring barriers to the wholly rational. But despite significant lags, we have now entered an era wherein most Americans look on disease as a natural phenomenon and on medical practitioners as men with knowledge and skill to deal with such phenomena rather than with access to occult powers. The relative recency and the incompleteness of these developments have prevented their full potential impact on traditional medical institutions. But the dislocating influences of fast-moving science and technology are far-reaching and are, even now, major sources of current problems in the organization and financing of medical care as well as in individual therapy.

NOTES

1. The two precursors of modern antisepsis, Theodoric and Henri de Mandeville, had no idea of the role of germs but advocated simple cleanliness in surgery and dressing wounds by removing all foreign bodies, suturing the edges and covering with pads soaked in wine. The contempt of their colleagues led to abandonment of the radical proposal.

2. Despite the fact that he was finally elected to the French Academy of Medicine in 1873 (11 years after his election to the Academy of Sciences) Pasteur had to struggle for many more years to win his colleagues to the view that the doctrine of spontaneous generation was invalid. Most of the medical profession considered the germ theory a heresy, which had to be suppressed; while others, disposed to admit the results of Pasteur's researches as laboratory work, opposed his experimental incursions into clinical medicine. René Vallery-Radot, *The Life of Pasteur* (1924), Chaps. 8, 9.

3. R.J. Godlee, *Lord Lister* (1917), p. 340. This type of controversy was not confined to Europe. As late as 1894, Dr. Lawrence F. Flick, one of the first doctors in the United States to specialize in tuberculosis, was severely censured by his colleagues in the Philadelphia College of Physicians for insisting that TB was contagious and that protection of the public called for compulsory registration. Ella M.E. Flick, *Beloved Crusader—Lawrence F. Flick* (1944), p. 285.

Selection 2

Grantsmanship and Stewardship: Federal Grants Management in Biomedical Research*

Unlike the gradual development of most public programs in the health field, federal support for medical research mushroomed after World War II with a speed and impact not unlike that of the Manhattan Project's development of the atom bomb, which indirectly helped to inspire the medical research programs. And, like that other mushroom, the fallout was more varied and complex than originally appreciated.

Along with the brilliant achievements, a number of negative effects were discernable by the early 1960s. Among them: the sharp skewing of medical education and a generation of young doctors to a preponderant emphasis on biomedical research with a concomitant neglect of patient care; the fracturing of responsibility for educational policy and administration in universities and medical schools; appropriations in excess of the "state of the art" resulting in waste; and exacerbation of the town-gown conflict in medicine.

One aspect, the impact of grants management on medical schools as seen in 1965, is discussed in the following selection. In recognition of several of the problems here noted, some shifts in emphasis took place in the next decade. Particularly noteworthy was the creation of national centers for research.

Conflicts arising out of federal grants management go to the heart of some of the thorniest and most portentous problems of public policy. In addition to the

---

*Excerpt from A.R. and H.M. Somers, "Grantsmanship and Stewardship: A Public View," paper presented to American Public Health Association and the Association of Management in Public Health, October 7, 1964; published in *Public Health Reports* 80, no. 8 (August 1965): 660-669.

long standing, but far from settled, issues of federal-state-local government relations, management of federal grants involves the newly emerging relationship of the federal government to higher education, a relationship so important and so complex that it has been called "the new federalism." It involves the relationship of government to science and of government to health, the relationship of public and private activities—a perennial issue in American society and an area where we have demonstrated a talent for pragmatic and nondoctrinaire compromise. It involves the relationship of the administrative process to substantive purpose and the relationship of the specialized expert to the generalist, who is responsible, at least in theory, for both policy making and general administration....

Here we concentrate on medical and health-related research, especially the programs of the National Institutes of Health, which account for nearly two-thirds of total federal expenditures in this field and for three-fourths of sponsored research in United States medical schools. NIH programs, procedures, and problems set the tone for all medical research. They also shed light on the broad general issues. On the recipient side, we focus our discussion on the medical schools, nearly half of whose total budgets are now underwritten by federal programs.

From 1947 to 1963 federal support of medical research increased at an average annual rate of 26 percent. The year of maximum increase was 1962, a 33 percent rise over 1961. With such rapid growth, it is not surprising that problems and controversies should have grown along with the programs and achievements. Everyone who has followed the investigations, reports, and debates of the past few years knows how highly charged the issues are. At first glance, it may appear that there is virtually no meeting ground between the opposing camps, often oversimply and misleadingly represented as those primarily concerned with adequate administrative controls to assure efficiency and those primarily concerned with full freedom to maximize scientific output.

To isolate the real issues of conflict, it is useful first to identify briefly the large and significant areas of agreement among the various interested parties:

1. The propriety and legal authority for federal financial assistance to medical schools and other nonprofit institutions engaged in medical research is fully established in public approval, in law, and in precedent.

2. The increasing costs of medical research and its large role in the national welfare have made it both desirable and inescapable that the broad taxing power of the federal government be employed to assist the medical schools and other nonprofit institutions to carry out this mission.

3. Such essential assistance must be, and can be, carried on in an atmosphere of complete academic freedom and in a manner to strengthen, rather than weaken, the recipient institutions.

4. Large scale federal support of research in medical schools has brought about a creative new relationship between the federal government and medical education which has, thus far, helped to enhance academic medicine.

5. This creative new partnership has already resulted in dramatic progress in medical research with breath-taking implications for the conquest of disease.

6. Thanks primarily to the intimate relationship between medical research and personal health, widespread public support for the federal programs appears certain to continue, and congressional appropriations will undoubtedly remain at a high level.

7. Despite the striking achievements, in part because of them, there is agreement that numerous problems and difficulties exist with respect to the new governmental-medical school relationship. Some are related primarily to the great speed with which the programs were launched, but others are inherent in the sheer magnitude of the funds or in the special circumstances of governmental-medical relations.

8. As research manpower shortages and other inhibiting factors become more pressing, the federal programs will probably increase at a decelerating rate, in accordance with the trend since 1962. This deceleration will serve to underscore the urgent necessity for rigorous analysis of, and attacks on, these problems by all interested parties if the future of the programs and the new government-medical school partnership is not to be jeopardized.

These are the major areas of agreement. We now try to identify some of the principal problems and issues.*

PROJECT VERSUS INSTITUTIONAL GRANTS

The project grant is a unique product of recent governmental experience taken over from private foundations. It has been popular with granting agencies, grantee institutions, and the scientific community. Its advantages are manifold and well known, including emphasis on individual excellence, selection by peer judgment through the scientists' advisory system, avoidance of a fixed formula for distribution of funds among institutions, minimization of political pressures, both national and institutional, and complete bypassing of the church-state issue.

The disadvantages are, largely, the obverse of the above. It is alleged that the project grant militates against the young investigator, who may not be known to the advisory groups, and against the less distinguished institutions. According to one critic, "Peer judgment is an elegant way of maintaining the academic *status quo*."

Primary reliance on study sections, panels, boards, and councils set up by federal agencies may have resulted in bypassing, to some extent, the institutional deans, research committees, and department heads representing the normal framework of academic administration and thus may have impeded more

---

*Discussion of two of the more technical issues—grants versus contracts and cost-sharing—is omitted here.

rapid development of institutional responsibility. The project system may have intensified the already highly developed individualism of the medical scientist and his resitance to any coordinating authority, even in his own school or institution.

Whatever the relative merits of the two sets of arguments, the project system has dominated the American scene from the outset. Starting a few years ago, however, increasing concern with the need to complement the project system with a mechanism that would provide greater latitude of decision and greater responsibility to the recipient institutions led to development of a new type of grant, known as the "institutional" or "general research support" grant. Under a general authorization permitting up to 15 percent of total funds to be spent in this form, NIH appropriations for its support grants have doubled in the past three years to a current level of 5 percent of total expenditures.

During the recent past, both types of grants have been increasing. While the general support grant has been growing at a faster rate, the level is still far too small to threaten the older project system. Nevertheless, as the predicted decelerating curve in total expenditures becomes more noticeable and both institutional and individual appetites continue to grow, competition between the two types will probably become keener.

Hopefully, both will be continued. The faults of one are the virtues of the other. Interestingly, in Great Britain, where the institutional grant has been dominant, the Franks Commission, taking testimony on the organization of research and higher education, has recorded strong support for a project-type system. This testimony suggests that a mix is desirable—a mix that we have approached from the project side, and the British, from the institutional side.

To achieve an optimum balance, given our present tremendous emphasis on the project system, we suggest special attention to the institutional grant. In the words of Dr. Donald F. Hornig, director, Office of Science and Technology, Executive Office of the President:

> The government-university partnership is changing and the focus is shifting from specific items of research to a more general support of the scientific area in which the interdependence of research, education, and the university as an integral institution is increasingly recognized. I think this is an important development. While fostering the creative initative and independence of individual faculty members, it seems to me that the university must also be more than an anarchic collection of talented individuals and students. It needs a soul of its own so that the whole is greater than the sum of its parts.

Hornig's words obviously apply equally to medical schools. The extent to which the development of institutional grants achieves this purpose, however, will depend on the ability of the less distinguished schools to improve their capacity for research performance and on the ability of nearly all schools to strengthen their own mechanisms for formulation of research policy and for research administration.

INSTITUTIONAL RESEARCH ADMINISTRATION

On all the issues just discussed—grants versus contracts, cost sharing, and project versus general support grants—we have favored the position that seems most likely to lead to the long run strengthening of the medical schools. None of the dichotomies is clear cut. In some cases, the immediate advantage may appear in conflict with the long run advantage. But a general theme appears throughout the entire discussion. On the one hand, businesslike unambiguous contracts with the *quid pro quo* clearly spelled out and with resonsibility focused on well-established individual investigators, regardless of their institutional or geographic location, may well provide the formula for the most effective federal research programs in terms of the rapid development of scientific knowledge and the speediest possible application of that knowledge to the battle against disease.

On the other hand, the less specific grant and a large delegation of responsibility to grantee institutions would appear the better recipe for long run strengthening of these institutions. Even if this analysis is correct, however, the question arises as to whether public policy will tolerate for long any situation that fails to produce less than optimal results in a relatively short time. The closer we come to actual breakthroughs in any of the vital biomedical research areas, such as cancer, the more feverish will be public pressure for quick results regardless of the price in terms of the welfare of medical schools, medical education, or other less immediate considerations.

In the face of this predictably increasing pressure, the schools that survive as first-rate educational institutions may be those that have not only the courage and the financial wherewithal, but also a mechanism for saying "no" to inappropriate or unbalanced proposals, regardless of whether these proposals come from the government or from one of their own scientists or faculty members.

At present, many schools do not have such mechanisms. This is not a lack unique to medical schools; but it is more serious than in other educational institutions, partly because the schools are more dependent on federal funds than education in general, partly because the pressures for large scale exploitation of research findings in the medical field are so great, and partly because the medical schools are so frequently understaffed at the administrative or managerial level.

The Public Health Service is currently conducting a significant experimental pilot project in delegation of administrative authority to seven institutions. But the success of this project and the eventual delegation of greater administrative discretion to all grantee institutions depends primarily on the ability of these institutions to develop and to demonstrate efficient research management. Money is not the principal problem. Medical schools, despite their financial difficulties, are not poverty stricken. They do not operate on subsistence budgets. Their faculty salaries are higher than those in other branches of American education. Lack of administrative facilities and leadership is not primarily a matter of money but of academic tradition and, especially, the traditions of academic medicine, including the extreme individualism of the medical profession and the autonomy of faculty members, many of whom are unpaid or employed part-time.

Many institutions have no special administrative machinery for handling research grants and contracts. Where the machinery exists, it may be little more than a clerical office for processing grant applications and writing checks. Research committees, while probably more common, may operate in the most perfunctory manner or even on a log-rolling basis. The idea of a research director or dean saying "no" to a project grant that seems likely to have NIH approval or of calling an investigator on the mat for inadequate attention to a research commitment or for improper travel on federal funds is highly repugnant to all concerned.

At this point we wish only to emphasize the necessity for more sophisticated and higher level research administration if the creative new partnership between the federal government and the medical schools is not to slide into a general nationalization of science and medical education.*

What is the minimal organizational framework that will permit a school to be master of its own destiny in the exciting but difficult years that lie ahead? This is not the place to attempt a catalog of administrative details. In general, however, it seems that any such institution must be prepared to assume responsibility for the following:

1. Clear definition and statement of its own research goals and their relationship to its other missions, such as graduate and undergraduate education, patient care, and community service.

2. Adequate institutional arrangements at the top policy making level to assure periodic reassessment and reformulation of these goals and to assure that the accepted goals are actually carried out. In most cases this arrangement will take the form of a research committee, but it must be a committee that combines sufficient expertise, institutional power, and staff facilities to be meaningful.

3. Adequate institutional arrangements at the administrative level to implement the accepted goals and policies, providing, among other things, procedures and staff for meaningful review of project grant applications (both originals and renewals), for development of institutional grant applications,

---

* Robert Gilpin of Princeton University, in a letter to the authors dated May 14, 1965, has called our attention to "... an analogous situation which contributed to the decline of French science in the latter part of the 19th century. The centralization of the French university system by Napoleon, which contributed to the excellence of French science in the early 19th century, at the same time destroyed the individual universities as effective decision-making institutions. Also, in contrast to Germany, there was little institutional rivalry in France which would have stimulated the universities to recognize new fields of research. As a consequence the universities had neither the will nor the capacity of overriding the natural inclination of scientists to pursue established lines of research rather than to open new areas. I wonder whether the project grant system might not have the same weakness?"

and for processing of periodic reports; responsible handling and accounting of all financial matters pertaining to sponsored research; and the fixing of terms of employment of research personnel on an institutionwide basis.

Development of such an administrative framework would help strengthen the educational institutions not only vis-à-vis government but also to meet their own general goals. In the words of the director of the Syracuse University Research Institute:

> Without administrative controls, a program [of sponsored research] can develop in an amoeba-like fashion, rendering long-range institutional goals almost impossible to attain.... Regardless of centralized or nominally decentralized general plans of research administration, a single review and approval check point, at a level high enough to provide the overall view, is the best insurance against disruption of university functions and shattering of its objectives by the fiscal and physical burdens of sponsored research.

ACADEMIC FREEDOM

The principle of academic freedom, rightly cherished by academicians throughout the world, was hammered out of the sufferings of the Socrateses, the Galileos, the Thomas Mores, and countless other scientists and scholars who paid with their lives, their jobs, or their fortunes for the privilege of advancing human knowledge. Academic freedom is recognized today throughout most of the free world as a protection for the scholar or scientist against arbitrary dismissal or other disciplinary action resulting from his scholarly activities, particularly the publication of findings that may be at variance with generally accepted values.

Academic freedom was not conceived and cannot be defended as a cloak for irresponsibility, fiscal or otherwise. Indeed, the existence of academic freedom depends upon academic responsibility in the use of freedom. Misuse of the principle can only end by discrediting the principle itself and thus contribute to weakening the position of the scholar and scientist in a world that is still often unsympathetic.

There are occasional cases growing out of the massive federal research programs that really involve academic freedom. In a few instances, federal agencies have objected to publication of specific findings. The problem in work on classified research is inherently complicated. But, by and large, such difficulties have been held to a remarkable minimum.

To often the battle cry of academic freedom has been raised over questions that have nothing to do with scholarship or scientific findings, questions such as accounting for funds or work time. These are real problems that require thoughtful consideration and perhaps negotiation. But that is far from the equivalent of saying they represent a threat to academic freedom.

The overall implications for academic freedom of the federal research program have been brilliantly analyzed by Dr. Charles V. Kidd, former associate director of NIH and now technical assistant, Office of Science and Technology, Executive Office of the President. Kidd firmly rejects any allegation of general restriction on academic freedom:

> Outside research funds, including federal funds, have extended the freedom of both individual investigators and the universities.... Scientists would be less able to do what they wish, under circumstances congenial to them, if large amounts of money were not available for research.

Kidd does not discount the real problems; but these, he insists, are different from, and more subtle than, those usually argued. One of the most important is the sometimes divisive effect of outside research on the recipient institution: "The outside agencies affect the distribution of power within universities whether they wish to do so or not, simply by the fact that they give money to someone." He concludes:

> A university which has avoided, or overcome, the potentially divisive effects of outside research funds has established the most significant prerequisite to maintenance of freedom. The attainment of a consensus, widely shared among the faculty and administrative officers of a university, as to [its] central purposes... the boundaries of its functions, and the standards of excellence expected of faculty and students, is the prime condition for receipt of outside research funds upon terms set by the university. And by setting the terms of acceptance the university remains free.

MEDICAL RESEARCH AND EDUCATION

Medical research and medical education are inextricably interrelated. Each is essential to the other. Contributions of federal research programs to medical education have been dramatic. Faculties have been strengthened, curriculums enriched, promising graduate students supported, and facilities and specialized resources supplied.

Despite this impressive record, however, it is now generally acknowledged that the relationship between research and education no longer remains in that subtle but essential balance necessary to continued progress. One dramatic illustration of the growing imbalance is the lopsided rate of growth between the highly specialized research programs and the skilled manpower competent to carry them out. Referring to federal support for research in general, not just medical research, the House Select Committee on Government Research recently pointed out that, while the annual growth in federal research and development has averaged 15 percent, the number of persons capable of performing R&D has increased by only 7 percent. The disparity is considerably greater in the medical research field.

Such comparisons cannot, of course, be taken literally; there are too many inconsistencies. They do not allow for the increasing productivity of the scientists, nor for the tremendous increase in the cost of specialized equipment. But even without benefit of statistical precision, there is increasing agreement on the part of the interested agencies, the scientific community, and the medical profession, that medical education and the application of research findings to medical practice are falling behind.

Some say that the research programs should be cut back; no doubt this is one of the reasons for the current and probable future deceleration in research expenditures. However, we would maintain that the primary problem is not too much attention to medical research but too little attention to medical education.

Fortunately, and belatedly, a beginning has been made to remedy this situation. The trend toward institutional grants already noted, is a move in this direction. So is the increasing NIH support of individual faculty members with teaching responsibilities. Even more important is the passage of the Health Professions Educational Assistance Act of 1963. But all of these are severely hedged by restrictions. The NIH general support grants still amount to only 5 percent of total NIH expenditures. The Educational Assistance Act limits federal support to construction and an inadequate student loan program. But it will accomplish little to expand the physical plant for education of health personnel if the high costs of that education fall entirely on the inadequate resources of institutions and individual students. If there is to be real hope of achieving the educational objectives that presumably underlay Congressional approval of this new law, problems of operating support must also be faced.

Hopefully, the political deterrents to forthright support of medical education will continue to decline while the continuing triumphs of medical research will proclaim to the nation at large the desirability of further strengthening this creative partnership between the federal government and academic medicine.

Part I

The Principal Actors and Some of Their Problems

Part I

The Principal Actors and Some of Their Problems

Selection 3

**Who's in Charge Here?—
Alice Searches for a King
in Mediland***

"Where in the world am I?" said Alice. She opened her eyes to a strange surrealist landscape that looked a good deal like the inside of a modern hopsital, only more so. To one side, as far as her eyes could see, stretched row upon row of little cubicles with seemingly thousands of people lying in bed and thousands of others rushing in and out doing things for and to those in bed. The center of activity was a huge operating room, brilliantly lit, with many tables, all kinds of elaborate equipment, and long queues of waiting people, some lying on stretchers, others hovering over them, all dressed—or undressed—in white or green.

On the other side was a great mishmash of stores and booths and mail-order houses, selling pills, potions, and drugs of all shapes and colors, eyeglasses, crutches, false teeth, hearing aids, bandages, aphrodisiacs, anything and everything that people could be persuaded to buy in the pursuit of health.

In between the beds and the stores were throngs of people sitting and waiting, some in little clusters as in a doctor's office, and others in huge lobbies as big as railway stations. In the background Alice could see long rows of people sitting at desks like in an insurance company, taking in and giving out checks, while still others sat on a huge raised dais trying to watch—obviously without success—all that was going on below.

"What's your name and address, child? What are your symptoms?" A woman in a white uniform shook Alice to wake her.

"My name is Alice. I haven't any symptoms. I'm not sick. I just don't know where I am."

"No symptoms?" the woman exclaimed in annoyance. "You must have! Everybody has. We'll send you to the multiphasic screening unit immediately.

---

*Excerpt from A.R. Somers in *New England Journal of Medicine* 287, (October 1972): 849-855.

The computer will find some symptoms. This is Mediland. Everybody here is either a consumer of medical care, or a provider, or a third party. You've got to be one or the other."

"But I don't want to be one or the other. I just want to go home," said Alice. "Please tell me how I can get out of here."

"You can't get out without a medical discharge, and since you don't yet have a diagnosis, you can't get a discharge. Imagine what the Utilization Review Committee would say to that! Anyway, Dr. Medipsyche will want to see you. You obviously have some serious negative hang-up about the value of medical care."

"Please," said Alice, "I have to get home. My mother will be very angry. Please take me to your king. Kings can do anything."

"King?" the woman snorted. "We haven't any king! Now someday we might have a queen. ..."

Alice started to cry when a deep voice interrupted.

"Rubbish, Miss Meddingale! You forget your place! Mediland may not be a monarchy. But when it comes to making important decisions, like who can be discharged or the size of the budget, I, Dr. Mediknife, am king!"

Alice looked up to see a large pair of hornrimmed spectacles peering at her between a surgical cap and mask. She was a little frightened, especially of the scalpel that Dr. Mediknife was waving under Miss Meddingale's nose. But she was so relieved to find someone who seemed to be in charge that she jumped up and started to curtsy when another man in a white coat came over.

"Silly child!" he said to Alice, ignoring Dr. Mediknife. "Don't take him so seriously. He talks big; but if you have a problem, I, Dr. Medicine, am the only one who can diagnose it. Follow me to my office at once."

Although Alice was confused, she was so anxious to find someone in charge that she immediately started to follow Dr. Medicine. But just then another man, in a business suit, stopped them both.

"I'm Mr. Mediplan," he said firmly to Alice. "Let me see your Medicard."

"Medicard? I haven't any Medicard. And I'm not sick. I just want to go home. I thought Dr. Medicine could help me."

"He can't even talk to you unless you have a Medicard."

Alice looked at Dr. Medicine, expecting him to object. But he didn't.

"I'm afraid that's right, child. You see we doctors are all paid by a plan. There's Medicare, and Medicaid, and Medishield, and Medihip, and so on. Unless you have a card from one of these, I can't get any medibucks for seeing you."

Alice was about to remonstrate that she hadn't really asked to see him when suddenly there was a big commotion. The nurses and attendants who were taking care of people in beds began to leave and started streaming out carrying union signs. Most went in the direction of two men sitting behind large desks, writing out cards and taking in medibucks. All the people around Alice—Miss Meddingale, Dr. Mediknife, Dr. Medicine, Mr. Mediplan—looked very angry but seemed helpless to do anything.

"Maybe I should go talk to one of those men," Alice thought to herself. "Maybe they are the ones in charge here."

But just as she started to join the crowds moving toward the two men, they both got up from their desks and started to fight each other.

"There go Vic and Leon again!" Mr. Mediplan chuckled. "We don't have to worry about them for a while."

At this point Alice gave up all hope of finding someone in charge who could help her and started to run, blindly. She was crying so hard now that she didn't notice she had run into another crowd of people listening to a handsome young man on a soapbox.

"My fellow citizens," he was saying, "I know you can't get good medical care. I know the plans you have now are no good. But I have a plan that will solve your problems. Vote for my plan and you'll get the best medical care in all of Mediland!"

"Hooray for Senator Kennymed!" shouted the people. "Hooray!"

An older man walked up to the soapbox and with one brush of his hand knocked Senator Kennymed off the stand.

"That's Representative Medimills," Alice heard someone whisper. "He's head of the Means and Ways Committee."

"My fellow citizens," Congressman Medimills said in a soft Southern drawl, "My distinguished colleague from the Senate forgets that any new mediplan must originate in my committee. When it comes to any new health plan, I am in charge."

"That's what you think, Congressman! Just wait until the plan becomes law!"

Alice looked up to the raised dais to see a large disembodied grin that reminded her of her old friend, the Cheshire cat.

"I'm a medicrat," the unctuous voice continued. "I administer the laws. I have the final say. Obviously, I'm in charge here."

But Alice was now beyond believing anything.

"I don't think you have a king at all! I don't think anybody's in charge! Is that any way to run a country?"

NO VILLAINS! NO FÜHRERS!

No wonder Alice was confused. It is not any way to run a country. But then Mediland isn't really a country. Of course, it is far bigger than most real countries. . . .

But despite its size, its complexity, and its life-or-death importance, no one really is in charge. Like Topsy, the United States health services industry "just growed"—without benefit of any conscious design or direction. Although this might be said of most industries in a nonsocialist economy, there is a difference, at least of degree. It would be hard to find another major United States industry (with the possible exception of organized crime) that has not had to submit to the discipline either of the marketplace or of public regulation. The result—uncontrolled growth and pluralism verging on anarchy—should not be surprising.

By the same token, the "massive crisis" referred to by President Richard Nixon in July 1969 cannot be attributed to any one factor—doctors, hospitals, the pharmaceutical industry, third party carriers, the government, unions, or patients. In the complex scientific, demographic, and economic calculus that has led to the current situation, all parties have played a part. All have contributed to the problem.

This does not mean that any are villains. The patient demanding the latest miracle drug or miracle surgery (to the neglect of routine diet and exercise), the medical specialist concentrating on one small orifice or area of the body (to the neglect of the whole man), the hospital seeking to meet all the complex and contradictory demands put upon it (to the neglect of rational organization and economy), the insurance carrier seeking to meet the buyer's most insistent demand for hospitalization benefits (to the neglect of ambulatory care), the politician uncritically espousing one legislative panacea after another, all are responding to the technological revolution in medicine and the popular revolution of rising expectations, each in his own way, each betraying his own humanity, which means a mixture of strength and weakness, good and bad.

If there are no villains in Mediland, neither are there many heroes. Of course, there are hundreds of thousands of heroic men and woman who are working long hours, often under difficult conditions and often with poor pay, to fulfill the obligations, as much of their own consciences as of any external authority. These are the true unsung heroes, and without them the whole industry would have collapsed long ago. But there are unlikely to be any great leaders on white horses—whether doctors, or politicians, or labor leaders—who will appear on the horizon to lead us to the promised land. Although this may be disappointing to a TV generation that likes to view all life as a series of confrontations between the goodies and the baddies, it is hardly surprising to anyone who takes the trouble to think about the nature of health and disease, the complexity of modern medical care, and the intricate professional and institutional structure needed to provide that care.

Where does all this leave us? As confused as Alice in a world of incredible cost and complexity but lacking villains we can blame for our problems, or führers we can turn to for deliverance? Possibly. But I prefer to think it strips away some of the nonsense we have been fed during the past few years and helps us to see the future—without illusions, without wishful thinking, without intellectual or emotional crutches to lean on, but with faith in the essential reasonableness and decency not only of our own fellow men but of ourselves, without any guarantees of either success or failure for our efforts. . . .

Chapter One

The Physician and Other Health Professionals

Selection 4

Dr. Smith and Dr. Jones:
Two Portraits*

In the process of accommodation to new and shifting technological and organizational imperatives, the medical profession was divided between those who were in the mainstream of the new trends, or could readily adjust, and those who resisted or found it too difficult or too late to change. Selection 4 (1962) presents the schism in terms of the human problems of individual physicians. It is perhaps noteworthy that the frustrations attributed to Dr. Smith appear to be the same that have since become commonly identified with the post-Medicare era. The painful consequences, for some, of rapid change and instability have been visible ever since World War II.

The strong differences of views and interests within the American medical profession are a sign of vitality. If there were no such differences, it would mean a static profession, whereas we know that the science and technology of medicine are dynamic in the extreme.

Many of these differences—including those between medical educators and the practicing profession—have been kept under wraps as if they were something to be ashamed of. Up to a point this is sensible. Family quarrels should be settled in private. But when the issues go beyond the family and involve public welfare, the latter is far better served by full disclosure and open debate.

The conflicts involve questions of salaried versus fee-for-service remuneration, full-time versus part-time educators, solo versus group practice, general practice versus specialism, closed versus open hospitals, quality controls, attitudes toward research and education, the role of government in medical affairs, and a whole host of related issues that go to the heart of the existing

---

*Excerpt from A.R. Somers, "Conflict, Accommodation, and Progress: Some Socioeconomic O' servations on Medical Education and the Practicing Profession," paper presented to Association of American Medical Colleges, Tenth Teaching Institute, 1962; published in *Journal of Medical Education* 38 (June 1963): 466-479, and 40 (January 1965): Part 2, pp. 258-272; condensed in *Medical Economics* 42 (April 19, 1965): 215 *ff.*

organization of medical care in the United States. The issues are partly economic, partly political, partly sociological, partly philosophical. Some might add ethical, but I prefer not to do so. I do not think these conflicts have much to do with moral values. There are good people and honest people on both sides.

Let's take a look at two of the principal protagonists in this fascinating drama: the medical educator and the practicing physician. I'm aware of oversimplification in the picture I'm about to present. For example, some of the most brilliant and open-minded doctors I have known have been older men, and some of the most tradition-bound have just emerged from medical school.

Start with Dr. Smith. This hard-working and conscientious general practitioner is 55. He graduated from medical school in 1932—when a hospital bed cost $3 to $5 a day and before penicillin, sulfa, and most of the drugs now in common use had been discovered.

It was also the depth of the greatest depression this country has ever known. Dr. Smith had wanted to be a surgeon, but his family could not afford the extra graduate work. He already owed $4,000 to various relatives and the father of his fiancee, and he had postponed his marriage for three years. So, after a year's internship in a community hospital, he borrowed the additional money necessary to set up an office, married and hung out his shingle as a general practitioner in his home town, a typical midwestern community.

When the war started, Dr. Smith was 35. Because of his age, his three children and the nature of his practice, his draft board decided that he was needed more at home than in service. He was one of a handful of doctors left to serve the entire community. Always a hard worker, he took on the extra load cheerfully, worked a 60 hour week, sometimes more, took few weekends, no holidays. His practice trebled; so did his income. The chief victim was his leisure and all that this much-abused word implies: leisure for recreation and relaxation, leisure to read and to think, leisure to visit and talk with people from different professions and with different interests, leisure to savor the life of the mind.

Even after the war was over, Dr. Smith never gave up his highly disciplined work schedule. Nor could he bring himself to give up solo practice and join a partnership or a group. Always individualistic and increasingly so as he grew older, the very thought of adjusting to a group made him uneasy. At 50 he cut down to 50 hours a week, taking off Saturday and Thursday afternoons. But by then, work had become a fixed habit, almost an addiction. He was not really happy away from it. He had virtually no other interests in life.

Dr. Smith is a member of the American Academy of General Practice and, with some grumbling, meets its minimum requirements of postgraduate work. But his heart is not really in the lectures or conferences. He complains that they are often too academic to be of much practical value. Although he readily acknowledges his debt to medical research, especially in the area of chemotherapy, he has no personal commitment to research. Since he already feels overwhelmed by the existing amount of medical knowledge, he is understandably less than avid about the continuing search for more and more new knowledge.

Dr. Smith is affiliated with a community hospital and takes many patients there. He is dependent on the house staff and fumes at the lack of sufficient interns. He is also dependent on the hospital's diagnostic services and on the drug companies' detail men—a dependency he hates to admit even to himself. A psychiatrist might say that this sense of dependency, of inadequacy in a rapidly changing world and profession, is the basic source of Dr. Smith's frustrations, especially his resentment toward the nearby medical school with its research orientation. But Dr. Smith himself has little time or inclination for self-recrimination. The next patient is always waiting.

Naturally, he has made a good deal of money—at least a good deal has passed through his hands. For a man with a good income, he may appear inordinately preoccupied with money—a fact that could stem from his heavy indebtedness when he first started practice. On the average, he grosses about $50,000 a year. Professional expenses cut the net to about $30,000. Federal income taxes take another $7,000. Lacking Social Security or any fringe benefits that would be available to a salaried doctor, he feels that he has to invest about $5,000 a year in retirement and insurance protection for his family. This leaves only about $18,000 in disposable income. Although this sounds adequate, he's found the going rough in recent years with three sons to put through college.

Dr. Smith worries a good deal about his children, partly because he sees so little of them. He worries about money and taxes and the national debt and "socialized medicine." Although his definition of the last item includes almost any type of medical practice that's unfamiliar, somehow government has become identified with all his myriad frustrations. He lashes out against it constantly.

If it's not government, it's Blue Cross, some insurance company, the hospital, a labor union, or the medical school that's expanding its clinical services and that he fears will attract some of his patients. It's always something big, impersonal, and apparently out to "get" him—not only his money but, as he sees it, his independence, his freedom, his very way of life.

Dr. Smith particularly dislikes the frequent discussions in the lay press over various forms of medical care and medical economics (although he reads avidly a certain journal by that name). Somehow these developments suggest that medicine is passing out of the hands of doctors into those of laymen. He is equally annoyed at some of the new full-time professors at the medical school, whom he holds responsible for the expansion of its services and for giving aid and comfort to the enemies of organized medicine who would like, as he sees the situation, to undermine the private practice of medicine.

During World War II, when there were few doctors left in the community, Dr. Smith was virtually drafted to hold office in his county medical society. He is now a trustee. He'd like to be more active but feels he cannot take the time to get involved in any specialized activities. He's never delivered a scientific paper at any professional meeting. In recent years, however, he's taken to attending the annual meeting of the AMA, partly because his wife enjoys the trip and it's at least partially tax-exempt. With little time for outside reading or community affairs, Dr. Smith finds that the AMA expresses quite accurately his worries, his frustrations, and his fears. He is a loyal member.

Now let's look at Dr. Jones. He is 43, only 12 years younger than Dr. Smith; but those 12 years were crucial. Thanks to wartime acceleration, Dr. Jones graduated from medical school in three years, married, rushed through his internship in nine months, and into the war and the most challenging practice that a young would-be surgeon could dream of. After the war, the GI Bill of Rights financed his remaining graduate work at a first-rate medical college—financed it in genteel poverty, it's true, but still it got him through. He served his residency at a famous eastern teaching hospital and became a board-certified surgeon at virtually no direct cost to himself or his family.

Personable and able, Dr. Jones soon became a member of the inside group at his school and was asked to stay on as a full-time faculty member, dividing his time among teaching, research, and patient care. The working conditions were superb. The university hospital was fully equipped with diagnostic and therapeutic aids. It provided him a private office at very reasonable rent. The capital investment necessary to furnish it was minimal, for the hospital itself is his real workshop, and the operating rooms are only ten minutes away.

Dr. Jones' salary is relatively modest by comparison with the earnings of outside surgeons. As a professor of surgery, he earns $25,000 a year. But he supplements this by another $20,000 in private practice.

With his academic reputation, Dr. Jones can easily attract the carriage trade. And, significantly, over two-thirds of his fees come from Blue Shield and other third parties. His professional expenses are far less than they would be on the outside. With a total pretax net income—academic salary plus practice net earnings—of about $40,000, his taxes are much higher than Dr. Smith's—around $12,000. But being eligible for Social Security and other fringe benefits, he feels that $2,500 a year is enough to invest in insurance and retirement. His disposable income is $25,000—$7,500 higher than Dr. Smith's.

I have taken no account of income other than professional, a factor that might well alter the picture. Nor have I considered the trend toward pooling of outside income in many medical schools, a trend that might affect Dr. Jones' total earnings to some extent. These omissions are not really important, however. What I am trying to show is that the American academic doctor, in material rewards as well as in status, is far from the unworldly, underpaid egghead claimed by some of his detractors. On the contrary, he's clearly acquiring many of the outward symbols of success that have long distinguished the European academic and have made the title of professor even more prestigious than that of doctor.

Like Dr. Smith, Dr. Jones is conscientious and hardworking. He puts in about the same number of working hours, but there's much greater professional variety in his work. Much of his time is spent in teaching, reading, conferences, and research. As part of a surgical group, with colleagues to cover for him when he is away, he is able to organize his work to provide for numerous professional meetings, a good summer vacation, and occasional weekends. Unlike Dr. Smith, Dr. Jones' work brings him frequently into contact with other professions and occupations. He does more outside reading and is better informed on national and world affairs. Having more time to spend with his children and being more relaxed himself, he worries less about them. He is, in short, a reasonably well-rounded, satisfied man.

In the last year or two, he has begun to worry about money—not his own, but the medical school's and the hospital's. Recently, there has been more and more talk in staff meetings about the size of the hospital deficit. A few months ago he was appointed to a joint staff-board committee to study this deficit. He plunged into a confusing mass of economic and financial data involving Blue Cross, Blue Shield, labor organizations, foundations, government, and so forth.

The image Dr. Jones formed of this complex world of medical care was quite different from Dr. Smith's. True, these lay organizations were frequently uninformed on purely medical matters. But they readily acknowledged this fact and deferred completely to the doctors in this respect. Their knowledge of socioeconomic data and statistical and actuarial techniques was clearly relevant. And they commanded sources of money, both private and governmental—money that his school and his hospital badly needed.

Dr. Jones remembers his own years in the army, his GI grants, his numerous NIH and foundation funds. He is well aware that the major portion of his practice income reaches him via third parties. He is confident of his own ability and has no doubt that he can hold his own in this complex new financial world. After all, the medical world he moves in is just as complicated as that of government or of health insurance. Indeed, somewhat to his own surprise, he has begun to find himself in occasional alignment with the lay groups and in opposition to the position taken by organized medicine. There have been some recent sharp disagreements over the reorganization of the school's clinical services and the operation of the intern-matching program in Dr. Jones' community.

As a surgeon, he has more contact with the local practitioners than some of his colleagues, especially those in the basic sciences. He is not unaware of the growing hostility to the medical school and personally shares some of the objections to its increasing research orientation. He often tells himself that something should be done about this rising town-and-gown antagonism. But his future is so clearly tied up with the school, and its financing is so dependent on research grants, that he hesitates to buck the dominant trend.

With respect to the AMA, Dr. Jones is thoroughly ambivalent. He respects the work of the Council on Medical Education and a number of other special groups. He has delivered an occasional paper at the scientific sessions of the annual AMA meeting. As to its general politics, however, he feels a growing sense of annoyance and embarrassment, tempered by a kind of detached amusement.

Nevertheless, Dr. Jones continues to pay his AMA dues regularly. Sometimes he feels he should resign in protest, but he hasn't. The issues never seem to be clear-cut, and the thought of initiating a public political debate is highly repugnant. He wishes that academic medicine were more adequately represented in such debates, but again he feels that he can spare neither the time nor the energy to take on any such crusades.

In this brief portrayal of Drs. Smith and Jones, I have tried to show two average men, neither heroes nor villains, but basically good, honest, and capable men tied together by the common bonds of a difficult and exacting profession, who now find themselves in reluctant conflict as a result of circumstances over which they have had little control. A novel could be written about this situation. The likelihood of suffering and even tragedy is considerable, but so is the potential for human growth and greatness.

But I'm no novelist, and this basically is not fiction. We are dealing here with a real-life conflict, one that's of utmost importance not only to the 230,000 doctors of this country but to their 185 million patients and, indeed, to the national welfare. The basic issue—the one that underlies all the others—is the future structure of medical practice in the United States.

What is it that is pushing Dr. Smith aside and propelling Dr. Jones to the center of the medical world? It is not government or labor or the Health Insurance Plan of Greater New York or Henry Kaiser or John L. Lewis. It's two things. First, and most important, it's medicine itself—the triumph of scientific medicine and its handmaiden, medical technology. The force that Dr. Smith is lashing out against, with such frustration, is the centripetal force of modern medical technology. The doctor who resists this force does so at the expense of his own technical competence. The second basic factor is the changing patient. He's a product of the new technological society—a better-educated, less fearful and far less dependent individual than he was even thirty years ago, when Dr. Smith graduated from medical school.

As a result of these two forces, each year the center of gravity of medical practice moves closer to the hospital, the medical school, or the organized group—in short, to institutional medicine. ...

Selection 5

Professional Licensure: Is It Effective?*

The many complex issues in medical, nursing, and allied health licensure have become even more controversial than they were in 1969, when this selection was first published. Some progress has been made. Spurred in part by the malpractice furor, by the end of 1976 at least 15 states had mandatory "continuing education" requirements for physicians in various stages of implementation. A number of states have broadened or strengthened the responsibilities

---

*Excerpt from A.R. Somers, *Hospital Regulation: The Dilemma of Public Policy* (Princeton, N.J.: Industrial Relations Section, Princeton University, 1969), pp. 81-93.

and powers of medical licensing boards (Selection 41). Despite such improvements, the essential problems, as then identified, remain unsolved: (1) Are personnel licensing laws adequate for consumer protection? (2) What effect do these laws have on institutional productivity and effectiveness?

PROTECTION OF CONSUMERS

In theory, the licensure laws protect the quality of health care in several ways: (1) by elevating standards of education through the requirement that candidates for licensure must have completed specified courses and curricula; (2) by requiring every candidate who wishes to practice in a given jurisdiction to obtain a license and, in order to obtain such a license, to pass an examination administered by a state board of examiners; and (3) by providing for the suspension or revocation of licenses under certain circumstances.

There is a wide gap between theory and practice, however, and the licensing laws are increasingly criticized as inadequate. Following are major points of criticism, particularly with reference to medical licensing:

1. *Rather than elevating standards of professional education, outmoded laws are now constraining educational innovation.* Dr. E.H. Forgotson, physician, lawyer, and authority on licensing, comments on this point:

> In the case of medicine, many specific statutory curricular requirements were prescribed in the pre-Flexner era to give physicians some exposure to certain pre-clinical and clinical subjects. Most specific requirements, however, were the product of implementation of the recommendations of the Flexner Report and were designed to close down or improve inadequate medical schools, diploma mills, and commercialized educational programs. However, these problems have long since been resolved and other problems such as requirements for curricular innovation in subjects ranging from medical genetics to community medicine have arisen while the statutes have been neither modified substantively nor given flexibility to respond to changing requirements by administrative rather than legislative revision.
>
> It should be noted also that there are no requirements for continuous coordinated education of allied and auxiliary health personnel with physicians and dentists. Such a requirement could elevate the qualifications of allied and auxiliary personnel and of the physicians and dentists who work with them. Such innovations need to be tried.
>
> Similarly, the statutory requirements for licensure of physicians in over 30 jurisdictions, specifying the internship as a separate entity rather than as part of a program of graduate medical education, can operate as a barrier to innovation in graduate medical education and more effective coordination of undergraduate and graduate medical education.

2. *One-time, lifetime licensure is grossly inadequate for many professions in this day of rapid progress in scientific medicine.*

Licensure laws evolved at a time when the amount of knowledge relevant to delivery of personal health care was clearly finite. These laws were enacted before the technological and information explosion which began in the late 1930's.... Laws did not recognize that development of new information would render a person's initial qualifications to practice obsolete unless they were upgraded periodically by a program of continuing education. The laws relating to medicine, dentistry, professional and practical nursing, and physical therapy have no requirements relevant to prevention of educational obsolescence through mandatory continuing education programs.

3. *Most medical licensing laws are too weak or too vague with respect to discipline and are particularly inadequate with respect to professional competence.* The principal ground for discipline is "unprofessional conduct" or some equivalent phrase. Generally included under this broad rubric are such specifics as criminal abortion, conviction of a crime involving moral turpitude, violation of narcotics laws, drug addiction, mental disability, fee-splitting, advertising, etc. Only a handful of states—South Dakota, Connecticut, Hawaii, Iowa, and Louisiana—specify incompetence as a basis for disciplinary action.

Horace Hansen, general counsel, Group Health Association of America, has criticized this situation as follows:

This means, for example, that a doctor of medicine could practice for 40 years without ever making any effort to keep abreast of advances in the science of medicine, and never expose himself to any form of discipline. In such cases, his lack of competency becomes more marked with the passage of time, with the result that his patients suffer unknowingly.... Such incompetence may constitute a worse form of malpractice than the deliberate use of doubtful technique....

The fact that current medical licensure acts are not serving effectively to protect the public is indicated from the type of complaints made against doctors to medical societies. The report of the AMA Medical Disciplinary Committee includes the results of questionnaires sent to medical societies throughout the country. In answer to the question, "What are the complaints in order of their greatest number?" the resumé by the Committee, of the answers received, reads, "Complaints about the size of fees are by far the most frequent received by medical societies. Next in order of frequency are the complaints of medical incompetence or the quality of care received. Closely following this are problems of narcotic addiction, complaints about unnecessary surgery, then problems of alcoholism and advertising."

When the first two largest categories of complaints are laid up against the grounds for discipline stated in the medical licensure acts currently in effect in this country, there is a notable lack of any tools to deal with such complaints. The proof of this may be shown in the same report. In a questionnaire to state licensing and disciplinary boards, the question was asked, "What are the causes usually involved in medical disciplinary cases?" The answers to this question: "In order of frequency mentioned, causes are narcotic addiction, alcoholism, mental incompetence, income tax evasion, abortion, falsifying insurance claims, aiding unlicensed persons to practice, and conviction of a crime involving moral turpitude." No mention is made of any cases involving "medical incompetence or the quality of care received," the second largest category of complaints made to medical societies throughout the country.

Even where incompetence is specified in the law as a basis for disciplinary action, disciplinary procedures in nearly all the states are so weak and so weighted in favor of the doctor that effective action is virtually impossible. In all but six states—Delaware, Illinois, Louisiana, Maine, Nebraska, Rhode Island—and the District of Columbia, the disciplinary bodies are controlled by the practitioners. The typical pattern is for the disciplinary board to be named by the governor from nominees submitted to him by the state medical society. In the seven states listed, disciplinary control has been assigned to the courts or some other public body.

Moreover, in most states, discipline is permissive, not mandatory. The word "may" is generally used instead of "shall" in connection with the statutory powers and duty of the board. In such cases, the board may fail to process complaints as it pleases, without any recourse or right of redress by the complainants or the public. Even assuming that a complaint is processed through the investigation, the hearing, and a determination that the stated offense has been committed, there is still no requirement that the board must suspend or revoke the license, or, in fact, do anything more than quietly reprimand the offending physician.

Hansen concluded this section of his study with these words:

> Consumers of medical services would do well to consider amending all medical license acts to make sure that lack of professional ability or competence is a ground for disciplinary action, and that procedures are provided whereby such a ground, properly and specifically defined, is effectively enforced.

The Hansen report failed to attract much attention, but the examples of malpractice and ineffective licensing continue to accumulate, and hopefully the complacency of both public and profession is being shaken. Two 1968 cases, while far from representative, illustrate the need for effective quality controls and the failure of licensing, as presently constituted, to meet this need—even in extreme cases:

1. A 56-year-old doctor, practicing in suburban Farmington Township near Detroit, Michigan, was convicted of manslaughter following the death of his part-time office assistant, to whom he administered a fatal overdose of sodium penathol in the course of treating her for a heart ailment. The state prosecutor condemned Michigan medical licensing practices as "sloppy" and for "failing to protect the public."

According to the prosecutor, more than two dozen complaints had been lodged against this doctor since 1954, either with the police or with the medical board. The complaints included molestation and rape in his office, unwanted termination of pregnancy, and excessive drug sedation. At least three patients died in his office, all because of poisoning.

Twice the medical board revoked his license on charges of moral turpitude. Twice he was arrested for practicing without a license, but he never served a sentence. Twice the board restored his license, once on the provision that he continue undergoing psychiatric care and the second time because he said he was going to Ghana as a medical missionary. A few weeks after leaving for Africa, he was back practicing in Michigan.

2. A surgeon in Beloit, Kansas, certified by the American Board of Surgery in 1949, had his license revoked for "extreme incompetency." This drastic step was ordered by the Kansas Supreme Court following this series of events: In 1963 he applied for membership on the staff of Community Hospital (name later changed to Mitchell County Hospital) in Beloit. His application was refused. He brought suit and the hospital was ordered to admit him. He performed eleven surgical operations in the hospital and three of his patients died. Examination showed malpractice in all three instances. Complaint was made to the state licensing board, which revoked his license, but this action was reversed by the district court because the state licensing law did not list "incompetency" as one of the specific bases for revocation. The licensing board then appealed to the state Supreme Court, which upheld the revocation. The doctor says he plans an appeal to the United States Supreme Court.

In the Kansas case, the state board obviously tried to go beyond the letter of the law, an effort that was condemned by one court and approved by another. The need to revise and update licensure statutes and to include competence as one criterion for the privilege of practicing medicine would appear so obvious as hardly to need pointing out. But apparently this is not so obvious to most state legislatures.

It is not suggested that medical licensure should take the place of specialty board certification, hospital medical staff requirements, or other nongovernmental procedures for raising the standards of medical practice or protecting the welfare of the consumer. On the contrary, it is generally acknowledged that licensure should represent a minimum floor below which standards should never be permitted to fall and above which professional groups and institutions should be encouraged to pursue their own standards of excellence. It seems clear, however, that the present licensing laws and procedures are not only failing to provide this minimum floor but, by providing a lifetime license to anyone who can pass an examination shortly after leaving medical school, may actually mislead the public into a sense of false security.

Another aspect of the Kansas case that should be noted is the fact that the surgeon obtained staff appointment at the hospital only under court order. The positive role of the judiciary in helping to eliminate racial discrimination and other unjustified causes for refusal to admit a physician to hospital privileges is well known. Here the opposite side of the coin is evident—a situation where the hospital's professional judgment was clearly correct and the death of three innocent patients may be, at least partly, attributed to the court's overriding of this professional judgment. Once again, this points up the need for an integrated, holistic approach to problems of regulating hospitals and the quality of care.

LICENSURE AND PRODUCTIVITY

With respect to the effect of licensure on hospital productivity and effectiveness, the consensus of informed opinion appears to be that the laws are thoroughly obsolete and more a hindrance than a help. Here again is Dr. Forgotson:

> By far the most significant issue affected by the licensure process is increasing the productivity of the physician by delegation of responsibilities to other members of the health manpower matrix. There is fairly unanimous agreement that any improvement of the gap between the supply and demand for medical care is highly dependent on obtaining the right kinds of manpower in the right numbers.... Studies are now being launched to determine optimal categorical mixes and numbers of manpower to optimize health care in various delivery patterns as part of the development of an overall manpower production strategy.
>
> It is quite clear that no such strategy can be implemented until present legal restrictions on allocation of tasks are identified and the problems they present are resolved.
>
> Analysis of statutory laws, administrative regulations, and relevant court decisions reveals that there is no coordinated governmental process for regulating the allocation of personal health care tasks among members of the health manpower matrix.... The situation is further complicated by a 1966 decision of the Supreme Court of the state of Washington which held that a statutorily unauthorized delegation of a task by a physician to a practical nurse was evidence of negligence

whether or not the task was executed diligently or with a high degree of care.... As a result, the delegation of authorized tasks is potentially liable for civil malpractice.

The situation is most significant because the status of new professions and occupations such as physicians' assistants or other categories that might be developed is unclear.... Since legal cases involving alleged unauthorized uses could result in penalties ranging from loss of licenses to fines to civil liability for malpractice, the problem is indeed serious.

A legal spokesman for the AMA, discussing licensure of paramedical personnel, agrees with the general point:

... Since this is an era of functional and knowledge specialization, the time may come soon when an individual will need four or five licenses to perform a limited service and his salary demands will increase accordingly if present trends are followed.

A particularly strong condemnation comes from Nathan Hershey, research professor of health law, University of Pittsburgh:

The major effect of our mandatory licensing system for professional and occupational specialists in the health field is to establish a rigid categorization of personnel that tends to interfere with the organization of services by health institutions to meet the demand of patient service....

Our present licensing system converts a question of whether it is safe and appropriate for a health worker with specified training to carry out a particular procedure or make a particular decision, to the question whether it is "legal" for that individual worker to do so....

The present situation with respect to the physician assistants makes clear the inhibiting effect of licensing legislation on innovation in health manpower. If the physician assistants who are already trained are to be employed in our health care system today at anywhere near the level of performance they are capable of, without being licensed, they will, of necessity, have to run the risk that their activities will be deemed the illegal practice of medicine, or of professional nursing, or of some other profession or occupation covered by a mandatory licensing law, or work within institutions that, because of their prestige, are insulated from interference by the state boards. Unfortunately, some of the institutions that have the most severe manpower shortages and could benefit the most from such innovation do not have such an aura of prestige.

The implications of this "professional narcissism" on the use of personnel, especially in an era of rapid technological change, are obvious, and the wonder is that hospitals have done as well as they have under such conditions. Only the low labor costs of the past made such a situation tolerable, from the point of view of hospital financing. With labor costs now rising dramatically it would seem evident that something will have to give.

In some of the best hospitals—those that are not afraid to break the law—something is giving, and it is the inflexible licensing codes. If the law had not been broken, we would not today have such indispensable new occupations as the intravenous or operating room technicians. Nevertheless, the threat of criminal prosecution, as noted by Hershey, or of increased liability to charges of malpractice, as indicated by Forgotson, are usually present in such situations; and it would be far better for all concerned to work out some procedure for doing legally what is now, of necessity, being done illegally. Either hospital management will be freed from these guild-like restrictions to run an efficient operation as American industry does, or the new levels of remuneration which are becoming competitive with industry cannot be sustained, or the whole inflationary "mess" will simply be passed on to the taxpayer via automatic full-cost reimbursement—leading to who knows what retaliatory and restrictive response.

The present situation might be justified, even though it is inordinately expensive and wasteful of scarce manpower, if it seemed to be essential to quality control. On the contrary, however, the system—with its built-in rigidities, its failure to provide for technological and educational innovation, and its virtual invitation to illegal maneuvering—does not offer effective quality controls either. ...

Selection 6

The Development of Professional Performance Standards*

While those resisting the trend toward the institutionalization of health care alleged it would lead inevitably to depersonalization and inferior quality, advocates claimed and attempted to demonstrate the opposite: It would now be possible, for the first time, to amass comprehensive patient records for different types of therapeutic facilities and procedures in aggregates large enough to per-

---

*Excerpt from H.M. and A.R. Somers, *Doctors, Patients, and Health Insurance* (Washington, D.C.: The Brookings Institution, 1961), pp. 111-119.

mit reliable measurement and comparisons. It would allow a broader range of skills and equipment to be brought to bear on patients' problems. It would make possible the development of quality assessment and, thereby, quality control. This selection (1961) summarizes the primitive "state of the art" and the "politics" of quality controls at the beginning of the 1960s. It also foreshadows the Professional Standards Review Organization (PSRO) and related developments.

Almost everybody alleges concern with quality, but what this means is usually vague. The definition of quality is as elusive as it is crucial, and rarely does it lend itself to precise measurement. The difficulties are especially acute in medical care. Despite great scientific advance, the many subjective factors and uncertainties in the etiology of illness and the nature of therapy do not allow complete standardization.

But this does not mean that no objective standards are available. Dramatic cures may occasionally follow a visit to a quack, but it is settled public policy that he cannot legally practice medicine. Nor is the care which licensed doctors render as mysterious or impalpable as the above may suggest. Dr. E. Richard Wienerman, a long-time advocate of quality controls in medical care, has said: " 'Good' medical care . . . is not simply a matter of physician ratios or aggregates of hospitals beds. [But] neither is it a semimystical attribute of the individual physician's bedside manner."

Medical science and technology have now progressed to the point that many particular aspects of medical care, many specific procedures and institutions, can be and are being subjected to increasingly rigorous measurement, testing, and control. The increasing acceptance of epidemiological concepts, progress in biostatistics, and the accumulation of records of patients, diseases, therapeutic facilities, and procedures, in aggregates large enough to permit meaningful comparisons, have all helped to facilitate the development of techniques for quality determination.

Thus far, the principal focus of quality control has been the hospital. Hill-Burton administrators consider the "development and practical use of standards" with respect to quality of services as well as quantity and distribution of beds, design, and equipment, to be one of the most important consequences of the entire program. The long struggle, started in 1918 by the American College of Surgeons, to improve the quality of hospital care and surgery culminated in the establishment, over three decades later, of the Joint Commission on Accreditation of Hospitals in which the AMA, AHA, the American College of Physicians, and the College of Surgeons all participate.

A recent survey lists 12 sources of "external appraisal" of medical care—Joint Commission on Accreditation, Council on Medical Education and Hosptials, Central Inspection Board of the American Psychiatric Association, etc.—and 16 methods of "internal appraisal"—tissue committees, medical records committees, autopsy reports, internal audits, etc. The tissue committee, for example, reviews the preoperate diagnosis side by side with the pathologist's diagnosis of the tissues or organs removed. Wherever such an audit has been introduced the amount of normal organs and tissues removed surgically has been significantly reduced. At the present writing numerous large scale research projects are attempting to develop additional techniques for the evaluation of hospital care.[1]

There is, of course, continuing controversy over the adequacy, appropriateness, and administration of particular standards and controls. But this is a different question from whether there should or can be standards at all. Furthermore, it is obvious that standards are not always adhered to. Only 58 percent of the nation's hospitals are accredited. Dr. Paul R. Hawley, director, American College of Surgeons, recently lashed out against the numerous "lavishly equipped" community hospitals which

> the local medical profession has been encouraged to use ... to the utmost, regardless of competence to undertake complicated procedures.... The results of such practices are evident to many qualified surgeons.... Only a few weeks ago, one of the most distinguished surgeons in the world ... told me that at least one-half of his practice now consists of attempts to correct the bad results of surgery undertaken in community hospitals by doctors inadequately trained in this field.

But despite these continuing lapses the various standards of hospital care stand out as acknowledged criteria by which performance can be and is being judged. Indeed, the hospital has become the most powerful standard-setter or police agent of the medical profession today—one reason that it has become so controversial.

The attempt to develop and apply qualitative standards to medical practice outside the hospital is still in its infancy.[2] The need is increasingly acknowledged, however. In the words of Dr. Roger Lee, past president of the AMA: "No one five years out of medical school is competent to practice medicine on the basis of only what he learned in medical school and on his internship."

A rigorous set of recommendations for professional quality controls came recently from Dr. Walter S. Wiggins, secretary of the AMA's Council on Medical Education and Hospitals. Addressing the American Cancer Society, Dr. Wiggins suggested four ways of inducing the practicing physician to keep abreast of new developments in medicine: (1) publication of the names of physicians participating in continuing medical education programs; (2) making membership in medical societies contingent on such participation; (3) making licensure renewal contingent on such participation; and (4) making licensure valid for a limited time only, with renewal by examination. Similar suggestions were made to the Federation of State Medical Boards by Dr. Gunnar Gunderson, then AMA president.

The practical problems in the path of such reform are formidable, however. It is to be expected that most active practitioners will remain strongly opposed.

The shortage of physicians, and the general loyalty of patients to their own doctors—whatever their merits—would make license revocation exceedingly difficult.

It appears that the major practical avenue for evaluation and control of medical care outside the hospital will be found in organizational arrangements such as group practice. There is impressive professional judgment on this point. For example, Dr. Alan Gregg, long-time director of the Rockefeller Foundation's Division for the Medical Sciences, said:

> The service given a patient by group practice gains in quality by the criticism of the other members of the group, whether the criticism be tacit or fully expressed. Whether we realize it or not, the presence of merely a competent trained nurse tends to raise the doctor's level of performance. Reluctant as an anxious patient may be to think that his doctor, above all people, might ever need the stimulus of competent critics, the fact remains that doctors do need, and usually respond well to, the realization that their work is observable and observed.

The reasons for the positive effect of group practice on quality are both obvious and subtle. The structural or institutional factors include medical center organization, higher standards of physical equipment and facilities, record-keeping, group standards of professional procedures, easier access to a larger range of specialized personnel, more frequent exchange of professional judgment, more time off for refresher and postgraduate courses, etc. Less tangible but important are such factors as the self-selection of physicians choosing group practice—a choice that generally implies the acceptance of both external and internal quality controls, and a preference for the scientific over the charismatic or personal elements in the practice of medicine. The frequent disposition of groups to submit themselves and their procedures to objective evaluation, often by outsiders, bespeaks both self-confidence and a continuing commitment to the pursuit of excellence.

While such factors help to explain the acknowledged excellence of such groups as the Mayo and Lahey Clinics, it does not follow that this form of organization provides automatic quality control. Group practice—especially in large urban clinics—is liable to certain abuses, not unlike those in other large corporations, which may reflect themselves in the quality of care—impersonality, factionalism, and favoritism in financial affairs. Overemphasis on business at the expense of patient care appears to be the chief complaint of doctors who have left group practice.

To guard against such perversion of the group practice ideal, to implement their concern with quality, and to help overcome the public relations handicap of the old image of the charity clinic, an increasing number of groups have formalized their administrative machinery for quality controls. In its 1959 group practice survey, the Public Health Service found that 63 percent of the groups reported some "formal method of maintaining quality of care." The proportion rose with the size of the group to 91 percent in the case of those having 26 or more full-time doctors.

The application of quality standards and controls to solo practice presents much greater difficulties than with group practice. Evidence is accumulating, however, that it can be done. The Tennessee Medical Society stated in 1953: "There are professional mechanics whereby we can judge good from the bad. There are rules and regulations that go far toward assuring a high quality of service and still zealously guard the patient-doctor relationship." The difficulties involved in the North Carolina study of general practice[3] were primarily political, not technical. The technique of evaluation was similar to that used in hospital standard-setting: the formulation of minimal criteria based on professional judgment and experience. In this case, the physicians were graded on the basis of clinical histories, physical examinations, laboratory aids, therapeutic measures, preventive medicine, and clinical records.

In general, it may be concluded that where qualitative standards are exceedingly difficult to establish, even harder to enforce, and need frequent adaptation, the technical problems of formulating and applying them are not insuperable. The profession itself has shown the way. True, there is reticence, even among those in the forefront of this work, with respect to general definitions of "good" medical care or general criteria for its measurement. According to Dr. Kenneth Babcock, director of the Joint Commission on Hospital Accreditation, for example: "The best that can be said is that coming up to or exceeding known standards undoubtedly helps improve medical care, and this indirectly helps in the evaluation and improvement of quality medical care."

Such caution is understandable in view of the professional disagreements in this area. But, if means can be found to assure "coming up to or exceeding known standards," a great advance in quality will have been made. The main question is now a political one: Are the doctors, through their own professional organizations, willing to assume responsibility for effective quality evaluation and controls?

Professional self-discipline does not, of course, reduce the need for personal self-discipline. As Dr. I.S. Ravdin told his colleagues, "Conscience has been and must remain the motivating force that controls our daily lives." Personal integrity is at the heart of effective organizational control—and the two are complementary. But personal discipline requires a standard against which to measure itself. And it must be recognized that a minority in any large group requires some external check. Significantly, it is precisely those sections of the profession which are already committeed to self-discipline that are the first to acknowledge the need for organized controls. The position of the American College of Surgeons has been repeatedly referred to. The American College of Physicians is now engaged in a long term project to develop standards of hospital practice with respect to internal medicine. The establishment, in a few medical schools or schools of public health, of graduate courses in medical care administration or "administrative medicine" is a hopeful development. So is the recent formation of medical society review boards and claims prevention pro-

38   HEALTH AND HEALTH CARE

grams in a number of states and localities. While designed primarily to deal with the threat of malpractice suits, these bodies could help to develop effective machinery for quality controls. ...

NOTES

1. One of the most ambitious is that of the Commission on Professional and Hospital Activities, sponsored by the American College of Surgeons and the Kellogg Foundation, which has been working since 1953 on an interhospital system of internal audits.
2. The feasibility of quality studies of general medical practice was demonstrated nearly 30 years ago by the Committee on the Costs of Medical Care. Professional evaluation of various forms of practice was made for the committee by a team of two doctors from the University of Pennsylvania. See, for example, the studies of the Endicott-Johnson medical program Committee on the Costs of Medical Care (Chicago: University of Chicago Press, Publ. No. 5, 1932); Roanoke Rapids (No. 20), and Union Health Services (No. 19).
3. O.L. Peterson, M.D., L.P. Andrews, M.D., R.S. Spain, M.D., and B.G. Greenberg, "An Analytical Study of North Carolina General Practice, 1953-1954," *Journal of Medical Education* (December 1956): Part 2.

Selection 7

Medical Education and The Community*

By the early 1970s, the trend to high technology and institutionalized care, discussed in Selection 4 as inherent in the dynamism of scientific medicine, had progressed to the point that many academic medical centers—increasingly citadels of superspecialty tertiary care—were failing in some of their important responsibilities. Some medical schools had become isolated from their communities as well as over-extended financially. Too often, education in the new rarified environment failed to provide appropriate training for ordinary medical practice and neglected primary care. While many medical schools have since added departments of family medicine and/or community medicine and are now experimenting with graduate programs in family practice/primary care, the central emphasis of academic medicine remains essentially the same. Selection 7 (1972) discusses these problems.

*Excerpt from A.R. Somers, "Medical Education and the Community: A Consumer Point of View," *The Pharos* 35 (October 1972): 149-155.

Of all the "communications gaps" in our complex pluralistic society, probably none is greater than that between academic medicine and the general public. Not surprisingly, each side sees the other at fault. To many a consumer the medical school doctor is associated not only with inordinate concern for money (an attribute which the public now associates with the medical profession in general) but also with an overriding interest in the esoteric and a contemptuous attitude toward ordinary patients, especially if they are poor.

Ignorant of what goes on in medical schools, the average consumer's image is largely based on sensational TV soap operas or paperback novels. Part of the image derives from the inner sanctum itself. Only a very few have read *Sickness and Society,* a bitter albeit scholarly critique of how patients were sacrificed—only a few years ago—to the learning process in a major teaching hospital. But for every individual who has skimmed the Duff-Hollingshead volume, millions have devoured Dr. William Nolan's dramatic autobiography, *The Making of a Surgeon,* which spells out in authentic detail just how many mistakes a young surgeon makes—even as a resident—before he acquires the necessary skill and experience. And now, thanks to George Scott and Paddy Chayefsky (lead actor and screenplay author of the movie "The Hospital") the image of the boozy, burned-out chief-of-medicine at a big city teaching hospital has earned its place alongside Willy Loman, Archie Bunker, and Portnoy as part of the American collection of nonheroes.

Scott's doctor is, of course, the antithesis of Marcus Welby, the ever-compassionate, never-hurried, never-billing family doctor whose only concern in life is the welfare of his patients. Small wonder that many consumers are frightened of medical students and oppose the whole concept of introducing undergraduate medical education into community hospitals and other community health care institutions.

Academic medicine, for its part, often seems to view the public as a mass of ignoramuses, always demanding instant cures, resisting payment of the funds necessary to carry on the research and education necessary for these cures, and more concerned with superficial amenities and a superficial freedom of choice than with the real quality of the care they receive. The nonacademic physician, the "local medical doctor (LMD)," is also often viewed as little better than his patient and often in cahoots with him in opposing serious quality standards and controls. In short, each views the other as a necessary evil.

THE NECESSITY FOR RAPPROCHEMENT

Whatever grains of truth there may have been in in these jaundiced views—even in the not-so-distant past—it is obvious that such attitudes are now a luxury that neither side can any longer afford.

Academic medicine is today enormously vulnerable. Along with the growing public criticism, it finds itself in trouble on numerous other counts. Most obvious, the costs of medical education have become almost prohibitively high.

With tuition averaging less than $2,000 a year, the balance that must be picked up from the taxpayer or some other outside source is formidable.

The comprehensive Health Manpower Training Act of 1971, with its generous three-year authorization of $2.8 billion was, of course, a lifesaver for many schools. It could signal not only a reaffirmation but strengthening of the old Congress-NIH-medical school love affair; or it could be its swan song.

Second, the schools' pools of indigent "teaching material" are drying up. With the advent of Medicare, Medicaid, the Office of Economic Opportunity (OEO) health centers, and other public and private fianacing programs, the number of poor people dependent on the medical schools and teaching hospitals for their health care is dwindling. A few schools say this is not a problem; that they have been able to obtain the "informed consent" of their private patients to participation the the teaching process. But the majority of academicians appear seriously concerned as to where and how the next generation of doctors, especially surgeons, will be trained.

In some cases, the decline in "teaching material" is also accompanied by a threat to the very existence of the medical school hospital. The cost of such hospitals has become so great, both in terms of construction and operating costs—$100,000 per bed and $150 per day are no longer startling figures—that new schools are finding increasing difficulty in securing the necessary financial support.

It might appear that the simultaneous disappearance of the university hospital and of the masses of poor patients they have traditionally served could be a happy coincidence. But this ignores the schools' needs to provide their students with the necessary clinical experience. To some the answer appears obvious—through affiliation agreements with community hospitals and other community institutions, a point to which I will return later. But to many schools, accustomed to virtually complete autonomy, the prospect of having to teach on wards and clinics which they do not fully "control" appears a fate worse than death.

Finally, there is the gradual shift in public emphasis from biomedical research to problems of the delivery system—the organization and finanacing of health care. The fact that the one has been rising rapidly during the past three or four years while the other is stationary (in an inflationary economy this amounts to a cutback) is enough to cause serious concern and even resentment on the part of some of the more traditional academicians who, again, see a threat to the future quality of care. Thus far, the schools have suffered far more from anxiety than actual deprivation. But it is probable that their fears are not unfounded. ...

If it now seems that the schools are going to have to adjust many of their attitudes and overcome much of their former aloofness—both from the community and from the practicing profession—the same is true on the other side. In the first place, it is now obvious that all of us—consumers, practitioners, allied health personnel academicians, and health care administrators—are going to have to participate in the teaching process. Second, it is going to call for some far-reaching reorganization of the delivery system at the community level. Third, it is going to mean additional upward pressure on health care costs, especially in community hospitals.

The combination of these pressures, plus his own increasing sophistication, may force the consumer to recognize the primacy of his own responsibility for his own health. This may be the most difficult of all adjustments in a society where too many doctors have long expected the patient to be a passive recipient of professional expertise and wisdom, where politicians are telling him that good health is a right guaranteed by the state, and where technologists and systems engineers now suggest that if he just queues up and follows directions from one health care station to another he will find utopia at the end of the road—rather, the flow-chart.

This, of course, is nonsense. But the habit of passivity has been so deeply engrained in millions of consumers, and the habit of "father knows best what's good for you" is so engrained in many providers, especially academic providers, that it is going to be excedingly difficult to turn the system around and put the consumer-patient back in the middle of the picture where he belongs, with all the burden of personal responsibility that this entails.

The rest of the selection will be concerned with three sets of problems involved in the turn-around.

THE PROBLEM OF "TEACHING MATERIAL" AND "CLINICAL EXPERIENCE"

Any effort to revive the traditional condescending concept of "teaching material" among paying patients is inevitably doomed to failure. The patient who is paying over $100 a day for a hospital bed and several hundred or even thousands more for his physician's services, or knows that these are being paid for him by a third party, is very likely to resist the prospect of being a "guinea pig" regardless of the consequences to medical education. A whole new approach to patient cooperation in the educational process is needed, an approach based on mutual need and mutual advantage in a completely new context.

A growing number of doctors are beginning to understand the importance of the patient's understanding of the nature of his illness and his active participation in his own cure or management. My husband and I have been saying this for years. [See, for example, Selection 10 (1961).] Now it is great to have such good company as John Millis,[1] Richard Magraw,[2] and that remarkable team of John Bjorn and H.D. Cross.[3] Dr. Magraw has listed four conditions which must be met if optimal care is to be rendered. These include:

> There must be agreement between the doctor and patient as to what is wrong. . . . There must be agreement between the doctor and patient as to what is to be done and why.

Drs. Bjorn and Cross go on to say,

> We, as physicians, must demand a change in the relationship between

the physician and his patient from an adult-child relationship toward adult-adult.... Patient co-operation is a measure of patient education. Dr. Millis writes,

> as health service comes to be viewed as also including health care and we focus upon the maintenance of health as well as the cure of disease, the physician alone becomes less sufficient. The behavior, the decisions, the habits, the understanding of the patient become as necessary as the physician.

If this philosophy is correct, as I believe it to be, then the medical school should welcome the opportunity to provide its students with clinical experience in a setting where patients do not have to forfeit their self-respect and dignity and where the emphasis has to be on active participation rather than passive compliance. In this context the paying patient becomes a colleague of the physician and the medical student on the health care team and should be approached as such by the student. If this attitude were adopted by medical educators, millions of paying patients would probably enter into the new relationship without resentment. The disappearance of the indigent patient could turn out to be a boon to medical education which would now begin to turn its attention to problems of "the whole man," to patient education as a basic component of patient care, and to developing in the medical student this new and more mature attitude toward his future patients.

The very term "teaching material" should be banned in favor of something like "participating patient," meaning that the patient is participating both in his own diagnosis and treatment and in the education of the medical student. "Service beds" could be renamed "participating beds," and patients who wish to participate in the teaching process would be permitted—never forced—to occupy them.

REDEFINING THE ROLE OF THE MEDICAL SCHOOL WITH RESPECT TO DELIVERY OF HEALTH SERVICE

Medical schools have always been involved in patient care to a greater or lesser degree. No school can carry on clinical instruction without patients. In the past, however, almost all of these patients were indigent. If inpatients, they were usually very sick; if outpatients, they were either very sick or pretty much social outcasts. The medical student usually had no exposure to middle-class patients. He had no experience with preventive medicine, or keeping people well, or even seeing sick people outside the hospital. He had no concern with the economics of health care, either how people could be helped to pay for their care or how care could be delivered more efficiently to large groups of people.

Among the first to identify the need for academic medicine to broaden its approach to patient care and to recognize the far-reaching implications for both medical education and the practice of medicine was Dr. Ward Darley. Shortly after World War II, as dean of the medical school at the University of Colorado, he set up, in cooperation with the city of Denver and with a grant from the Commonwealth Fund, a teaching program in comprehensive care at the Denver General Hospital. Later as excutive director of the Association of the American Medical Colleges, Dr. Darley brought his concern for comprehensive care, family medicine, and the delivery system in general to center stage. The theme of the 1960 Association of American Medical Colleges (AAMC) Teaching Institute, "Medical Education and Medical Care: Interactions and Prospects" might have been formulated today.

I mention this bit of history because it is important to realize that this is not a brand new problem and that it is not necessary to start from scratch in seeking solutions. Americans have a frightful habit of ignoring history—meaning almost anything that happened over two years ago. Throughout the past decade, we have rediscovered the wheel a number of times. Almost every year has witnessed a major conference or report dealing with the redirection or redefinition of medical education in one aspect or another. The Coggeshall report,[4] the two Millis reports,[1,5] the Debakey report,[6] the Evans report,[7] the report of the Commission on Community Health Services,[8] the report of the National Advisory Commission on Health Manpower,[9] the 1970 report of the Carnegie Commission on Higher Education[10]: these are only a few of the better known.

Although the emphasis differs from document to document, the common theme is obvious: Medical education must get out of its ivory tower—must look outward to the community—for its own sake as well as that of the community. Millis stated as one of the three overriding priorities for medical education:

Initiate the organization of a local system of health science education and interdigitate that system with a regional system of health service.

The Carnegie report is particularly explicit: The "Flexner Model"—emphasizing self-contained instruction and especially research in the basic sciences—is no longer adequate. The commission recommends development of a new model—not for all but for most schools—"the health care delivery model where the medical school, in addition to training, does research in health care delivery, advises local hospitals and health authorities, works with community colleges, and comprehensive colleges on the training of allied health personnel, carries on continuing education for health personnel, and generally orients itself to external service."

The commission's dichotomy is not entirely felicitious. Having known Abraham Flexner slightly many years ago and remembering him as a compassionate humanitarian as well as a scholar, I don't like the negative connotation attached to the so-called "Flexner model" Nor do I like the implication that, because the medical schools should be more concerned with delivery than they have in the past, delivery should now be their primary concern. A careful reading of the Carnegie document makes clear that this is not the intent. But the juxtaposition of "research model" versus "delivery model" will inevitably lead some—both friends and foes of the report—to such a simplistic conclusion.

The danger of oversimplification at this point is great. A case in point is the current extraordinary emphasis on HMOs (health maintenance organizations). I am a long-time friend of prepaid group practice. I have belonged to two plans and am a special admirer of Kaiser. But I do not think the HMO is the panacea for all our delivery problems; nor is it a panacea for all the problems of academic medicine. In his "Caveats for Medical Schools," Dr. Ernest Saward,[11] one of the founding fathers of the Kaiser system, wrote,

> No model system should be expected to be universally applicable, for our society is too diverse.... The generic purpose of prepaid group practice is other than to subsidize the teaching program of a medical school. Educational costs must be identified as such and directly funded, not vicariously or by subterfuge.

The school that reaches headlong into the HMO business as a way to pick up easy federal money and recapture a captive patient population is in for some very stormy days. The embarrassment now being felt by some schools with respect to their OEO centers, as federal support dwindles for some of these projects whose innovative image is already beginning to fade, could be multiplied manyfold. The public relations consequences alone could be serious.

At the risk of being hoist on my own petard—of rediscovering a few wheels of my own—I admit that I have my own formulation of a practical approach to redefinition of the medical school role with respect to our evolving health care delivery system. The first and overriding objective shoud be to give full recognition to the importance of the organization and financing of health care in the education of all future physicians, in the continuing education of those already in practice, and in the institution's departmental organization, its financing, its general reward and status systems, and in its relations with provider institutions and personnel throughout its area of influence.

Second, it means improving and strengthening the relationship between the medical school and university hospital, on the one hand, and the community hospitals, doctors, and other community health providers, on the other. Most crucial, of course, is the relationship of the medical school with the community hospital, which is becoming the de facto center of community health services.

THE NEW MEDICAL SCHOOL-COMMUNITY HOSPITAL AFFILIATIONS: OPPORTUNITIES AND PROBLEMS

There was a time, not so long ago, when these two institutions scarcely gave each other the time of day. "Ivory tower" and "LMD workshops"—each eyed the other with a mixture of fear and contempt. Fortunately, these attitudes are beginning to disappear.

Throughout the nation, today, we see a growing network of medical school-community hospital affiliations. There is probably not a school that does not have some such relationship, although its importance in the different institutions varies greatly. I understand that the University of Indiana School of Medicine now has teaching affiliations of one kind or another with fifty-one separate hospitals throughout the entire state. Michigan State University is now fully accredited as a degree-granting medical school and in June 1973 will graduate its first class without owning or controlling any hospital. At the other end of the spectrum, a few traditional schools still do almost all of their teaching in university-owned or controlled hospitals.

Factors that enter into these different relationships include the pressure of new enrollment; the organization and primary interests of the faculty; the adequacy of existing clinical facilities under direct medical school control; the extent of local town-gown conflicts; the medical school's own financial strength and the extent of its reliance on the research dollar; its responsiveness to changing public needs and demands; the closeness of legislative involvement; the quality and organization of community hospital administration and leadership, especially of the state or regional hospital association; the strength and attitudes of state and local medical societies; and the effectiveness of state and regional health planning and regulation.

Obviously, the varying combinations of factors in different localities will—and should—produce different patterns of medical school-community hospital affiliations. This area is still one of intense and exciting experimentation. In fact, there is no reason why the affiliation movement should be limited to hospitals. Prepaid group practice organizations, medical society foundations, clinics and health centers of various sorts, even the office of the individual practitioner, are already, in a few instances, being used as sites for portions of the clinical clerkship.

For example, Mount Sinai School of Medicine and the Health Insurance Plan of Greater New York (HIP) are jointly developing an educational program in one of the HIP groups. The Pennsylvania State University College of Medicine at Hershey uses individual doctors as preceptors. The hospital affiliation is stressed in this selection primarily because it offers the broadest and most widely available opportunity for clinical experience in a context that can be readily monitored for quality.

Overriding the many local and regional differences, there seems little question but that this relationship will be increasingly important in the future—both to the medical school and to the hospital. One factor alone is now close to being decisive—the cost of building and equipping a new university hospital. Even where the decision has been made to proceed with a new hospital, the size and scope are frequently being curtailed with the result that the medical school cannot rely exclusively on its "own" hospital for clinical instruction but must supplement it by affiliation agreements.

As to the community hospital, the implications of the phasing out of the internship and the requirement of medical school affiliation for approved residencies are becoming clearer and will be for many, probably most, community hospitals a potent force leading them to seek formal affiliation.

The possibilities in these developments for improved medical education as well as for upgraded patient care are enormous. The implications for improved care are familiar but so important that they bear repeating: better communications and working relations between the nation's major academic and research centers and the providers who are actually giving most of the care; the importance of regional health planning and the concept of concentric rings of less specialized institutions and personnel surrounding the academic hub; better regional distribution of physicians and other health manpower; more and better trained housestaff; the possibility of turning out more doctors faster at less cost; etc.

The advantages from the point of view of the medical school seem equally great. Dr. Robert Ebert, dean of the Harvard Medical School, recently said,

> Some thoughtful professors of clinical departments are beginning to wonder if other clinical settings are not needed to complement the university teaching hospital. Ambulatory care, which represents the largest part of medical practice, is often poorly taught in the university hospital, and the medical student has little opportunity to see the more routine medical care that predominates in the community hospital. Medical schools and medical centers will need to expand their own facilities to include a much larger proportion of primary care or will have to affiliate with the community institutions which offer such services.

Along with all these advantages, however, there are obviously a number of difficult problems. We have already talked about the issue of patient acceptance. A second problem has to do with the relation between the hospital's house staff program and its undergraduate teaching program. Hospitals that have no approved residencies or can attract only foreign-trained residents will probably have special difficulty in establishing and maintaining a good student program. On the other hand, it is obviously difficult to attract good residents to an institution that has little or no teaching facilities.

How to break the cycle of mediocrity should be a major challenge not only to the community hospitals but also to the medical schools in their area or region. The need for a cooperative approach to the hospitals' problems in seeking to upgrade their standards is essential. Any suggestion of arrogance or condescension on the part of the academics could be fatal and drive the community hospitals away from the educational enterprise altogether. Similarly, undue defensiveness or fear of academic surveillance on the part of the community hospital's medical staff could destroy the new partnership.

Here again the Indiana plan with its simultaneous emphasis on graduate and undergraduate education and its concept of the "communiversity" or "university without walls" in which both the core campus and the community institutions are accorded equal importance, appears highly promising.

A third problem is the one inherent in all collaborative undertakings: maintenance of responsibility. "What is everybody's business tends to become nobody's business!" The danger of dilution of responsibility applies both to the student and to the patient. In a situation where the student is rotated from institution to institution, between his academic professors and a series of clinical instructors, there is some danger that he may end up feeling as badly fragmented as the patient often feels today in a world divided up among specialists.

This obviously presents a special challenge to the director of medical education (DME) in the community hospital. Some say the DME is not the appropriate person to assume this coordinating responsibility on behalf of the community hospital and that there must be a full-time chief of staff for every department where undergraduate teaching is conducted. Undoubtedly, different solutions will emerge in different situations, depending at least in part on the personalities involved. But one thing we can be sure of. It will cost a great deal of money!

Who *is* going to bear the expense of clinical instruction in the community hospital—the hospital itself or the medical school? In this respect widely varying patterns appear to be developing. One school of thought, for example, insists that the affiliated hospital must bear full expense and that all salaries—that of the full-time chiefs, and anything that may be paid to the attending physicians, as well as the director of medical education—must be paid by the hospital. The concept of "geographic full-time" could help, in some situations, to relieve part of the burden on the hospital. But this is not always possible.

Another view is that the affiliation agreement is an integral part of the school's teaching responsibility and should be financed, in part at least, by the school. In Indiana, for example, the new program includes state funding, via the medical school, for salary supplements to directors of medical education, who assume responsibility for undergraduate as well as graduate education in their hospitals, for visiting professorships in these hospitals, and for grants-in-aid to the hospitals for intern and residency programs.

Some may say that, since ultimately the public pays in any case, it doesn't matter too much how the financing is handled. Most economists would reject this argument.

Many additional problems involved in development of the new affiliation agreements could be raised. Some critics fear the emergence of a new form of "diploma mill," with almost exclusive emphasis on numbers of students and totally inadequate attention to quality. At the other extreme, some fear that the affiliated community hospitals will turn out to be carbon copies of the university teaching hospitals—just as impersonal, just as remote from the community in which they are located, and just about as expensive. To quote Dr. Ebert again:

> Community institutions often fear that they will be taken over by the university, and staff physicians fear that they will gradually be forced out to be replaced by members of the clinical faculty. These are not idle

suspicions because too often in the past this is precisely what has happened; and yet, to transform the community hospital into a university hospital would, at the present time, defeat the purpose of affiliation.

The same general point was made by Dr. John Evans, president, University of Toronto, in 1970. Discussing the question of cost and its relation to control, he asked: "Can the academic health center afford to become involved with the full spectrum of health services?"

Then he answered himself:

> This should be a financial problem *only* if it [the academic center] insists on controlling these services as has been the case with university hospitals. But control by the academic health center carries with it several perils. First, the services controlled and operated by the center may become sufficiently different from those of the community system as to be irrelevant; experience to date with university hospitals does not allay this fear. Secondly, with the major responsibility for operating health services, the academic health center could lose its objectivity, become defensive about criticism, and resist change, thereby jeopardizing its innovative role in education and health care research. Finally, the substantial commitment of resources required to control and operate its own health services would limit the scope of involvement of the academic health center with health care delivery and would seriously curtail its capacity to respond to changing needs.

There is obviously danger in any new approach. But there is greater danger in doing nothing, in simply pretending that there is nothing wrong with medical education in the United States today which a few more billions of dollars can't cure.

To those who invoke the memory of Abraham Flexner to justify uncritical adherence to the status quo, I must remonstrate that Flexner's entire life and personality cry out against any such misuse of his name. Indeed, he anticipated, many years ago, the very things we are talking about today:

> The reconstruction of our medical education is not going to end matters once and for all. It leaves untouched certain outlying problems that will all the more surely come into focus when the professional training of the physician is once securely established on a scientific basis. At this moment the social role of the physician will generally expand and, to support such expansion, he will crave a more liberal and disinterested educational experience.

For a number of years, medical historians have wondered what the new post-Flexnerian revolution in medical education would look like and when it would come. I submit that it is almost here and that its name is "communiversity." Like any other serious revolution, it will evoke a combination of hope and fear and produce a combination of pain and progress.

NOTES

1. John S. Millis, *A Rational Public Policy for Medical Education and Its Financing* (New York City: National Fund for Medical Education, 1971).
2. R.M. Magraw, M.D., *Ferment in Medicine* (Philadelphia: W.B. Saunders Co., 1966).
3. John C. Bjorn, M.D. and H.D. Cross, M.D., *Problem-Oriented Practice* (Chicago: Modern Hospital Press, 1970).
4. Lowell T. Coggeshall, M.D., *Planning for Medical Progress through Education*, Report to the Association of American Medical Colleges (Chicago: Association of American Medical Colleges, 1965).
5. Citizens Commission on Graduate Medical Education, John S. Millis, Chairman, *The Graduate Education of Physicians* (Chicago: American Medical Association, Council on Medical Education, 1966).
6. The President's Commission on Heart Disease, Cancer, and Stroke, Michael E. DeBakey, M.D., Chairman, *A National Program to Conquer Heart Disease, Cancer and Stroke* (Washington, D.C.: U.S. Government Printing Office, 1964).
7. Lester J. Evans, M.D., *The Crisis in Medical Education* (Ann Arbor: University of Michigan Press, 1964).
8. National Commission on Community Health Services, Marion B. Folsom, Chairman, *Health Is a Community Affair* (Cambridge, Mass.: Harvard University Press, 1967).
9. Report of the National Advisory Commission on Health Manpower, J. Irwin Miller, Chairman (Washington, D.C.: U.S. Government Printing Office, 1967).
10. Carnegie Commission on Higher Education, Clark Kerr, Chairman, *Higher Education and the Nation's Health* (New York: McGraw-Hill, 1970).
11. A.R. Somers, ed., *The Kaiser-Permanente Medical Care Program: A Symposium* (New York: The Commonwealth Fund, 1971).

Chapter Two

The Consumer-Patient

Selection 8

Death and Disability Among
American Workers*

Occupational disability and death have historically been among the nation's major health problems. Over the years, many of the conditions described in Selection 8 (1954) have been substantially ameliorated, but other dangers have replaced them. The hazards of the workplace are still very much present, not only in mining, transportation, and heavy industry, but also many lighter industries where exposure to radiation, noxious fumes, and toxic chemicals have emerged as a new threat. The most dangerous occupations were generally among the first unionized, so it was not surprising that organized labor became a principal spokesman for consumers with respect to general, as well as occupational, health problems.

Picture the vast army of American labor, about 62 million men and women, going forth each morning to do the nation's work: into the mines, the mills, the factories, the shops, the offices, the stores, and onto the farms, the stockyards, the railways, the highways, and construction sites. Imagine this army returning from work, and count the casualties of one work day. Include only those who were injured *on the job*.

Consider only those hurt badly enough to lose time beyond the day in which they were injured. Even with this limited count, in the course of an average work day about 62 workers will have been killed, 350 will have suffered some permanent impairment, and 7,600 more will have suffered injuries which will keep them from work for an average of about 18 days.[1] Another way of putting it would be that one American worker will have been killed or crippled every three minutes. Another will have been injured every 11 seconds.

Multiply the daily casualty list by the 260 days which constitute an average American work year and you arrive at the annual human toll which modern industry exacts: about 16,000 fatalities, 91,000 permanent disabilities—of which

---

*Excerpt from H.M. and A.R. Somers, *Workmen's Compensation: Prevention, Insurance, and Rehabilitation of Occupational Disability* (New York: John Wiley & Sons, 1954), pp. 1-3, 6-9.

some 1,600 are "total" such as paraplegia, broken backs, blindness, or double amputations; the others representing loss, or loss of use of, an arm, a leg, an eye, a finger or a part thereof—and nearly 2 million temporary disabilities.

The totals represent both occupational accidents and diseases, including silicosis, lead poisoning, dermatitis, industrial deafness, and occupational cancer.[2] Great progress has been made in industrial safety and occupational health since the early part of the century. But as these data demonstrate, the production and wealth of the nation are still paid for in blood and tears.

VARIATIONS AMONG INDUSTRIES

Some occupations are far more dangerous than others. Loggers, coal miners, and stevedores will, on average, be killed or maimed far more frequently than workers in other occupations. In 1950 loggers suffered 97 disabling injuries per million employee-hours worked (the *injury frequency rate*); stevedores, 59; coal miners, 53; structural steel and ornamental ironworkers, 60. On the other hand, the frequency rate in the communications industry was 2; in business services, 4; in the ordnance industry, 6; in retail trade, 14. The average injury frequency rate for all manufacturing was 15; for construction, 41.

There is also a wide variation in the intensity of injuries and in the resulting loss of work days. In 1950 the *severity rate*—the average number of days lost through occupational injuries per thousand employee-hours worked—was 8 in the coal mines, only 0.1 in communications, and 1.2 in manufacturing as a whole, the lowest year on record. Time lost per injury—the *severity average*—in the logging industry averaged 129 days; in coal mining, 150 days;[3] in trade, 45 days. In some industries, although the severity rate is low, the number of days lost per injury is high because, although there are relatively fewer accidents, those which occur are more serious, with a high proportion of fatalities and/or permanent disabilities. Thus, for example, in aircraft manufacture the severity rate was 0.9, but the average number of days lost per injury was 280. In blast furnaces and steel mills the severity rate was 1.2, but the average number of days lost per case was 219.

Contrary to popular opinion, accident rates in agriculture are relatively high. The death rate from accidents in agriculture is more than three times the rate in manufacturing, and the injury rate appears to be increasing.

OCCUPATIONAL CASUALTIES AND WAR CASUALTIES

War is commonly regarded as the most destructive of human events. But the statistics indicate that occupational injuries cause far more casualties than war. They occur with a monotonous and relatively unpublicized regularity.

E.H. Downey, a leading authority on industrial accidents, summed up the comparative statistics, before World War II, as follows:

Of deaths [from occupational injury] alone the twelve months' total is four times the number killed and mortally wounded in the battle of Gettysburg; of permanent injuries the annual sum surpasses the yearly average of the Civil War. The total casualties of the American Expeditionary Force in the World War [I] did not equal the casualties to American workmen in peaceful employments between April, 1917, and the signing of the Armistice. The toll of life and limb exacted by American industries during the second decade of the twentieth century exceeds the nation's losses in battle from the Declaration of Independence to the present day.

During World War II there were 20,500 major amputations in the Army, Navy, and Air Forces; while in the same number of months in industry there were 65,000 amputations. After more than three years of war in Korea, the Department of Defense announced in August 1953, after the truce, a total of 25,604 killed and 8,529 missing, "the fourth bloodiest conflict in the nation's history." During the same period about 48,750 civilians were killed on the job.

To be sure, these are totals rather than rates. If exposure rates could be computed, the rate for war would far exceed that for occupational injury. Yet, the comparative losses to the nation, in total, are significant and insufficiently considered. Speaking during World War II, Ned H. Dearborn, of the National Safety Council drew another comparison:

> Those who have lost sons or other loved ones in the war have at least the pride of knowing that they gave their lives for a cause as big as human freedom. But no death is so pointless, so brutal, so wholly devoid of compensation for survivors as is death by accident.

ORIGINS OF THE PROBLEM

Work has always been dangerous. Eolithic cave men and Pharaoh's slaves, the road builders of Imperial Rome, and Queen Elizabeth's intrepid sailors—all paid with life and limb for their day's sustenance and the wealth they created. But the mechanization of industry and its more recent "chemicalization" have increased the hazards of labor. Modern technology makes use of stupendous forces—steam, electricity, chemical agents, and the most powerful of all forces thus far discovered, ionizing radiation—that multiply human power and effectiveness a thousandfold when under control, but are equally destructive when out of control. Even when controlled, they may cause serious injury through gradual and undramatic erosion of vitality or body damage.

The human organism is imperfectly adapted to its new mechanical-chemical-radiological environment. Downey has described the titanic agencies of modern production as a:

> vast aggregation of machinery which the individual workman can neither comprehend nor control, but to the movements of which his own must closely conform in rate, range, and direction. Nor is the worker's danger confined to the task in which he is himself engaged nor to the appliances within his vision. A multitude of separate operations are united into one comprehensive process, the successful consummation of which requires the co-operation of thousands of operatives and of innumerable pieces of apparatus in such close interdependence that the hidden defect of a minor part or the momentary lapse of memory or of attention by a single individual may imperil the lives of hundreds. A tower man misinterprets an order and a train loaded with human freight dashes to destruction. A coal miner tamps his "shot" with slack and a dust explosion wipes out a score of lives....

To the physical hazards of mechanized production there were added, especially toward the end of the 19th century, two other modern phenomena—the impersonal corporate organization of industry, and a plethora of cheap labor resulting from heavy immigration.

Prior to 1900 the owner of a plant usually operated it, was regularly in the plant, and generally felt a sense of responsibility toward his employees. The "trust" movement introduced the absentee owner, with resulting decline in sense of responsibility. Processes were speeded up, greater energy was used to operate heavier machines, and operations became steadily more dangerous. "It was said of many plants that they were slaughterhouses."[4]

The steady stream of penniless immigrants, frequently helpless and willing to work under any conditions, contributed to the debasement of the price of human life. The "double standard" which resulted, and its effect on early attitudes toward safety and hygiene, were emphasized many times by early investigators. Sample two illuminating incidents told by Dr. Alice Hamilton, one of the pioneers in the industrial hygiene movement in this country, which occurred during her studies of lead poisoning in 1910 and 1911:

> Because enamelling tubs was notoriously hard, hot, and dangerous, most American men shunned it and I found in Pittsburgh and the surrounding towns, in Trenton, and in Chicago, foreign-born workmen, Russians, Bohemians, Slovaks, Croatians, Poles. I remember a foreman saying to me, as we watched the enameller at work, "They don't last long at it. Four years at the most, I would say, then they quit and go home to the Old Country." "To die?" I asked. "Well, I suppose that's about the size of it," he answered.

There were always more to take their place.

A few months later, after visiting Leadville, Colorado, Dr. Hamilton wrote:

> I am amazed to see how lightly lead poisoning is taken here. One would almost think I was inquiring about mosquito bites. When I asked an

apothecary about lead poisoning in the neighborhood of the smelter, he said he had never known a case. I exclaimed that that was incredible, and he said: "Oh, maybe you are thinking of the Wops and Hunkies. I guess there's plenty among them. I thought you meant white men!"

We have grown more civilized. Such attitudes no longer prevail, and it is difficult to realize how large a role they played in our early neglect of human safety.

The peak in industrial accident rates was reached during the first decade of the century, probably about 1907-1908. In the year ending June 30, 1907, 4,534 workers were killed in railroading alone; 1907 was also the blackest year in mining: 2,534 men were killed in bituminous mines alone.

The usual explanations offered, in addition to the factors already mentioned, are the unprecedented acceleration of industrial activity during that period, the complete absence of any organized safety effort, the prevalent 12-hour day in dangerous trades, and child labor.

Against this background the record of improvement is remarkable and heartening, but the previous black period should not be forgotten both as explanation and as a caution.

NOTES

1. Averages are based on a ten-year period of experience, 1943-1952. Because of inadequate accident reporting in many states, these estimates tend to understatement.

2. Compensable occupational diseases constitute, on the average, about 3 percent of all occupational disabilities.

3. Over the period 1900-1950, 93,000 soft-coal miners were killed, an average of over seven per working day.

4. A.H. Reede, *Adequacy of Workmen's Compensation* (Cambridge, Mass.: Harvard University Press, 1947), p. 345. Fortunately this was not enduring. The large corporations are now, relatively, the safest places to work. The period here referred to, in which an increasing accident rate is partly attributed to development of the corporate structure, precedes the birth of the safety movement in which big business played a leading and effective role.

Selection 9

The Fragmented Patient*

It is ironic that widespread criticism of the medical profession and medical care institutions should develop precisely at the time when such care is technically better and more accessible than ever before. Indeed it is precisely the knowledge of the high quality and partial availability of superb medical care that causes the patient so often to feel let down, frustrated, dehumanized—in short, abandoned.

The patient's plea for personalized care is heard in many accents and with varying degrees of sophistication. His complaint is probably the most widely expressed criticism of medical care today, more urgent in the minds of many than even the rising costs of care. When the two are linked together in personal experience—high costs for ineffective impersonal care—the result is often a bitterness that bodes ill for patients and providers alike. The plethora of journalistic exposés, bearing such titles as "Cruelty in Maternity Wards," "What's Come Between You and Your Doctor?" "The American Doctor: Death of a Legend in an Era of Miracles," all echo the now familiar themes of impersonality, haste, no time for sympathy, no time to treat or even to know the patient as a human being.

No doubt, some of this criticism is the result of an oversell of the personal physician-patient relationship, a propaganda backfire. Some of it involves nostalgia for a past that never really was. Yet even this yearning for an ideal that was always more myth than fact is not without meaning. Partly, there is an intuitive grasping for a human being to translate the impersonal vocabulary of the computer, the x ray, and the autoanalyzer into terms that the patient can understand. Partly, too, there is the instinctive realization that the patient must be viewed as a whole if effective management of his illness is to be achieved. And this can only be done by a human being who can sort out and integrate all the information and advice provided by the various specialists and translate the results into meaningful directions for the patient.

In brief, this yearning for a personal physician and a personal doctor-patient relationship, while partly nostalgic and partly the product of propaganda, has a firm basis in the realities of good medical care. It is a legitimate demand and a quintessential ingredient of such care.

Unfortunately, however, it is increasingly a missing ingredient. In 1950, there were 116,400 doctors engaged in family practice, i.e., general practice, internal medicine, and pediatrics. In 1965, this number had fallen to 98,000. The ratio

---

*Excerpt from A.R. Somers, paper presented to Ohio Academy of General Practice, Family Practice Seminar, April 1968, Columbus, Ohio; published as "The Missing Ingredient," *Medical Opinion and Review* 5 (August 1969): 27-35.

fell from 76 per 100,000 to only 50 per 100,000. Commenting on this situation in *Journal of the American Medical Association* (April 4, 1966), Surgeon-General Luther Terry wrote:

> Growth in the number of specialists ... has been going on at such an increasing rate, that today 80 percent of the country's medical graduates study for specialty practice. The necessity of this development of specialized care in every field of medicine is not to be disputed .... But if we reach the point—as I think we have—at which the specialist is crowding the generalist off the scene, then there is reason for very serious concern.

THE STORY OF RUTH

In October 1967 *McCalls* carried an article entitled "With a Life at Stake," by Edward Brecher. He and his wife, Ruth, were talented medical journalists who collaborated on dozens of popular articles describing the miracles of modern medicine. A year previously Ruth died of cancer, after a protracted illness. They were a devoted couple, and I know that Edward would never have brought himself to write of her trials and anguish had it not been for his conviction that something must be done about the impersonality of modern medicine. Here is part of that story:

> During the weeks after Ruth's operation, questions multiplied—and so did our doubts concerning the quality of the care she was receiving at the medical center we had selected (reputed to be one of the country's best). Doctors came and went; no one of them was in command. One of them told Ruth one thing, the same doctor or someone else gave me an altogether different report, and there was no one to whom we could turn to tell us which version was true. Like many other patients we came to know during those stress-laden days and nights, we felt as if we were floundering in a quagmire of medical confusion. When things went wrong, as they not infrequently did, there was no one in authority to listen to us. One capable young hospital resident—the friend of a friend of ours—did take a personal interest in Ruth's problems at one point; but because he lacked status in the hosptial's rigid hierarchy, no one would listen to *him*, either ....
>
> We first became aware of [a conflict over radiation] when the surgeon who had operated on her recommended immediate radiation therapy. "Don't worry about it," he told me. "The dose will be small, only twenty-five hundred units, and only to a limited region of Mrs. Brecher's abdomen. Hence she need not fear any subsequent radiation damage. Since the tumor has already spread beyond control, there is no point in

adding to her discomfort by too much radiation. The important thing is to get the treatments started as soon as possible—next Monday morning. I will remain in personal charge."

The surgeon's associate underlined some of these points to the two of us a little later. "You're fortunate," he added to Ruth, "to be here where we will give you continuing personal attention. At many medical centers the surgeons would just turn you over to the radiation therapists and forget all about you. We'll get your treatment started Monday morning; every day saved is a day gained."

Bright and early Monday morning, as the surgeon had promised, Ruth was wheeled to the radiation therapy department. I accompanied her. She was photographed, handed a paper to sign waiving claims against the medical center, asked a few questions about her hospital insurance, then wheeled into a small room dominated by a linear accelerator—an imposing ultramodern device that looked like something out of a science-fiction television show.

Ruth and I were alarmed. So far, she had not been examined by, or even introduced to, a physician specializing in radiation therapy. Was her treatment to be in the hands of one of the nonmedical attendants we saw wandering aimlessly around, apparently none too sure of what they were supposed to be doing?

Our alarm was not relieved when a young woman attendant threw a switch. Soft music began to play. "You'll have to leave the room now," she told me. "We're going to start the treatment." I left and went in search of a radiation therapist. None was in sight. A few minutes later, Ruth was wheeled out of he linear-accelerator room, still untreated, and returned to her own room. Something, apparently, had gone wrong; we were never told what.

Later that day, a radiation therapist examined Ruth, studied her record and gave her a talking to. "I have ascertained," he told her in a voice meant to carry conviction, "that this is a tumor of a kind which can be totally *eradicated* by radiation if we deliver a large enough dose over a large enough portion of your body—your entire abdomen and chest. Hence I propose to eradicate that tumor." He was careful not to say "cure"; that would have been unethical. But the impact on a naive patient would surely have been the same. "We'll start your treatments," he concluded, "next Monday morning." This was precisely the delay the surgeon and his associate had warned against.

The two departments concerned with Ruth's care were thus in basic disagreement about almost everything—time when treatment should begin, the amount of radiation, the area of her body to be irradiated and the probable outcome. Which was right? There was nobody we trusted to tell us or to explain the reason for the disagreement. We could only wait helplessly to see which department would win the tug-of-war in which Ruth's future was the stake.

"I feel like the character in a novel by Kafka or in a play written by Ionesco for the Theater of the Absurd," Ruth wrote in a note to a physician-cousin of hers that evening. She was a Quaker and much more tolerant than I of human and institutional shortcomings.

I do not know how representative this case is. I know that specialism has brought great progress to medical science. But what a cruel irony: that modern medicine in its grasping for life and healing should bring added terror and loneliness to dying. Surely the very least we can do in such cases is to make sure, *very sure,* that the patient has a personal physician.

WHAT WAY TO PERSONALIZED CARE?

The problem of the fragmented patient is now recognized by both the practicing and the academic physician. The American Academy of General Practice and the state academies have done a great deal to bring this matter to the attention of the profession. Thanks to the Coggeshall Report, the Millis Report, the Willard Report [see notes to Selection 7], and others, organized medicine is now on record as recognizing the need for a new specialty of family medicine. Indeed, such a new specialty has now been officially established.

But can the new specialty of family medicine fill the need we face? Should the personal physician be a new type of specialist in family medicine or should he be a pedi-internist, or whatever name they invent to designate the man with the proposed dual certification? Or, should he be a sort of minidoctor, with less than the standard baccalaureate plus MD degrees? We have heard many proposals to this effect.

Or should we take a different route altogether? There are numerous non-MD candidates for the job. In Denver, Chicago, and elsewhere, specially trained pediatric nurse-practitioners, under the general supervision of an MD, are rendering continuing care to children. In a few teaching hospitals in New York City and elsewhere, nurse-midwives are doing the same thing for pregnant women. One of the most interesting experiments is the one at Duke University Medical School—the well-known two-year program for training exmilitary corpsmen as "physician's assistants."

Interest on the part of young people in these new experiments is intense. Dr. George Harrell, Dean of the new Pennsylvania State Medical School at Hershey, reported over 1000 applicants for the 40 places in their first class, and nearly 2000 for 48 places in their second class, at which point applications were cut off. This school specifically emphasizes family medicine. Duke University reports 500 applications for the ten places available for the second year of their program.

In some situations the shortage of trained personnel is now so great and the demand so intense that all sorts of persons, trained or untrained, are being thrown into the breach. Public health nurses, social workers, and even home health aides (a new category of indigenous personnel with three to six months of training who are widely used in the Office of Economic Opportunity neighborhood health centers) are all helping to bridge the chasm between scientific medicine and the bewildered patient. In at least one OEO center, the director, a courageous young internist, has decided not only that there are not enough MDs to maintain a one-to-one relationship with patients, but that the practitioner should not even be head of the health team. Every team has a physician, but the team leader who maintains a continuing relationship with the patient is the nurse. The MD has been relegated to the role of expert technician, well paid, indispensable, but no longer the primary contact with the patient.

This seems the ultimate destination of the route that professionals and medical educators are traveling today. It is the role already chosen voluntarily by pathologists, radiologists, and increasingly by surgeons and many of the superspecialists. These physicians still talk about the sacred doctor-patient relationship, but their meaning is quite different from what the patient reads into this phrase—a friend in need who understands and cares about the patient's total needs.

If our society is forced to turn for medical care to 18-year-old high school dropouts or middle-aged grandmothers who have been given three months of catch-as-catch-can training, if this is the best we can do in this affluent nation, so be it. It is probably better than nothing. When a man is dying, he does not question the training of the hand that holds his own. It is the human warmth that counts. And the ghetto mother with seven small children and a persistent backache may get more practical help from a home health aide who can direct her to needed social services than from an orthopedic surgeon who can only report that the x ray shows no spinal pathology. ...

Selection 10

The Changing Doctor-Patient Relationship*

"Doctor-patient relationship" is both a serious reality and a vaporous slogan. Professionals and patients, conservatives and liberals, all have appealed to the

---

*Excerpt from H.M. and A.R. Somers, *Doctors, Patients, and Health Insurance* (Washington, D.C.: The Brookings Institution, 1961), pp. 457-467, 470-482.

concept when advocating or resisting a significant change in the organization or financing of health care. Traditionalists in the medical profession have claimed, at one time or another, that health insurance, group practice, HMOs, PSROs, and almost every other innovation would destroy the "sacred doctor-patient relationship." In recent years patients have increasingly complained of impersonality, lack of continuity, and deprivation of an alleged former special relationship. But for all this emotional appeal, rarely are we told just what it is, what it was, or what it should be.

Selection 10 (1961) tries to sort out the nostalgia and the propaganda from the reality, past and present, and the need.

THE PERSISTENT MYSTIQUE

The popular concept of the doctor-patient relationship is a mixture of fact and fancy. Until World War II the general practitioner family doctor was still in the majority. The one-to-one relationship of a personally chosen physician—where economic and other factors permitted any choice—with his patient was the most common form of medical practice. In big cities the doctor had an office, usually mahogany and leather, sparsely equipped with simple diagnostic aids, a few surgical tools, and some antiseptic drugs. But, especially in rural areas and suburbs, he was more often found in the homes of his patients doing his rounds, working at the bedside of the sick and injured. His black bag held almost all his equipment.

His records were kept partly in a small notebook, mostly in his mind and heart. He appeared indefatigable, compassionate, and available wherever and whenever needed. It was not his fault—nor was he blamed for the fact—that he was better acquainted with suffering and death than with diagnosis and cure. His limitations were tacitly understood.

This doctor of the past has been idealized in story, picture, and legend. One of the most publicized by the medical profession is the gloomy portrait by Sir Luke Fildes. In this, a little girl lies desperately ill—apparently with diptheria. Her parents stand by, humble and fearful, but trusting. The entire room bespeaks poverty. Beside the improvised bed sits the doctor, clothes rumpled, head bowed. It is obvious that he is keeping a solemn vigil—that he will stay with her until either the crisis has passed or death has claimed her. It is equally obvious that there is little else he can do except offer his comfort, friendship, and prayers.

This touching picture is patently irrelevant today. An American child so desperately ill would usually be in a hospital. Between her and her parents, if they were present, would be an oxygen tent, perhaps a transfusion machine or even a heart-lung device, not to mention hospital regulations and personnel. Her personal physician might or might not look in on her during the night; his instructions would long since have been delivered to the nurse and hospital resident doctors. It could be expected that his decisive contributions would be penicillin, sulfa, surgery, or other specific medical intervention rather than devotion alone.

It is also relatively improbable that a child would have so critical a disease. Thanks to scientific medicine and public health measures most American children are now successfully immunized in early years against diptheria, whooping cough, tetanus, and smallpox.

Despite its apparent anachronisms, the picture still appeals to people's sentiments—even to those fully aware of its use as a public relations device. It has the warmth and intimate concern that no hyperdermic needle—no complex of steel and tubing—can replace, however effective they may be. Although medical miracles may be performed successfully between strangers, doctors and patients both believe that the absence of continuity, personal concern, and individual attention are detrimental to the best medical care. This is not without foundation.

The origin of the "traditional" doctor-patient relationship reaches deep into the past. From the beginning of medical history, the practicing physician has been part priest, part technician, part personal or family counselor. In early days when medicine had very little in the way of scientific knowledge to rely on, it was inevitable that the subjective priestly element should be dominant. In the words of the pioneer anthropologist, Bronislaw Malinowski, "Magical beliefs and practices tend to cluster about situations where there is an important uncertainty factor and where there are strong emotional interests in the success of action. ..."

In modern times medicine has become more scientific. But the traditional reliance on mystical forces and a highly authoritarian doctor-patient relationship persists to a degree unknown in other contemporary human relations, with the exception of priest-parishioner in certain religious groups. There is no general acknowledgment or acceptance of the significant change that has, in fact, been taking place in the doctor-patient relationship. Of the manifold and complex reasons, only a few of the more important can be noted here.

First and basic is the persistence—in spite of scientific progress—of large elements of uncertainty and fear regarding illness and medical care which are conducive to continued reliance on hope, faith, confidence, and other subjective factors on the part of both doctor and patient. "Honor thy physician because of the need thou hast of him." So said Ecclesiasticus to the Hebrews thousands of years ago. Still, today, patients yearn to have confidence in their doctors, to idealize them, to endow them with superhuman powers.

As the boundaries of medical ignorance and uncertainty are pushed back, one would expect this resort to supra-scientific factors to decline; and, indeed, it has in the case of bacterial and other diseases where the cause and cure are clearly established. But the reduced role of subjective factors in the treatment of specific cases has been more than offset by an increasing interest in the role of the emotions in illness. A widespread increase in psychotherapy and psychosomatic medicine has renewed the emphasis on a personal doctor and a personal doctor-patient relationship of a type that permits knowledge of the "whole man."

As part of this growing interest, it is now often said that the old-fashioned leisurely family doctor, the "folksy" chiropractor, and the sophisticated psychiatrist have something in common—even that "the chiropractor's table is the poor man's couch." Moreover it is now widely believed that illness, *per se*, tends to create—even in the most intellectual of patients—an attitude of dependence, of "regression" to helplessness, and perhaps to childlike behavior. In this state, confidence in the authority and benevolence of the doctor, as well as in his scientific knowledge and technical skill (the now-familiar "father-image") is generally desired and often desirable.

Finally, there is the impenetrable mystery of death. The physician's relation to this event—however helpless he in fact may be—has endowed him in the eyes of centuries of patients with an aura of the mystery. To the extent that the physician identifies himself with this priestly role and takes on himself the burden associated therewith, or at least appears to do so through the gravity of his personal demeanor and behavior, his supra-scientific role continues to be respected and perpetuated, reinforcing in the eyes of individual patients and society at large his status as a dispenser of increasingly scientific medicine.

OSLER: THE MAN AND THE SYMBOL

Perhaps the outstanding exemplar in United States medical history of such a doctor was William Osler, chief physician of the Johns Hopkins Hospital from 1888 to 1905. His portraits, his voluminous lectures, essays, and letters, especially those emphasizing the ethical and historical aspects of medical practice, the picture which emerges from his chief biography,[1] indeed his whole life, testify to the wise, dedicated, righteous, and—as far as his patients were concerned—autocratic father.

The piercing deep-set eyes, the exceptionally high brow, the grave, almost forbidding, demeanor, unrelieved—at least in his public pictures—by any sign of levity bespeak a man who has looked deep and long into the face of death,[2] who has not shrunk from what he has seen but, on the contrary, has dedicated his life to the pursuit of truth and the alleviation of suffering. *Noblesse oblige*—the aristocratic concept that a privileged position, no matter how well earned, imposes a sense of obligation to those less fortunate—was the basis of his philosophy. He had outspoken contempt for doctors "among us who serve for sheckels, whose ears hear only the ... jingling of the guineas." Similarly, he belittled the pursuit of fame. Like Plato, another of his lifelong heroes, Dr. Osler held an elite, intellectual, detached view of life, medicine, and humanity. "Mentally," he once said, "the race is still in leading strings .... In the childhood of the world we cannot expect people yet to put away childish things."

With this view of man's intellectual and emotional immaturity, Osler's patient relationships were naturally authoritarian. He had relatively little interest in private practice. The idea of a doctor-patient relationship based on a rational discussion and a free economic contract was utterly alien to one whose professional life was centered in hospital wards and dispensaries. But he was never patronizing. In the words of a former patient, quoted by Dr. Harvey Cushing:

> The moment Sir William gave you was yours. It was hardly ever more than a moment, but there was curiously no abrupt beginning or end to it. With the easy sweep of a great artist's line, beginning in your necessity and ending in your necessity, the precious moment was yours becoming wholly and entirely a part of the fabric of your life. He made you respect his time, but he also respected yours. If he said: "I will come at two," and the hands of the clock pointed to ten minutes after, you knew that he could not come. And if that rare thing happened—a broken appointment—he never failed to send a few lines of explanation.... One other thing he safeguarded, and that was your purse. If a conscientious secretary sent a bill, it had to be a very moderate affair.

The noble Oslerian tradition became a symbol in American medical practice, influencing greatly the attitudes of both doctor and patient, touching the former with an aura that made him a saint as well as a scientist.[3]

A THEORY AFTER THE FACT

Nearly half a century after Dr. Osler left Johns Hopkins for Oxford and knighthood, Talcott Parsons of Harvard University set down on paper an elaborate "theory" of the doctor-patient relationship which articulated and systematized the relationship which Osler and other great doctors of the late 19th and early 20th centuries had exemplified. Briefly, the Parsons theory is as follows: The patient (and usually his family) is, by definition, characterized by helplessness, lack of knowledge, and profound emotional involvement. As a result of this combination of factors, it is almost impossible to expect him (or his family) to exercise rational judgment with respect to his illness or his treatment. He must, therefore, have complete "confidence" in his doctor and accept his judgment unquestioningly "on authority."

The physician, also by definition, is required to "'do everything possible' to forward the complete, early and painless recovery of his patients," and must do so in the face of "large factors of known impossibility and of uncertainty," which inevitably impose a great emotional strain on him, over and above the strain of dealing with the patient as a human being and his family. Moreover, he must assume this heavy burden entirely out of professional obligation and social altruism, without any thought of personal gain on his part. The situation of the medical profession, according to Parsons, is entirely different from that of the

> ...business world, where each party...is expected to be oriented to the rational pursuit of his own self-interest... "caveat emptor."...

The general picture is one of sharp segregation from the market and price practices of the business world, in ways which for the most part cut off the physician from many immediate opportunities for financial gain which are treated as legitimately open to the businessman.

Like many other socioeconomic theories in this fast-moving world, this one appeared after the reality had changed rather substantially. But again, like many theories and ideas that happen to fit the emotional and/or economic needs of important segments of society, the idea or "image" of such a relationship has acquired an independent force of its own.

THE TARNISHED IMAGE

To what extent did that image really represent the prevalent pattern of the past?

It was not until the 20th century that any but a tiny fraction of mankind—even in the most advanced civilizations of the past—had access to a personal doctor. The very concept of a personal doctor-patient relationship was inconceivable for most people. In part this was due to the almost universal poverty and ignorance; in part to the low state of medical science. But these were not the only reasons.

Historically, medicine has been a means of livelihood as well as a humanitarian vocation. Sometimes the periods associated with the most dramatic scientific advances have also been noted for callous disregard of individual suffering. Greek medicine—even in the days of the idealistic Hippocrates—was largely a privilege of the leisure class. The first result of the 18th century development of teaching hospitals and clinical research was to close the hospitals to cases that did not appear scientifically "interesting." The most popular medical handbook of that century, *Primitive Physic,* was written not by a doctor but by the evangelist John Wesley. In it he attacked both doctors and hospitals for lacking touch with the people. The notorious "gold-headed cane" of the 18th century English doctor symbolized not only his ostentation but his fear of contamination and dislike of poor patients. Whatever else one may say about the "traditional" doctor-patient relationship, one must recognize that, for the vast majority of mankind, it never existed.

The barriers to a good relationship, especially the economic ones, are less extreme today than they used to be. Nevertheless, they still exist. Rapidly changing conditions have brought conspicuous maladjustments and anomalies in their wake. The scientific development of medicine was not an isolated phenomenon but part of a general advance in science, technology, income, and education. As the doctor grew more capable, his patients also became more knowledgeable—less dependent on his devotion, and more demanding of the specialized skills of his profession.

Consider, first, the typical American patient around 1960. He is likely to be older than in Dr. Osler's day.[4] He is better educated and has a higher income. He usually sees the doctor not when he is flat on his back but in the doctor's office or clinic. One out of four visits is made when he is not sick at all, but for preventive purposes. The extent of his medical knowledge is still very limited, but it has increased rather dramatically. His own attitudes are more scientific. In many, if not the majority of, cases he knows enough to recognize ignorance or gross incompetence on the part of a doctor. On average, death is further removed and fear hangs less pervasively over the atmosphere.

He expects to pay for services rendered—directly or through a third party—and does not feel that he owes the doctor any special gratitude after the bill has been paid. His health insurance probably does not cover the doctor's visit, but the knowledge that he has hospital and surgical insurance reassures him in case serious illness and high costs develop. While the role of uncertainty, fear of suffering and death, and the emotional regression of sick people have certainly not disappeared, it is evident that the average American patient is now far less dependent, better informed, and less frightened than he was in Osler's day.

On the doctor's part, he is now rarely confronted with penniless patients. His collection ratio is running 90 percent or better. There is clearly neither the need nor the opportunity there used to be for philanthropy or *noblesse oblige* on his part. Little outright charity is expected or bestowed.[5] He knows that most people can and are willing to pay for medical care. If they cannot, a public or private agency is likely to do so. The practice of medicine has become highly profitable, and the medical doctor is now the best paid professional in the country. He is not only making money but is becoming a successful businessman—in terms of managerial techniques and even temperament.[6]

There is little time for friendly conversation with the patient or family counseling. The next patient is always waiting. The brisk impersonal atmosphere of office and hospital combined with the typical five-to-ten-minute consultation are effective inhibitors of social intercourse or of tales of woe—financial or emotional. The following picture of some harassed doctor's patient relationships, written to us by a prominent physician, may not be typical but is prevalent enough to cause grave concern:

> The busy doctor finds he can give less and less time per office, home or hospital service. I have seen a busy surgeon with 15 to 20 patients in a hospital, running between the rooms, with no time to hear of the postoperative problems or questions of his patients and no time to give them either the moral support they need or to determine whether or not the medical situation requires his attention. The jamming of so many doctors' offices with 20-30-40-50 or more patients per day is not uncommon—and the result, of course, is no time really to *listen* to a patient and learn what his problems really are, no time to get to know the patient and his family, no time to work up the case to arrive at a proper diagnosis and give sufficient thought to what is the best treatment . . . .

Time is money to the physician—the less time per professional service, he calculates, means more income to him. For too many physicians this is true.

Dr. Ward Darley, executive director of the Association of American Medical Colleges, presents a more restrained, but equally critical, picture:

> The present patterns of medical care present barriers to the concept of continuing, comprehensive care because of the fragmentation of patient care that has resulted from specialization, practice habits that limit interest to the episodic care of illness, and efficiency measures that limit the amount of time a physician gives to the individual patient.

"DOCS AND CROCKS"—THE WIDENING GAP

Related to this situation is the distaste of the average practitioner for patients whose problems are mainly emotional or where the organic disease is complicated by emotional involvement. This attitude starts in medical school where the young doctor acquires a strong bias against "neurotics," "hypochondriacs," and other "crocks."[7]

The North Carolina study of general practice (see Selection 6, note 3) found that only 17 percent of the physicians surveyed recognized and treated emotional problems with any competence. The authors concluded:

> Emotional problems appear to constitute an enigma for the practicing physician; many physicians completely failed to recognize these problems in their practices. Others, while recognizing the problems, were either indifferent to them or appeared to be made uncomfortable by patients with such problems. References to malingering, hypochondriacs, "problem patients" or "getting them out of the office quickly" were frequently heard, all indicating that some physicians were not prepared to deal sympathetically with these patients.

The concept of the "uncooperative patient" has become deeply imbedded in medical mores. A recent study in the outpatient clinic of a teaching hospital, for example, found that students, faculty, and other medical personnel readily agreed on the definition: a patient is "uncooperative" "when he is stubborn," "when he won't recognize that help is being given to him," "when he refuses to accept his condition," or "when he fails to appreciate the effort that has been expended on his behalf."

Unfortunately for the doctor's peace of mind, however, the desirability of a completely passive patient is now widely challenged, not only by many patients but also by leaders of the profession. It is increasingly recognized that the patient's active cooperation is frequently essential to effective therapy, whereas too great a dependence on the doctor—emotionally, financially, or otherwise—can be disastrous. Large reliance on placebos—intellectual as well as physical—is frowned upon.

A hundred years ago Dr. Oliver Wendell Holmes might, or might not, be forgiven for the following well-meant deception:

> Some shrewd old doctors have a few phrases always on hand for patients that will insist on knowing the pathology of their complaints without the slightest capacity of understanding the scientific explanation. I have known the term "spinal irritation" serve well on such occasions, but I think nothing on the whole has covered so much ground, and meant so little, and given such profound satisfaction to all parties, as the magnificent phrase "congestion of the portal system."

But this attitude today appears unjustifiable. Consider this quotation from a respected contemporary British doctor and author:

> We doctors are far more modest about our knowledge of physiology, pathology, and pharmacology than are these patients who desire to be told precisely how the medicine we have just ordered them is going to act on their illness. Yet because it is with their bodies that we are dealing, they have an undeniable right to be given some simple, if entirely insufficient and inaccurate, explanation of what we are hoping to do. Nor is it profitable, either to the patient or the doctor, for the doctor to be as modest on these occasions as the author has been in this book, for patients as a class do not want to be treated by a modest doctor but by a super-intelligent wonder-working one. The prescription must not, therefore, be handed over by the doctor casually, as though it were problematical whether it would do any good, but presented to the patient with the reverence owing to a magical formula.[8]

* * *

The justification for an optimistic "bias" and the importance of hope and confidence in medical treatment have been and will continue to be fully acknowledged. But the sort of treatment that consciously deceives the patient and that continues to recommend contrived emotion and magic formulas will be, we submit, increasingly resented and resisted by patients and doctors alike.

The patient may not only run out on his doctor, but he may come back with a malpractice suit—a symptom of deteriorating relationships that has been spreading ominously. According to the AMA Law Department, about 18,500 living physicians—one out of seven AMA members—have been the target of a malpractice suit or claim. In California the figure is one out of four.

The growth in malpractice claims has been attributed to many causes, including the persistence of a small but increasingly documented amount of genuine malpractice. Most recent studies of the problem, however. blame poor doctor-patient relations. A study made for the California Medical Association,[9] which attracted nationwide attention, declares, "The malpractice suit is a symptom of the breakdown in the doctor-patient relationship" and "most suits grow from the interaction of suit-prone doctor and suit-prone patient."

The suit-prone patient, according to this study, is likely to be a mild neurotic, dependent, lacking in understanding of his own emotions. "He leans unrealistically on the doctor—he wants the doctor to have godlike powers, but simultaneously distrusts what the doctor can do for him." He does not sue primarily for financial gains. He is generally angry at the doctor and sues to punish him as a child might try to punish his father for failure to help with his emotional difficulties. The view that such suits are primarily stimulated by lawyers appears false. Most patients thought of taking action themselves. In only one tenth of the cases did a lawyer advise suit. In just as many cases another doctor gave the advice.

The study also revealed that doctors who have been sued—especially those who have faced multiple suits—differ significantly in personality from doctors who have not. The suit-prone doctor wants patients to be dependent and grateful, he prefers not to call in consultants, is defensive and resentful of offers of help. He tends to blame others for things that go wrong; he dislikes and fears his patients, yet wants to be like a father to them.

The study contends that the doctor who is sued resembles psychologically the suing patient. Both are "suspicious," "immature," have low "self-esteem," and cannot handle emotional difficulties. "The patient expects powers that medical science cannot offer. The doctor, in his efforts to bolster his self-esteem, tends to promise more than medicine can deliver . . . . The feelings of inadequacy that both patient and doctor feel erupt into disputes, despair, and mutual recriminations."

> Perhaps the most significant categories of replies . . . center on how—in the patient's view—the doctor could have prevented him from suing . . . . Very few patients actually want to sue . . . . In no case was a doctor sued who told the patient directly and honestly that he made a mistake and that he was sorry for it . . . . Two out of three suing patients said the doctor could have prevented their suing if the doctor had discussed the matter with them in a plain and candid manner. A third said that they would not have sued if the doctor had not merely sent the bill with no reference to the incident and no indication of concern for the patient.

If the Blum thesis is correct (in spite of the furor the study caused in California medical circles no serious effort at refutation was attempted) it would appear that the underlying cause of the vast increase in malpractice claims and suits is the tension and conflict resulting from the effort to maintain an anachronistic 19th century form of human relations in the mid-20th century. This appears consistent with the surprising statement attributed to a leading medical management consultant that half his firm's work is trying to help doctors improve their patient relations.

These charges may involve a great deal more than inconvenience, irritation, or legal battles. According to Dr. Ward Darley, "the time has come when illness as it may be caused or aggravated, and health as it may be perpetuated, by iatrogenic factors, should be subjected to careful and intensive study." This is a point long emphasized by psychiatrists and specialists in psychosomatic medicine. "We still are not sufficiently aware," says Dr. Flanders Dunbar, "that the physician himself is often pathogenic. He is so when he concentrates on symptoms without adequate attempt to ascertain or remove their causes." He is so, according to this school of thought, when he permits the patient's craving for dependence and his own craving for admiration to dominate the diagnosis and choice of therapy. By refusing to help or even force the patient to assume some responsibility for his own cure, he may, it is alleged, be contributing to a prolongation or "fixation" of the physiological symptoms and thus injure him physically as well as emotionally.

> The risk of fixation is increased whenever treatment becomes very intensive, very elaborate, or very impersonal, and today, when ever-growing facilities are available for mechanistic diagnosis and therapy, there is a danger... of inducing "fixation invalidism" on a scale hitherto unknown.

This is a very serious indictment, and it is, of course, deeply resented—just as was the charge made a hundred years ago by Drs. Semmelweis and Holmes that hospital obstetricians were often pathogenic. In that case the critics were correct, and present-day aseptic childbirth is as much a tribute to their courageous and unpopular perspicacity as to the work of Louis Pasteur and his followers.

If today's critics are correct, it can only be concluded that the image of the "traditional" doctor-patient relationship is not only inaccurate, but that it has lost most of its beneficent value and may now have become injurious to doctor and patient alike. Dr. Osler's benevolent authoritarianism was appropriate for his day and type of practice, but it is out of harmony with the realities of 1960. The image appears to have degenerated into a public relations stereotype, potentially harmful to patient and doctor—therapeutically, ethically, and financially. These developments are not due to financial and organizational mechanisms that improve access to modern medicine. They are more likely related to futile attempts to perpetuate the past—a past which, for the great majority of sick people, never existed.

TOWARD A NEW KIND OF RELATIONSHIP: THE DOCTOR AS EDUCATOR

"Educational" may suggest the essence of the newly emerging relationship of doctor and patient just as the "traditional" relationship is frequently identified as "authoritarian." The terms are not mutually exclusive; the overlap is also evident in the types of relationship they suggest. Yet the differences are fundamental.

Where the authoritarian relationship assumes—and does not discourage—the continued dependence of the patient on the doctor's superior knowledge and wisdom, the educational relationship aims to help the patient understand his illness or problem, to assume maximum responsibility for his own recovery, and to overcome his dependence. Where the old relationship was one of unbridgeable inequality, the new is essentially democratic, although never quite reaching the point of equality. The doctor remains in full charge of the diagnosis and treatment, but makes of his patient an informed, active participant, with full knowledge of the facts and the probable consequences of alternative courses of action. The relationship is basically secular, although it cannot fully dispel the elements of mysticism and faith that overhang the continuing uncertainties and fears surrounding life-and-death situations.

The doctor's attitude is humane and sympathetic; his attention highly individualized; but he stops short of personal involvement. Just as the wise Hippocrates warned against too intimate an interest in individual patients, the modern doctor refrains from involving his own ego in the patient's problems and responses. He attempts to combine scientific neutrality with human warmth into a quality larger than either.

While this new relationship has not yet, to the authors' knowledge, been formulated precisely, practical evidence indicates it to be the present trend. Increasingly common is the experience of many patients of being trained by the doctor to assist him in his diagnosis and treatment. Mothers are asked to use the thermometer on their children before calling the pediatrician; maternity patients are asked to time their own labor pains before going to the hospital; the general public is urged to examine itself frequently for possible cancer symptoms. Many doctors and health plans require new patients to answer self-administered questionnaires such as the Cornell Medical Index with its 195 questions concerning bodily symptoms, past illnesses, family history, and "behavior, mood, and feeling." While the index was designed primarily as a convenience and aid to the doctor, the experience is educational for the patient. It compels him to probe his own need for treatment even before the doctor begins his examination and strengthens the patient's role in the relationship.

In the fields of preventive medicine, industrial medicine, rehabilitation, and psychiatry, greater stress is often placed on the patient's participation than on the doctor's activities. For example, Dr. Karl Menninger, one of the nation's leading psychiatrists, says that the turning point toward health is reached when a patient "begins to feel that it is his own responsibility to take charge of his life, and not the analyst's function . . . ."

In rehabilitation, the doctor's emphasis on patient responsibility and effort and the patient's response to the doctor's challenge represent extraordinary departures from past views and practices. Even paraplegics, the blind, the legless, and other seriously handicapped persons are not coddled; they are challenged to become self-sufficient and self-supporting. Dr. Howard Rusk, the world famous rehabilitation specialist, points to the vastly expanded scope of the physician's task:

> Regardless of the type of disease or disability, the responsibility of the physician to his patient . . . cannot end when the acute phase of the disease or injury is over. It ends only when . . . proper referral has been made to those agencies and institutions which are equipped to rehabilitate and retrain the patient with a physical disability. Medical responsibility is not met until the patient has been trained to live within the limits of his disability but to the hilt of his capabilities.

Dr. Lemuel C. McGee, a specialist in industrial medicine, has shown the courage as well as the insight to submit himself publicly to this self-examination:

> I am disturbed . . . at my use of drug therapy as a crutch for the patient (either a frank placebo or one of the many and notoriously inadequate synthetic spasmolytics) whose gastrointestinal problem is rather obviously and fundamentally one of emotional origin. I am not sure but that I undo the beneficial effect of my explanation to him of the basis and mechanism of his illness by trying to control symptoms at the level of the autonomic nervous system while further and necessary investigation is made of his emotional situation and other factors back of his illness.

How different this attitude toward the placebo, medications in general, and toward the education of the patient from that previously recounted!

The attitudes of doctors specializing in pediatrics, obstetrics, preventive medicine, rehabilitation, and psychiatry are increasingly relevant to the general practice of medicine as we move from an era of acute episodic illness into one dominated by chronic disease. Patients with diabetes, ulcers, high blood pressure, arthritis, heart conditions, and glaucoma are increasingly taught to understand their diseases and to handle routine treatment themselves. It could hardly be otherwise: no doctor could conceivably expect the diabetic to come to his office for daily insulin injections. Again, this in no way relieves the physician of responsibility for overall management of the case, but it clearly alters the nature of the supervision and his relation to the patient.

An interesting statement, suggesting that this new educational type of relationship, is beginning to be accepted in the traditional specialties, comes from Dr. Dana W. Atchley, professor of clinical medicine, Columbia University College of Physicians and Surgeons:

> In his ignorance the medical man of previous generations often assumed a self-protective and rather arrogant remoteness that discouraged all questions; he knew too little to dare say, "I don't know." Treatment was smothered in secrecy, prescriptions were wholly in Latin, and no clue as to the whys or wherefores was offered. Of course, the warm-hearted, sympathetic practitioner managed to evade this convention of unapproachability, but many patients still apologize before they make a thoroughly justified query as to the results of their examination. The modern physician takes pride in exposition. He avoids dogmatic authoritarianism. He feels that his prime responsibility is to teach the patient all that he can comprehend about his illness; exposition, not dictation, is his concern.... The atmosphere is that of an honest and candid interchange, the patient responding to the penetrating interest that is implicit in a modern diagnostic study and the physician reacting with a confidence and humility that comes from scientific insight.

Dr. Atchley makes clear that, "In contrasting the physicians of today and forty years ago, I speak only of the best of the profession." He acknowledges that "there are many doctors who have not changed with the progress of their discipline." Yet, he insists, "The vigor and freshness of a profession rest primarily on the quality of its leaders." It may be protested that examples from the "best of the profession" are hardly representative of what happens to the average patient with the average doctor. Nor, of course, is it necessarily true that the "best of the profession" are also its leaders. Nevertheless, as in the case of Dr. Osler, who was certainly not typical in his own day, such outstanding doctors may in time establish the ideal image for the whole profession. ...

Obviously, not all patients are prepared for this new type of relationship. Just as many students prefer to be told "the answers" in black and white rather than being taught to think for themselves, so many patients still want and need an authoritarian relationship with their doctors. In many cases this may be the only means of rapport. An example is the different patient reaction to the old problem, "Should cancer victims be told?" But the wish for honesty appears to prevail. In the effort to study patient reactions, a British medical team discussed their cases frankly with 231 patients (93 men, 138 women) with curable cancers. There were four types of reactions: 153 approved of learning the truth. They said it helped them face treatment better; that ignorance might have worried them more. Seventeen (all women) were sorry; 17 had no definite opinion; 44 denied they had ever been told they had cancer—a protective reaction.

Alongside the wide variety of patient attitudes, there is the notable fact that two-thirds approved of a completely honest relationship.

Not all studies are so encouraging. According to a 1958 survey of reading habits by the National Association of Science writers, a large proportion of popular medical articles does not really sink in or is garbled in the patient's mind. In spite of all recent publicity on the Salk vaccine, for example, only 40 percent of those surveyed understood it in some detail; only half knew that fluoridation had something to do with teeth; and one-third said they had never heard of radioactivity.

A better educated and more responsible patient is essential, not only for his own sake, but for the improvement of medical care in general and to keep the national cost of medical care within manageable bounds. It has been said that "patients tend to look for a physician more or less in their own image, at least in what they believe to be their own image." It is primarily up to the doctor to set the "tone" of the relationship. But he cannot be too far ahead of his patients without losing them to someone less qualified but less demanding.

The modern doctor cannot depend on a single inclusive formula for dealing with patients. He must recognize the existence of individual differences and the corresponding need for different therapeutic attitudes on his part. He takes on himself the burden of diagnosing the type of patient he has, just as much as he assumes the burden of diagnosing the nature of the physical ailment. Clearly, his job is far more difficult than in the past—in terms of human relations as well as in technical competence.

NOTES

1. Harvey Cushing, M.D., *The Life of Sir William Osler* (London: Oxford Univ. Press, 1925). Osler was the youngest son in a family of nine born to a Cornish Anglican missionary in an austere two-room parsonage on the edge of the Canadian wilderness. His original expectation of entering the ministry was deflected only by an even greater interest in natural science, which led him into "the ministry of healing." But his attitude toward his vocation was symbolized by his lifelong favorite book, Sir Thomas Browne's *Religio Medici (The Religion of a Physician)*.

2. He once described himself as "a student for many years of the art and the act of dying." *Ibid.*

3. "From the Atlantic to the Pacific, he [the European visitor] will find a picture of Osler hanging on the wall in almost every doctor's house.... A myth is beginning to accrete round his figure." H.E. Sigerist, M.D., *The Great Doctors* (2nd ed., 1933; republished, 1958).

4. In 1820 the median age of the population of the United States was 17; in 1958 it was 30.

5. There are exceptions, of course. Dr. Lonnie Coffin of Farmington, Iowa, the doctor chosen by AMA as the "GP of the Year 1958," said that he still sent his patients no bills. "If they aren't able to pay, then I don't want 'em to pay. If people are honest, they'll pay eventually. If they're not honest, they won't pay—I don't see that it's worth worryin' about." (W.B. Furlong, "On the Rounds with the G.P. of the Year," *New York Times Mag-*

azine, January 11, 1959, p. 30.) The poignancy of this story derives not only from the fact that the Dr. Coffins are as rare today as the horse and buggy but also from a conviction—even among the severest critics of the profession—that such quixoticism is unnecessary and largely irrelevant in a day when most patients expect to pay. A few months after his selection as "G.P. of the Year," Dr. Coffin died. He had been actively seeking a doctor "with a sense of mission" to take over his practice. But every young man he asked "grinned sheepishly and turned me down."

6. Reporting to the Fourth Teaching Institute of the Association of American Medical Colleges on a survey of personality characteristics of medical school applicants, D. Lowell Kelly, professor of psychology, University of Michigan, summarized as follows:

> Essentially, our medical students are persons who, if they were not becoming physicians, would be planning to become manufacturers, big businessmen, production managers, engineers; they are not the kind of people who would become teachers, ministers, social workers, i.e., professional persons interested in doing something for the good of mankind. As a group, the medical students reveal remarkably little interest in the welfare of human beings.
>
> All of the evidence available to us leads to the conclusion that the *typical* young physician has little interest in cultural aspects of the society in which he lives, has very little sensitivity to or feeling for the needs of the community, and is generally not inclined to participate in community activities unless these contribute to his income....
>
> As I see it, medical practice today, as characterized by the people going into it, is the last stronghold of individual economic competition, a stage through which big industry has already passed. It is my impression that the typical young executive in big industry today has a far greater sense of community needs and sensitivity to his role in helping society solve its problems than does the young physician who is still essentially an entrepreneur. ("Multiple Criteria of Medical Education and Their Implications for Selection," *Journal of Medical Education* (October 1957): part 2, pp. 195-196.)

7. A "crock" has been defined as "a patient from whom the diagnostic sheen has been worn." A questionnaire given to approximately 500 fourth-year students at Cornell, University of Pennsylvania, and Western Reserve medical schools revealed an almost unanimous preference for patients with organic as opposed to emotional illness. William Martin in R.K. Merton, G.G. Reader, and P.L. Kendall, eds., *The Student-Physician* (1957), p. 192.

8. Kenneth Walker, M.D., *Patients and Doctors* (London, 1957). The fact that similar obscurantist attitudes are held by doctors operating under such dissimilar economic systems as United States private practice and the British National Health Service suggests that its basis is less financial than critics of the profession often alleged.

9. Richard H. Blum, *Malpractice Suits—Why and How They Happen: A Summary of a Report to the Medical Review and Advisory Board of the California Medical Association* (1958).

Selection 11

The Future of Demand: Some Influential Factors*

When people speak of "adequate medical care" they do not have in mind any finite or defined quantity or quality. The meaning varies with the "state of the art" as seen by professionals and patients, the availability of health services, and people's perceptions of what is illness and its responsiveness to medical therapy. The possibility of excessive demand was not of wide concern or discussion in the early 1960s, when observers were still almost exclusively concerned with "need"—a far more indefinite concept than was acknowledged—and removal of economic barriers to meet such need. Since then, the rapid rise in demand has led to widely articulated fears that if economic barriers are further removed the flood of demand unloosed could exceed our economic and professional capacities. But the problem appears more complicated.

Recent experience does indeed indicate that reduction of financial barriers increases utilization. But more than financing has changed. The introduction of new medical technologies, shifting cultural values, revised perceptions of "illness," and changed individual attitudes toward pain or discomfort are all contributing to demand. These are not easy to measure, but should be seen as a caution to those engaged in predicting future need and/or demand.

Selection 11 (1961) summarizes a number of contemporary studies of consumer attitudes and behavior and evaluates their significance.

SOCIOECONOMIC AND INDIVIDUAL DIFFERENCES IN THE PERCEPTION OF HEALTH AND ILLNESS

We have discussed the broad change in general attitude toward sickness and medical care. Within this overall picture there are, however, many important differences among social groups and within them. Even individual variations may be significant. Here are a few examples derived from representative case studies.

1. The late E.E. Koos' *The Health of Regionville* (1954) reports the divergent attitudes toward illness, health, and medical care in a "typical" small town in upstate New York in the late 1940s.[1] The population of Regionville was divided into three major groups or classes, based primarily on the occupation of the head of the family. Class I comprised families whose heads were business or professional men, with a modal annual income of slightly over $4,000 (in 1946). Class II included skilled or semiskilled workers (average income $2,374) and

---

*Excerpt from H.M. Somers and A.R. Somers, *Doctors, Patients, and Health Insurance* (Washington, D.C.: The Brookings Institution, 1961), pp. 150-165.

farmers (average income $2,722). Class III consisted of laborers, both village and rural, with an average income of about $1,700. Class I accounted for about 10 percent of all households, Class II for 65 percent, and Class III, 25 percent.

On almost every question involving attitudes or behavior in health and illness there was a significant difference among the three social groups. Among these differences were the following:

The perception of illness: Given a list of 17 specific symptoms medically recognized as danger signals—chronic fatigue, shortness of breath, lump in breast, blood in urine, etc., and asked which should be called to the attention of a doctor, over 75 percent of Class I respondents checked all but two. Class II showed less sensitivity, while Class III showed a marked indifference to most symptoms. Fifty percent checked only three—all involving unexplained bleeding.

Incidence of disabling illness and use of medical care: About 50 percent of Class I were reported to have had a disabling illness, and two-thirds of these had sought medical care. In Class II, 54 percent reported such an illness, and 82 percent of that number had had treatment. In Class III, illness was reported by 67 percent, two-thirds of whom were treated.

Use of a family doctor: In Class I, 82 percent reported having a family doctor, and only 10 percent had changed since the household was established. In Class II, 73 percent had a family doctor; 16 percent had changed. In Class III, only 32 percent had a family doctor, and 63 percent had changed.

Group practice: Over 90 percent of Class I families favored group practice as opposed to solo practice, but only about 50 percent of Class III felt similarly.

Use of druggists and chiropractors as a substitute for regular physicians: Fifty-eight percent of Class III families were prepared to use a chiropractor for any illness, but only 2 percent of Class I. Class III sought medical advice from the druggist to a much greater extent than Class I or II.

Medications: Among Class I families, 91 percent kept an antiseptic at home; Class II, 88 percent; Class III, 52 percent. With respect to "liver pills," the proportions were: Class I, 10 percent; Class II, 21 percent; Class III, 66 percent.

All classes were found to be lacking in perception or concern for community health problems. A uniform 82 percent said there were no special problems in their community.

2. *Social Class and Mental Illness* (1958) by A.B. Hollingshead, a sociologist, and Dr. F.C. Redlich, a psychiatrist, both at Yale, concentrated on New Haven, Connecticut, in 1950-51.[2] The population was divided into five classes, based on occupation, years of schooling, and area of residence. The median income of families (with only one wage earner) varied from $10,000 for Class I down to $2,700 for Class V. In addition to the income variable, extreme differences among the groups were reported with respect to ethnic and religious

backgrounds, accumulated wealth, family and community life, recreation, and attitudes toward illness in general and mental illness in particular. These were among the specific findings:

A distinct inverse relationship between social class and treated mental illness. The lower the class, the greater the proportion of patients from that class. Class V, in particular, contributed more than twice the percentage of patients as its proportion of the population warranted. On the other hand, Class I had only one-third as many as might have been expected on the basis of population. Classes II, III, and IV were also underrepresented among patients, but not to the same extent as Class I. This relationship prevailed even when other influences like sex, race, religion, age, and marital status were taken into account.

A definite relationship between class position and type of mental illness. The higher the class, the greater the proportion of neuroses; the lower the class, the greater the proportion of psychoses. This was particularly dramatic in the case of schizophrenia: the rate was found to be 895 per 100,000 population in Class V, as compared with 111 for Classes I and II.

A great difference in the method, place, and expense of treatment of similar disorders. In general, psychotherapy, especially psychoanalysis, was limited to Class I and II patients. Organic therapy, especially shock treatment, was the standard therapy for the lower classes. Many Class V schizophrenics did not get any treatment, at least for any length of time, but were relegated to the "hopeless" wards of state hospitals.

Lower-class persons did not understand psychiatry and went to a psychiatrist only under compulsion, usually of police or social agencies. Upper-class individuals went voluntarily, although they often concealed the fact in one way or another.

A tentative conclusion suggests a significant relationship between neurosis and upward social mobility, the moving of persons or families from one class and sociocultural milieu to a higher one.

The authors, angered at society's treatment of mental illness among lower-class citizens, conclude that this all adds up to "deep social fissures in psychiatric treatment, such as we do not encounter in the rest of medicine, with the possible exception of peacetime cosmetic surgery." Clearly the fissures also exist in the attitudes of consumers. ...

3. During the course of a Baltimore study of chronic illness,[3] 1,292 "representative Baltimorians" were invited to have a complete physical examination by the staff of the Johns Hopkins Hospital at no expense to themselves. Appointments were offered at convenient times, transportation by taxi was provided, and no effort was spared to insure their comfort. Nevertheless, 41 percent refused to participate. No clear-cut explanation for acceptance or refusal was discernible. There were these differences, however: The best response came from the highest and lowest income groups; the poorest response from among

those with family incomes between $2,000 and $3,999, and those who would not or could not tell their income. There was a more favorable response among non-whites than whites. There was a much higher rate of refusal among older people.

In general, the commission concluded that people's attitudes toward health and medical care were "major obstacles to the application of available therapeutic measures." Of a selected high disability sample, more than half were said "to need to adjust their attitudes toward their disease, and more than one-third toward recommended care of the disease." Included in the noncooperative group were the seriously obese who refused to diet, diabetics who refused to take insulin or follow the prescribed regimen, and those with occupational diseases who refused to try to change jobs.

IGNORANCE, IRRESPONSIBILITY, AND THE MAGIC BOTTLE OF MEDICINE

The wide disparities in health attitudes and behavior indicated in these studies are confirmed by national surveys, which show that while 6 percent of the population see a doctor 20 or more times during the year, 28-37 percent do not see a doctor even once. Included in the first group are 1.5 percent who report 50 or more visits a year.

Part of this variation is readily attributable to differences in incidence of illness, which are as conspicuous within particular economic and social groups as among them. But, some of this difference in real illness is also a product of individual and cultural variations in attitudes and behavior. The number of physician visits is not directly correlated with illness. Failure to see a doctor for 12 months is not necessarily proof of good health, any more than a weekly visit demonstrates serious illness. Hypochondria and apathy, ignorance and knowledge, irresponsibility and concern are all aspects of consumer demand.

Many Americans are highly casual, even irresponsible, in respect to personal indulgences that are known to be serious threats to health. It has long been known, for example, that excess weight is a serious hazard that is linked with consistently higher mortality rates. Yet it is estimated that the average American is 20 pounds overweight. According to doctors' reports even the obese patient who is specifically instructed to reduce is likely to return a little heavier for the next visit. Although a probable causal connection between cigarette smoking and lung cancer has been pointed out repeatedly by the highest authorities, cigarette sales have increased steadily—helped, no doubt, by the self-comforting gesture of changing to a filter brand.

When prevention is made easily available, millions of people who denounce the lack of "cures" fail to respond. Even after the tremendous public interest generated by the development of the Salk vaccine, as late as September 1958, some 40 million Americans in the susceptible under-40 age group had not been vaccinated against polio. Similarly, effective prophylaxis and penicillin therapy for venereal disease are now easily and inexpensively available. Although great progress has been made in reducing its incidence, a substantial case reservoir of unknown size still exists, and reported cases are no longer declining.

On the other hand, we observe some peculiar expressions of real concern in the pursuit of quackery in its many forms, the purchase of food nostrums and useless drugs, and in misuse of genuine pharmaceuticals. The drug fetish is nothing new. From time immemorial people have searched for magic herbs, potions, and elixirs that would free them from pain and disease and restore health and youth. Opium, cinchona, and other valuable botanicals were discovered in the course of this search. But along with the positive results, there has been widespread misuse.

Historically there have been cycles in liquor and drug addiction, related in part to the severity of external pressures in a society, in part to the availability or absence of legitimate medical care, and in part to the emphasis (or lack of it) on self-discipline in the national culture. The patent-medicine era in the United States was probably due primarily to the impotence of the poorly trained doctors in our 19th century frontier society. It declined as scientific medicine developed and leading physicians like Holmes and Osler took a firm stand against "dosing."[4]

Then came the genuine pharmaceutical triumphs which transformed the drug industry. But alongside the $2.2 billion annual sales (1959) of prescription drugs, over $1 billion is spent for self-medication. This includes not only aspirin, antiseptics, and other standard home remedies but thousands of questionable items—the ever-popular liver and stomach pills, pain-relievers, tranquilizers, energizers, and undifferentiated vitamins—sold (often illegally) over-the-counter or peddled from door-to-door.[5] On all sides, we are told, not only health but happiness, peace, serenity, and even religious experience are available—at least temporarily—for the price of a little pill. "When an American goes to the doctor," says the *Journal of the Iowa Medical Society*, "he expects a prescription." If he does not get it, he is disappointed or even angry. So "more and more doctors" are prescribing "more and more medicine." Dr. E.M. Popper of Columbia University reports that tranquilizers are now taken by one out of every seven Americans "as an escape from anxiety."

The problem of the use and abuse of drugs is clearly one of great national as well as individual significance. Tighter professional and public regulations have been advocated. Others agree with Dr. Milton Roemer that "The greatest abuses of America's drug consumption are due to factors that cannot be legislated away." He believes that the major factor is "an inadequate provision of medical care that forces people to resort to the corner drugstore as a cheap substitute for medical attention." But the general availability of medical care is not in itself a solution to the problem, although it may alter its dimensions. Even nations with universal health insurance or a national health service are troubled by "overprescribing." According to Richard Titmuss of England, "Every country with a modern system of medical care is now faced with the question of 'controlling' the supply and consumption of drugs."[6]

CONSUMER "RIGHTS" AND "RESPONSIBILITIES"

In recent years epidemiologists and social scientists have been devoting increasing attention to sociocultural factors in illness and in attitudes toward medical care. Ecological studies have sought to correlate categories of illness and forms of medical care with specified cultural characteristics. The potential value of this work is apparent. If, for example, a scientific epidemiology of mental illness could be developed analagous to the epidemiology of tuberculosis, similar results might be achieved. At present, most of these studies are exploratory and suggestive. Together with the basic demographic and economic information, however, they help to provide some useful hypotheses regarding demand in a society moving toward increasing accessibility of medical services through both voluntary and statutory measures.

1. The wide differences among groups and individuals in perception of illness and demand for medical services—running from extremes of indifference to frenetic hypochondria—are well documented. Nonetheless, the responses of the large majority of consumers appear "rational" and generally consonant with the apparent realities. The "problem areas" are represented by numerical minorities. This is not to minimize their importance. On the contrary this chapter has been devoted to the idea that it is essential to understand the "special factors" as well as the general picture.

Clearly, it is inaccurate to think of the whole American population avidly awaiting access to better and more comprehensive medical care. It is also inaccurate to assume that there is not a considerable inherent potential for abuse. Those responsible for programming medical care services cannot afford to overlook either fact.

Yet a substantial portion of these "aberrations" appears due to a time factor, a cultural lag, already in the process of change. They are hangovers from less prosperous days, from sharper economic divisions, from a time when most medical care was provided through luxury services or charity wards, with little in between. It is likely, for example, that as the three classes in Regionville all improved their economic status during the past prosperous decade, and as health insurance became more widespread, the medical attitudes and mores of Class I became more widely accepted.

Similarly, it is interesting to speculate on the Baltimore experience, which showed that the lowest income group responded well to the invitation to a physical examination while the next higher group did not. The fragmentary information suggests that in the past the lowest income people in a city like Baltimore have known fewer barriers to medical care and are accustomed to the services offered at free clinics. Having seen friends and relatives cured at such clinics, they are medically more sophisticated and more inclined to cooperate in health matters than their somewhat higher income neighbors, who did not qualify for free care but were not able to buy their own. The latter's apathy was probably a product of ignorance and fear, including the fear that, if the examination found something seriously wrong, there would be no one to pay for the cure.

If these explanations are valid, they suggest that the shrinking economic barriers to medical care, rising levels of income and education, and more universal familiarity with good health services will steadily reduce and minimize the apparently irresponsible attitudes of the apathetic groups. This type of "underutilization" will be characteristic of a declining number.

In addition, we must take note of the general ethos of American society, which takes stronger hold as the population becomes more homogeneous. Titmuss has pointed out that attitudes toward illness and medical care rest ultimately on

> the significance that death holds in a given culture at a particular time. The more that a society as a whole values success in life and fears death, the higher may be its demand for medical care in some form or other. The more that the individual personality is sensitive and self-conscious about the roles he thinks he is expected to play in society the more demanding may be his perception of what constitutes "efficient function" or wholeness for himself and for others. What man himself regards as sickness and as his role as a sick or well person are the critical factors for, as Charles Lamb observed, "sickness enlarges the dimensions of a man's self to himself . . . supreme selfishness is inculcated upon him as his only duty."[7]

Few cultures have placed more value than ours on "success," or made its citizens more conscious of "efficient function," or feared death more. Balancing these many factors, it appears clear that the pressures will be toward a steadily increasing volume of demand per capita.

As "overutilization" appears to be conditioned to a significant degree by psychological and emotional factors, the future of this type of demand will depend in large measure on the evolving nature of the doctor-patient relationship and the presence or absence of institutionalized restraints.

2. The degree to which potential demand is constructively harnessed and prevented from improperly dissipating our limited medical resources depends in large measure on the medical profession. The Koos and Hollingshead-Redlich studies both emphasize the role of the doctor as molder of consumer attitudes. Koos makes it clear that the typical Regionville doctor did not try to improve the health understanding of his patients. On the contrary,

> He tends to perpetuate [their] perceptions. . . . There is little evidence that the Regionville physician has broadened his own interests to take into account all the factors, psychological and social, which have affected or brought about the illness. . . .

Hollingshead and Redlich find that psychiatrists as a whole have made little effort to cope with the mental problems of low-income people. They indicate that most psychiatrists are themselves "upper class" and find effective communication with lower-class people almost impossible. They are outraged by the treatment generally meted out to Class V psychotics and indicate that the dread of the "bughouse" is probably justified. They do not believe that classical psychoanalysis can ever be made practically available on a mass basis and plead with their colleagues to develop some new form of psychotherapy to meet the ever-growing need and to adopt a more sympathetic attitude toward lower-income people.

Such examples suggest that the irresponsibility or irrationality of medical consumers results, in not inconsiderable measure, from experience with medical practitioners. The doctor who is too busy, or too lazy, or opposed on principle to explaining to his patient the precise nature of his illness, including any relevant mental or emotional factors, or the ingredients of his prescription, is not helping him to develop a sane, critical attitude toward illness and medical care. On the contrary, he is helping to create a "fall guy" for some persuasive nostrum peddler.

With respect to preventive medicine, the ambivalence of the consumer is matched by that of the profession. For example, a 1955 survey found that 80 percent of the people believe they should see a doctor for a regular checkup even when they feel well, but only 29 percent do so. Among family doctors, 80 percent also said that people should have such checkups, but only 45 percent make a point of recommending it to most of their patients.

The fact that patients make extensive use of unaccredited hospitals and frequently permit themselves to be operated on by doctors who are not trained surgeons[8] may reflect simply the insufficient availability of the higher quality care in a particular locality, or it may mean that that many patients are being misled by their doctors as to the adequacy of the care they are receiving. In part this probably reflects the *mystique* nurtured by licensed professions, such as medicine and law, that the mere possession of the license is proof conclusive of adequate competence in any aspect of the field, behind which those outside the profession have no right to probe—also a form of group irresponsibility.

3. Acceptance of the view that access to good medical care is a "civic right" has an implicit corrollary obligation: the rational and responsible use of that right. This obligation has long been emphasized by those in the forefront of the "rights" movement. The European epidemiologist, Dr. René Sand, for example, insisted, "Health cannot be simply given to the people; it demands their participation."

In the past, the medical consumer's actions were, except in the case of contagious diseases, considered his personal business. But, as we move toward greater risk-sharing of the costs of illness and note the increasing pressures on a scarce supply, there is growing concern about responsible consumer behavior.

As "third parties" increase their stakes in health practices and medical care, and as representatives of second parties become better organized and more professionalized—union and management representatives, health and welfare fund officials, etc.—they will be less satisfied to depend exclusively on either the self-discipline of the individual or his physician. They are likely to seek means of controlling at least the more costly forms of irresponsible health behavior and demand.

NOTES

1. The study was based on a series of 16 household interviews with 514 families, approximately 20 percent of the total community, over a four-year period.
2. This ambitious study, supported by the National Institute of Mental Health, involved: (1) household interviews with 3,559 families constituting 5 percent of all households; (2) a complete census of all psychiatric patients in the New Haven metropolitan area during 1950; (3) an intensive study of 25 neurotic and 25 psychotic patients; and (4) interviews with 40 local psychiatrists.
3. Commission on Chronic Illness, *Chronic Illness in a Large City* (1957).
4. Consider Dr. Holmes' well-known aphorism, "If all the medicines in the world were thrown into the sea, it would be so much the better for mankind and so much the worse for the fishes." Osler, as usual, spoke more somberly:

> "Upon us, whose work lay in the last quarter of the nineteenth century, fell the great struggle with that many-headed monster, Polypharmacy—not the true polypharmacy which is the skillful combination of remedies, but the giving of many—the practice of at once discharging a heavily-loaded prescription at every malady, or at every symptom of it. Much has been done and an extraordinary change has come over the profession, but it has not been a fight to the finish. Many were lukewarm; others found it difficult to speak without giving offense in quarters where on other grounds respect and esteem were due. As an enemy to indiscriminate drugging, I have often been branded as a therapeutic nihilist.... I bore this reproach cheerfully, coming, as I knew it did, from men who did not appreciate the difference between the giving of medicine and the treatment of disease...." [Harvey Cushing, M.D., *The Life of Sir William Osler* (London: Oxford Univ. Press, 1925).]

5. No account is taken here of expenditures for illegal narcotics. However, it has been estimated that the underworld reaps a profit of $400 million a year from this source. *Time*, June 1, 1959, p. 63.
6. R.M. Titmuss in Foreword to J.P. Martin, *Social Aspects of Prescribing* (London: 1957). This study found that regional custom and local tradition continue to play a major part in the wide variation in prescription frequency even after the coming of the National Health Service.
7. R.M. Titmuss, *Essays on the Welfare State* (London: George Allen and Unwin, 1958).
8. A nationwide survey of patients hospitalized for surgery found that 22 percent of the operations were performed by doctors without any surgical specialization, mostly GPs. Another 27 percent were performed by doctors who specialized in surgery but were neither board-certified nor Fellows of the American College of Surgeons. O.W. Anderson and J.J. Feldman, "Distribution of Patients Hospitalized for Surgery in the United States 1952-53," *Bulletin of the American College of Surgeons* (September-October 1958).

Chapter Three

The Modern Hospital

Selection 12

Bigger, Better, and Beleaguered*

The role of the hospital in modern health services can hardly be exaggerated. Physical and intellectual center of the medical world, it is the doctors' indispensable workshop, where the three essential elements of scientific medicine—patient care, research, and teaching—are increasingly focused. The hospital is also gradually becoming a community health center, the one institution with the potential for encompassing and integrating the wide range of comprehensive medical services—prevention, treatment, rehabilitation, and after-care.

EXPANDING ROLE IN MEDICAL CARE

The hospital has not always been so important. Until the late 19th century, it was primarily a hostel for the sick poor, where the physical and economic derelicts of society usually found compassionate but ineffective care until death relieved them of their misery.

However, with the development of scientific medicine and its handmaiden, medical technology, the hospital changed radically. It became preeminently a place for medical service rather than custody. Modern surgery and anesthesiology could not have developed without such an institutional setting. Modern obstetrics and pediatrics take for granted the aseptic delivery room, the incubator for prematures, and other standby equipment for emergency treatment of mother and baby. Recently, though still incompletely, the hospital has begun to employ an array of electronic, radiological, biochemical, and other diagnostic techniques for the detection and prevention of disease.

Other services to ambulatory patients are also being extended. Previously these services, if available at all, were largely restricted to emergencies and the indigent. Today they are more and more a part of regular medical care. More

---

*Excerpt from H.M. and A.R. Somers, *Medicare and the Hospitals* (Washington, D.C.: The Brookings Institution, 1967), pp. 43-55.

doctors find it effective and convenient to see their patients at the hospital and often establish their own offices within the hospital complex to make better use of its advantages.

The teaching hospital is the principal setting for the nation's clinical research. It conducts, or is the site for, a dozen or more educational programs—in undergraduate, graduate, and postgraduate medicine, nursing, x-ray and laboratory technology, physical therapy, medical social work, hospital administration, etc. Community hospitals are also increasing their research and teaching activities.

Most recently and somewhat reluctantly, the hospital has found itself entrusted with considerable responsibility for developing relationships with the growing network of community health facilities and consequently involved in community health planning. Some of the better hospitals now provide or supervise nursing home care, home care, and other "parahospital" services.

GROWTH AND CHANGE

These professional developments have been accompanied by vast increases in hospital use, costs, and in the hospital's share of the national health dollar. Hospital care consumes a far larger portion of national expenditures for health than any other category, about 33 percent in 1965. If construction and research costs are included, the figure would reach 40 percent, almost twice as much as the next largest category, physicians' services. If we were to add the expenditures for medical services received in the hospital, but allocated to other categories, the hospital portion would be on the order of 55 percent, and all these ratios are rising steadily.

In 1872 the ratio of total hospital beds (short term and long term) per 1,000 population was less than two. In 1945, because of the World War II expansion in military beds, a peak of 13 per 1,000 was reached. During the past decade the figure has leveled off to a little over 9, representing about 1.7 million beds in over 7,100 institutions. Of these, some 5,700 with 741,000 beds are nonfederal short term hospitals. They account for 92 percent of all admissions, 71 percent of employees, and 71 percent of total hospital expenditures. They contain only about 40 percent of the occupants on the average day, however, because most of the other hospitals are long term institutions, often of a custodial character, with relatively little turnover. Actually, long term hospitals play a gradually declining role, since short term general hospitals provide care formerly given in mental and tuberculosis institutions, and because of the increasing availability of nursing homes and other parahospital institutions for custodial care.

The nonfederal short term hospital is the place where more than one out of every seven Americans, on average, was hospitalized last year. The number of beds per 1,000 population increased 15 percent over the 15-year period, 1950-65. Inpatient admissions per 1,000 rose 25 percent to a 1965 high of 137.9. Both these rates have shown steady increase throughout the period.

The Modern Hospital   87

Average length of stay—7.8 days in 1965—declined about 6 percent between 1950 and 1960, but a reversal has taken place since that time so the net reduction for the 15-year period is only 3.7 percent. Because of the long term decline, patient days per 1,000 population rose less than admissions, 19 percent; but the reverse has been true in the more recent experience. However, the inpatient population in absolute numbers (average daily census) has continued to rise.

Outpatient care is an increasingly important hospital activity. Unfortunately, comparable data are not available for these services. Incomplete statistics indicate a steep rise, especially in emergency room and private diagnostic services. The 93 million outpatient visits reported for 1965 represent a 40 percent increase over 1957, the first year for which roughly equivalent data are available. This was a 50 percent more rapid rate of increase than inpatient admission, and the trend appears to be continuing.

Full-time personnel (or their equivalents in part-time workers) rose 109 percent from 1950 to 1.4 million in 1965. The personnel-patient ratio rose 38 percent to a 1965 high of 2.5 employees per patient. Despite the rise in personnel and higher wages and salaries, payroll as a percent of total expenses advanced relatively little over the 15-year period and actually declined slightly during the last five years, indicating that other costs were rising faster than payrolls.

Total expense per patient day, the hospitals' average per diem cost, rose steadily throughout the entire period, a total of 185 percent to a high of $44.48. The shorter length of stay was not nearly enough to offset such increases, and the average expense per patient-stay advanced 173 percent to $347.

An important indicator of changing hospital operations is the rising number of institutions with specialized technical facilities. Between 1946 and 1965, the percentage of nonfederal short term hospitals with a clinical laboratory rose from 76 to 98. For diagnostic x-ray the rise was from 86 percent to 98. Batteries of laboratory tests and x-rays, once reserved for unusual cases, have become routine in the early stages of hospitalization. In 1946 patients averaged only four laboratory procedures per admission, but in 1965 the average varied from eight in hospitals with less than fifty beds, to sixteen in those with 400 or more beds.

Not surprisingly, such developments have produced important changes in hospital architecture and space distribution. In the average new hospital only about one-third of the area is designed for in-patient bed and nursing service, less in teaching hospitals. If the research space in advanced medical centers is counted, the bed and nursing space may be as little as 15 to 20 percent.

THREE MAJOR CATEGORIES

The term "hospital" is widely embracing. Even within the designation, "nonfederal short term," there are numerous classifications. The 1965 distribution, according to ownership and relative size, is as follows:

	Percentage		
	Hospitals	Beds	Assets
Voluntary	60	70	76
Proprietary	15	6	3
State and local government	25	24	21
TOTAL, nonfederal short return	100	100	100

The state and local hospitals are owned and operated by municipalities, counties, or states. In larger areas they tend to serve mainly the indigent and low income patients. Charges are usually scaled to income. However, in some localities, especially in the west and midwest, the county hospital is the only one within a broad geographic area and serves the entire population.

The proprietary hospital is an entrepreneurial enterprise, often owned and operated by groups of doctors, usually in connection with their medical practice, sometimes as a separate business activity. Such hospitals may also be owned by lay investors.

The voluntary hospital, which derives its now rather obsolete and misleading name from its historic origins, falls in a twilight zone. Ownership is vague, as the original capital is usually raised through community drives or philanthropy. A substantial number are controlled by Catholic and other religious groups. The hospital is legally operated by a board of trustees, usually composed of prominent community figures. Its distinguishing features are: (1) it is considered "private" in that it is not owned or operated by government; (2) it is generally not accountable to any public instrumentality; (3) but it is a "not-for-profit" undertaking of a quasi-public character, with privileges and emoluments that befit public institutions.

As in some other sectors of the American economy, traditional distinctions between public and private are being blurred, particularly with respect to patient population and sources of revenue. For example, while government hospitals are still mainly supported by taxation and designed for the indigent, they are increasingly accommodating Blue Cross and other paying patients. The "voluntaries" receive an increasing portion of their patient revenues from tax-supported programs of many kinds. Moreover, the voluntaries receive substantial and increasing support from government through subsidies and grants for construction, research, and education.

The proprietaries are usually guided, in what they do and what they charge, by financial considerations similar to those of other entrepreneurial activities in the economy. Normally they confine their care to full-pay patients, avoiding the indigent. However, with government payment of full "reasonable costs," on behalf of the former indigents, proprietaries will be opening their doors more widely.

Even the nonprofit status of the voluntary hospital is losing some of its distinguishing characteristics, as it sheds its eleemosynary functions and character. The nonpaying patient is a disappearing phenomenon. Increasingly, the voluntary hospital expects to be paid, and receives costs or better for nearly all its patients. Both proprietaries and voluntaries hope to produce a "profit" in the sense of current operating revenues exceeding costs. The difference lies in what is done with the surplus. None of the voluntaries' surplus can be distributed to the nonexistent "owners"; it is all eventually reinvested in expansion, renovation, or improvement.

The American culture has long favored the voluntary institution. Government hospitals have suffered in reputation from their identification with the "dole," and financially pressed local officials have been glad to avoid these investments to the extent that others were willing to assume them. As to proprietaries, the general feeling appears to be that "profit in health" is improper, although it is not entirely clear why this attitude has been confined to the hospital field and not carried over to pharmaceutical production, nursing homes, or even medical care—probably a matter of historical accident. Moreover, because proprietaries tend to be smaller, lacking in medical school affiliation, and often inadequately equipped for serious cases, the group as a whole does not enjoy much prestige in the medical profession.

The Voluntary Hospital: Organizational Anomaly

Due to its beginnings as a community charity for the poor and hopelessly ill, the voluntary hospital has inherited a unique and ambiguous organizational structure that is proving increasingly troublesome in its new role as a modern health center. It is a tripartite arrangement of trustees, administration, and medical staff, with the formal lines of authority often in conflict with the realities.

The roots of the design go back to 18th century Britain. There is generally no such three-cornered dispersion in the major continental hospitals, usually run in a hierarchical fashion by full-time chiefs of medical services. A central feature of the Anglo-American institution (which can now be considered American only, as the British have abandoned the old structure) has been its use as a place for the private practitioner to bring his private patients for treatment, but where he had no administrative or financial responsibilities. In return for this privilege, the doctor usually donated care for the indigent who constituted the majority of the hospital's patients.

The hospital's changed role and function and its altered financial base have made the old structure an anachronism. Health insurance, public medical programs, and new patterns of hospital use have, as indicated, transformed the large majority of admissions into paying patients. The dwindling proportion of indigent cases is now generally paid for, in part at least, by public funds. The hospital is being changed into a community service organization.

Ultimate responsibility for policy has always rested with lay trustees. In the past, this usually meant fund raising and—all too frequently—making up operating deficits out of their own pockets. In recent years, however, the tremendous rise in hospital costs, the increasing role of government in capital funding, the decreased likelihood that hospitals will end the year in the red, the growing size and complexity of hospital operations, and the growing professionalization of hospital administration have all tended to down-grade the trustee vis-a-vis the administrator. While the trustee's legal responsibility has not diminished, his role and status have.

Conversely, these same factors have greatly enlarged the job of the administrator. Traditionally untrained and content to play a passive role, the old-style administrator is being replaced by trained men and women with increased confidence and authority. A few of the most prominent hospital directors are MDs.

Despite his enhanced authority and status, the typical administrator has a trying and often anomalous job. The old tensions between the medical staff and administration, built into the structure of the voluntary hospital, remain. In the eyes of most physicians, the administrator is in charge only of the nonmedical aspects of the hospital's operations.

Aside from the impossibility of segregating the medical from the nonmedical, the dichotomy involves divided authority over individual personnel, many of whom are engaged in a variety of duties. For example, nurses are the hospital's employees and, therefore, accountable to the administrator. But they are responsible to the doctor for the individual patient—meaning to many doctors at once—in their medical duties.

In relation to his patients, the doctor is supreme, an unchallenged authority (except that clearly improper professional conduct is subject to discipline). With his high professional status he can, in most hospitals, countermand administrative orders and defy lay authority with relative impunity. When a doctor claims that a patient's health is at stake, an administrator will not often quarrel over prerogatives or invoke the rules of proper institutional conduct. This remains true despite the fact that the courts are increasingly emphasizing the hospital's corporate accountability for medical care.[1] Thus far, this legal trend has served primarily to increase the hospital's liability to suit without affecting the real authority structure.

Medical responsibility is divided among individual doctors and the collective staff. The staff has collective responsibility for medical policies (or making recommendations to the trustees). Some hospitals have "open staff" privileges; its facilities are available to any doctor in the community. Others have a "closed staff;" only those doctors elected by the staff (or trustees) may use its facilities, although such hospitals may extend courtesy privileges to additional physicians who may use the hospital without becoming members of the active staff. In metropolitan areas, many doctors have staff appointments in two, three, or more hospitals and, of necessity, wear their staff duties lightly.

The medical staff also has collective responsibility for the conduct of its members. In practice, this is usually quite loose. The staff is primarily a professional fraternal order, not an organization. To some extent the activities of the staff will depend upon whether the hospital has full-time chiefs and whether the administrator is a physician. The staff's power is generally pretty much what it wishes to make of it. The trustees are laymen, serving part-time without compensation, but the institution is there to render professional health services. The doctors make a special point that the hospital cannot practice medicine, that the patient is the doctor's, not the hospital's—a precious distinction that dilutes the unity and authority of the hospital.

The doctor's relationship to the hospital has become increasingly contradictory as its place in his professional life grows. Although the degree of his dependence varies with type of practice, probably at least 50 percent of the average physician's income is earned in the hospital. A surgeon or radiologist may earn up to 100 percent of his income there. In any case, even with staff duties, the physician who is the key and indispensable figure in the hospital, with wide authority and latitude, is not a real part of the administrative or financial organization.[2] On the other hand, a united and aggressive medical staff can effectively take over an entire hospital and conduct its affairs almost independently without any of the financial risks or responsibilities that would otherwise be expected. ...

These are, in the main, internal problems with an old history. Recently, however, modern technology and its high costs have emphasized the importance of external relationships with other health institutions. Construction, the character of services to be offered, personnel policies, and the range of equipment are no longer matters of concern to the individual hospital alone, but affect the quality and cost of health services throughout the community. This requires, at a minimum, some joint planning on a community basis. But hospitals are autonomous, and autonomy is rarely surrendered voluntarily in any field. Moreover, any sacrifice of institutional autonomy threatens the physicians' independent authority over the hospitals. Dr. Martin Cherkasky, director of Montefiore Hospital in New York City, has said, "Resistance to planning reflects a little-publicized but bitter struggle over who shall control our hospitals and for what purpose."

The community has begun to express its discontents vigorously, and the hospital is increasingly a subject of public debate. This was an inevitable consequence of spiraling costs. Annoyance and criticism have been mounting. Trustees are accused of "failing to represent the public interest," but it is not often made clear how they might go about doing this or what public they are supposed to represent. The administrator, a favorite target, is accused of "inefficiency" and "lack of concern for productivity," but his limited jurisdiction is not clearly understood and the resistance of the medical staff rarely acknowledged.

NOTES

1. For example, *Darling v. Charleston Memorial Hospital,* 211 N.E.2d 253 (1965); *cert. denied* 383 U.S. 946 (1966).

2. There are, of course, other patterns. A few excellent hospitals operate with a full complement of salaried physicians. This description is confined to the more typical institution.

Selection 13

The Rise in Hospital Use*

Americans have steadily increased their use of medical services since World War II. Since hospitalization is the most costly element in medical care, and hospital prices have been rising more rapidly than other medical prices, hospital utilization has attracted much concern. Between 1931 and 1958 the annual rate of admissions to general hospitals rose nearly 2.5 times. Recent increases have been smaller, but admissions continue to rise in both absolute terms and in proportion to the population (Table VI). However, the length of stay has decreased over the years, which means that total patient days in relation to population have moved up at a much slower rate, most recently appearing to plateau.

Selection 13 examines the major factors in the rising utilization as they appeared in 1960. It should be noted that, despite the common assumption that Medicare and Medicaid were the principal causes of rising hospital use after 1965, all the forces contributing to such acceleration were operative long before these programs. For example, the influence of an excessive number of beds, the effects of the imbalance in types of available health insurance, and the influence of health insurance per se were already apparent.

The movement to hospital cannot be regarded as an isolated phenomenon. The greater hospital use is at the core of the expansion in almost all forms of medical care, including physicians' services, drugs, nursing, and the use of all sorts of paramedical personnel. Identification of several major factors may, however, help to illustrate the intricate web of influences in the creation of effective demand.

Both doctors and patients now prefer the hospital as a setting for serious medical care. The emergence of the general hospital as the good doctor's favorite "workshop" is the primary cause of the "trend to hospital." The elementary fact is frequently overlooked that, except in case of extreme emergency, no hospital admission or discharge can take place without a physician's authorization. In addition to the obvious technical advantages of hospitalizing a seriously ill patient, the physician's preference may be influenced by the greater convenience and saving of time, the inadequate facilities of the typical solo office, the method of physician remuneration, and other factors.

There is virtually no resistance to this trend by the patient. On the contrary, the American public has acquired almost unquestioning confidence in the modern hospital both as symbol and embodiment of the scientific revolution in medicine. There is scarcely a trace left of the old stereotype of the hospital as a

---

*Excerpt from H.M. and A.R. Somers, *Doctors, Patients, and Health Insurance* (Washington, D.C.: The Brookings Institution, 1961), pp. 174-181.

place "from which no one returns." The hospital stands for the oxygen tent, the blood bank, the aseptic operating and delivery rooms, anesthetics, and the other miraculous devices through which modern medicine has demonstrated its lifesaving capabilities.

A comparison of the reasons people are admitted to hospitals today and 30 years ago indicates the important changes in the role of the institution. Maternity cases account for much of the increase—although, since mothers now stay a shorter time, the effect on total days of care is relatively small. Twenty years ago less than two-fifths of all American babies were born in hospitals. The figure is now over 95 percent. The accident toll has increased both admissions and days of care. Children are now hospitalized less often and older people more so. Among the surgical categories, tonsillectomy and appendectomy rates have fallen, while those for more complicated procedures, notably heart surgery, have increased. Mental cases, once entirely segregated, are increasingly admitted to general hospitals. In general, the hospital is now used, not as the extreme recourse when all else has failed, but as the normal site of treatment for any illness the doctor cannot handle on an ambulatory basis.

Supply creates demand. We live in an era of manipulated demand, manipulated primarily for the benefit of the vendors—and the medical care field is no exception. This applies to the increased availability of both hospital services and insurance for hospitalized illness. In the words of Dr. Milton Roemer and Max Shain,

> Of all the determinants of hospital utilization arising from the patient, the hospital, or the doctor, probably the most fundamental is the supply of beds available to the population.... Quite regardless of the amount of illness, the attitudes of people, or other influences, the rate of hospitalization depends directly on the ratio of beds per 1,000 population available for use.... The effect of bed supply in placing a *ceiling* on utilizaton rates will be readily acknowledged—that is, no more days of care can be provided than there are beds to provide them in—but, with payment assured through insurance, the bed supply likewise tends to set a *floor* on utilization. For the relative supply of beds... is bound to influence the decisions of doctors on admission of patients to hospitals.

The authors document this thesis with data showing a positive correlation between bed-population ratios and utilizaton rates in various sections of the world, especially Saskatchewan, Canada, and the United States. "When new beds are built," conclude Roemer and Shain, "they are quickly filled with people." But the decision to build additional beds depends on all sorts of influences—philanthropic, political, religious, ethnic, business—which bear "only the crudest or most irregular relationship to illness-need in a community."

Recent historical data suggest only partial support for this thesis. From 1948 to 1958 there was an increase of 9 percent in nonfederal short term general and special hospital beds per 1,000 population, the category most relevant to this dicsussion. When compared with the data on increased use, it appears that greater bed availability probably plays a contributory role, but it is one among many others.

In addition to the supply of beds, use is further influenced by the efficiency of hospital operation, the nature of hospital financing, and the availability of alternative custodial and outpatient facilities. On the question of method of payment, Roemer and Shain are particularly outspoken:

> As long as hospital income is derived from patient-day payments (whether from individuals, insurance plans, or government agencies) an empty bed means a loss of income. Under the circumstances, the administrator will naturally try, consciously or unconsciously, to maintain in his institution the highest possible occupancy.

The pressures are even greater with respect to currently prevailing patterns of health and disability insurance. Cash disability policies often pay benefits only if the patient is hospitalized. This is also generally true of medical expense coverage. Recent studies are consistent in pointing to the decisive influence of insurance in raising admission rates to general hospitals. ...

Common sense inferences from these data indicate that the insured go to the hospital sooner and for less serious situations; the uninsured wait, go only for more serious cases, and hence frequently have to stay longer. Despite such generalizations, however, we do not know whether there is "overutilization" by the insured, "underutilization" by the uninsured, or some combination of both. The experts are in wide disagreement on these questions.

There is, however, a general consensus as to the built-in tendency toward higher hospital utilization in the dominant pattern of health insurance. This conclusion is reinforced by evidence that where the insurance covers outpatient as well as inpatient care, hospital utilization rates are usually lower than where only hospital and surgical costs are covered. In the most thorough study of this type, a 1955 comparison of matched groups of New Yorkers insured under Blue Shield (BS) and the Health Insurance Plan of Greater New York (HIP), both with identical Blue Cross (BC) coverage, the annual admission rate for HIP/BC enrollees was 77.4 per 1,000 compared with 95.8 for BS/BC. The number of days of hospitalization per capita was 0.6 for HIP enrollees, 0.7 for Blue Shield.

Without passing judgment as to the "abuse" of hospital services implicit in such statistics, it is hardly surprising that, in the general absence of coverage for ambulatory care, both patients and physicians would try to stretch the available hospital expense protection to cover portions of their uninsured costs. A disproportionate supply of one type of insurance can lead, at least temporarily, to a distorted demand for the insured service.

Insurance of nonhospitalized medical care is not, by itself, a guarantee of lower inpatient utilization rates, however. A 1958 study of two "comprehensive" plans in New York City, HIP (a group practice plan) and Group Health

Insurance (which insures solo fee-for-service practice) suggests that the organization of the insured physicians' services may be as important as the fact of coverage. The hospital admission rate for GHI members was 11.0 per 100; for HIP 6.3. The number of hospital days per capita was 0.9 for GHI; 0.4 for HIP. As in the previous study, both groups had the same Blue Cross coverage.

A third exceedingly important factor is the increased longevity of the population. [The discharge rate from general hospitals, per 1,000 population, rises steadily and sharply (excluding the effect of child-bearing on females) with age. For example, in 1957-58, the rate rose] from an average of 53 per 1,000 for persons under 15, to 124 per 1,000 for those 75 and over—approximately 134 percent. The rise in hospital days per year is especially impressive. From a low of 295 for those 15 and under, both male and female curves go up to nearly 2,000 at 75, an increase of 555 percent. The average number of days per capita in general hospitals was twice as great for those 65 and over as for persons of all ages, 1.8 and 0.9, respectively.

In recent years the aged have been going to the hospital with increasing frequency. Comparative surveys in 1952 and 1956 found that their number in general hospitals per 1,000 increased by one-third during that brief interval, with a relatively greater increase among *uninsured* aged males and among *insured* females. The 65 and over age group appears to be the only one in which insurance does not play the controlling role.

Other factors known to influence hospital utilization include sex, income, education, and the availability of alternative community facilities. Contrary to popular belief male utilization of hospitals is greater than female at all ages in spite of the higher female admission rate during the child-bearing years. This is contrary to the sex differential in other areas of medical care and reflects primarily the men's substantially longer hospital stays, especially in mental and other long term hospitals. When the comparison is confined to short stay hospitals, however, the female dominance during the child-bearing years is obvious.

Income continues to influence hospital utilization, but where there is hospital insurance the historical relationship has changed. Among the insured, the lower the income the higher the admission rate, and the greater the number of hospital days used. Similarly, insurance appears to reverse the traditional rural-urban variation. When prepayment is provided, rural hospital utilization rises up to or above the level of the cities. An illustration of the effect of socioeconomic difficulties on hospital admissions is revealed in a recent study of a group of Alabama patients with extremely high multiple admissions under the United Mine Workers Welfare and Retirement Fund. In almost every case, it was found, there was no employed breadwinner in the family. Most of the patients subsisted on inadequate diets in rural slum dwellings. In no case was there evidence of a satisfactory doctor-patient relationship. Low income also continues to restrict utilization indirectly through its effect on health insurance coverage.

The effect of increased education, closely associated with income level, also differs from the past but is still unclear. From the limited data available, it appears that more education is probably associated with higher admission rates but shorter stays. An important British study found that marriage appears to be a safeguard against hospitalization.[1] The same phenomenon appears to prevail in this country among older men, whether insured or not. This and the generally longer length of stay for men of all ages suggest the important role of home care and community facilities. The general home environment, lack of adequate home care, nursing home, and other domiciliary facilities, even sheer loneliness, all contribute to hospital lists, especially of the aged. During the past few decades, the hospitals have been called on increasingly to provide services that other facilities might have provided more economically and more suitably.

From these various factors it appears that the growing demand for hospital care is warranted by its increased technological importance in modern medicine, by the frequent necessity for hospitalization of the aged, and by the backlog of need on the part of many people to whom it was denied until fairly recently. To some extent, however, demand has been artificially raised by the greater availability of hospital beds as compared with outpatient facilities and alternative community services, by the financial need of hospitals to maintain maximum occupancy rates, by the frequent limitation of insurance to hospitalized illness, by inadequate physician and consumer appreciation of the importance of preventive medicine and comprehensive care, and by the failure of large segments of the medical profession to discourage hospital use where it was not medically in order.

It is conceivable that some signs of deterioration in hospital standards—the staphylococcus episode of the late 1950s, the serious overcrowding in some public institutions, the growing shortage of interns and residents—could signal the beginning of a reversal in popular and professional attitudes. But this does not seem likely. The forces in the other direction are too compelling. Nor would one wish to turn the clock back. What is indicated is a rationalized system of community and regional hospital facilities with the general hospital as specialized center of a network of appropriate medical and paramedical institutions. Such a system, long advocated by leading hospital and medical authorities, could relieve the financial pressure on the inevitably expensive general hospital without denying the legitimate demands of doctors and patients alike.

NOTES

1. B. Abel-Smith and R.M. Titmuss, *The Cost of the National Health Service in England and Wales* (Cambridge, England: Cambridge University Press, 1955). It was reported that, in relation to their number in the total adult population of the country, the single, widowed, and divorced make about double the demand on hospital facilities.

Selection 14

Those Who Ignore History*

Despite the intense opposition of the American Hospital Association and most of the industry (the Hospital Association of New York was an exception), the National Labor Relations Act was extended to hospital employees in 1973. The legacy of bitterness growing out of the long exclusion, the ineptness of much hospital personnel administration, and the belated third party effort to introduce some controls into the prevalent cost-plus reimbursement: all have contributed to rising labor tensions and augur more intense disputes for the future.

The urgency of the problem becomes more critical at the conclusion of each so-called negotiation. It is time for a complete reappraisal of collective bargaining in the hospital system. We can no longer afford to push the square peg into the round hole. Unless the Federal Government actively pursues a program of research, investigation and finally, legislation in the area of hospital labor relations, we may yet witness the destruction of the voluntary hospital system in our country.

In these concluding words to a case study of hospital labor relations in New York City, Norman Metzger, vice president for personnel, Mt. Sinai Medical Center, New York City, and senior author of this important book, emphasizes not only the need for a national hospital labor policy, but the relationship between labor relations and the viability of the industry.

"Those who ignore history are condemned to repeat it." It seems almost incredible that 35 years after the great labor upheavals of the 1930s, the adoption of the Wagner and Taft-Hartley Acts as national labor relations policy, and the acceptance of unions as integral parts of American society, one of the largest and most vital industries in the nation should be condemned to relive all the turmoil, the trials, and errors of that period.

The reasons for this anachronism are complex. They include the nonprofit status of the majority of hospitals which apparently led the Congress to exempt them from coverage under the National Labor Relations Act, the special difficulties of hospital management in adapting—either in terms of corporate structure or increased productivity—to new socioeconomic and industrial developments, the large proportion of female and minority group employees who historically have shown little militance, the lack of concern by the leadership of organized labor for this hard-to-organize group, and public opposition to

---

*Excerpt from A.R. Somers, Introduction to Norman Metzger and Dennis D. Pointer, *Labor-Management Relations in the Health Services Industry: Theory and Practice* (Washington, D.C.: Science and Health Publications, 1972), pp. xxii-xxiv.

any development which could further exacerbate the rise in health care costs or the possibility of hospital strikes.

But, as the authors make clear, the time has long since passed when these circumstances could be considered extenuating. Many of the same factors that inhibited earlier organization of hospital employees now contribute to especially militant unionism. The absence of the National Labor Relations Act (NLRA) is conducive to bitter representational strikes. The large number of black and other minority workers has produced a volatile marriage of unionism with the civil rights movements. This, in turn, along with their alienation from the main centers of AFL-CIO power, has contributed to a brand of political unionism more akin to that of the 1930s than the business unionism that has emerged in the last two decades of union "respectability."

The nonprofit status of the voluntary hospital, which has too often been equated with "unbusinesslike" procedures, and the currently dominant method of hospital payment—cost reimbursement by third parties—have led hospital unions (along with many administrators, physicians, and other hospital personnel) to adopt a cavalier attitude toward rising costs which, it is assumed, will simply be passed on to third party payers without any real hardship to the institution or even a challenge to increased productivity. It would be hard to conceive of a situation less conducive to responsible collective bargaining. ...

The authors claim that no matter how hard the individual hospital administrator may try (Metzger himself is "Exhibit A") to make collective bargaining work, he is unlikely to be successful until Congress and the states provide some workable ground rules. At the same time, they make clear that under the best of circumstances, collective bargaining is a difficult specialized skill, that it involves a whole new "life style" for the hospital, and that the leadership of the institution has much to learn—not only with respect to labor relations but also in personnel administration in general and productivity and cost controls—if it hopes to survive in the new environment.

Looking back once again to the "labor revolution" of the 1930s, that experience was obviously a major factor in changing and shaping modern corporate management. There are those who feel that the imminent labor revolution in the American hospital will play a similar role in that institution's future.

Selection 15

Democratizing the Hospital*

... My second suggestion concerns the relation of health professionals to each other. I am distressed by the internal warfare between, and even within, some professions. I am distressed by the unscalable walls of professional privilege and credentialism that you erect against each other. I am appalled at the growing power struggle between the medical staff and the administration in many hospitals.

And I am dismayed at the spread of unionism among American physicians—the best paid professionals in the world today. This is not because I am against unions or collective bargaining, as such, but because I see doctor unions leading to even greater fragmentation of the health professions, and hence of the patient, and even greater loss of professional and institutional autonomy.

With or without unions, the average hospital is in serious trouble today. It is a house divided against itself, and Lincoln's famous words apply to this indispensable institution just as they apply to the larger society.

The solution to the problems of hospital governance, hospital finance, and interprofessional relations lies not in a competitive power struggle between the various professional and occupational groups. Such a struggle can only end in irreparable damage to the quality of patient care, in making team care impossible, and—ultimately—forcing the federal government to step in as the only arbitrator capable of dealing with nationwide organizations of doctors, nurses, nonprofessional workers, etc.

The solution, I submit, lies in a new and real—not just lip service—commitment to team care and in a revitalized and democratized form of self-government for the hospital and all its employees and affiliated professionals. Elsewhere I have suggested that all first-class hospitals be franchised by the state and held responsible and accountable for comprehensive health care for a defined population (see Selection 31).

I am now adding to this model the proposal that the structure of the hospital's governing board be modified to give equal or at least significant voice to its employees and affiliated professionals. For years doctors have been asking for representation on hospital boards. For years they have been denied this on the grounds of conflict of interest. I think this was wrong. Instead of exercising their legitimate authority overtly, they have generally exercised it covertly. I am suggesting that not only the medical staff but nurses and all other hospital-based professionals and employees be represented on the governing board, either directly or indirectly.

---

*Excerpt from A.R. Somers, Commencement Address, Health Sciences Center, State University of New York, Stony Brook, June 17, 1973; published in *The Bulletin of the American College of Physicians* 14 (September 1973): 545-546.

I also think that we should devise a better way of electing or appointing the consumer representatives on the boards. And some way must be found—through financial incentives, legal requirements, or otherwise—to force all members of the hospital staff to recognize that they constitute a mutually interdependent team with a recognized goal—the best possible care of their patient population at a feasible price.

In short, I am suggesting that the hospital should become a more democratic institution—both with respect to its own staff and to the community it serves. It should also become a more cohesive organization, with greater professional, emotional, and financial identification on the part of affiliated professionals and employees.

The development of such democratically controlled, self-governing units within a framework of public accountability, spelled out in the state franchise, offers the possibility of a way out of our current professional and institutional impasse. It offers the possibility of rescuing our principal health care institution from what now appears an inevitable slide toward federal control and restores it to local governance and understandable human dimensions. It also offers a professional and financial climate within which the individual patient care teams can grow and multiply. Both provider and consumer would benefit—which is as it should be. ...

Selection 16

The Rising Costs of Medical Care*

Medical care costs are measured in a variety of ways: prices *(unit cost of a particular good or service);* total costs *for a nation, community, or other population group; or* per capita *expenditures. Any of these, standing alone, may be misleading. A change in price level is not in itself informative as to whether the cost burden is greater or lower. An individual whose charge for a physician's visit has been raised from $10 to $15 is no worse off if, at the same time, the number of required visits has declined proportionately. On the other hand, the physician's definition of a unit of service may have changed, e.g., by charging separately for an injection which had previously been included in the visit charge. Similarly, a rise in total costs may reflect primarily an increase in population, or the use of more medical services, or a rise in price, or any combination of these. In the United States all have contributed to increased medical costs, particularly price rises which have accounted for more than half the total increase in recent years.*

---

*Excerpt from H.M. and A.R. Somers, *Doctors, Patients, and Health Insurance* (Washington, D.C.: The Brookings Institution, 1961), pp. 193-196, 212-217.

The spectacular rise which attracted so much attention in the late 1960s and 1970s, was already quite evident by the late 1950s. The relative inflation attributed to the later Medicare and Medicaid programs is frequently exaggerated. Although both general and medical prices inflated far more sharply in the mid-1970s the relative rise of medical prices was no greater than in the 1950s (Table XIV). This selection summarizes some aspects of this enduring phenomenon as seen at the close of the 1950s. The purpose of its inclusion is to emphasize the long history of the problem.

THE PRICE SPIRAL

Since the end of World War II medical care prices have spiraled upward more rapidly than the general cost of living or any of the other major consumer price index categories. From 1945 to 1959 all prices rose 62 percent, but medical care prices increased 81 percent.

Percentage Increases in Prices of Selected Items in the Consumer Price Index, Selected Periods 1929-59

	1929-59	1935-59	1945-50	1945-59	1950-55	1950-59	1955-59
All items.....................	70	112	34	62	11	21	9
Food	80	138	47	72	10	17	7
Apparel	—	113	29	41	6	10	4
Rent........................	—	79	20	54	20	28	7
All services (excluding rent) ..	—	103	24	70	20	36	13
Medical care	105	111	28	81	21	42	18
Medical services (excluding drugs)....................	119	126	30	90	23	46	19
Hospital rates.............	—	344	78	224	44	82	27
Physicians' fees............	—	92	20	68	18	36	15
Dentists' fees..............	—	97	29	62	14	26	10
Drugs and prescriptions	—	48	18	39	7	18	10
Prescriptions..............	—	—	—	—	10	14	25
Other drugs	—	—	—	—	3	9	12

Source: Computed from U.S. Bureau of Labor Statistics, Consumer Price Index.

In recent years the differential has been increasing conspicuously. Most of the increase in general prices occurred in the immediate postwar period, while medical care has been making its relatively more rapid advances since about 1950. The more current the comparison the more sharp the comparative rise in medical prices.

Between 1945 and 1950 general prices advanced 34 percent and medical care only 28. But from 1950 to 1959 medical prices advanced twice as fast as all prices, 42 percent compared with 21. Between June 1958 and June 1960, they rose three and one-half times as fast.

As medical care is composed primarily of services, it is important to compare medical care prices with other services. The movement of service prices often follows a different pattern from that of commodities. To make this comparison we use the index for medical care services, exclusive of drugs, and compare with all services, excluding rent. From 1945 to 1959 medical service prices advanced 90 percent, while all services rose 70 percent. According to this measurement, also, the differential is increasing; from 1955 to 1959 medical service prices advanced 19 percent as compared with 13 percent for general services.

It is apparent, by any measure, that medical prices have run ahead of other prices in recent years. It is sometimes argued, however, that concentration on postwar data may cause one to overlook the fact that medical prices had advanced relatively slowly during the previous decade. Indeed, it is occasionally claimed that medical prices have just been catching up with the relative lag into which they had fallen before the war. It is true that medical prices increased only 16 percent from 1935 to 1945, while general prices advanced 31 percent. From 1935 to 1959 medical care prices rose 111 percent and general prices gained 112 percent.

This comparison overlooks the fact that during the depression almost all prices—particularly food, rent, and clothing—declined sharply, but medical prices held firm. From 1929 to 1935, while all prices declined 20 percent, medical prices fell only 3 percent. The argument can be made with equal persuasiveness that, from the end of the depression until about 1950, general prices were simply catching up with ground lost relative to medical prices during the depression. On the other hand, taking a 30-year span—from the predepression peak of 1929 to 1959—all prices advanced 70 percent, but medical care prices went up 105.

All this demonstrates the well-known fact that statistical base periods tend to be arbitrary, and different selections will appear to furnish quite different results for partisan exploitation. There is no particular point of time during which it can be said that prices were in some correct or proper relationship to each other as compared with any other period of time. One can only speak correctly of trends and relationships of one period to another. At present, the most significant picture is derived from concentration on the postwar period because it is now long enough to reveal significant contemporary trends, because in terms of economic and social developments it is an era to be viewed differently from the war and prewar periods, and because the farther back one goes the less reliable and comparable are the data. In presenting the postwar period, however, we have taken pains to make percentage comparisons over several periods of time to clarify differential movements within the period.

Hospital Rates

The overall index of medical care prices conceals wide variations among the components. Since 1945, rates for room, board, and general nursing in nonfederal general hospitals have more than tripled. They have advanced almost four times as fast as physicians' and dentists' fees, six times as fast as the price of drugs, more than three times as rapidly as the index for all services or for all items. No matter what the time period of comparison, there is no item in the consumer price index—either service or commodity—that has moved up as sharply or persistently as hospital prices. Since the war, hospital rates have risen at an annual average of almost 9 percent.

Just as important as the extraordinary rises that have already taken place is the almost universal expectation of hospital administrators and experts that costs will continue to rise 5 to 10 percent annually. Since hospitals play a progressively larger role in the lives of Americans, this is a menacing prospect. As the spread between hospital services and other prices continues to grow, year after year without promise of surcease, and the resulting costs of insurance spiral from moderate to painful, consumer resentment has gradually been converted into public protest. ...

PER CAPITA EXPENDITURES

It is, of course, the combination of price and utilization that determines the comparative costs of medical care to the consumer over periods of time. These costs in relation to income then determine the comparative strain on the family budget.

Consumers are spending a much larger proportion of disposable personal income for medical care than ever before—and this does not take into account the greatly increased public expenditures financed through tax dollars. In 1929 the proportion of disposable personal income spent for medical care was 3.5 percent. In 1946 it was 3.8 percent; by 1956, 4.9; and in 1958, 5.2. The increase between 1946 and 1958 was thus 37 percent.... Between 1948 and 1958 per capita expenditures for personal medical care increased from $52.68 to $95.65, about 82 percent. In constant dollars the rise was 51 percent....

Especially interesting is a Health Information Foundation-National Opinion Research Center (HIF-NORC) finding that the expenditure differential associated with insured status is even greater than it used to be. In 1952-53 the average for an insured individual was 35 percent higher than for the uninsured; in 1957-58 it was 49 percent higher—$106 and $71, respectively. This should not lead to the conclusion that insurance alone caused the higher expenditures. The evidence is that those more likely to make large expenditures for medical care are also more likely to buy insurance.

THE UNEVEN INCIDENCE OF COSTS ON FAMILIES

According to HIF-NORC, while the average American family spent $294 for medical care in 1957-58, 17 percent spent $500 or more, and 5 percent spent $1,000 or more. On the other hand, 17 percent spent less than $50.

The historical persistence of this pattern of uneven incidence is noteworthy. The Committee on the Costs of Medical Care found, in 1928-31, approximately the same distribution as did the 1952-53 HIF-NORC survey. Three decades ago 10 percent of American families incurred 41 percent of total annual personal medical costs. Precisely the same distribution held for the 1957-58 survey. In 1952-53, 50 percent of the families with the highest costs accounted for 90 percent of all expenditures; in 1957-58 they incurred 88 percent of the total. While, in general, higher income families have higher expenditures, the outlays are rarely proportionate to family incomes. The heavier proportionate burden falls on the lower income families. ...

The real tragedy of medical costs can never be told through averages. No family, no individual, can foretell how much will be imposed on it and when. In the main, expenditures are not discretionary. Nor can one budget intelligently for a contingency that is largely unpredictable and uncontrollable in time and amount. Medical care not only imposes unusual expenditures, but if the illness hits the breadwinner, it also may cut off his income. The authors are personally acquainted with a case costing $22,500.

A father, in his 60s, has a stroke. He was hospitalized for four months, with round-the-clock nursing, expensive medications, and specialist services. He appeared to recover and was brought home. For two more months he continued with a practical nurse and medications. He then had another stroke and died. His wife and son, both of whom work daily in the family drugstore, lost all their savings. The father, a small businessman with a heart condition, was unable to buy health insurance. The $22,500 did not include the services of the family doctor (donated) or medications obtained through the family drugstore. When medical costs do strike with their full potential weight on the unfortunate minority, the burden can be so staggering that no amount of foresight would have made a real difference.

These are some of the reasons that the costs of medical care—which are still not staggering when averaged across the nation—cause insecurity, anxiety, and discontent.

It is often pointed out to the disgruntled consumer that while he is paying more, he is getting a better buy for his money than ever before; he is receiving a better quality of medical care and more of it. This has not proved sufficient assuagement. Even if he appreciates the fact that he is receiving a far better product, it does not necessarily make it easier to pay for. The intelligent consumer may be well aware that compared to its predecessors the new medical product is as a new Cadillac to an old Model T. But unlike the Cadillac, the purchase of which is optional, modern medical care is essential, irrespective of one's means. This makes the difficulty all the more aggravating. As science and technology continue to serve us with ever-improving medical care, and as consumers become more conscious of its essentiality, the concomitant higher costs become a sorer and sorer point.

The problem is almost universally recognized, and a steadily mounting volume of public debate has been generated. Fortunately, the increasing clamor has been accompanied by a considerable amount of action—public and private. Many new institutions have been created. Common to all is the search for a mechanism for effective pooling of risks and sharing of costs.

Part II

Assuring Access: Central Aim of Public Policy During the 1950s and 1960s

Part II

Assuring Access: Central Aim of Public Policy During the 1950s and 1960s

> Access to the means for attainment and preservation of health is a basic human right.
>
> President's Commission on the
> Health Needs of the Nation (1952)
>
> Our first concern must be to assure that the advance of medical knowledge leaves none behind. We can—and we must—strive now to assure the availability of and accessability to the best health care for all Americans, regardless of age or geography or economic status.
>
> Lyndon B. Johnson (1966)

During the Johnson years, the United States had an identifiable and virtually explicit health policy, representing the climax for activities and proposals that had been gathering momentum for at least two decades. The clear goal was to assure access to the best health care for all Americans. The operational strategies were interrelated: (1) remove all or most financial barriers to health care; and (2) increase health manpower, facilities, services, and biomedical research to meet the new demand.

The policy had already been implicitly accepted by the American people long before Medicare, as evidenced by the phenomenal growth of private health insurance during the 1950s and early 1960s, and industry's ability to absorb or pass on the cost of such insurance in the price of its products. Presidents Truman and Kennedy translated implicit assumptions and ongoing practice into explicit public policy aspirations. President Johnson turned them into operational programs.

The dramatic Medicare breakthrough arrived in a period of great national ebullience, characterized by unprecedented prosperity and a euphoric faith that all social problems would yield to sufficient expenditure of money. With compassion and generosity, the Great Society could be achieved. Medicare and Medicaid were soon followed by numerous additional programs and enlargement of old ones. The Johnson years produced more health legislation than any previous period in our history.

Results were soon apparent. The country experienced dramatic increases in research laboratories, in hospital beds and nursing homes, in number of admissions and patient days in hospitals, in outpatient visits, physician visits, expansion of medical schools and medical school graduates, nurses and other health personnel; indeed, in virtually all indices of medical care availability and utilization (Tables IV to VIII, X to XIII).

Much good was accomplished. Our biomedical research capability was substantially enlarged, and some dramatic achievements were obtained in both the basic life sciences and their application in sophisticated diagnostic and therapeutic procedures, chemotherapy, and other areas. More people attained regular access to health services than ever before. A backlog of long-neglected needs, especially among the elderly and the poor, was specifically addressed, although their special problems were not fully resolved. There were substantial improvements in the quality of health care institutions and facilities.

But there were also unanticipated and not-so-happy results. Medical care prices, which had already been rising much faster than all other prices, accelerated rapidly and unremittingly (Tables VI and XIV). Almost totally lacking in any financial discipline, the health care economy expanded beyond the boundaries of demonstrable need and attracted a variety of dubious enterprises and questionable activities. Demand for services rose to meet or exceed every increase in supply with no apparent natural limit. The fragmented industry became further disjointed as problems of organization were disregarded in the drive to open access.

Implicit in the unbridled expansionary impulse were some widely accepted assumptions: (1) that the demand for medical care and the need were more or less the same; (2) that an increased supply of physicians and facilities would almost automatically control prices; and (3) that more medical care was virtually synonymous with improved health. Experience was to lead to questioning of such assumptions.

Although some of the selections in Part Two were written before or after the Great Society era, most were the product of that period. The reader will note a persistent undercurrent of caution, concern, and even warning: (1) that the phenomenal growth of private health insurance concealed serious weaknesses in both the financing arrangements and in health services that required correction; (2) that public programs required adequate provision for effective and responsible administration; (3) that expansion of the industry required attention to more rational and effective organization; (4) that voluntary planning alone probably could not cope with such problems; (5) that inflation would not automatically yield to increasing supply; and (6) in general, that the available lessons of history were being ignored.

Nevertheless, the general mood was upbeat. In the main, we shared the optimistic expansionist philosophy of the time. Our proposals for corrective action still stressed the opportunities for voluntary control and self-discipline by the providers themselves. The disappointments and the search for other kinds of reform are left to Part Three.

Chapter Four

Private Health Insurance

The large and influential role of private health insurance in the United States, in contrast to most other developed nations, is attributable to a variety of factors. Among them: affluence; an historical preference, even on the part of labor organizations, for private as opposed to governmental enterprise; the divided authority between federal and state governments; the ingenuity and resourcefulness of the major carriers; a fortuitous marriage between medical care and industrial relations bargaining in the 1940s and 1950s; the reaction to a real or perceived threat of national health insurance; and, for a long time, the unusually strong and effective resistance of organized medicine to governmental intervention.

Between 1940 and 1957, the heyday period, annual premium payments rose from $100 million to $4.2 billion, a rate of growth (25 percent per annum compounded) unprecedented in insurance history. During that period the proportion of Americans with some type of coverage (predominantly hospital insurance) rose from 10 percent to about 70 percent. The industry has continued to grow although, inevitably, at a slower pace (Tables VIII, IX, X). By 1974, nearly 80 percent of the civilian population had at least basic hospital coverage, and 98 percent of these had some surgical insurance. Total premium income exceeded $28 billion. But insurance still met only a third of consumers' costs for personal health care.

Involved in the overall growth were a wide range of insurance institutions and consumer groups as well as a multiplicity of differing contractual arrangements. It was difficult to see the forest for the trees. During the halcyon 1940s and 1950s, steady expansion generally obscured the serious difficulties already making their appearance just below the surface. The problems grew more apparent over the years and progressively more difficult to resolve.

In a sense, private health insurance, although far from guiltless, was a victim of its own success. Having helped to open the door of access to medical care for many millions, it increased impatience with all shortcomings and heightened the sense of inequity for the less privileged. Public expectations rose more rapidly than the industry could meet. It could not cover the whole population. Passage of Medicare in 1965 proved a substantial boon, relieving it of its most formidable burden—coverage of the aged—without inhibiting growth. But the difficulties—both the problem of reaching the "unreachables" and providing adequate and balanced benefits at a feasible price—have persisted.

For these and a variety of other reasons, private health insurance has become the "whipping boy" for numerous critics. There is even a common belief that great profits are being reaped. On the contrary, the industry as a whole has regularly experienced net underwriting losses, although there is substantial variation among different components and part of the loss is compensated by investment of reserves.

Inflation has, of course, been the major villain. With health care costs rising more than 10 percent a year, the additional premiums required are a formidable obstacle to broadening benefits or enrolling more of the uninsured. Large deductibles and coinsurance, one way of offsetting the need for higher premiums (often advocated by economists), appear unacceptable to a large part of the public. Major medical, originally the insurance companies' answer to the public demand for broader coverage, has enjoyed steady growth. But major medical is administratively very cumbersome for the consumer, is always accompanied by substantial cost-sharing, and rarely meets a satisfactory proportion of the family's health costs.

Organized labor and business management, the primary purchasers of health insurance, have become increasingly disenchanted with this ever more expensive "fringe benefit." By 1970 it was estimated that 85 percent of all benefit payments came from employee benefit plans, and that 50 percent of all premiums were paid by employers. Labor maintains it is paying for the insurance, directly or indirectly, since it assumes that the employer's payments are in lieu of wages. On the other hand, employers face progressive escalation in costs without commensurate benefits or satisfaction to employees. Both are assuming more activist roles in attempts to control the problem. Labor's resentment is expressed by the AFL-CIO insistence that private carriers be excluded from participation in any future national health insurance program.

Thus the continuation of private health insurance as a major force in financing health care is in some jeopardy. Most of the major carriers have not been unaware of this, and some have made a real effort to remedy the situation. This called for a significant change of attitude.

During most of the period of ebullient growth, the industry maintained that it was merely a "fiduciary institution" serving to facilitate payment of health care costs. Policing costs or trying to influence the character of the delivery system was not its jurisdiction. As we observed in 1961 in this connection, "Practical convenience often gets elevated to ideological status." By the late 1960s the "principle" had become nonoperational. Led by Blue Cross, portions of the industry tried to become active in cost containment, supporting health care planning, utilization review, HMOs, consumer health education, and other measures which, it was hoped, would help to mitigate the relentless inflation.

Some progress has been achieved. But the power of insurance alone to control costs, or the practices in health care which lead to high costs, is limited. To harness the many underlying forces indicated in this volume requires authority and action that necessarily go far beyond the scope of insurance mechanisms.

Even remedies for some internal industry deficiencies require the aid of government, for example, the excessive fragmentation represented by some 1,700 carriers, the inordinately weak insurance regulation in most states, and the legal restraints against Blue Cross and Blue Shield mergers. The success or failure of such measures as planning, rate regulation, and refashioning of health care processes will influence insurance costs more than anything the industry itself can do. Even more decisive for the future role of the carriers will be the scope and character of any significant moves toward national health insurance.

Despite this array of difficulties and problems, it should be clear that private health insurance remains a large and formidable influence throughout the health care economy—with legislatures, purchasers of insurance, and providers of care.

Selections 17 to 22 describe some of the more interesting and unconventional programs of health insurance as well as some of the industry's practical problems. A number of reforms and adjustments are proposed with a view to maximizing the contributions of private health insurance in a balanced and pluralistic system. Some of the reforms advocated, as far back as 1961, have been at least partially adopted. For example, the federal Health Maintenance Organization Act of 1973 requires that an HMO option be offered, wherever one is available, by all employers of 25 or more. In May 1974, the New York Superintendent of Insurance approved a merger of the Blue Cross and Blue Shield plans of Greater New York, a move that has been emulated by several other states.

Selection 17

A Mid-1950s Perspective: Some Definitions and Problems*

The carriers have exhibited great energy and ingenuity, but equally important is the extraordinary degree to which the industry is conditioned by a variety of technological and economic developments outside its control. As Professor Kulp put it, the health insurance industry has been

> both the beneficiary and victim of these events. It has had presented to it not only a group of potential buyers commanding the largest volume of mass purchasing power in our history but, for a considerable part of the decade [during World War II], buyers with few other goods or services on which to spend this purchasing power, and—very impor-

---

*Excerpt from H.M. and A.R. Somers, "Private Health Insurance, Part 2: Problems, Pressures, and Prospects," *California Law Review* 46 (October 1958): 508-533.

tantly—official encouragement of the purchase of group insurance.... In large part this new business has been manna from heaven or Washington or Mars.

The manna has continued to descend, but growth is slowing down; now the difficulties, internal contradictions, and external pressures besetting the industry are daily more prominent. The current rapid changes in both the technology of medical care and the sociology of medical demand are major sources of the instability of the industry. Like a circus rider, trying to keep his balance with one foot on one horse, the other on a second, the animals both galloping forward but not necessarily in step, health insurance must seek to keep its balance astride these two rapidly changing movements. Moreover, all three areas—consumer demand, the organization of supply, and the insurance programs themselves—are affected by cultural and institutional pressures and resistances which further complicate the problem of adjustment.

MAJOR HEALTH INSURANCE CONCEPTS AND TRENDS

Space permits only a few highlights of the vast and complex health insurance industry.

Health insurance plans are usually classified as either "service" or "indemnity." A service plan provides specified services when required by an insured person. The insured receives no bill since the plan pays the hospital or doctor directly. Under an indemnity plan, specified amounts of money are provided to reimburse the insured, usually in part only, for the cost of the services he purchases. Most Blue Cross plans provide service benefits, usually a semiprivate or ward room for a specified number of days and all or most "extras," such as use of the operating room, prescribed drugs, etc. They reimburse the hospital, rather than the insured, in accordance with a contract which may be based on hospital costs or charges, in the latter case usually with a "wholesale discount," or a formula combining elements of both. In turn, the hospitals guarantee fulfillment of Blue Cross subscriber contracts.

By contrast, commercial carriers usually have no contractual relations with the providers of service—hospitals and doctors—and their benefits are almost always in the form of indemnity. Their hospitalization policies usually provide a specified number of dollars a day plus specified allowances for "extra" charges.

Surgical and medical plans usually indemnify, according to a specified fee schedule, a list of allowances payable for different surgical procedures. The first Blue Shield plans were primarily service contracts, and the attached fee schedules constituted full payment for the various surgical procedures by the insured to his doctor. If the insured earned more than a stated amount, the doctor was permitted to charge more than the scheduled fee—presumably on the basis of ability to pay—but in California, for example, the income limit in the early California Physicians Service (CPS) plan excluded only about 10 percent of the population from full service benefits.

The doctors found this type of contract unsatisfactory and gradually abandoned the service principle, primarily by permitting income limits to become obsolete in the face of rising incomes, but also by switching to straight indemnity insurance. ....

*Events and experience have a way of confounding theories and blurring ideological distinctions. The practical difference between service and indemnity is now frequently unclear. Virtually all service plans, including the direct service group, have added some indemnity features; and many indemnity plans have adapted some service concepts.

"Major medical" (originally called "catastrophic" insurance) is not limited to a single type of expense but applies broadly to almost all kinds of medical care. Such policies are usually classified as "supplementary," that is, added to "basic" hospital and surgical coverage, or "comprehensive" when the entire package is incorporated into one policy.

Another major distinction is that between "group" and "individual" policies, a distinction maintained to some degree by all types of carriers. Volume and administrative savings make possible lower rates in group insurance. Under this method, a large proportion—usually 75 percent—of the employees of a firm, members of a union, or persons covered by a trust fund, are enrolled as a group. The high proportion reduces overhead costs and minimizes adverse selection of risks. Group enrollment is usually facilitated by bulk payment of premiums by the employer or fund. Individual insurance is sold directly to the covered individual. Lacking the economies of the group enrollment technique, it costs considerably more than group insurance. Over 65 percent of all health insurance enrollment in the United States is under some kind of group coverage.

PRICING POLICIES

Among the many variables affecting the price of health insurance are (1) type of carrier, (2) type of policy, i.e., group or nongroup, (3) range of benefits, (4) geographic differences in hospital charges and doctors' fees, and (5) characteristics of the particular group or individual risk. The last factor has become especially important in recent years. Accompanying the relative expansion of commercial insurance and the trend to indemnity benefits there has been a movement away from communitywide pricing, originally employed by all the Blue plans, to differential pricing or "experience rating" techniques developed by the insurance companies.

Under "community rates" premiums are set on the basis of the medical costs of a cross section of the community—the good risks help pay for the poor risks. Differential or experience rating means that good risks—e.g., a group of younger-than-average employees with fewer-than-average women in a non-

---

* The following three paragraphs are excerpted from Somers and Somers, *Doctors, Patients, and Health Insurance* (Washington, D.C.: The Brookings Institution, 1961), pp. 250-54.

hazardous occupation—are rewarded for their own anticipated or actual low claims experience by lower initial rates, annual refunds, dividends, or other downward adjustments from the standard premium. The result is lower prices for preferred risks and higher prices for poorer risks. It increases the difficulty of covering the aged, the self-employed, and those workers employed in small groups or in dangerous occupations.

Despite this drawback, the intense pressure of competition for the big and profitable group policies has resulted in a steady trend to experience rating. Many Blue Cross and other nonprofit plans have reluctantly fallen in line.

THE "INDEPENDENTS"

The "independents" constitute a third category of insurance carriers, including some 300-odd plans with a total enrollment variously estimated at 5 to 9 million, or 4 to 7 percent of all United States health insurance enrollment. The strength of the independents is greatest in four states—New York, Ohio, Connecticut, and California. About the only characteristics they have in common are that they are self-insurers, they are nonprofit, and they are not part of a national organization like BC or BS. They are generally classified as industrial or nonindustrial. The former confine their membership to a particular employee group, e.g., members of a union, employees of a railroad, public utility, or other industrial concerns. The nonindustrial plans are open to the general public and include community plans such as the Health Insurance Plan of Greater New York and the Kaiser Foundation Health Plan, private group practice clinics such as Ross-Loos in Los Angeles, and a number of smaller consumer-sponsored plans.

The most significant distinguishing aspect of this type of carrier is the extent to which comprehensive benefits are provided. This is related to the fact that nearly two-fifths of independent enrollees receive medical care through group practice. [For further discussion of this type of plan, see Selection 19.]

MAJOR PROBLEMS TODAY

The history of voluntary health insurance during the past 15 years might be summarized briefly in these terms: phenomenal overall growth accompanied by rapid changes in underwriting practices, a *de facto* rapprochement among the principal types of carriers under the impact of common problems and pressures, with a current lead for the commercial companies, and now deep foreboding about the future. The reasons for this foreboding can be subsumed under three major problems which embody the principal challenges to the industry today: (1) Can the enrollment gap be significantly reduced? (2) Can benefits to the insured be made adequate in relation to the enlarged concept of medical needs? and (3) Can these goals be achieved at a practical price? The answers to these questions may determine the future, not only of individual health insurance carriers but also of the business as a whole.

Health insurance is an important cost factor in at least three ways. The net cost of insurance overhead has added about 5 percent to the nation's medical bill, the pattern of health insurance affects the rate and type of utilization, and there is evidence that the availabiltiy of insurance has contributed to price inflation of unit costs.

It would seem that any significant reduction in hospital costs will have to come from a reversal of the present trend toward ever-greater utilization of inpatient services rather than from any substantial reduction in unit prices. "Abuse" is virtually built into the present insurance pattern. When the patient has insurance only for hospitalized illness, and the doctor's convenience is also served by sending him to the hospital, and the hospital itself has no control over admissions, what incentive or instrument is there for substantial reform of admissions policy? Some tightening up there may and probably will be. But it is not likely that any substantial results will be achieved until there is a basic reorientation of health insurance away from its present overconcentration on hospitalized illness.

Selection 18

What Consumers Expect from the Blues*

In spite of a rapidly growing population, it is quite evident that the era of relatively easy expansion of enrollments is about over. There will be mounting criticism of private health insurance for failure to reach the remaining, and exceedingly difficult to cover, portion of the population. More attention will be directed to the value of what is being purchased for the premium dollar in terms of the amount of benefits purchased and the quality.

Most of the scientific and technological factors that have contributed to forcing up premium levels at a rate of about 7 to 10 percent per annum, and to making costs a national issue, will continue to operate at a probably accelerated pace. Even more clearly, predictable changes in demographic and morbidity patterns will cause a greatly expanded, and far more expensive, rate of utilization.

The new consumer has thrown off most of the inhibitions his father or grandfather had in respect to medical services. In addition to his higher level of education and income, health insurance has helped to acquaint him with the

---

*Excerpt from H.M. Somers, "What Consumers Expect from Prepayment," presented to National Blue Cross and Blue Shield Enrollment Conference, 1961; published in *Modern Hospital* 98, no. 4 (April 1962): 91-92.

value and importance of modern medicine and has generated expectations of freer access. ... The consumer spokesman is growing more sophisticated and technically competent in what was once an area enshrouded in mystery. He is beginning to understand what he wants and is no longer hesitant to push for it.

In the recent past, organized labor has been the primary spokesman for the consumer. But the trend for management to assume the total costs of employee health insurance plans has important significance. Management is becoming sensitive to its heavy stake in participating in the organization and financing of medical care. It is entirely possible that it may organize itself to speak with a more effective voice in this field.

The management and labor spokesmen are themselves likely to be under severe pressure from workers. What they will ask for first is *more* protection. They will not be satisfied with insurance that meets one-third or even 40 percent of their medical costs. Second, they and their representatives are already recognizing that there are differences in the quality of medical care available and that, in addition to its intrinsic merits, quality also affects long range costs. Moreover, it is no longer a secret that the manner of organization of health services influences both quality and cost.

During this decade, private health insurance plans will be under severer criticism and public scrutiny than ever before, because costs are bound to rise substantially. This will quicken competition within the industry. The chief opportunity to counteract the discontents will be to satisfy the demands for more comprehensive services, improved quality of care, and a better doctor-patient relationship.

If private health insurance is to act in its self-interest and self-protection, it will move toward a more aggressive attempt to influence the factors in the medical services picture that can determine whether it can meet the conditions of demand during the next decade—or whether the demand will be channeled through a new medium. It seems fairly clear that the "good old days" when the industry could say it was merely a financial conduit to join consumers and suppliers are over.

The industry has a direct stake in the adequacy of the supply of physicians and paramedical personnel that will be forthcoming in the years ahead. It has a large stake in the amount and character of planning of hospital and other health facilities in American communities. It has a growing stake in the rationality and efficiency of the organization of health services. Only if these goals are achieved will it have adequate opportunity to meet successfully its responsibility to reorganize itself to meet the challenge. Its future may well depend upon the way in which this responsibiltiy is met.

Service plans still have the best opportunity for meeting the consumer demand of the next decade for comprehensiveness and better quality at the most reasonable cost. Comprehensive service protection can be furnished, and is being furnished, in different parts of the country, either through physicians in solo practice or group practice, or through complete service hospital-clinics. This must be made a primary objective.

Second, it is now increasingly recognized that comprehensiveness and prepayment can best be combined with high quality care and improved doctor-patient relationships when offered through group practice.

Private health insurance is here to stay. However, some very important matters for the future of private health insurance will be determined in this decade:

1. A redistribution of business—enrollment and premium volume—as among different types of carriers will take place.
2. The decade will determine whether private insurance will carry the major and basic part of the business with government fulfilling a supplementary role, or whether private health insurance will provide mainly the supplementary coverage.

In the first matter, the service contract organizations have both some apparent disadvantages and a vast opportunity. In a market of continuous and rapid cost inflation, such as this decade firmly promises, service plans will increasingly be at a competitive price handicap. If they offer what appears to be substantially an undifferentiated product—or perhaps even a thinner product—there is every reason to forecast a continuation, and probably an acceleration, of the relative loss of business to the indemnity carriers.

But there is also opportunity. In a general high price market, with consumer representatives restless and impatiently searching for improvements, the potential demand for a significantly differentiated product is enormous.

The days of the 1930s and 1940s—days when the buyers still naively believed that medical care was medical care and that there were no qualitative differences, or that in any case there were no reliable criteria for determining quality—or the days when any form of health insurance represented an improvement or even a breakthrough—or the days when this type of plan had a virtual monopoly—these days are now over. The fight will be more rugged from here on.

Clearly, it is not easy to develop comprehensive outpatient as well as inpatient coverage; there is influential and shortsighted resistance. It is not easy to underwrite group or clinic arrangements when they may not even exist in many communities. And it will not be cheap either. But the future is likely to belong to those who not only act as vehicles for the purchase of medical arrangements that already exist but who also influence the character of medical services and arrangements to be made available—who help create what they have to sell—because that may be the way to stay in business.

Of course, there are and will continue to be a considerable number of employee benefit plans, wherein the employer simply seeks the lowest possible price for the minimum plan he can get away with. But this will not be true of the large and powerful leaders in the field, the significant corporate enterprises. They are beginning to understand and to be aggressive about the nature of the product they are buying. And they will pay more if that is the way to get the product they want.

Experience shows that the large corporate interests are always pragmatic. If they cannot get what they want in basic protection from private carriers, they too will turn to government, as was shown in the pension field in 1949-50.

Private insurance may soon get a financial boost in government's assuming—through Social Security—the disproportionately weighty burden service plans have been carrying in enrollments of the aged. Many administrators are recognizing the great boon this would represent for the service plans, but it is considered bad form to say so. ...

Selection 19

Comprehensive Prepayment Plans: The Original HMOs*

The term "comprehensive prepayment" refers both to an ideal goal and to an operating reality. To some experts, comprehensive prepayment means that form of health insurance which provides the full gamut of needed health services—prevention, diagnosis, treatment, rehabilitation and long term care.

No existing health insurance in the United States meets this exacting concept. The working definition of the 50-odd plans, generally known as comprehensive prepayment organizations, is much more modest. Although they vary greatly in many respects, all have this in common: they emphasize service benefits for ambulatory physicians' care and coverage of routine or early stage medical bills. Other benefits, including hospital services, dental care, and drugs, may or may not be covered.

Proponents of this form of prepayment believe they are on the right track toward eventual achievement of truly comprehensive coverage. They believe that the physician is the indispensable key figure not only in the provision of medical care but in its economics. Only when regular physicians' services are fully covered under a service benefit contract, they say, can we seriously begin to incorporate prevention, rehabilitation, and effective management of chronic illness into the prevailing patterns of medical care organization and financing. Only thus can we improve the totality of availabile medical services while minimizing the costs of hospitalization and other highly expensive forms of treatment.

---

*Excerpt from A.R. Somers, "Comprehensive Prepayment Plans as a Mechanism for Meeting Health Needs," *Annals of the American Academy of Political and Social Science* 337 (September 1961): 82-91.

Other authorities disagree with this view. They maintain that the plans are too ambitious in their goals and too limited in their achievements. Indeed, the comprehensive plan has long been the stormy petrel of the health insurance field, controversial as to sponsorship, organization, financing, and future prospects.

SOME ILLUSTRATIVE PLANS

The comprehensive organizations may be classified according to sponsorship—whether limited to one industry or industrial group or open to the community at large. They can also be distinguished according to the way in which physicians' services are provided—through group practice or solo practice.

Historically, a number of farsighted employers led in the development of comprehensive prepayment. Today, however, most of the leading industrial plans are identified primarily with organized labor, although they may be administered by joint union-management trustees. The largest and most influential is the medical care program of the United Mine Workers (UMW) Welfare and Retirement Fund. This organization provides an exceptionally board range of service benefits to nearly a million potential beneficiaries in 26 coal-mining states. In fiscal 1960, over $61 million was spent for hospital and medical benefits.

Other leading industrial plans include the Labor Health Institute of St. Louis, Missouri (16,000 enrollees), the American Federation of Labor (AFL) Medical Service Plan of Philadelphia (72,000), the Chicago Union Health Service (10,000), and the numerous health centers sponsored by the International Ladies Garment Workers Union and the Amalgamated Clothing Workers of America.[1]

The most prominent of the community organizations are the Kaiser Foundation Health Plan on the west coast and Hawaii (815,000), the Health Insurance Plan of Greater New York (HIP) (617,000), and Group Health Insurance (GHI), also of New York City (650,000). [See Selections 21 and 32.]

Unlike Kaiser and HIP, Group Health Insurance (GHI) is not a group practice organization. Like Blue Shield, it has no official concern with the organization of medical care and pays doctors on a fee-for-service basis. The 10,000 GHI doctors are virtually all in solo practice. Unlike Blue Shield, however, GHI requires that all participating doctors accept its fee schedule as full payment for outpatient care, regardless of the patient's income. For inhospital services, semiprivate accommodation rather than income is used as the determinant of service benefits. In effect, therefore, GHI provides comprehensive coverage—provided the patient uses a participating doctor. Its control is divided equally between doctors and laymen. Like HIP, GHI generally relies on Blue Cross for hospital benefits.

GHI is illustrative of a new medical care hybrid—the comprehensive solo practice plan. The first to attract general attention was Windsor Medical Services (WMS) of Windsor, Ontario. WMS is sponsored by the Essex County

Medical Society and now has about 175,000 subscribers, 85 percent of the local population. Over 90 percent of Windsor doctors participate. Like GHI and unlike Blue Shield, WMS provides full service benefts for physicians' care regardless of the patient's income.

Altogether, the comprehensive plans have a total enrollment of some 4 to 5 million. Perhaps 2.5 million are in the group practice organizations; another million in the solo organizations; the UMW accounts for most of the balance.

ADEQUACY OF BENEFIT COVERAGE

A 1958 survey of HIP and GHI by the Health Information Foundation-National Opinion Research Center found that these plans were meeting, on average, about one-third of the total medical care expenditures of their members: HIP—35 percent, GHI—34 percent. This was over 40 percent better than health insurance as a whole. (The average benefit-expenditure ratio for all enrollees in 1958 was only 24 percent.) But it is still a long way from the comprehensive ideal.

On the insured portions of medical expense, however, the study found that the plans' record was excellent—especially HIP. This organization, together with Blue Cross, met 88 percent of the subscribers' average hospital costs, 92 percent of surgical costs, 87 percent of obstetrical costs. HIP alone covered 80 percent of the costs of all physicians' services. GHI and Blue Cross together met 78 percent of hospital costs, 63 percent of surgical, and 71 percent of obstetrical. GHI met 59 percent of all physicians' services.

The proportion of all physicians' services covered is especially impressive when compared with the comparable figure for all health insurance enrollment—18 percent in 1958. If surgery and obstetrics are omitted, the proportion covered declines to 7 percent. Here, then, is one major distinguishing feature of the comprehensive plans—the feature that has earned many the right to be called comprehensive, on a relative if not an absolute basis.

ECONOMICS OF PREPAYMENT

Prepayment is not cut-rate health insurance. Premiums are generally higher than the more usual surgical-medical policies. Furthermore, the claim to "first-dollar" coverage is no longer entirely valid. To avoid even greater rate increases, many of the plans have added numerous supplemental charges to patients. In most cases, these charges are modest—for example, Kaiser and the Community Health Association of Detroit (CHA) charge $1 for office visits; HIP $2 for night home calls; GHA charges $50 for maternity cases. Nevertheless, they now constitute a sizable portion of the plans' income, ranging in some cases from 15 to 25 percent of the total.

Despite the similarity of competitive rates, proponents of comprehensive prepayment believe that this type of coverage is potentially far more economical, both to the individual and to the nation. The most expensive form of medical care today is hospitalization. Any health insurance program which discourages unnecessary hospitalization and emphasizes less expensive types of care should be conducive to economy.

The group practice plans, in particular, have concentrated on this problem. Every effort is made to keep patients out of the hospital unless absolutely necessary from a medical point of view. Their medical centers or clinics are equipped to provide most diagnostic tests. Ross-Loos, with its own anesthesiologist and recovery room, does tonsillectomies on an outpatient basis. As a result, many plans report significantly lower rates of hospital utilization than is true for other health insurance enrollees. The differential is generally claimed to be about 20 percent.

Thus far, the individual member has not greatly benefited financially from this lower utilization. The Kaiser plans, with their own hospitals, have been able to pass part of the savings along to subscribers in lower premium rates. But this is not true of plans that do not have their own hospitals, where the member has to buy hospital coverage at regular rates.

So far as the community and nation are concerned, the potential savings are very great. For example, E.A. Van Steenwyk, executive vice president of the Philadelphia Blue Cross, estimates that a reduction of one-half day in the average length of stay of his enrollees would save that plan $3 million a year in 1960 dollars. Donald Straus, vice president of HIP, has calculated that a 20 percent reduction in general hospital use would save New Yorkers $156 million in current bed replacement costs and $35 to $44 million in annual Blue Cross hospital payments.

PROSPECTS FOR THE FUTURE

The comprehensive prepayment plan occupies an anomalous position in current health insurance developments. Long supported by leading medical educators, it has received the repeated protection of the courts, including the United States Supreme Court.[2] Also, in 1959, following a four-year study by the American Medical Association Commission on Medical Care Plans (Larson Commission), it obtained the unenthusiastic but on-the-record endorsement of the AMA House of Delegates. Its national press has been highly favorable, and, in those areas where the plans operate, the local press has usually been friendly.

Nevertheless, comprehensive prepayment has not kept pace with the general increase in health insurance enrollment. The larger plans have continued to grow, but, as a general mechanism for meeting health needs, comprehensive prepayment remains limited to a few geographical areas, primarily along the eastern and western seaboards, and probably covers no more than 3 percent of all health insurance enrollees. Why?

There appear to be two main reasons for the slow growth: the opposition of organized medicine and slow public acceptance. The many practical obstacles, including legal restraints and financial difficulties, are primarily consequences of these two.

Professional Opposition

At first glance, the hostility of large portions of the medical profession to comprehensive prepayment is difficult to understand. Medically, its orientation is in line with the most progressive professional thought. Economically, it appears to offer a practical method of restraining the spiraling costs of hospital care and, hence, reducing the pressure for governmental intervention in the health insurance field. Nevertheless, the opposition, particularly at the state and local levels, has been intense.

Publicly, the issue has been presented by the profession primarily in terms of free choice of physician by the patient. This is a matter of considerable importance and one which the author has dealt with elsewhere.[3] It is not, however, the crux of the opposition. Nonfree choice programs such as workmen's compensation have long been supported by organized medicine, while comprehensive solo practice plans, such as San Joaquin and Windsor, which provide complete free choice, continue to be opposed. The heart of the opposition is the matter of controls—controls over fees, utilization, and quality.

Significantly, those doctors who are associated with teaching hospitals and other institutions where quality controls are taken for granted are also most likely to be friendly to comprehensive prepayment. The antagonism comes primarily, although by no means exclusively, from the rugged individualists in the profession—those who have been away from medical school for some time, who are used to operating completely on their own, and who have profited from this type of practice.

As opposed to this individualistic approach, the comprehensive prepayment plans maintain that, in order to make optimum use of our modern medical resources, doctors must accept some voluntary limitation on their fees and must submit to some degree of continuing qualitative supervision by their professional colleagues—an extension of the principle of hospital audit to general medical services.

In practice, the nature of these limits and controls varies widely. The group practice plans generally impose greater financial controls than do the solo plans. In some groups, all the doctors are on salary; in others, they operate through partnerships and divide up their income in any way they wish. Some plans permit their doctors to handle private patients without any restrictions—a device to enable them to earn additional income. Other plans exercise various degrees of control over such outside practice.

The solo plans exercise far less control. Generally, they have a panel of doctors who agree to accept a schedule of fees as full payment for services rendered. The panel may be practically coextensive with the total number of doctors in the locality, as is true in San Joaquin and Windsor, or it may constitute a relatively small proportion. In any case, they differ from Blue Shield in that there are no income limits on service benefits and, hence, there can be no extra charges to enrollees.

The extent and effectiveness of the qualitative controls also differ greatly. At HIP, a Medical Control Board, consisting of 11 outside and seven HIP doctors, sets the basic standards which all groups are required to meet. These standards relate to physician qualifications, group organization, services, facilities, and equipment. The board also reviews individual applications for appointments and makes periodic surveys of the groups' work.

In all cases, as far as the author is aware, the qualitative controls over doctors are exercised by other doctors. There is no sign of any drift toward lay interference in purely professional matters. This was attested to by the Larson Commission, which also endorsed the quality of care in the plans investigated. This has not significantly removed local medical society opposition, however.

Over the years, this opposition has been expressed in many ways—through state legislation outlawing lay-controlled medical care plans, through invocation of legal prohibitions against the corporate practice of medicine, through boycotts of plans and expulsion of plan doctors from medical societies, through refusal to extend hospital privileges to these doctors, and so on. Partly as a result of 20 years of legal defeats for organized medicine, the more flagrant of these restraints have now been ended. Nevertheless, many of the obstacles remain.

Public Attitudes

For many years it was virtually impossible to determine public attitudes with any precision. In most communities, no comprehensive prepayment plans existed, and there was no way for the public to express its preference. In communities where they did exist, it was frequently on an embattled basis, with members never knowing when they would be denied admission to a hospital or otherwise penalized for belonging to this type of plan. During the last decade, however, a number of the plans have achieved sufficient strength and status to permit the public to join with a reasonable sense of security and "respectability." Moreover, the new technique of "dual choice" or multiple choice has enabled people insured under a number of public and private employee benefit programs to choose between a comprehensive plan and a different type of health insurance on a reasonably informed basis. For the first time, we have some measure of public opinion.

The most extensive choice program—covering 5 million persons—is that operated by the United States Civil Service Commission under the new Federal Employees Health Benefits program. In the first election, June 1960, employees were offered a choice of 38 plans as follows: a governmentwide Blue Cross and Blue Shield program, a governmentwide indemnity program, 13 comprehensive group practice plans, eight comprehensive solo practive plans, and 15 employee organization plans.

In the areas where they were available, the group practice plans obtained 16 percent of the total enrollment; the solo plans 8 percent. The percentage choosing group practice varied from about 35 percent in the San Francisco area down to 1 percent in St. Paul. Kaiser, which had a considerable number of federal employees before the new program began, did especially well. The plans as a whole attracted younger employees and those with more dependents.

During the spring of 1961, the commission conducted a sample survey of employees to determine levels of utilization and satisfaction as an aid to the renegotiation of contracts and preparation for the next election, November 1961. Eighty-three percent of the comprehensive plans' enrollees reported they had used their plan, compared with only 36 percent of the total. While satisfaction was high among all users—82 percent of the total said they were generally satisfied—it was particularly high for the comprehensives—92 percent. The commission also reports that the comprehensives are getting more than their original share of new enrollees.

The rapidly accumulating results of dual choice elections on the west coast, in New York City, Detroit, and elsewhere, deserve careful scrutiny by all students of comprehensive prepayment. Pending such quantitative analysis, a few hypotheses appear in order. Public acceptance of this method of providing medical care is still limited to a minority. Given equal access to a comprehensive plan and an opportunity for reasonably informed choice, the minority can be very substantial—a third or more. Whether public acceptance will increase or not appears to depend primarily on three factors.

1. The extent to which a particular plan is able to establish itself as a "respectable" and secure institution in the community.

2. The extent to which potential enrollees become sophisticated with respect to medical practice and medical economics. Contrary to the expectations of many group practice enthusiasts, low income groups, when first given a choice, tend to prefer traditional forms of medical practice. A survey of attitudes toward medical care in the mid-1940s reported that over 90 percent of the upper income group preferred group practice—the prepayment issue was not involved—but only half of the lowest income group. The latter also had little concern for preventive medicine or the early detection of disease. This group still tends to think of medical care primarily in terms of acute illness requiring hospitalization. (See Selection 11.)

Both scientific and economic considerations are, however, causing a rapid transition in such attitudes. Moreover, it is clear that familiarity does not breed contempt. On the contrary, most comprehensive plans can demonstrate a high degree of enrollee satisfaction. Despite their relatively high cost, there is little attrition. Their problem is to persuade the public to try the unfamiliar in the first instance. In this respect, the solo plans may be serving a particularly useful function in communities like New York, where the tradition of the neighborhood family doctor is so deeply rooted. This fact may explain GHI's remarkable recent growth. Given the encouragement of the medical profession, there is reason to believe that comprehensive solo plans would probably mushroom across the nation.

3. The attitude of the medical profession is probably the most important direct influence on the development of these plans. In addition, doctors exert

tremendous indirect pressure through their influence on consumer attitudes. ...

NOTES

1. Some of the older or smaller union programs provide diagnostic services only, stopping short both of family doctor care and hospital care. Although frequently identified with comprehensive prepayment, these programs serve a different and more limited purpose.
2. *American Medical Association v. United States,* 317 U.S. 519 (1943).
3. H.M. and A.R. Somers, *Doctors, Patients, and Health Insurance* (Washington, D.C.: The Brookings Institution, 1961), pp. 409-413, 487.

Selection 20

Self-Regulation: Can Voluntary Controls Work?*

The dramatic rise in the costs of medical care is well known. In part this was due to increased use of medical goods and services. To a larger degree, however, the rise is attributable to a 43 percent advance in medical prices, which were spiraling upward far more rapidly than other prices. Indeed the most disturbing aspect of the price rise is its acceleration and the increasing disparity with general price trends. Between 1947-49 and 1959, medical care prices rose twice as much as the general cost of living.

This persistent rise is the major factor in the ever-increasing loss ratios of which all carriers and plans complain and in the extreme finankial difficulties of many Blue Cross plans. It threatens both the comprehensive major medical and comprehensive prepaymentplans with retrenchment at a time when both should be expanding and has generally made it more difficult to expand benefits (not to mention being a major cause for increasing government intervention in the problem of the aged). For all these reasons many experts feel that costs have become the greatest single issue facing voluntary health insurance today.

Not everyone agrees with this view. Some take the position that there really is no cost crisis as yet—at least so far as group insurance is concerned. In spite of all the rate increases, they say, health insurance still represents an insignificant item in industry's overall budget, perhaps no more than 2 to 3 percent of total

---

*Excerpt from A.R. and H.M. Somers, "Coverage, Costs, and Controls in Voluntary Health Insurance," in *Public Health Reports* 76 (January 1961): 1-9.

labor costs, and less than pensions. Furthermore, they say, as costs rise, it simply means that employees will take a little less of their next pay increase in the form of direct wages and a little more in the form of medical benefits. And since the total cost can be spread so easily and painlessly throughout the consuming public, so runs the argument, nobody really has to worry.

Indeed there seems little doubt that Americans are destined to, and probably should, spend more than they now do for medical care. Not only is scientific advance making more and better health protection available, but rising living and educational standards and the aging of the population are making the demand larger and inexorable.

But if the price of medical care continues to rise at its current rate, and health insurance even faster as it must to keep up with the greater rise in hospital prices, still the major component in insurance benefit payments, then we may find that all the additional money is absorbed in maintaining the present level of benefits. In fact, premiums could continue to rise substantially, while benefits actually decline.

The price of health insurance is primarily, of course, a problem of medical, not insurance, prices. Group health insurance has become largely a "cost-plus" operation, and when we talk about the rise in cost of health insurance we are inevitably talking about the rise in cost of medical care.

The matter is not quite that simple, however. It is increasingly recognized that the presence of insurance is not a neutral force in the medical marketplace however much its proponents may wish it to be so. The influence of various types of insurance on subscriber utilization and expenditures has frequently been noted. Consider, for example, the effect of the HIP type of coverage in reducing hospital use and, therefore, costs. At one point, before it undertook necessary reforms, the United Mine Workers medical care program faced financial disaster, so great was the increase in the costs of hospital and surgical services by its beneficiaries.

It seems clear that health insurance, originally designed to ease problems of medical costs, has actually contributed, by its effect on utilization and on prices in a scarcity market, to intensification of the problem. This is not to deny the great good which insurance has already accomplished. However, if it is to continue to play a constructive role in the easing of medical costs for consumers and in the stabilization of income for producers, it must acknowledge, more forthrightly than heretofore, its influence on costs and be prepared to accept the corollary responsibilities.

Fortunately, the same insurance mechanism which has aggravated the cost problem also appears to contain the possibility for an equitable solution: an administrative mechanism for reconciling the three great objectives of economy, quality, and free choice.

As already indicated, the "closed panel" is one reasonably effective method of controlling some forms of medical cost. The HIP record, for example (even in this decade of inflation, it has not raised its premiums since 1953), is impressive. This fact, made possible by the plan's capitation method of payment to affiliated groups, has undoubtedly resulted in some hardship to individual doctors, especially the best and most dedicated of them. But, it is not likely that it could have held together an organization of 1,000 physicians, with the reputation they have established, if any inordinate economic sacrifice had been required. The HIP experience, of course, is not definitive; not all closed panel plans have such a record.

SAN JOAQUIN COUNTY FOUNDATION

It is not necessary, however, to confine the discussion to closed panel practice. There are examples of effective cost controls among doctors in solo fee-for-service practice. Among those are the San Joaquin County (California) Foundation for Medical Care and two Canadian plans, Windsor Medical Services and the Saskatchewan Swift Current program. Let us sketch briefly the functioning of the San Joaquin program.

The foundation is not a carrier. It is the brainchild and a legal subdivision of the San Joaquin Medical Society. It was organized in 1954 partly as a countermeasure to the success of the Kaiser Foundation Health Plan. Its officers are appointed by the county society, and it is housed in the same building as the society in Stockton. The relations between the foundation and the society could hardly be closer. Nevertheless, in practice as well as in philosophy, it has construed its role as a protector of consumer interests as well as those of the physicians.

The functions of the foundation include the setting of benefit standards for all policies marketed as foundation approved, the review and payment of claims, and the establishment of maximum fee schedules for physicians' services. The actual underwriting and sale of policies is left to insurance companies which are willing to accept the foundation's liberal benefit standards and vigorous claims procedures.

Participating physicians, about 98 percent of all in the county, practice on a solo fee-for-service basis, but they agree to accept the foundation's fee schedules as full payment, thus guaranteeing service benefits and certainty-of-costs to the insured and eliminating the whole problem of income limits, which plagues Blue Shield. The physicians must reapply annually for membership.

The key to the foundation's control is its insistence on handling all claims itself. Each one receives a twofold review—a contractual review by specially trained clerks and a medical review by a rotating committee of physicians who give an hour a week to this work and who, as members of a committee of the county medical society, have the authority to call up a colleague and insist on an adjustment, if necessary. This review is directed as much at the quality of care as the price. It represents an extension of the principle of internal medical audit, familiar to most accredited hospital staffs, to outpatient care. The results, according to foundation officials, are generally educational rather than disciplinary. But enough discipline has been applied, including refusal to readmit one physician, to act as a powerful influence on the whole program. The San Joaquin experiment has received the compliment of imitation by 13 other California counties.

PHILADELPHIA BLUE CROSS

Another illustration, from the hospital insurance field, is Blue Cross of Philadelphia. This plan, one of the oldest and largest of the Blue Cross group, has experimented over the years with numerous institutional devices for exercising some discipline over the rising costs of hospital care and hence its own subscription rates. One is a negotiated hospital reimbursement formula, which does not pay on the basis of the individual hospital's costs or charges, however discounted, nor on the basis of a flat community rate, as was done originally. The present formula is a complex one which attempts to incorporate the best features of all these approaches. Its aim is to build in incentives for more efficient hospital operation by rewarding, within limits, the more efficient institutions and penalizing the less efficient.

One especially interesting feature divides the affiliated hospitals into ten categories according to their patients' average length of stay and then adds, within these categories, differential payments, varying from 200 percent of the basic rate for the first day to 75 percent for all days over the average in the appropriate category. The purpose is to create a financial incentive for the hospitals to discharge patients as soon as possible. To try to cut down possible misuse of hospital services by consumers, this plan has also introduced a deductible contract, outpatient diagnostic benefits (now carried by about 60 percent of the enrollees), and visiting nurse services for older subscribers.

In 1958 a physicians' review board was created with the backing of the Philadelphia County Medical Society to check on practices of physicians that might lead to unnecessary admissions, overuse of ancillary services, and unnecessarily prolonged stays. The board is composed of 34 outstanding local doctors, with a leading surgeon and an internist as cochairmen and an advisory council of six, which includes such nationally eminent physicians as I.S. Ravdin and John H. Gibbon, Jr. The doctors, divided into seven groups, are continuously engaged in review of hospital records, and the plan's new electronic equipment makes the data available in detail for every case admitted to every hospital.

The cases mentioned are, of course, conspicuous exceptions to the general policy of *laissez faire*—of allowing the seller to charge what he will. Indeed, even these plans have encountered bitter opposition. A portentous policy conflict is currently taking place in Philadelphia over the Blue Cross reimbursement formula. In 1959, about half the affiliated hospitals refused to renew the existing contract. This issue is currently being investigated, at the request of Blue Cross and most of the hospitals, by a committee of the American Hospital Association. Meanwhile, eight Catholic institutions served notice, in January 1960, that they would cancel their Blue Cross affiliation on March 31 if their demand for reimbursement based on individual charges was not met.

The nature of their demand, while complicated by secondary factors, goes to the heart of the control issue. They insist that Blue Cross' function is solely to pay the bills of its subscribers. They deny that it should have any favored position on rates, or the right to negotiate terms and conditions, or to check their books, records, or administration.

Blue Cross maintains that capitulation to such a demand would remove incentives to more efficient cost-conscious hospital administration and would inevitably lead to higher hospital rates. This would force a further rise in Blue Cross rates and might result in the loss of subscribers. Some of these would switch to indemnity contracts; others would lose coverage altogether. In either case, the hospitals would have to carry a larger proportion of nonpay or part-pay patients. In brief, the plan maintains that by exercising reasonable protection of subscriber interests through attempts to keep prepayment rates within bounds it is also serving the best interests of the hospitals.

In a statement to the press, the "lay representative" of the disaffiliated hospitals—a Philadelphia insurance broker—accused Philadelphia Blue Cross of a "conflict of interest." The plan is acting in a dual and conflicting capacity, he claimed, as a seller of hospital insurance and "as a social agency with power to dictate the administrative procedures of hospitals." Herein is the crux of the issue: overlooking the political hyperbole in such debating terms as "power to dictate," are these two functions really in conflict or are they complementary? Was Philadelphia Blue Cross going beyond its proper function or discharging a necessary duty? Does the plan, which provides about 70 percent of patient days in Catholic hospitals and serves 70 percent of the city's population, have the responsibility to represent its subscribers as well as the hospitals, or not?

Officials of the Philadelphia plan believe that if they can establish this broad authority it will mean a notable victory for the entire voluntary health insurance movement. It will mean that it has the authority to keep its house in order, balance its books, and tackle with some assurance of success the problem of extending benefits. If the authority cannot be established, if the majority of providers and subscribers do not sustain it in this challenge, an important test case for the future of voluntarism will have been lost, including the possibility that the plan may have to abandon its traditional responsibiltiy for the aged. A big step will have been taken toward abdication of responsibility by the voluntary agencies and the likelihood of public intervention. [Blue Cross lost in its conflict with the eight hospitals. Sixteen years later, however, the underlying issues still plague the industry in general and the Philadelphia area in particular.]

It is a truism in this country that the government is generally permitted to do only what private enterprise cannot or will not do satisfactorily. The initiative still rests with the voluntary movement. But it may not indefinitely. It is inescapable that public financing, in one form or another, will increase in the medical care field.

There are, however, at least two big questions which are far from settled. One involves the future boundaries of public financing; the other, the relationship between public financing and private administration. At this particular juncture of affairs, one would expect the medical profession and the health services industry as a whole to be enormously concerned with strengthening the voluntary institutions, not only to make sure that they can discharge their own responsibilities effectively, but also to enable them to play a responsible role in the administration of the new public programs.

This cannot be accomplished without responsible, community-conscious leadership and strong management. It also calls for determined support from the majority of the providers and consumers of medical care. The ability of voluntary health insurance to meet successfully the challenge of the "3 Cs"—coverage, costs, and controls—and hence ensure its own survival, will probably be determined as much by the leaders of the medical profession and other health services as by the plans and carriers themselves.

Selection 21

A Successful Past and Uncertain Future*

In 1968 private health insurance organizations had a total subscription or premium income of $13 billion; paid out 88 percent in benefits; used 14.8 percent for operating expenses; and had a net underwriting loss of nearly 3 percent. The only segments of the industry that appear to be thriving financially are the dental societies, whose plans produced a net surplus of 11 percent, and Blue Shield, with a 5 percent surplus. Losses were heaviest—nearly 7 percent of premium income—in the insurance company group business, where it was at least partially offset by investment income (although data on this are not available), as well as by profits from more lucrative types of group insurance frequently sold in the same package. Blue Cross sustained a net loss of 2 percent.

It is evident that, aside from the notoriously inefficient insurance company individual policies (in this category, operating expenses or "retention" consumed nearly half of income; even so, the companies failed to show a profit), there is not much room for administrative savings. Private health insurance has, in effect, become largely a cost-plus operation except that, ironically, for most of the industry, the "plus" has become a "minus." It may be significant that the smaller independent plans, with their emphasis on out-of-hospital benefits, appear to be at least holding their own.

---

*Excerpt from A.R. Somers, *Health Care in Transition: Directions for the Future* (Chicago: Hospital Research and Education Trust, 1971), pp. 48-55.

Unlike the insurance companies, Blue Cross plans in most states must obtain the approval of state insurance commissioners for rate increases. In at least two states, New York and New Jersey, the increases requested in 1969, averaging 49.5 percent in New York and 44.3 percent in New Jersey, precipitated bitter political battles. The press, the politicians (especially in New York City), the unions, and millions of individual Blue Cross members waxed indignant and swore publicly and privately throughout the summer. The city of New York requested a court order directing the state insurance department to show cause why the increases should not be barred. The city also threatened to set up its own "Blue Cross" on a self-insured basis.

Despite all the tumult and the shouting, however, no one had any effective remedy for the underlying inflation in provider costs. The bitter drama was marked by a pervasive atmosphere of futility and frustration. Faced with the undeniable fact that the plans could not stay in business without a substantial rise in premium income, the insurance commissioners had little choice except to grant most of what the plans were asking. New York Blue Cross got 43.3 percent; New Jersey an emergency 28.5 percent in December and another 21.9 percent in May 1970. It was understood that a further increase would be required by mid-1971.

A particularly poignant casualty of the current inflation was the long standing Montefiore Medical Group, HIP's showcase affiliate since the start of the plan in 1947. The hospital claimed that it could not provide services for the payment HIP was able to make for its members. HIP claimed it could not pay more. A 40 percent subscriber rate increase had already been put into effect early in 1969.

By summer of 1970, the problems facing Blue Cross in many parts of the country were reaching crisis proportions. The honeymoon between Blue Cross and the hospitals was generally at an end. Forced by subscriber pressure and state legislatures to put the screws on hospitals, Blue Cross was even fighting implementation of the new American Hospital Association (AHA) reimbursement policy. Presumably the long run advantage of putting more teeth into planning was outweighed by the immediate cost of a capital factor based on current cost replacement and sharing the cost of indigent care. In several eastern states, the renewal of Blue Cross-hospital contracts was being approached with growing hostility on both sides.

Meanwhile, the era of relatively good feeling between Blue Cross and the commercial carriers, the product of the phenomenal postwar growth enjoyed by all, was also coming to an end. In several states Blue Cross was being sued by insurance companies as an "unlawful monopoly;" in others, the carriers were stepping up pressure on state legislatures to revoke Blue Cross exemption from the usual premium tax. In turn, Blue Cross was demanding that the insurance companies be brought under greater state regulation. In the growing atmosphere of tension and pessimism more and more carriers, as well as hospitals, were looking—anxiously if somewhat surreptitiously—to government to provide a way out, a posture already held by numerous consumer groups.

In the growing disappointment over the inability of the private carriers and health insurance funds to insure the entire population adequately and to meet the growing crisis in health care costs, however, it would be a serious error to overlook their many impressive achievements.

First, there is the basic fact that millions of people have obtained access to good medical care for the first time. For example, the United Mine Workers Welfare and Retirement Fund reported a 30 percent gain in the average life expectancy of bituminous coal miners between 1946, when the fund began, and 1967. At the earlier date, miners died at a median age of 57.4, more than eight years earlier than the average United States male. In 1967, the average age of a miner at death was 74.7, over six years older than the general average. Allowing for the possibility of some exaggeration and the fact that health benefits were not the only cause of the increased longevity, nevertheless the improvement must be at least partially attributed to the union health program. The same, to varying degrees, could be said of many other insurance or prepayment plans.

Second, it has been possible, by spreading the risks and costs of care, to develop a much broader and stronger financial base for our rapidly expanding medical care economy. The fact that the private sector has been unable to cope adequately with the special problems of the aged and the poor should not obscure those areas where they have proved both innovative and successful.

Perhaps it was too easy to translate relatively modest contributions from thousands of employers and millions of employees into $50-, $60-, and even $100-a-day hospital payments. There are those who fault the carriers for not controlling these costs more effectively. The fact is that they were unable to do so, an inability that Medicare and Medicaid have similarly demonstrated. This latter should give pause to those who believe that national health insurance would provide a magic instrument of control.

INNOVATIONS AND IMPROVEMENTS

Among the most innovative programs, one thinks immediately of prepaid group practice, associated with Kaiser, HIP, Group Health Cooperative of Puget Sound, and others. The obstacles faced by these organizations, especially in their early days, were very great. Not all have been successful in overcoming them, but several have been spectacularly so. What has come to be known as the "Kaiser Formula" can now be accepted as an experiment that has fully proved itself over a period of 26 years.

The essential ingredients of this formula, as defined by the medical director of its Portland clinic, include (1) prepayment, usually by monthly dues; (2) group practice; (3) a unified medical center, including both hospital and satellite clinics; (4) voluntary enrollment, based on the choice of two or more different kinds of health plans; (5) payment of physicians and hospitals on the basis of capitation or fixed fees per time-period for each enrollee, regardless of the amount of care provided; and (6) coverage of the full spectrum of comprehensive care, starting with prevention.

Nor has success been confined to prepaid group practice. Group Health Insurance (GHI), with 1.3 million enrollees in New York and New Jersey, and the much smaller San Joaquin County Medical Foundation, have both demonstrated that something approaching comprehensive coverage can be provided even without group practice, without a hospital base, and without capitation payment to the provider.

Despite these differences, however, there are some basic similarities among these programs. The common ingredients in Kaiser and GHI, for example, can probably be identified as the *sine qua non* of a successful health insurance program today.

1. Both view their responsibility primarily as providers of health care, not just as conduits for medical expense dollars.

2. Both assume some responsibility for the cost and, to a lesser extent, the quality of such care. GHI doctors are all in private independent practice, but they must accept a fixed fee schedule without income limits. This has been maintained despite pressure from Medicare and other sources. GHI quality controls are not so direct as under Kaiser, but their claims are constantly scrutinized for appropriateness as well as price.

3. Both plans are distinguished by strong, independent management, making full use of computer capability and other modern managerial tools.

Blue Cross, through the Blue Cross Associaiton and individual plans, has long been in the forefront of efforts to strengthen private health insurance. In its 1970 Member Hospital Reimbursement Formula, the Associated Hospital Service of New York, the largest Blue Cross plan, has introduced, in accordance with New York State's 1969 Hospital Cost Control Law, several important new features, including a productivity incentive payment, a utilization control incentive payment, and a trusteed community pool of depreciation funds. A few Blue Cross plans are underwriting prepaid group practice and other innovative programs.

The commercial insurance industry, long a bastion of conservatism, has now become a champion of progressive developments in the delivery system, developments aimed at both better cost controls and more comprehensive coverage. Several companies are underwriting prepaid group practice experiments.

THE FEDERAL EMPLOYEES PROGRAM

Perhaps the most interesting program in the entire field of private health insurance is the Federal Employees Health Benefits Program (FEP). This huge plan, which has been in existence for ten years and is successfully insuring over eight million persons, including nearly 450,000 retirees, constitutes a creative, pragmatic mix of public and private initiative.

Indeed, it is difficult to be sure of the correct way to classify it, whether public or private. In the various federal reports, however, it is classified as private, even though it is statutory, since its benefits are entirely underwritten by private carriers and the government participates principally in the role of employer.

Under FEP, federal employees choose, at specified intervals, from among a number of different types of carriers and different benefit packages carrying different price tags. There are strict limitations on the number and qualifications of carriers. The 38 currently approved organizations include a governmentwide Blue Cross-Blue Shield Plan, a governmentwide consortium of insurance companies administered by Aetna Life and Casualty, a group of employee union plans, a group of comprehensive group practice plans including Kaiser and HIP, and a few comprehensive individual practice plans such as GHI and the San Joaquin Foundation Plan. All are permitted to sell the best program they can underwrite. Most sell a "low" option and a "high" option, providing broader benefits at a higher price. Enrollment under the high options has steadily increased since the program started, until today about 85 percent of enrollees are so covered.

All plans provide a wide range of benefits, exceeding by a substantial margin the insurance available to most Americans at comparable prices. Under the high options, the following benefits are generally available, although with some variation as to adequacy: inpatient hospitalization, most physician services, most hospital ambulatory services, psychiatric care, prescribed drugs, and some appliances. The principal gaps involve physical checkups, dental care, and long term care.

Premiums vary widely. Originally the government, as employer, contributed to all plans an amount equal to half the premium of the low option Aetna plan. This resulted in the government paying about 38 percent of total costs. The difference between the government contribution and the actual premium of the plan selected by the employee is paid by him, thus providing a brake on rising costs and an incentive to intercarrier competition. In recent years, the rising costs of all health insurance resulted in a decline in the government proportion to 24 percent. Congress is currently debating how much to raise the federal contribution—probably 40 to 60 percent.

The program is administered by the U.S. Civil Service Commission, which approves the various benefit packages and the prices charged for them, conducts the various "open enrollment" periods including approval of the informational material distributed by the competing carriers, collects the required contributions, and funnels them to the participating carriers.

The distribution of enrollees among the various plans has been relatively stable, although with some significant changes, over the years. Following are the percentages for 1960 and for March 1970:

	1960	1970
Blue Cross-Blue Shield	54.2	60.8
Aetna	26.9	18.0
Employee plans	13.2	14.6
Group practice plans	4.2	4.9
Individual practice plans	1.5	1.7

It must be kept in mind, of course, that the two latter categories are local and not available in many parts of the country.

One of the interesting aspects of FEP is the opportunity it affords to compare utilization of health services under the different types of insurance. Consistently, the comprehensive plans have demonstrated lower hospital use, in terms of both admissions and days, than the more conventional programs. For example, the rates for nonmaternity inpatient hospitalization under the different plans, both options, in 1966 were as follows:

	Utilizers per 1,000 Covered Persons	Hospital Days per 1,000 Covered Persons
Blue Cross-Blue Shield	98	876
Aetna	85	884
Employee plans	93	808
Group practice plans	46	408
Individual practice plans	71	499

The total cost of FEP has increased over the years from $343 million, or $59 per capita, in 1962, to $826 million, or $104 per capita, in 1969. While some significant benefit improvements have taken place during this period, clearly FEP has not been immune to the general inflation. Nevertheless, $104 is still low for the coverage provided, and satisfaction among FEP enrollees is generally high. This is a program to be studied carefully in any movement toward national health insurance.

AN AGENDA FOR REFORM

Rather than issue either a blanket condemnation or a total endorsement of private health insurance, it is essential to sort out the different experiences of different carriers, to distinguish the successful from the unsuccessful, and to seek ways of assimilating and generalizing the positive. Among the reforms that have been suggested are the following:

1. elimination or reduction of the usual statutory limitations on Blue Cross and Blue Shield benefit coverage, including merger of the two programs;
2. establishment of minimum state benefit standards for all carriers, with special emphasis on out-of-hospital benefits;
3. repeal of all state laws restricting the establishment of prepaid group practice plans;
4. a requirement that, in all states where such plans now exist, tax-exempt employee benefit plans include in their health benefits a prepaid group practice option;
5. provision in state laws for the self-employed and other individuals who lack access to group coverage to be treated as groups to obtain the benefit of group rates;

6. compulsory coverage of part-time and temporarily employed workers and of those temporarily laid off;
7. noncancellability of policies in effect for a year and convertibility from group to individual coverage at equitable rates;
8. public subsidy to carriers sponsoring experimental programs, such as prepaid group practice;
9. prohibition of duplicate benefits, especially for hospital confinement;
10. prohibition or strict control of mail-order insurance;
11. reduction in the number of carriers, from the present 1,700 or more to a comparatively few with the size and adminsitrative strength to match the problems.

Some of these proposals have been recommended in recent Department of Health, Education, and Welfare reports, including the National Conference on Private Health Insurance (1967), the Secretary's Advisory Committee on Hospital Effectiveness (1968), and the Secretary's Task Force on Medicaid and Related Programs (1970).

The final result of pursuing this approach to its logical conclusion would be designation of a limited number of carriers as "chosen instruments"—operating under private management but under strict public regulation, which might or might not permit competition. The transition from such regulated private health insurance to certain types of compulsory health insurance would not be a large one.

Regardless of the ultimate outcome, however, many of these proposals could be extremely useful as devices for improving existing insurance coverage and strengthening the private sector against continuing default to public programs.

Selection 22

Blue Shield: Special Problems, Special Remedies*

I agree completely that the question of an appropriate rate increase cannot be considered solely, or even primarily, on the basis of actuarial considerations. It cannot be sensibly considered apart from the value of the insured package that Blue Shield is selling. This, in turn, opens up the whole question of the price, adequacy, and quality of physicians' services and the extent to which consumer needs are being met.

---

*Excerpt from A.R. Somers, Statement on Blue Shield Reform, Hearings before Commissioner H.S. Denenberg, Insurance Department, Commonwealth of Pennsylvania, Philadelphia, September 25, 1972, unpublished.

This is a formidable problem, not likely to be disposed of through any one set of guidelines or one set of hearings. In *Health Care in Transition: Directions for the Future,* I presented a list of 11 reforms of private health insurance which were intended not only to help improve immediate performance but also to strengthen the private carriers for future responsibilities under national health insurance (Selection 21). ...

As far as Blue Shield's immediate performance is concerned, there are two overriding and legitimate consumer complaints: (1) inadequate coverage of out-of-hospital services, and (2) the uncertain degree of protection for even those services that are nominally covered.

Physician complaints heard most often include: (1) where fee schedules are used as the basis of payment, they are frequently obsolete, not only in terms of current fee levels but of current medical procedures, especially in the nonsurgical areas; (2) where the "prevailing fee" or "usual, customary, and reasonable" basis of payment is used, there is widespread confusion and lack of clarity as to what fees are acceptable and what are not; (3) excessive paper work in connection with claims; and (4) excessively slow payment of claims.

I know of no currently meaningful studies indicating the percentage of subscriber medical care costs being met by Blue Shield benefits. There was a time, a decade or so ago, when some Blue Shield leaders spoke valiantly of trying to assure at least 75 percent coverage of subscribers' surgical-medical expenses. My guess today is that even within this restricted area—mostly inpatient, of course—the national average is probably less than 50 percent. This varies in different parts of the country, depending in part on the strength of local consumer bargaining units. In Michigan, I am told, the ratio may be as high as 80 percent; in some localities as low as 35 percent.

The low levels result from three factors: (1) the extremely low income limits on service benefits for most subscribers, (2) the fact that many doctors are nonparticipating, and (3) unrealistically low fee schedules.

At Rutgers University, for example, a spokesman for the Personnel Department told me that the $5,000 and $7,500 New Jersey limits exclude at least 90 percent of their 8,000 employees from service benefits. In these cases, the physician can charge the patient any additional amount that he wishes.

As an extreme case, but an actual one, a member of the Rutgers faculty recently paid $1,840 to a nonparticipating surgeon for a serious operation on one of his children (for which he was reimbursed $500), plus $215 to the anesthesiologist (for which he was reimbursed $65). His out-of-pocket expenses of $1,490—73 percent of the charges—were incurred in precisely the area that Blue Shield is supposed to be most effective—inpatient surgery. It is perhaps no coincidence that this individual is a prime mover in the effort to establish an HMO at Rutgers.

As to nonparticipating doctors, the New Jersey plan claims, for the state as a whole, that three-quarters of all doctors are participating. But in Princeton I know of only one. Anesthesiologists, I understand, are generally nonparticipating throughout the state.

Thus far, I have been considering only the traditional Blue Shield areas, especially surgery. If you compare all Blue Shield payments to doctors with total expenditures for physician services in 1970, Blue Shield accounted for less than 18 percent. If you think in terms of the whole gamut of typical family health costs, Blue Shield protection is simply negligible—meeting less than 4 percent of United States personal health care expenditures.[1] A few of my more sophisticated academic colleagues have decided to drop Blue Shield, preferring to rely on a combination of Blue Cross and major medical.

Is this uncertain and limited coverage inevitable? I think not. In the first place, several million Blue Shield subscribers, who are members of large interstate groups such as the Federal Employees Program or the auto and steel workers, have much better contracts, with fairly comprehensive coverage and no income limits. Second, a few individual plans are much better.

Let me cite one example. I have just returned from Hawaii where I looked into the Hawaii Medical Service Association (HMSA), the Blue Shield plan for our fiftieth state. HMSA covers both hospital and physician services, outpatient as well as inpatient. It emphasizes ambulatory care beginning with home and office visits, preventive services, diagnostic services, outpatient surgery, and outpatient psychiatric care. It has recently started to cover prescription drugs, vision care, and dental care. It has also taken the lead in establishing a health maintenance organization (HMO) on the island of Maui, as a subscriber alternative to fee-for-service care.

Hospitalization is well below the national average. For Hawaiian FEP subscribers in 1968 the number of hospital days per 1,000 covered persons was only 433, less than half the 924 reported for all Blue Cross-Blue Shield FEP members nationwide.[2] This is still higher than the 357 days reported for members of the Kaiser Health Plan in Hawaii, but it is in the same ballpark. With an expense ratio of 6.8 percent of dues income, HMSA claims the lowest expense ratio of any Blue Shield plan. The national average is 11.0. It also claims to be the fastest growing in proportion to population.

In short, it is possible for Blue Shield to operate an effective program. But the prerequisites seem to include: (1) effective competition (in Hawaii, Kaiser undoubtedly provides the spur); (2) effective administration, which must include the willingness as well as ability to monitor price and utilization; and (3) the willingness as well as ability to underwrite both inpatient and ambulatory benefits. Whether this joint underwriting is accomplished through a merger of Blue Cross and Blue Shield or as a result of one or the other plan assuming responsibility for underwriting both types of benefits is less important, from the consumer point of view, than that the net result be a single responsible carrier. Under these circumstances, improved coverage in the outpatient area can often be paid for by the lower costs of hospitalization.

This suggests that the first and most urgent reform that state government could undertake with respect to Blue Shield in particular or private health insurance in general would be a requirement that all health insurance policies sold in the jurisdiciton must include a specified and balanced minimum range of benefits, covering both hospital and physician services, inpatient and outpatient, and that it be sold for a single inclusive premium. This would force Blue Cross and Blue Shield to merge, or make other provision for joint underwriting, or force the more aggressive of the two plans to take over the whole business, as in Hawaii.

Such a requirement would, of course, also apply to the commercial carriers so that neither they nor the Blues would have a competitive advantage. By requiring all carriers to sell balanced benefits, it would probably improve the competitive position of HMO-type organizations. It might also assist in reducing the deceptive and socially wasteful mail order business in cash hospitalization benefits.

The rationale for such a measure relates as much to sensible health care as to economy. Separation of the two kinds of care impedes reform of the delivery system. Removal of this traditional "iron curtain" between the two kinds of health insurance would do as much for the promotion of sensible comprehensive health care as it would for economy. It is an essential element in attacking our current overemphasis on hospitalized illness rather than exclusive dependence on promotion of capitation plans.

The second most urgent Blue Shield reform is abolition of the arbitrary and inequitable income limits on service benefits. I understand that, nationwide, about 30 percent of Blue Shield subscribers are now covered by policies that do not have such limits. Why permit discrimination against the rest of us? It is possible that abolition of the limits would follow, almost automatically, from implementation of the comprehensive benefit requirement. Blue Cross never had such limits and would, I think, find it almost impossible to impose them. To make sure that this reform is effective, however, it would probably be necessary for the states to prohibit this type of discrimination.

Third, there is the question of physician payments. Commissioner Denenberg's Guidelines suggest that payment be made on the basis of the sixtieth percentile in the current range of fees in the community rather than the ninetieth. Quite possibly, the ninetieth does result in overpaying some doctors. The sixtieth would probably underpay a good number. Any such underpayment would be almost certain to weaken the effort to improve the quality of Blue Shield medical care.

One figure is as arbitrary as the other. And why give the state "seal of approval" to the "prevailing fee" or "usual, customary, and reasonable" method at all? After years of observing the operation of this method, I find there is only one conclusion from the public's point of view: It is inevitably inflationary and thus a threat to the value of any policy that depends on it as the basis of physician payment. If continued much longer, it will, almost certainly, lead to even more rigorous federal control over physician fees than we have yet seen under the Economic Stabilization Program.

Moreover, it is unnecessary. Historically, Blue Shield operated on the basis of fee schedules, and many of their subscribers are still under policies that pay on the basis of a schedule. It was not until Medicare put its "seal of approval" on "usual and customary," in 1965, that the concept became prevalent. The error was perhaps excusable at that time. Few realized just how inflationary it would turn out to be. But now we do. Why continue the same mistake and end up by discrediting fee-for-service altogether?

What is needed is a schedule that is equitable, understandable, and administrable:

- not one that rejects the concepts of "usual," "customary," or "reasonable" as factors to be taken into consideration in the development of an equitable fee schedule, but one that reduces the end-product of such consideration to a formal document which all parties can read and understand and which the carrier can administer with relative simplicity and without exorbitant costs;
- not one that is biased in favor of one branch of medicine, but one that is fair to all doctors and recognizes degrees of education, responsibility, and essentiality to the total care of the patient;
- not one that imposes identical fees throughout a state with significant geographical and/or socioeconomic differences, but one that allows for reasonable variations;
- not one that is imposed unilaterally either by the carrier or the doctors, but one that is negotiated by the carrier with the medical society;
- not one that will remain inflexible for years but will be reviewed at least every two years.

My third suggestion, therefore, is that the state require of any policy, which provides for payment of doctors on a fee-for-service basis, that such payments be on the basis of a negotiated fee schedule, to be reviewed no less than biennially, and to be available to providers and consumers on demand.

I recognize that there could be problems for the providers in negotiating with a number of different carriers. It might be advisable to provide by law for joint negotiations by all carriers operating in the state with the state medical society. The general use of a relative value scale, with variable factors, would greatly simplify the problem of regional variations within the state and interstate variations for national accounts.

Finally, I urge that the insurance departments of the various states work closely with Blue Shield, other carriers, the medical societies, and responsible consumer respresentatives to develop greatly simplified and standardized claims forms. This would reduce costs, speed payments, and obviate much of the current irritation on the part of the individual doctors. It would redound to the benefit of consumers, providers, and the carriers.

Taken together, these four reforms—combined underwriting of hosptial and medical benefits, abolition of income ceilings on service benefits, a requirement that fee-for-service payments be on the basis of a negotiated fixed fee schedule, and simplified standardized claims forms—would go a long way toward meeting the most frequent consumer and provider complaints against Blue Shield.

We are not starting from scratch and cannot erase the mistakes of a quarter century overnight. But such adjustments would help the plan to provide far more adequate benefits at a predictable, controllable cost. They are, I believe, philosophically in tune with the commitments and aspirations of the top leadership of both Blue Cross and Blue Shield.

NOTES

1. Derived from reports of the U.S. Department of Health, Education, and Welfare. Total Blue Shield claims expense, 1970: $2.4 billion. M.S. Mueller, "Private Health Insurance in 1970," *Social Security Bulletin,* February 1972, p. 18. Total personal health care expenditures, 1970: $62 billion. D.P. Rice and B.S. Cooper, "National Health Expenditures, 1929-71," *Social Security Bulletin,* January 1972, p. 13. Total payments to physicians in 1970: $13.6 billion. *Ibid.,* p. 7.
2. These are not age-specific rates.

Chapter Five

Public Programs

> Public health is purchasable. Within natural limitations, a community can determine its own death-rate.
>
> Herman Biggs, M.D., Director
> N.Y. State Department of Health (1911)

The United States has differed from most advanced nations in the absence of general public health insurance or a national health service. Nonetheless, we have, since the 1930s at least, followed the worldwide trend of ever greater government financing of health services.

In the years following World War II until the coming of Medicare and Medicaid, the government share of rapidly rising personal health care expenditures hovered consistently at a little more than 20 percent (Table X). Then the public, particularly the federal, share began to rise sharply. By 1975 the public outlay was about 40 percent of the expanding total. The federal government paid about two-thirds of that portion; state and local governments the remainder (Table XIII).

Public and private differentiations are, however, becoming blurred. Crude public expenditure data do not mean that a comparable proportion of health services is rendered in, or controlled by, the public sector. Government typically purchases from private providers the health care it finances. For example, most government payments for hospital services are made to privately owned and operated hospitals. These payments are generally made through private insurance instrumentalities. Many private hospitals also receive various types of government subsidy for construction, research, and other purposes. A large portion of the private sector is represented by not-for-profit institutions of a quasi-public character. In short, our health services constitute a mixed pluralistic economy with indeterminate boundaries. Overlaps are great, joint action common, and clear distinctions are often difficult to make.

However, categorization within this wide variety of public programs, which are generally lumped under a single heading, is essential for analytical purposes, even if the categories are necessarily general and somewhat overlapping. We have found helpful a classification developed in 1961:[1]

1. direct provision of services by the responsible agency, as in the Defense Department's programs for servicemen, the Veterans Administration hospitals, and hospitals operated by state or municipal governments;

2. purchase of services directly from providers by a government agency, as in most federal-state public assistance or Medicaid programs, the Veterans Administration "home town" program, rehabilitation, maternal, child health and crippled children's programs;

3. government purchase or payment for specified services through fiscal agents, as in Medicare and in the program for dependents of Armed Services personnel (CHAMPUS);

4. mandatory purchase of insurance by employers, for covered employees, from private or state carriers or through self-insurance, as in workmen's compensation;

5. government purchase of insurance, rather than direct services, from private plans or carriers, as in state "buy-in" arrangements for Medicare insurance for aged welfare recipients and in some parts of the CHAMPUS program. This is the pattern also used for the FEP and similar programs of state and local governments, but since these are operated exclusively for the governments' own employees they are not usually considered public health insurance.

There have been a few programs that do not easily fit any of these categories. For example, the neighborhood health centers, originally developed by the Office of Economic Opportunity, were, in the main supported by federal grants (Selection 32).

The arrival of Medicare and Medicaid, which together now consume over 60 percent of public expenditures for health services, stimulated demand for additional government activity in all aspects of health care, research, and resource development. New programs proliferated, with further fragmentation. On top of actual service programs, a variety of funding, planning, and regionalization agencies were created throughout the country, which were intended to bring order out of the confusing bits and pieces. Within five years, proposals for universal national health insurance were multiplying, and a protracted debate over "how" and "what kind" had begun.

Selection 23 (1954) describes an earlier period of medical administration by the states in workmen's compensation, the first of our social insurance programs and the first to undertake a form of public health insurance (except the short-lived program to provide hospital care for merchant seamen, legislated by Congress in 1798). Selection 24 (1954) appraises some problems and conflicts which beset the attempt to make vocational rehabilitation available to victims of occupational disability. The conflict over the concept of "total medical care," herein described, anticipates the more recent debates over "comprehensive health care." Both these historical pieces offer some cautionary lessons in problems of public supervision and administration of health care programs. The relevance to more recent Medicaid and other welfare experience will be apparent.

Selection 25 (1967) relates the final legislative maneuverings and dénouement of the Medicare breakthrough. It also describes the early administrative activities in setting the program in motion. Most people in the health field soon acquainted themselves with the principal legislative provisions and the more important administrative regulations. But relatively few troubled to understand either the legislative or administrative processes from which such decisions emerged. This they generally regarded as mere "politics," and their interests lay elsewhere. But if health professionals and reformers are to do more than complain of their limited influence on public decisions it is essential that they understand better how such decisions are arrived at—a far more complex process than is generally appreciated.

Selection 26 (1967) presented an early warning of the inevitable inflationary troubles inherent in Medicare's methods of reimbursement to providers of care. Over the ensuing years these difficulties have been aggravated with little effective corrective action. Medicaid, as Selection 25 pointed out, slipped into the Medicare legislative package relatively unnoticed. In Selection 27 (1966) we indicated that it could be the "big sleeper," as indeed it turned out to be.

Selections 28 (1976) and 29 (1971) attempt to clarify the major issues in the national health insurance controversy, presenting some history, criteria, and an original proposal.

NOTE

1. H.M. Somers, "The Interrelationship Between Public and Private Medical Care Programs," in Iago Galdston, M.D., ed., *Voluntary Action and the State* (New York: International Universities Press, 1961), pp. 95-101.

Selection 23
Workmen's Compensation: Medical Administration*

The record of administrative incompetence, chicanery, and fraud described in this discussion of state medical administration in workmen's compensation, as of 1954 (and strongly suggestive of current abuses under Medicaid), should be balanced against the very real benefits received by millions of workers who did obtain needed medical care through this program, care that would not have been otherwise available. However, the history should heighten several cautions that we frequently reiterate: (1) legislation is not self-administering; (2) transferring responsibilities to a public authority does not automatically ensure that the necessary administrative motivation and competence will be forthcoming; and (3) the complex problems of human relations that prompted the legislation will not evaporate. It should remind us that public purposes are unlikely to

---

*Excerpt from H.M. and A.R. Somers, *Workmen's Compensation: Prevention, Insurance, and Rehabilitation of Occupational Disability* (New York: John Wiley & Sons, 1954), pp. 166-177.

be achieved if administrative authority and machinery consistent with the objectives are not provided.

The professional services of the doctor are essential elements in the entire compensation process from the first treatment after injury to the final stages of rehabilitation. In addition, compensation administration depends upon prompt and correct medical reports throughout the period of disability, accurate testimony from doctors in contested cases as to the nature and degree of disability, and determination of fair medical fees.

The material resources for fully adequate medical care are now potentially available, at least in two-thirds of the states. Medical expenses consume about one-third of all benefit payments. Theoretically all the modern techniques of surgery and other medical specializations are available under compensation laws. Nevertheless, administration of the medical and rehabilitation aspects of workmen's compensation has probably come in for more sharp criticism than any other aspect of the program. The Medical Committee of the International Association of Industrial Accident Boards and Commissions (IAIABC) reports that "little, if any, progress has been made to date, in the vast unexplored field of compensation medical care and administration."

Admittedly, the problems are highly complex. To the variety of administrative difficulties already discussed and the conflicting laws and interpretations are added numerous medico-legal complexities.

MEDICAL TREATMENT

Among the major issues are choice of physician and supervision of treatment and medical costs. Originally, it was an almost universal custom for the employer or carrier to choose the doctor. This remains the practice in the majority of states. However, the trend has been moving away from this original procedure, and many states now specify other methods of selection. According to a 1949 survey, in at least eight jurisdictions the worker may select the doctor he wishes. In North Dakota and Washington the administrative agency makes the selection. Wisconsin permits the worker to choose from a panel of doctors drawn up by the employer or carrier. New York has experimented with employee selection from a panel established by the compensation board. There are other variations.

Supervision of medical treatment by the administrative agency has been generally absent in the United States. Most agencies lack either the authority or the facilities for such a task. Less than half have any sort of medical department, and most of these do not employ even one full-time physician.

Whether the choice of doctor is made by worker or carrier, serious and frequent abuses have been discovered. In former days, a frequent source of difficulty was "contract practice," under which employers or insurers committed all injured workers requiring medical treatment to a physician, hospital, or hospital association for a fixed periodic fee. The worst abuses connected with contract practice arose out of the incentives presented to the doctor or hospital to cut corners to achieve lowest possible cost. Investigations almost invariably indicated that medical care under this system was of a dangerously low quality. "As one of the physicians... observed, it is sometimes cheaper to amputate a leg than to try to save it, and to let a man die than to attempt a cure."

The quality of medical service rendered by the majority of "insurance company doctors" has also been severely criticized. Walter Dodd, a leading authority, concluded in 1936, that

> most of these doctors are selected or retained for their legal ability in defeating employees' claims rather than for their medical skill in healing their injuries.... A few of the larger insurance companies take a more intelligent view of medical problems arising in compensation and regard it as not only good ethics but also good business to supply the best of medical attention for the period it is needed, but the number of these companies is unfortunately small.

More has been heard recently about abuses in states where the employee is permitted "free choice." This is not entirely new. Dodd also pointed out that, where the employee can go to his own doctor at the expense of employer or carrier, the doctor is likely to be paid for his services only if the case is compensated.

> A series of hotly contested cases... in which the employees were treated by their own physicians... showed that there was a 100 per cent correlation between the findings of the employees' physicians and the conclusion most favorable to the maximum claim of the employee for compensation.

Selig Greenberg, a well-known medical writer and investigator, reports that in Rhode Island, a free-choice state, about 30 doctors, 4 percent of the total number in private practice in the state, are guilty of

> collecting exorbitant fees in compensation cases, prolonging treatment far beyond the patients' needs, resorting to unnecessary forms of treatment, padding their bills, winking at malingering, and helping chiselers—sometimes under oath in court—to exaggerate their injuries.... Some fee-hungry general practitioners hang on for many months to patients whom they are incompetent to treat. Such delays in referral to specialists or to the Rhode Island Curative Center not only tend to prolong the period of disability and to jack up costs, but frequently aggravate the condition of patients and occasionally cripple them for life.[1]

Shortly after these reports were published, the Rhode Island Medical Society announced its own legislative reform program, including appointment of a full-time medical adviser to the Division of Workmen's Compensation who would review all medical reports on injured workers, and the requirement of more complete reports from treating doctors. It did not, however, agree with an earlier commission recommendation that medical fees should be fixed by a medical director or that he should have authority to select doctors eligible to treat compensation cases.

In theory, the New York panel system was supposed to resolve conflicting interests by placing the basic selection of physicians with an impartial administrator, aided by professional medical societies, yet leaving to the patient a large degree of final choice. This policy was adopted in 1935 in an effort to correct abuses which had developed under the previous practice of employer designation of physicians. It did not take long to discover that New York had not found a solution to its problems and that the results were quite different from those envisioned. A president of the Casualty Actuarial Society pointed this out as early as 1937.

> It was originally intended that the medical societies would be very careful in the admission of qualified men and approve applications only for those best fitted to do the work. Unfortunately in actual practice the method adopted was to admit all or nearly all applicants to the compensation practice and to rely upon future occurrences to exclude those who were not competent. It appears, however, that disbarment is a difficult proceeding, requiring in each case a set of definite incontestable facts with the possibility of quasijudicial and judicial review, so that removal from the panel of incompetent doctors, while in theory desirable, in practice would prove to be extremely difficult of realization.

Difficulties rapidly materialized, and criticism was soon as widespread as under the previous system. In 1944 the Bleakley-Stichman Report described the existence of "rings" of "licensed representatives," lawyers and doctors, with reciprocal arrangements for referring cases, fee-splitting, bill padding, and kickbacks of numerous varieties; all of which was said to constitute "a secret and illegal medical tax adversely affecting a large part of the citizens of this state," and which resulted in dissipation of a substantial part of the millions paid to physicians under compensation benefits. The report did not, however, assign all the blame to what was now in effect "free choice," but claimed that some carriers and employers still influenced the worker's selection of a physician, occasionally under threat of discharge, or controlled the doctor's judgment directly or indirectly.

New York has made strenuous efforts to correct such conditions. In the four counties where abuses were most prevalent (Bronx, Kings, New York, and

Queens), applications for compensation practice by doctors, medical bureaus, and laboratories and recommendations for revocation of such authorization must now be approved by a special medical practice committee, composed of three qualified physicians, appointed by the chairman of the compensation board, and paid by the state. In all other counties (those with a population under a million) such recommendations are still made by the county medical societies.

The chairman is directed to bar doctors found guilty of any of a long list of malpractices, including solicitation, fee-splitting, etc. While any doctor still has the right to appeal to the Medical Appeals Unit, made up of three physician members of the Industrial Council appointed by the governor, its recommendations are now advisory only, and the chairman has final authority. Authorization of four doctors, out of 25,347, was revoked in 1952.

No claim for payment of medical treatment in New York is valid unless it is reported within 48 hours of the first treatment with a follow-up report within 15 days. Most fees are fixed by schedule. Disputed medical bills are decided by the medical practice committee in the four counties under its jurisdiction and by special arbitration procedure in other counties. If abuses are still prevalent in New York, and accusations are still plentiful, the fault cannot be laid to lack of effort on the part of the legislature or the compensation board.

The IAIABC has devoted a great deal of time and attention to the problem of medical supervision. This reflects the rapidly growing role of medical care in the total compensation picture, the increasing complexity and specialization in medicine, and increasing recognition that rehabilitation, the ultimate objective of a proper compensation program, must begin during the first stages of medical care. General concern has also been fostered by the American Medical Association's campaign against health insurance, in which it eloquently dramatized the importance of free choice of physician, thus throwing a spotlight on the fact that most compensation laws provide for no choice at all by the patient.[2] So sensitive has the public become to this principle that many employers and carriers forego their legal rights and permit the worker to choose his doctor.

The IAIABC medical committee presented a detailed report in 1949 which was reaffirmed by the association at its 1951 and 1952 meetings. With regard to choice of physician, the committee adopted two principles: (1) limited free choice by the patient, and (2) control and supervision of medical care by the compensation authority. Said the committee,

> Unrestricted free choice... is not compatible with the best of care—most people choose their physician or surgeon because of a friend's advice, a liking for his personality... if not for his availability and location alone. Thus... the man who directed the last family confinement may be called to treat a spinal-cord injury.... On the other hand, the family physician, the trusted friend of the claimant, can frequently attain results in cases within his competence far beyond those of his more skilled but unknown brother.

The committee was obviously influenced by the impressive example of Ontario practice, where initial free choice by the patient is combined with commission responsibiltiy for supervision of surgery and other specialized care.

The trend which the IAIABC claims to see is more conspicuous in Canada than in the United States, and it seems rather doubtful that state legislatures will move rapidly toward increasing the medical supervisory powers of the agencies. Basic to the problem of supervision and control is the relative strength of the administering agency in its own political milieu. The Canadian agencies appear to hold an influence role in relation to the medical societies, employers, and labor which far exceeds that of their United States counterparts. They do not have to consider the interests of private carriers, for they are state fund systems. The statute books may say "supervise," but, if the agency does not have *de facto* power exceeding the parties it is to supervise, the words remain empty, as the New York experience demonstrates.

Thus, the present difficulties may at least partly stem from the conflicts of interest inherent in the compensation program, which place almost intolerable pressures on medical standards without the presence of any socially adequate authority to cope with such pressures. This is not resolved merely by passing a new law.

Fortunately, some abuses could be remedied, and probably will be, simply through higher professional standards. Much that tends to be called chicanery is only incompetence. The emergence of industrial medicine as a specialized profession has helped to underscore the inadequacy of much that goes by the name of compensation medicine and is likely to exert a beneficial influence on professional standards in this whole area.

MEDICAL CONTROVERSIES

"Courthouse medicine" is the contemptuous epithet applied by the famed expert on compensation medicine, Dr. Henry H. Kessler, to the "psuedo-system of medical jurisprudence" practiced in connection with the determination of extent of disability. He describes the typical medical hearing as follows:

> There are many participants in the daily dramas that take place at these hearings in every state: the injured worker, the adjuster for the insurance company or employer, the employer himself, the treating physician, the physician representing the employer or the insurance company, the physician representing the state industrial accident commission, perhaps the lawyer for the insurance company, the lawyer for the injured worker, the union representative with his lawyer, to say nothing of a dozen or more satellites that have crept into the picture. Out of the welter of selfish interests arrayed in this economic tower of Babel arises a series of dilemmas from which there is no escape.
>
> The injured worker starts out with the simple expectation of having his injury treated and his return to work expedited.... A chance state-

ment by a physician, apparently magnifying his disability, the deliberate machinations of an ambulance chaser, the efforts of the union representative to get a square deal for his client and thus justify his own position, the intransigence of the insurance adjuster—all these factors soon transform a simple case of injury to a cause requiring months of litigation and a persistence of the incapacity beyond all normal expectation. Expert medical opinion is dragged on the scene to add a macabre touch.... Talmudic scholars, the medieval philosophers, the dialecticians of Greece never carried on abstruse discussions such as take place in compensation hearings. The relationship between injury and disease and the fine mathematical evaluations of disabilities are pure speculation that has no relation to every-day working conditions. Yet this is the stuff which compensation hearings deal with. They have become an arena where emotions and passions are arrayed with the same intensity as at the race track, the boxing bout, and gambling table.

Many who view such proceedings from the point of view of the worker or the administrator concur with Dr. Kessler's evaluation. For example, Marshall Dawson, the U.S. Department of Labor's authority on workmen's compensation, has said:

If some injured workers are not already "shell-shocked" or neurotic before they attend a hearing and listen to the medical testimony, they are indeed hardy and non-suggestible if they leave the hearings other than in a hopeless state of mind. It is a common occurrence for medical witnesses, in order to obtain a maximum disability rating for the worker, to testify loudly and emphatically that the injured man will never be able to resume his accustomed occupation, that he is seriously and permanently disabled, that the condition will get worse instead of better, and as an occasional climax that the worker may die soon.

Permanent-partial injury schedules were, of course, intended to minimize the need for such controversy by the simple application of an anatomical slide rule. Clearly they have not succeeded in this purpose. In Illinois

the much-publicized amputation schedule... is only the beginning of inquiry; whether the workman has lost one of the listed members, or whether he has not, the question arises as to what other injuries he has. Conversation with adjusters and attorneys in the workmen's compensation field produces endless accounts of battles of the expert witnesses, as though no schedule existed.... The chairman of the Illinois Industrial Commission reported a proceeding in which one side produced 12 expert witnesses, and the other side, 11. ...

Perhaps the most disturbing exposures have come from Rhode Island, where Greenberg asserts that perjury is not uncommon in medical testimony. He quotes a claimant's attorney as follows:

> 'Neither side will bring a physician into court unless it knows that his testimony will be favorable from its own point of view. The insurance companies shop around for doctors, and so do we.'

> 'For almost any doctor you can get to say black you can get another one to say white,' declared another lawyer. There was a case recently where two physicians read an x-ray in the courtroom and gave diametrically opposed opinions as to what it showed. One said it showed wrist fracture and the other said it didn't.

Little wonder that the head of the Rhode Island agency gave a cynical illustration of the problem facing the compensation official. He told the IAIABC 1951 convention:

> As a young lawyer... walking out of the courtroom with the trial justice, I said, 'Judge, tell me, how can you determine which side was telling the truth, and which side was lying?' His answer was, 'That is not *my* problem; *mine* is to determine which side is lying the most.'

NOTES

1. Among his exhibits, Greenberg describes: a doctor who charged for 32 visits in a case where only two visits were made; a general practitioner who charged for 76 hospital visits at $3.00 each to a patient operated on by another doctor; a practitioner who charged $1,827 for treating a man suffering from hysteria following a brain contusion, for two and a half years, although he admitted he could not cure him and should have referred him either to a psychiatrist or to the Curative Center; a doctor suspected of coaching people to fake back injuries. *Providence Evening Bulletin,* January 28, February 2, and February 3, 1953.

2. However, the doctors apparently do not feel that unrestricted free choice is good in compensation cases. Dr. C.O. Sappington, the executive secretary of the AMA's committee on workmen's compensation, said: "What does a sick or injured man know about what physician he should choose? Is he in any position mentally to choose what doctor he should have?" He approved a "supervised form of free choice... such as the practice in Wisconsin...." United States Bureau of Labor Standards, IAIABC, *Proceedings 1949,* Bulletin 119, pp. 16-17.

Selection 24

Rehabilitation: The Trauma of Administrative and Professional Adjustment*

Civilian rehabilitation was originally the child of workmen's compensation. The positive social and economic relationship between the two has long been evident. During the Congressional debate on the first civilian rehabilitation law, the main pressure for action came from spokesmen for industrial workers, with support from social work groups. The federal law gave special attention to the industrial worker by requiring that the state vocational education boards cooperate closely with the state compensation agencies to obtain federal funds. In spite of this preachment and apparent interdependence, relations between the two programs have not been notably close in most states. Vocational rehabilitation still reaches an inadequate proportion of the industrially injured, including compensation recipients, who could profit from it.

A joint statement issued by the United States Department of Labor and the Office of Vocational Rehabilitation (OVR) in 1950 estimates that at least a tenth of the two million injured annually on the job need medical rehabilitation, and some 12,000 of the permanently disabled need full rehabilitation (medical, vocational, and placement) to assist them in returning to work. But the federal-state program is currently rehabilitating not more than half of the 12,000 and reaches a very small percentage of the group in need of medical rehabilitation.

A good part of this failure can be attributed to inadequate appropriations by Congress and state legislatures. There is, however, considerable evidence that compensation and vocational rehabilitation officials do not see eye to eye regarding the best use of available funds and are not working in close coordination.

Some compensation people allege that the OVR program, still under control of vocational education in the states, gives preference to young people with congenital or chronic diseases who are easier to train as opposed to older industrial workers, many of whom have little formal education, and who frequently present difficult and expensive surgical problems.

Rehabilitation officials offer a counteraccusation that workmen's compensation agencies are not referring, or adequately encouraging through their administrative procedures, the industrially injured to seek rehabilitation.

It is significant that of the 3,700 cases involving compensable work in-

---

*Excerpt from H.M. and A.R. Somers, *Workmen's Compensation: Prevention, Insurance and Rehabilitation of Occupational Disability* (New York: John Wiley & Sons, 1954), pp. 254-266.

juries referred to state rehabilitation agencies... in 1949... only 1,600 were referred by workmen's compensation agencies or insurance carriers. The other 2,100 reached rehabilitation agencies through other sources or after compensation benefits were exhausted.

Failure to make effective referral from workmen's compensation to rehabilitation is especially conspicuous where lump-sum payments are readily allowed and in cases involving prolonged litigation.

All concerned agree that early referral is essential for effective rehabilitation at reasonable cost, but the timing of compensation agency referrals has been remarkably lethargic. The average time lag between date of injury and referral for those referred by a compensation body and rehabilitated in 1951 was seven years, as compared with an average of 6.4 months at the Liberty Mutual Center. Such delay represents the loss of years of productive labor as well as waste in medical expenses and renders the job of rehabilitation infinitely more difficult, if not impossible.

The lack of coordination sometimes takes on the appearance of jurisdictional conflict. In 1950-1951 the IAIABC and the Vocational Rehabilitation Council, composed of 87 state rehabilitation agencies or commissions for the blind, undertook at the instance of the council to find some mutually acceptable basis for cooperative action. The 1951 report of the IAIABC Rehabilitation Committee casts light on the nature of the impasse:

> The ultimate goal for which this organization of compensation boards should strive in the field of rehabilitation is that all of these activities for the care, cure, maintenance, and restoration to work of the injured employees should be under the direct control and supervision of the workmen's compensation agency from the day of injury until the worker is gainfully employed in the occupation for which he is best fitted.... your committee urges better and closer co-operation between the compensation agencies and the rehabilitation agencies without, however, surrendering any of the direct control and supervision over the restoration of the injured workers through physical rehabilitation.

In the absence of rehabilitation units and facilities attached to the compensation agency, which is now generally the situation, this position would appear to create a virtual stalemate between the two groups.

SOME BASIC DIFFICULTIES

It would be unfair to interpret these difficulties as stemming merely from capricious rivalries of bureaucratic officials. The causes of lack of cooperative action, frequent irritation, and misunderstanding are substantive and substantial. Unless these inherent conflicts are faced forthrightly, rehabilitation cannot develop as an integral part of workmen's compensation, which in terms of present-day requirements would mean a progressive deterioration in the adequacy and suitability of the entire compensation program.

The problem is more than one of early or late referral, or of easy as against difficult cases, although both of these are significant symptoms. Two of the basic problems are inherent in the present OVR program. First, since it can accept cases only when the disability has become fixed or static, the broad type of rehabilitation program carried on so successfully in Ontario, Puerto Rico, and on a limited scale by the Liberty Mutual Insurance Company is automatically ruled out. By setting an arbitrary line between medical care during the acute stages of an injury (during which the later need for rehabilitation might well be prevented or minimized) and rehabilitation after the disability has become fixed, the whole process is made more difficult for the worker, more expensive for the employer and society, and far more complicated for the rehabilitation specialists. It also tends to diminish in the minds of compensation officials the imperative need for early referral.

Second, the means test required for the medical aspects of the OVR program appears to be a substantial deterrent to many injured workers who, rightly or wrongly, believe that they are confronted with a choice between attempting to maximize their legal claim to needed cash benefits, which they regard as a "right," or giving up this right for the uncertain results of rehabilitation "on the dole." Compensation officials tend to be sympathetic to the workers' view.

There are also many impediments in the current workmen's compensation programs. The current overriding emphasis on legal processes in workmen's compensation with all its uncertainties, the long delays involved in many serious cases, the increasing resort to lump sum settlements, and the poor quality of much of the medical treatment which is rarely supervised or related to the ultimate rehabilitaiton of the worker, all represent substantial deterrents to rehabilitation. To undertake rehabilitation while his compensation case is pending will often appear to the worker to jeopardize a maximum award, since awards are related to the degree of disability. The legal settlement is also interpreted by most compensation officials as their primary responsibility.

Money awards are tangible and easily understood; rehabilitation often appears intangible and uncertain, and in most communities is simply nonexistent. Compensation officials reflect the attitude of the majority of workers when they insist that, in the absence of anything like adequate rehabilitation facilities, and the uncertainties attendant upon them, the worker can best be protected by assuring him his utmost legal rights. This is a reflection of the compensation laws' failure to provide, as promised, prompt, adequate, and *assured* benefits. Too often the benefits must be fought for, and the worker understandably feels that he cannot forsake any of his weapons in the battle.

As a result of all this, compensation law and administration stand in an ambivalent relationship to rehabilitation. Although the importance of rehabilitation is widely acknowledged by compensation officials, and enthusiastically advocated by some, actual compensation procedures represent one of the major stumbling blocks to the goal of industrial rehabilitation.

The question of worker incentives is a thorny one. Some rehabilitation people appear to feel that adequate levels of benefits may conflict with incentives for rehabilitation, "a crutch to impede the patient's recovery." This is a problem even more frequently attributed to the veterans' program, where it is alleged that "pensionitis" has had a deleterious effect upon rehabilitation of some veterans. On the other side it is argued that it is better to encourage a disabled person to concentrate on the rehabilitation task before him, having been assured a modicum of security for himself and his family, rather than to dissipate his energy in unproductive worries over his own and his family's maintenance in case he should fail.

Not enough is known about the entire problem of incentives or motivation. There is considerable evidence, however, that people who have a minimum security show greater morale and initiative toward improving their economic status than those totally devoid of resources. It has been noted by rehabilitation experts that a great deal of the cooperation essential for successful rehabilitation depends upon the worker's sense of security regarding provisions for his wife and family and the anticipated job outcome of the rehabilitation process. Furthermore, income is not the sole motivation for work. For the vast majority of men, a job is essential for dignity, fulfillment, and community status. Lack of assurance to the disabled that they will be provided for until they have been able to reobtain gainful employment has caused workers to concentrate first upon their legal rights to compensation. Professor E.H. Downey pointed out many years ago that

> Very much that passes by the name of malingering is, in reality, a well-founded fear of forfeiting compensation without being able to hold a place in industry. Much of the reluctance manifested by industrial, as by war, cripples to undergo retraining, is due to the maladroit device which rewards the victim's zeal therein by cutting off his indemnity. The way to promote rehabilitation is not to penalize it.

A reconciliation is possible by strengthening both links of the chain. Assured income maintenance is essential for injured workers as a legal right, as a social necessity, and because the security it offers can under proper circumstances assist in the rehabilitation process. By furnishing the economic means to make rehabilitation effective, compensation agencies can press the injured worker to an understanding and acceptance of his share of responsibility for his rehabilitation. But this is contingent upon the assurance of adequate rehabilitation facilities for all disabled workers, a matter which is largely outside the powers of either the compensation or rehabilitation agencies, but in the hands of legislatures.

TOWARD A NEW CONCEPT OF MEDICAL CARE IN OCCUPATIONAL DISABILITY

The implications of the rehabilitation movement are wide-ranging, offering a challenge to many past practices and social arrangements. This may be one of the reasons why some people are suspicious and even balk at it. This is especially true in the medical field. By creating a new concept of "total medical care"[1] and by placing a premium on "multidisciplined" analysis and action, the doctor is removed from his accustomed niche of relative isolation and is obliged to work cooperatively with other restorative elements in the community: social workers, psychologists, vocational educators, employment counselors, private welfare agencies, government officials, employers, insurance companies, and unions.

The goal is no longer confined to accurate diagnosis and expert treatment of trauma or some other acute condition. The goal of rehabilitation is no less than the restoration of the whole man to a useful function in society, involving manifold skills and techniques. This implies as great a revolution in medical care, medical thinking, and training[2] as it does in social insurance legislation and techniques. The revolution has been under way for some time but at a slow and hesitant pace. Social insurance, and social security generally, are moving away from confinement to the eleemosynary concept of "meeting need" toward the broader economic necessity and social value of redeeming men and labor. Society's task is being recognized as the maximization of effort to remove or reduce need, as much as meeting it when it arises.

The urgency of getting on with this new and positive approach is clear from the statistics of increasing proportions of disabled and aged in our society, an annual increment with which present rehabilitation resources are in a constantly losing race. The nature of the medical problem requires not only highly specialized rehabilitation facilities accessible to patients in all parts of the country but, equally important, a new orientation on the part of individual doctors. It is said that some practitioners refuse to permit their compensation patients to undertake rehabilitation, possibly for fear of losing a source of fees or lack of faith in the new techniques. Since the family doctor generally makes the decision, "free choice" may, in fact, mean that the patient will never know that rehabilitation is available to him.

Compensation medicine presents the medical profession with some extremely challenging and basic problems. It is becoming increasingly clear that rehabilitation cannot be made an effective part of the compensation program without the full cooperation of the doctors. If this cooperation is not secured voluntarily by the profession, the result is likely to be necessary public action which will cause many to complain that freedom is being threatened. The new theory of "total medical care" offers a basis for voluntary cooperation to the advantage of all concerned, but to make it broadly effective will require a large degree of professional self-discipline and education.

Fortunately, leadership in this direction appears to be emerging. The "Basic Principles for Rehabilitation of the Injured Worker," recently approved by the Board of Regents of the American College of Surgeons, states:

> Rehabilitation and restoration to gainful employment of the injured worker must begin with first aid and continue through the period of

158 HEALTH AND HEALTH CARE

disability. In order for a physician to carry out this responsibility, it is essential for him to recognize the total medical problem of the patient in addition to his injury, as well as his personal problems. The physician must bring to bear on these problems all the skills and disciplines that science and society can offer, and utilize all community resources which can assist him in the accomplishment of these objectives.

Scientists can provide leadership, but success requires the understanding and support of politicians and administrators. This will not be achieved by mutual pointing of fingers.

NOTES

1. "... more and more, medicine is beginning to recognize that medical care cannot be considered complete until the patient with a residual disability has been trained 'to live and work with what he has left.' " Howard A. Rusk, M.D., "Total Rehabilitation," *Journal of the National Medical Association* (January 1953): 1-2.

2. "Failure to comprehend the value of adequate aftercare stems largely from our basic training. The modern medical school devotes its time largely to the field of diagnosis and treatment of the acute lesion. Rarely is any instruction given, either in the field of medicine or surgery, to the treatment of the individual once the emergency has passed." A.P. Aitken, M.D., "The Need for Adequate Aftercare in Complete Rehabilitation of the Disabled," *Surgery, Gynecology, and Obstetrics* (September 1952): 318.

Selection 25

Medicare: Legislation and Administration — The Seamless Web*

The Medicare breakthrough was heralded as "revolutionary" by both advocates and opponents. Many years of tempestuous controversy over the proposed legislation contributed to that view. In fact, it was neither a sudden nor a radical departure from the march of events in the organization and financing of medical care and the federal government's growing involvement. No existing institutions were overturned or even seriously threatened by the new program. On the contrary, Medicare clearly responded to the needs of providers as well as of

---

*Excerpt from H.M. and A.R. Somers, *Medicare and the Hospitals: Issues and Prospects* (Washington, D.C.: The Brookings Institution, 1967), pp. 12-42.

consumers. It was primarily a financial underpinning of the existing health care industry—with all that implied in terms of strengths and weaknesses.

Medicare's immediate importance lay in its ability to provide a viable mechanism for financing a substantial portion of health care for a large and growing sector of the popualtion. Its greater significance was its potential direct and indirect effect on the entire pattern of medical care in the United States— organizational as well as financial—however unintended. In that sense it might be said that it was indeed a conduit for revolutionary transformation.

MR. MILLS' TOUR DE FORCE

The elections of 1964 were decisive for Medicare. President Lyndon Johnson's campaign featured his determination to push such legislation. Senator Barry Goldwater was explicit in his opposition. Many congressional candidates pinpointed it as a major campaign issue. Organized medicine and its political action committees focused their energies and money on the defeat of some 40 selected incumbents who had supported Medicare. The National Council of Senior Citizens, established in 1961, was equally determined in its backing of Medicare supporters. Organized labor made it a primary concern.

The 1964 returns were understandably interpreted as a victory for Medicare. Candidates who had made support of Medicare a key campaign issue were successful in almost every instance. Particularly telling was the fact that three members of the Committee on Ways and Means, who had consistently opposed the program, were not returned.

The year 1965 opened with the Report of the Advisory Council on Social Security. The report concluded that health insurance was an indispensable element in providing the security for which the Social Security system had been established.

On January 4, the president's State of the Union Message gave high priority to "hospital care under social security." Three days later, he delivered his first message to the 89th Congress, "Advancing the Nation's Health." In a series of wide-ranging proposals, top priority was given to the hospital insurance program.

In February, the Committee on Ways and Means was again holding executive sessions on a revised King-Anderson bill, the Administration's measure. By this time, virtually all interests had accepted the inevitability of some legislation. The only significant opposition continued to come from organized medicine. Other formerly critical groups, including the American Hospital Association and Blue Cross, were either silent or actively engaged in trying to influence the character of the final program. The committee's hearings were no longer directed to the question of whether an insurance program should be established but toward seeking views on the specific content of such legislation. For the first time the House would have an opportunity to vote on such a measure.

Chairman Wilbur Mills would not permit his committee to sponsor a bill with only marginal support or any substantial risk of House disapproval. He wanted to make clear that sufficient time and opportunity had been allowed for full expression of AMA and other criticisms and that every attempt had been made to accommodate reasonable objections. He wanted to be sure that a formula would be found to assure that the hospital program could be made actuarially sound, one that would remove all alleged threats against the funds of the existing Social Security program.

The Republican leadership had also responded to the new climate. Representative John W. Byrnes of Wisconsin, the ranking minority member, introduced a countermeasure accepting the insurance principle and administration by the federal government. But there were fundamental differences. The King-Anderson bill provided for compulsory contributions as an adjunct of the Social Security system and was confined to hospital, nursing home, and home health care. The Byrnes Bill provided a separate system outside Social Security with voluntary participation and a government subsidy. However, the range of benefits was far more comprehensive, including physician services in and out of hospitals. It was modeled after the high-option indemnity plan available under the Federal Employees Health Benefits Program.

The wide publicity given the Byrnes bill centered on the claim that the Administration proposal was a puny pittance, that the aged needed far more than just hospital benefits. This view was also advanced in a massive promotional campaign by the AMA, which opposed both the Republican and the Administration measures, or any other government insurance plan. But it, too, had read the election returns and apparently concluded that a posture of sheer opposition was no longer tenable. Its hastily devised alternative, "Eldercare," was only a modest liberalization of the existing Kerr-Mills program, the federal-state Medical Assistance for the Aged; but it was thrown into the legislative arena with a tremendous publicity campaign. It purported to pay doctors' bills and other medical costs not covered by the Administration bill.

Eldercare also broke the remaining Republican front against the Social Security plan. But its chief effect, together with the Byrnes bill, was to focus attention on the limited benefits of the Administration program. The outcome, however, was altogether different from what the AMA intended.

Mills himself had been uneasy about the limited scope of the Administration bill, although this was apparently related to fears that demands would soon arise for expansion of benefits and thus raise the ultimate cost. Polls indicated that most people, including the elderly, thought the pending measure did cover far more than was actually provided. To meet the challenge of a larger benefit package, made necessary by the counterproposals, and yet honor a commitment he is alleged to have made at the time when only hospital insurance was under consideration—that physicians' services would not be covered under the basic Social Security plan—Mills came up with an ingenious surprise. He proposed combining the King-Anderson, Byrnes, and AMA bills into one comprehensive package.

The resulting bill called for two new Titles—XVIII and XIX—to be added to the Social Security Act. Part A of Title XVIII was substantially the King-Anderson bill, offering hospital, nursing home, and home health services in a program financed by compulsory contributions of employers and employees through the Social Security system, with a separately earmarked payroll tax and trust fund. Part B of Title XVIII, modeled substantially after the Byrnes bill, created a supplementary medical insurance program on a voluntary basis, financed in equal amounts from premiums paid by the insured and a contribution from general federal revenues.

Title XIX provided a third layer, encompassing the AMA Eldercare plan. It was an enlargement of Kerr-Mills, not only broadening the scope of benefits but extending protection beyond the aged to needy recipients of other federal-state public assistance programs and ultimately to all the medically indigent.

Mills' package, which *Fortune* magazine promptly labeled "Elder-Medi-Bettercare," caught the Administration by surprise, just as it did everyone else. It increased enthusiasm for the measure and made it more difficult to oppose, although considerable resistance remained as evidenced by the fact that Byrnes' motion to recommit was defeated by only 45 votes. The House passed the bill itself by a vote of 313 to 115.

The Senate Finance Committee again held extensive public hearings and then spent nearly a month voting on individual provisions before finally approving the bill with some 75 amendments. On July 9, after an exceptional amount of floor discussion and amendment, the Senate passed the bill, 68 to 21, with some 513 additional changes, most of them minor.

The Conference Committee devoted nine days to reconciling differences and came up with an agreed compromise on July 21. The following week the Conference Report was ratified by both Houses by one-sided votes similar to the original versions. With President Johnson's signature on July 30, 1965, Medicare became part of Public Law 89-97.

CONFLICT AND COMPROMISE: THE LEGISLATIVE PROCESS

The legislative history tells us a great deal more than the final outcome. Nor is "final" the correct term. Enactment of the law was merely one stage in a long historical development that will continue through administrative decision making and legislative amendments with the gathering of experience and changing conditions.

The legislative gestation period for Medicare was longer than ordinary. But path-breaking programs are usually a generation in the making in the conservative and deliberate American legislative process. Except in times of acknowledged crisis, significant change is legislated only with a wide consensus. President John Kennedy was fond of quoting Jefferson on an enduring American conviction: "Great innovations should not be forced on slender majorities." A contemporary scholar, Clinton Rossiter, points out, "The imperatives of American pluralism, indeed the very dictates of our time-tested Constitution, require us to muster a 'persistent and undoubted majority' " before taking decisive legislative action.

Certain it is that Medicare—generally regarded as bearing profound implications for our daily lives—was a product of at least 20 years of thorough and widespread public and legislative debate. The Committee on Ways and Means conducted more days of public hearings on hospital insurance than on any other matter in its jurisdiction over the same period.

Not surprisingly, the final product was different from any of the early proposals. Equally unsurprising, Medicare proved no exception to the rule that the legislative process rarely produces large or sudden upheavals, that it rarely imposes programs out of context with the existing social and economic environment. Almost inescapably, for good or ill, Medicare had to be adapted to existing medical care and financing practices and institutions.

The long legislative debate was itself a significant influence in altering the environment in which it was taking palce. This, in turn, caused adjustments of posture for protagonists on both sides. President Harry Truman's drive for national compulsory health insurance did not result in legislation, but it gave initial impetus to the development of private health insurance as a major force in medical care financing in this country. The debate throughout the 1950s and early 1960s continued to stimulate innovation in this field. This development, while it reduced interest in a universal government program, contributed to the understanding of, and receptivity to, the need for a program for the elderly.

The spectacular growth of private health insurance took place largely among the employed and their dependents, its natural market. The experience demonstrated that similar success could not be expected in covering a high risk, low income group, such as the aged, who were mainly out of the labor force. But by making more people acquainted with the wonders of modern medicine, by opening wider the door to such care, and by making the general public aware of what was potentially available through improved financial mechanisms, private health insurance increased intolerance of remaining barriers and stimulated interest in the Medicare type of proposals.

By 1960, the AMA supported the Kerr-Mills welfare legislation, although only four years earlier it vigorously opposed a similar step. By 1964, significant portions of the health insurance industry were quietly admitting that their attempts to offer adequate insurance to the aged were ineffective and that the industry might be better off with the Medicare plan.

Public focus on problems of paying for health and its rising costs led to many other new and expanded federal measures, including aid for construction of hospital facilities, for medical research, for medical education, etc. Throughout the debate, Congress, while not yet willing to accept the insurance approach, kept acknowledging the reality of the underlying problem by legislating new and liberalized medical care financing under public assistance programs.

The empirical and cumulative character of legislation and program development was also evident. There is little doubt that the successful 30 years of Social

Security experience was a steadily growing asset to the Medicare advocates. When the nation was debating the original Social Security scheme, in the early 1930s, cries were raised that it was socialistic, unnecessary, restrictive of freedom, actuarially unsound, and inevitably tending to bankruptcy. But by the 1960s, Social Security was an established and extraordinarily popular part of the American scene. Millions were beneficiaries, and almost everybody else expected to be.

Its effective operation had brought a degree of dignity to the dependent aged instead of the humiliation of the dole, and none of the dire predictions of yesteryear materialized. Its conspicuous public acceptance and efficiency made it a popular program with Congress. Attacks on health insurance for the aged under Social Security often assumed the character of an attack upon the Social Security system itself. This now sounded hollow and unpersuasive at best and, at worst, ominous to those already or potentially dependent on the system.

This was also a factor in the proposal always being advanced as a Social Security measure rather than a health program. Within the executive branch, the active leadership for the proposal came from those identified with Social Security. The Public Health Service was generally passive and unengaged. The advocacy was not presented on ideological grounds, but as a necessary extension and improvement, based on experience, of an ongoing program.

Impatient proponents will argue that this deliberate evolutionary process is too slow, permits excessive blocking power to dissident minorities, and encourages log-rolling in legislation. Trading is indeed the price that must be paid for conciliation and agreement. The law is replete with evidence that it is a product of many compromises.

A Dual Program

Throughout its legislative history, the advocates of Medicare exhibited political flexibility on almost every feature of their proposal—coverage, omission or inclusion of particular benefits, deductibles, administration, etc. Only on the basic principles of financing through the Social Security mechanism and opposition to private underwriting were they adamant. This was the crux of the matter for them. The protection against medical expense had to be an earned right, like cash benefits; and the right had to be firmly established through mandatory contributions during working years.

However, throughout the years of debate on the King-Anderson bills, the assumption was that the program would not cover general physicians' services This addition was a last-minute surprise bonus. It was then too late and, for a number of other reasons, probably impractical to demand that financing of the additional benefits be amalgamated with the basic program. As it turned out, therefore, the Medicare program is a dual structure comprising two separate insurance programs, distinct as to benefits, coverage, financing, and administration. Part A, hospital and related benefits, is incorporated within the existing Social Security patterns. Contributions are universal and mandatory. After a transitional period, eligibility will be a right only for persons 65 and over who meet the conditions required for cash Social Security benefits.

Part B, the supplementary medical benefits plan, is voluntary and open to any person aged 65 or over irrespective of Social Security status. Premiums are paid on a current basis. Benefit payments under the two plans are made by different administrative "intermediaries," called "carriers" under Part B.

The history of the legislative compromise that led to this complex dual structure has been indicated. A similar pattern is evident in the growth of private health insurance. Many people combine a basic hospitalization policy with a separate medical or "major medical" policy. It is not uncommon for families to carry two, three, or more separate policies.

Critics point out that it was unwise to carry over this unfortunate fragmentation, itself a legacy of fortuitous historical development, to the new public program. But others reply that the public program did not evolve *in vacuo*, but is itself part of the long historical process of development in a pluralistic society. In any case, it is better to have medical expense protection under a Part B pattern than not at all, and certainly the dual pattern is a net gain over the King-Anderson proposal. The evolution will continue, and it is quite possible that eventually the two programs will be merged in a single comprehensive plan, as indeed may be the trend in private health insurance as well.

Deductibles and Coinsurance

These subjects have been controversial since the beginning of health insurance in this country. The $40 deductible—roughly the cost of one day's hospitalization in 1965—in the Medicare Part A plan is a departure from prevailing practice. Most Blue Cross policies do not require any deductible. The $10 a day coinsurance for the 61st to 90th days, is somewhat more common. The $50 deductible and 20 percent coinsurance in Part B are in keeping with the conventional "major medical" pattern.

Little objective evidence is available as to the actual effect of deductibles or coinsurance on utilization of health services, but convictions and sentiment run high. One group feels strongly that a sizable deductible is essential to restrain unnecessary utilization. Representatives of medical societies argued for a larger deductible and earlier copayment in the hospital provisions. Other groups favored a larger deductible because they believed insurance should be designed for catastrophic illness and not routine anticipatible events. For that reason, some congressmen favored a deductible running as high as $200 or more, but with much longer, or even indefinite, periods of eligibility for hospital service at the other end.

On the other side are those who opposed all deductibles as deterrents to early attention to medical problems and preventive care. Blue Cross representatives, for example, testified that the deductible would create the danger of underuse, as serious as overuse, and even suggested that, if necessary, duration of benefits should be cut down to make up for the additional cost that might result. The final decision on hospital deductibles may be considered an arbitrary compromise, with no scientific evidence to go by. To a major extent the decision was based on cost.

The coinsurance on the final 30 days of hospital eligibility faced similar arguments. Here the problem was less one of costs, since the average stay is far less than 60 days, than a question of whether it was needed to discourage unnecessarily long stays. Some argued that it was, while others felt strongly that protection was most needed by the long stay cases and that the penalty should not be put at that end. Few were entirely pleased with the final outcome, and many were quite unhappy, although for quite diverse reasons.

UNFINISHED BUSINESS

Many similarly delicate decisions had to be reached to reconcile conflicting viewpoints and interests, to support continuing improvement in quality of care but not to direct changes in care, to cover expensive needs but not to create incentives to use one form of service when another less expensive one would do as well, to try to safeguard the expenditure of public funds but not to involve government in the establishment of physicians' fees, to provide for utilization review procedures but not to involve the government in medical judgments, to cover institutional health service for a period of time sufficient to meet medical needs but not so long as to encourage hospital use for custodial needs, etc.

The answers to these dilemmas left many perfectionists grumbling about the price of compromise. They frequently forgot that had compromise not prevailed, the solution might have been quite different from the one they preferred. Yet it is probable that the law which emerged is more satisfactory and durable than anything that might have been pushed through more forcefully. None could doubt that a full hearing had been given to all concerned; and few, even among the remaining opposition, could justify further belligerence.

By the final stages of the legislative process, the hospitals had made clear that they anticipated substantial advantages from the proposed legislation. The American Hospital Association had broken away from its customary collaboration with the AMA. The American Nurses' Association had endorsed the proposal quite early, when such an independent position took considerable courage. Blue Cross and, to a lesser degree, private insurance carriers withdrew from active opposition and, indeed, made some quiet contributions to the law.

Even the views of AMA, the only important interest group that remained unreconciled to the end, were accommodated on important particulars, although less than might have been the case had their stubborness not been carried to excess. The process had minimized the possibility of any tenable mutinous behavior. In fact, within a few months after passage, Medicare was receiving praise from formerly hostile sources.

It is impossible to be sure which of the many compromises will be enduring burdens and which may actually prove to have some advantages. Medicare's basic, and long run, problem is probably more profound. The program's assumption was that only monetary means were needed to purchase additional access to services. Complementary legislation was directed toward increasing the volume of available services: subsidies for hospital and nursing home construction, subsidies for medical education, etc. Legislation has been mainly devoted to easing the financial problems in health services.

Money, however, is only one part of the problem, and probably the easiest to handle. The profounder, thornier, and more complex difficulties are likely to derive from maladjustments in the structure and organization of medical care, already a subject of wide controversy. These, Medicare will probably aggravate, and they are likely to harass the program's progress. The government, as mass purchaser and subsidizer of the health establishment, cannot be neutral as to its character, cost, and conduct.

ADMINISTRATIVE POLICY MAKING

Legislative policy is rarely completed when legislation is enacted. The legislature must assign to the administering agency the formidable tasks of rule making, standard setting, and specific interpretations. Such rules and standards have the force of law and are a form of delegated legislation. It may be said to be part of a larger process of continuous legislation, without the need for frequent amendment and without making the formal legislative process impossibly protracted.

If an effort were made to include all "guidelines" in the basic law, not only would the law prove impossibly cumbersome, but very probably no significant law could be passed at all. Controversies over numerous details would exacerbate divisions and diminish, if not obliterate, areas of general agreement. A law must be clear in its purposes, but the inevitable disputes regarding details must be postponed and transferred to another arena—the administrative process. A law must also afford sufficient latitude for administrative regulation and policy to meet changing needs.

The elaborate preparations for administering Medicare may be described in two broad, but overlapping, categories: (1) the development of mechanical procedures for record-keeping, eligibility determination, bill paying, premium collection, and a multitude of other processing functions; (2) policy development in the form of rule making, standard setting, and interpretation of the law. We are here primarily concerned with the second category.

Administrative policy making in the health field is exceptionally sensitive and unavoidably political. Special pleading, pressure, and negotiations now moved into a new arena, circumscribed by the boundaries of the law but just as intensive. For many the stakes were high.

Unlike the systems and data processing job, where the Social Security Administration's (SSA) own expertise and experience were formidable, in the substantive field of health the SSA needed and actively sought expert guidance and counsel from many sources. Moreover, the launching of so influential a program required widespread understanding of the issues inherent in its administration if misconception and suspicion were not to impede its early implementation. It was at least wise, and probably necessary, to involve intimately as many affected interest groups as possible. Public policy in this country cannot be made without the participation of the "publics" most concerned, whether in legislation or administration. Congress, in several parts of the law, stated explicitly that this was intended; but it was only underlining a normal and inevitable pattern of administrative behavior.

The process of wide consultation began long before there was a law to administer. But in the "tool-up" period of August 1965 through June 1966, the process moved into high gear and reached over the entire nation. The process will continue indefinitely, although at a lower pitch of intensity. Many of the issues to be resolved do not lend themselves to permanent solutions, only to temporary operating agreements.

Among the major issues to be resolved were: a set of principles for reimbursement of "reasonable costs" of providers of care; methods of determining "reasonable charges" of physicians; minimum standards of participation for providers of care; standards for operation of utilization review committees; qualification standards and selection of intermediaries for both parts of the program; determining the division of payments between physicians and hospitals for medical care provided by hospital-based physicians; and a host of others. Where precedents existed, as in the case of hospital accreditation standards and reimbursement formulas, the agency had a reasonably firm working base. In other areas, however, the agency had to start from scratch. For example, the standards for qualifying home health agencies were among the first to be developed anywhere in the world. The problem was only a little less difficult for extended care facilities, although the New York state licensing law for nursing homes was helpful.

Where a preponderant consensus of expert and professional opinion could be shown to exist, standards could be developed and supported with reasonable confidence. But there were many areas where no such consensus obtained, e.g., personnel qualifications for independent laboratory staffs, and appropriate payment formulas as between residents and supervisory physicians in teaching hospitals. Even where an effective consensus dictated the nature of the decision, the aggrieved party-in-interest could not always be accommodated. Needless to say, where financial stakes are involved, feelings run high and interests are articulated through every conceivable channel of pressure.

Consultation and Negotiation

A variety of devices was established and used to foster orderly consultation with the many organizations and groups with a vital stake in the program, as well as those with professional or administrative competence to contribute to it. Even the mechanical processing and systems phase of administration cannot be decided by the agency alone. Although the decisions deal mainly with internal operations, many affect other interests. For example, each step in the development of systems flow was discussed and checked with the Blue Cross Association, insurance companies, hospital representatives, and other affected parties. Such questions as whether individual record-keeping would be centralized in the SSA or established in the field were controversial, as was the character of the teletype network. The extent to which the activities of intermediaries would be subject to centralized policy, especially under Part B, was also disputed.

Technical advisory groups were established to identify issues and to offer technical and policy advice in nine broad areas: conditions of provider participation, role of physicians, reimbursement policies, role of administrative intermediaries, costs of intermediaries, psychiatric services, services of hospital-based physicians, operational systems, and training and information. The groups consisted primarily of representatives of interested organizations—the health professions, health insurance industry, etc. Independent experts were also added. The members of the groups, in their lively exchanges, soon recognized the complexities of the decisions that the SSA had to make, and they often found that the decisions were even more difficult because of the large disagreements they had with each other.

However, the groups were not asked to arrive at agreed recommendations unless they wished. They were asked to furnish knowledge, experience, ideas, and viewpoints. Different recommendations, none representing a majority position, might emerge on a single problem. All of this was helpful to the SSA in drafting rules and standards. Detailed summaries of all the meetings were passed on to the statutory Health Insurance Benefits Advisory Council (HIBAC) to help guide it in making its higher level recommendations. The members of the groups knew that they were genuine participants in administrative policy formation.

While all this was in motion, Congress exercised administrative oversight in several ways. SSA and HEW officials were in frequent contact with the chairman of the Committee on Ways and Means at their own or his instigation, to check on delicate issues in negotiations, interpretations of the law's intent, or even just to keep him informed. The staff of the Senate Finance Committee kept in close touch and articulated its views.

GOVERNMENT BY CONSENT AND PARTICIPATION

The protracted, often embittered, and highly vocal battles that raged over the proposed legislation visibly affected the early administrative stages, but not always in the way expected. Many a bystander who thought of legislative disputes as winner-take-all affairs—which they seldom are—also expected that the opponents would be omitted from participation in designing the administrative arrangements. This would have been unwise and, in practical terms, impossible.

Not only were the specialized knowledge, skills, and experience of all the health and health financing fields needed, but the program could never be viable without widespread participation, cooperation, and understanding. These had to be won, not by exhortation or propaganda, but by active and honest involvement of all major interests in decisions that would affect them.

From this viewpoint, the administrative tooling-up period was successful, although the reasons are more numerous and complex than can be reviewed here. Predicted rebellions in the medical profession did not materialize, despite disproportionately advertised threats by a small group. In fact, virtually all groups that had fought long and hard against the legislation soon adopted cooperative postures. Gradually, even the medical press began to find favorable things to say about the law. In October 1965 one of the long-time leaders of opposition, Dr. Morris Fishbein, a former editor of the *Journal of the American Medical Association,* gave his blessing in a Baltimore address: "When conditions become so severe that they can no longer be handled by private initiative, government must step in." *Medical World News* published a report that month describing the program as a new bonanza for physicians. *Time* magazine ran a detailed story, on October 22, 1965, with this general message: "Most insurance companies now realize that Medicare, far from being the disaster they once predicted, may prove to be a welcome pep pill for their industry."

Participation slowly diminished fears of the unknown and relaxed hostilities and suspicions that had built up over the years. Most important, through intimate working relations, the affected parties developed confidence in the competence and integrity of the SSA. By the end of the year, there were few exceptions to the general praise for the agency's fairness, dedication, and ability.

This is not to say that controversy disappeared or the pursuit of self-interest subsided. Nor can one say that th$_t$ decisions that emerged were always wise or in the best public interest. The point is that the procedure of negotiations and collective participation enabled the parties to work together, to resolve disputes, at least temporarily, and to accept decisions. The law was made administrable.

Many dissatisfactions remain; many interests feel aggrieved by particular decisions; some are committed to come back to fight another day. But none can claim he has been denied his day in court. At one extreme, the government has been accused in some quarters of "purchasing" consent—always in some degree inevitable. At another extreme, a small group of unregenerate physicians accuses its colleagues of "selling out" to the government by its cooperation. Such discontents will continue. There is no universally acceptable or permanent solution of conflicting interests and conflicting ideologies.

The net result was that on "M-Day," July 1, 1966, administrative arrangements for the opening of the program were in order at all levels, far beyond most people's expectations. Some remarkable achievements were recorded. Ninety-two percent of the approximately 19 million older citizens had voluntarily signed up for the supplementary benefit program under Part B. Nearly all had their identification cards for Part A and could be assured that doctors and hospitals were prepared for them. But many problems and hazards lay ahead, not only for the program but also for the whole national medical care establishment within which it must operate, and which it would vastly influence. ...

Selection 26

"Reasonable Costs" and "Reasonable Charges": Early Warning; Trouble Ahead*

Medicare is less than a year old. Posthospital extended care benefits have been in effect less than six months. Data are still only fragmentary and tentative. But even the limited knowledge we now have permits us to derive a few reasonably secure conclusions. It is also sufficient to indicate some large issues confronting not just Medicare, but the whole medical care economy, issues that demand prompt and serious attention.

THE HOSPITAL "REASONABLE COSTS" FORMULA

Medicare has undertaken to pay for the costs of care for beneficiaries who are expected to consume about 30 percent of the bed-days of American hospitals. It thus has responsibility for a major share of costs of one of the country's most rapidly growing industries and the one that has shown, over the past two decades, the most striking and consistent inflationary tendencies. The implications of such relentless cost increases are potentially grave, not only for Medicare but also for the whole health services industry. The dangers have been increased by the government's massive entrance into the hospital economy, giving to some the misguided comfort of apparent "easy money."

Into this explosive situation Medicare has entered with commitment to pay costs for its beneficiaries. Medicare payments made directly to hospitals and related institutions (Part A) are expected to account for over 70 percent of total 1967 benefits of the program. In addition, perhaps 60 percent of payments made to physicians (Part B) will be for services rendered in such institutions. In total, substantially more than 80 percent of all payments will be for services delivered either in or by hospitals or related institutions. The method and amount of payment will determine far more than the cost of Medicare. They will significantly influence standards of payment for all other hospital programs, as well as those of Blue Cross and other third party payers. They will also influence the prices paid by individual purchasers.

Congress, following the precedent of most Blue Cross organizations, legislated that providers should be paid "the reasonable costs" of services for individuals covered by the insurance program. Many Congressmen may not have realized how elastic the concept of "reasonable costs" could be, that it was as

---

*Excerpt from H.M. Somers, "Medicare and the Costs of Health Services," presented to the Princeton Symposium on the American System of Social Insurance, June 1967; published in W.G. Bowen *et al.*, eds., *The American System of Social Insurance* (New York: McGraw-Hill, 1968), pp. 119, 122-141.

much an issue to be resolved by bargaining as by the data, complicated by the generally backward state of cost accounting in most hospitals.

While the immediate content of the reimbursement formula may have less long term significance than the basic question of whether a straight cost reimbursement for individual hospitals is viable, certain aspects of the formula do have important implications. [Of the three factors discussed at this point—apportionment, depreciation, and the "plus factor"—only the last two are included here.]

The Depreciation Factor

Nobody questions that depreciation for the use of hospital facilities is a "reimbursable cost," but there is little else respecting depreciation on which the parties fully agree. Under accepted accounting principles, depreciation is based on original or "historical" cost. Hospitals, however, assert that accounting principles should yield to economic principles which, they say, means that the basis should be current replacement cost, to recognize both price increases and technological improvements.

The financial implications of the disagreement are substantial. Depreciation based on historical cost is assumed to represent about 6 percent of total reimbursement. Estimates of the difference between that and a replacement base range from 50 percent upward to over 80 percent.

Actually, historical depreciation can, in practice, make available, at the time of replacement, far more than the original investment, especially since the hospitals won a major concession permitting the use of accelerated depreciation, although this had not been included in the actuarial assumptions of the program. Investment of accelerated depreciation payments, under the sum-of-the-years-digits method, at a 4 percent return, would ordinarily yield after 20 years approximately the same amount as a fair replacement formula.

Unfortunately, the fact is that hospitals have generally failed to set aside and invest depreciation money, or have paid no attention to depreciation at all in their accounting. The hospitals are really trying to solve a different problem through the vehicle of depreciation. The AHA *Principles of Payment* was amended significantly after the passage of Medicare to state "the capital requirements of hospitals necessitate a reimbursement allowance based on current replacement costs."

The statement is, of course, a *non sequitur*. Whatever the capital requirements of hospitals, and they are substantial, it does not follow that depreciation should be transformed into something for which it was not designed. Depreciation, in its customary and accounting sense, has nothing to do with replacement of assets, let alone meeting new capital needs. It is an expense for assets already used. It is an expense of institutions that have no intention of replacing, or will replace only partially, as well as those that will replace fully or even expand. The depreciation allowance cannot be based on an assumption that every institution is or should be perpetual. On the other hand, the logic of the AHA position would mean that depreciation would be denied to institutions willing to admit that they may be going out of business.

The depreciation decision of the government was liberal. In addition to accelerated depreciation, the hospital is permitted to use one method of depreciation for one asset or a group of assets and another for others, in whatever combination is most advantageous. It may change from one method to another, although only one such change is permitted with respect to a particular asset. Depreciation on assets being used at the time a hospital enters the program will be allowed even though such assets may be fully or partially depreciated on the hospital's books.

In addition, depreciation is allowed on assets financed with Hill-Burton or other federal or public funds. Since these assets do not really represent a cost incurred by the hospitals, it may be said that the government was here accepting a replacement principle in depreciation. But there is in fact little reason to believe that when present Hill-Burton assets are consumed, the government will not be back with grants to replace them.

In its objections to this provision, a staff report of the Senate Finance Committee made a point that seems basic to the entire depreciation issue. "Such depreciation," it said, "can only be justified if all depreciation allowances are funded in accordance with a plan approved by ... an agency designated by the state and the funds used in accordance with such plan." The Social Security Administration (SSA) argued that it could not legally require this.

No one wishes to deny hospitals the resources genuinely needed for modernization and expansion. If it could be reasonably assured that the use of depreciation and other capital payments to hospitals would be related to real hospital and community needs, then the question of the size of such payments might become secondary. This is distinctly not the case, however.

If hospitals do not fund depreciation and expend the money on other items not subject to any judgment of community health needs, the depreciation money becomes inflationary for Medicare and for all other consumers. When the need for replacement or modernization arises, the hospital will turn to traditional fund raising sources, philanthropy and government; and they will get the money. Use of depreciation money as a kitty for individual hospital replacement or expansion also ignores the fact that movement of population and new technology may make it desirable that certain institutions shut down, that others be contracted, while still others should be encouraged to expand rapidly. There may be an inherent dichotomy between the interests of the individual hospital and social policy in respect to hospitals generally.

At the May 1966 Senate Finance Committee hearings on the reimbursement formula, both Senators and Administration participants appeared to agree that funding was necessary, but that funding by individual institutions has as many, or more, dangers as advantages, unless controlled by an area or state hospital plan. The planning objective, however, could probably only be achieved if all depreciation moneys were treated in this way, not only the Medicare portion.

Meanwhile, at least one happy result may emanate from the dispute: it has brought the problem of depreciation and funding forcefully to the attention of hospital administrators and trustees and seems likely to induce some modernization of their accounting practices and to lead to a more orderly financial way of life.

The "Plus Factor"

Simultaneously with their demand for replacement depreciation, hospitals also sought a provision for a return on equity capital as a "cost." The two demands had the same motivation, finding a road to generate new capital from operating revenue; and in large degree they were interchangeable. Traditionally hospitals have not created capital in this way. In recent years only about 30 to 35 percent of capital has been internally generated.

Is the value of capital a "cost"? Under generally accepted accounting principles it is not. In ordinary business enterprise it is not recorded as a cost, nor does the Internal Revenue Code recognize it as a cost of doing business. It is conceded that Congress had not anticipated the inclusion of such an allowance for nonprofit institutions.

Accounting cost, however, is admittedly different from economic cost. Invested capital is an economic cost. The argument was made that the absence of a reasonable return on capital would cause a flight of capital elsewhere. This point is germane to proprietary institutions, which represent 6 percent of the beds in nonfederal general hospitals, and for which the Congress did provide a generous return on equity capital in an amendment passed in November 1966. But nonprofit hospitals do not receive capital (other than that which is borrowed) from sources that expect either a profit or a direct return of any sort.

The money already invested is mainly public money—philanthropy and government. What the hospitals are really seeking is an assured means of generating new capital for the future. The questions arising, therefore, are: (1) Is generation of new capital a current "cost," economic or otherwise, of doing business? (2) Is cost reimbursement by insurers, including Medicare, an appropriate means of producing such revenue?

The answer to the first question is patently no and needs no elaboration. The answer to the second seems also clearly negative, but this will be elaborated. The SSA did hold out strongly against this type of payment—commonly and significantly referred to in the trade as a "plus factor," sometimes as an "override"—to the time of the preliminary official announcement of the reimbursement principles. But in the end, the pressure was too great, and a compromise was struck. An additional allowance of 2 percent of all other allowable costs except interest expense is to be paid to voluntary hospitals.

A percentage "add-on" is by any available criterion a dangerous element in a reimbursement formula. Even if one accepts the idea of paying a return on equity capital, or a payment to generate new capital, it is a poor way of doing it.

That the "plus factor" represents a payment in excess of actual cost seems evident, but that is not the most important problem. More important is the fact that the method gives no assurance that the extra money will contribute to any net improvement of facilities or new facilities when and where they are needed. The money goes to each and every hospital in direct relation to the level of its current operating costs. Presumably those hospitals which have the least difficulty generating funds will get the most, the impoverished hospitals the least. If the nation were to try to meet all the costs of hospital facilities and equipment by an across-the-board grant to all existing institutions proportionate to their present size and lavishness, enormous waste and misdirection of moneys would be inevitable. Equally important is the fact that such a payment, being an override on all other costs, offers a small bonus on every other increase of expenditure. You get that back, plus 2 percent. This turns incentives upside down.*

IS COST REIMBURSEMENT VIABLE?

Important as the specific provisions of the reimbursement formula are, far more fundamental is the question of whether the basic concept of individual cost reimbursement has long term viability. In the tense controversial atmosphere that characterized the legislative struggle, Congress probably had little practical choice. It was anxious to make clear that government had no intention to overhaul the institutional structure of health services and intended only to provide the financial means for medical care for the aged. Individual costs were the prevailing basis for third party reimbursement, and this was generally accepted.

If, however, payment of costs, whatever they turn out to be, is virtually guaranteed (and Medicare, under present regulations, is practically open-ended in that respect), where are the financial incentives for cost control, difficult enough in any case, to come from? If this form of payment applied only to Medicare's 30 percent share of hospital expenses, and the other 70 percent had to be collected from patients in some kind of competitive system, protection might be built in by the guarantee representing only a minority of cost. But we are moving into a period where most hospital revenues come from third party payers, in some states already 80 percent or more. The result has been summarized by economist Gerald Rosenthal of Harvard:

> The payers exercise little control over prices and offer little or no resistance to increases.... This automatic "cost-pass-through" from hospital to payer, together with the decreased relevance of price to the patient, provides a basis for the considerable inefficiency of the hospital system as a whole.

---

*The plus factor was rescinded in 1969.

In no other realm of economic life are payments guaranteed for costs that are neither controlled by competition nor regulated by public authority, and in which no incentive for economy can be discerned. This is a case where the existing method is almost certain to prove inappropriate, and we must be prepared for the necessity of change.

But there are no readily apparent substitute methods to turn to. Is it possible to develop monetary incentives for institutions without a profit motivation? Some economists have recognized the dangers. But in the main their suggestions have relevance to the more conventional economic model with which they are familiar, one in which there is an identifiable unit product, profit motivation, or some competitive factors.

Hospitals have many ways to reduce costs without improving efficiency by relatively invisible reductions in quality, if they are forced to in order to avoid a penalty. Also, monetary rewards in the form of any excess over actual costs are most likely to find their way into additional investment in facilities or in higher salaries, thus raising costs for the next go-round unless accompanied by productivity increases for which there is no apparent present incentive.

Ideas with respect to possible alternatives are emerging. Most are still nebulous. But full exploration and, wherever possible, experimentation with alternatives should be undertaken. Specifically, the SSA should be authorized and urged to enter into agreements with hospitals to try out any new ideas that offer real promise. Other agencies engaged in research in the socioeconomic aspects of medical care should consider sponsoring experimental projects of this type.

One prominent proposal calls for prior external budget review and approval. ... A second suggestion may be identified as the "target rate" concept. Under this proposal, an annual "target" *per diem* rate is established for each hospital based on a projection of its experience during the preceding three years. In addition, a maximum and a minimum are set for each institution. If a hospital's expense proves less than the target rate it will be paid its actual expenses plus a variable incentive bonus, the total coming to less than the target rate but not less than the minimum. If a hospital's actual expense is greater than its target rate, it will be paid less than actual expenses, although more than the target rate, but no more than the maximum.

A third idea, involving "capitation" payments, has already received encouraging experimentation in Colorado and is under serious consideration for an early limited trial by the Health Insurance Plan (HIP) in cooperation with New York City Blue Cross. Under this version, Blue Cross would pay a designated hospital, which agrees to come into an integrated HIP-Hospital Program, on a capitation basis rather on the customary bed-days of use basis. It may be noted that under the "target rate" plan, the emphasis is primarily on incentives for controlling *per diem* costs, while in the "capitation" system the accent is on incentives for utilization control.

The sophisticated critic will readily find weaknesses and inadequacies in each of these ideas. Some allege that the target rate concept is not administrable and that it represents a threat to quality. For example, a hospital could lower its *per diem* costs simply by keeping patients an additional day, which involves very little additional service. Thus the hospital could receive a bonus while it was actually increasing total program costs. Others claim the capitation method encourages underutilization just as much as fee-for-service and cost reimbursement tend to overutilization.

In brief, it should be clear that a reimbursement formula not only determines what costs will be reimbursed but also has a significant influence on what the actual costs will turn out to be. It should also be emphasized that important as the payment mechanism is, one cannot expect too much from it alone, whatever form it may take. There are many strong inflationary drives in hospitals quite aside from sources of revenue. Efforts to discipline these tendencies entirely, or even primarily, through a reimbursement formula, however designed, are doomed to failure because they ignore the institutional peculiarities of the hospital economy. Costs will have to be tackled directly as well as indirectly through the payment formula.

PHYSICIANS' FEES

According to the law, doctors must be paid, or the beneficiary reimbursed, in relation to a "reasonable charge" for each service, defined as not to exceed the doctor's "customary" fee or that "prevailing" in the community, and not be more than the intermediary would pay for its own insureds.

The doctor is limited to the "reasonable charge" only if he accepts assignment from the patient and is therefore paid directly by the intermediary. If the patient pays the doctor himself, the doctor may charge anything he can collect; the intermediary will, however, limit its reimbursement to the patient to 80 percent of the "reasonable charge." (The law requires 20 percent coinsurance.) Estimates indicate that assignment is taking place in about half the cases. Beneficiaries are resentful of the requirement that unless the doctor will accept assignment, they must send the carrier a receipted bill, for which they often must go into debt or seek welfare assistance. Indignation at this requirement is particularly great among former low income Blue Shield members whose doctors were paid directly by the plans.

Carriers are having trouble determining "customary" fees. There is nothing in the law to prevent a doctor from raising his "customary" fees. "Prevailing" fees, which had been rising about 3 percent a year between 1960 and 1965, took a sharp jump of 8 percent during 1966. It does seem clear that the medical costs of the program are going to run much higher than anticipated.

An inescapable basic question emerges: is it feasible for the government to guarantee to any group or profession payment at any level the group may unilaterally elect? The answer appears increasingly self-evident. The entire fee-for-service system is being called into doubt. But alternatives are not easily available. The medical societies are resolutely opposed to fee schedules or fee controls of any sort.

Clearly, Medicare faces stormy days ahead in the entire field of payments to providers of care. Present arrangements are so vulnerable it seems unlikely that they can be lived with very long. Yet any basic reforms will invite strident controversy. They will be slow in coming and the expense of delay will be high.

Selection 27

Medicaid: The Big Sleeper*

In October 1965, months before the new program took effect, Medical Economics *interviewed one of the authors on the subject of Title XIX, the last-minute addition to P.L. 89-97 which was receiving very little notice. Virtually all public attention had been concentrated on the dramatically disputed Title XVIII—Medicare. No one had yet suggested that Title XIX might become as costly and as explosive as Medicare. Although the term "Medicaid" had not yet come into general use, for clarity, it is substituted in this selection for terms like "new" or "revised Kerr-Mills," as the program was identified in the interview. Some provisions of the original legislation here mentioned were later amended or dropped. The interview form is retained.*

Q. Professor Somers, you've predicted that the broadened benefits of the Medicaid program will give it a substantial impact on the private practice of medicine. How so?

A. Because virtually every added benefit will entail a doctor who, in most cases, will be a private physician. Under the original Kerr-Mills welfare program, a participating state had to provide merely "some institutional and some noninstitutional care"—and in most states, benefits were minimal. But after July 1, 1967, a participating state must cover all physicians' services—whether furnished in the office, patient's home, hospital, or nursing home. Moreover, the state will have to provide extremely broad benefits that include inpatient and outpatient hospital care, nursing home care for adults, lab work, and x rays. In addition, the federal government will help finance many optional benefits: prescribed drugs, prosthetic devices, diagnostic and preventive services, and the like.

Q. How many doctors will the new program affect?

A. A large majority of the private physicians in the country. That's because of the program's increased patient load. Kerr-Mills used to cover only 2.4

---

*Excerpt from H.M. Somers, "The Big Sleeper in the Medicare Law," Interview by Howard R. Lewis, *Medical Economics*, January 24, 1966, pp. 110-122.

million needy old people. But if every state enacted just the first stage of the revised program, more than 7.4 million people would be immediately eligible for benefits. You see, participating states must cover all 5 million recipients of the federally assisted welfare programs for families with dependent children, for the blind, and for the permanently and totally disabled—regardless of age. This, of course, is not all a net addition, since many of these people already receive some medical benefits under state programs.

Q. You say that's just the first stage. Who else would be added to the patient load?

A. Millions of medically indigent people. The original Kerr-Mills Act provided benefits for only those medically indigent persons over age 65. Now the states will also cover medically indigent patients *under* 65. They include patients whose incomes are too high for the federally assisted programs for families, the blind, and the disabled—but who still can't afford medical care.

Q. How's the expanded program likely to affect doctors in private practice?

A. In many ways. The volume of patients is likely to go up fast for many of them. They'll perform many more services that will be paid for by government. Welfare discount rates will give way to full payment of charges consistent with prevailing rates in the community. There will be far fewer free services and nonpaying needy patients. In short, the typical doctor's income is likely to be augmented by Medicaid as well as by Medicare. And he'll be able to offer better care.

Q. Why better care?

A. Many doctors report that they're often hesitant about prescribing medically indicated procedures if they know the patient cannot stand the financial strain. With the financial barrier gone, doctors can be free to follow their best medical judgment. And patients are likely to seek care earlier than they used to. Thus the patient's condition won't worsen because he's afraid of the cost of treatment.

Q. But what about the drawbacks? Many doctors liked the original Kerr-Mills program because it left lots of leeway to the states. Now with all the federal requirements as to eligibility and benefits, how much local autonomy will be left?

A. A great deal, actually. A doctor will still deal solely with the state agency or, if the state chooses, with an intermediary like Blue Shield. And each state will continue to determine allowable fees and how much of each type of required benefit it will provide and what eligibility test it will set. All administration remains with the state. The federal standards mainly say that the state cannot be unreasonably restrictive in its medical benefits and that the state cannot shortchange the doctor with unreasonably low fees.

Q. Still, isn't the state agency apt to interfere with the way a physician makes his charges under the program?

A. Only if you think it's interference for a third party to review what it's paying for. Questions concerning fees will be a source of perennial controversy as long as we have third party payments. Government agencies generally review doctors' fees as fairly as private third parties do. I think the broadened benefits and liberalized fees will reduce the area of potential conflict.

Q. How does the new Medicaid system compare with the "Eldercare" program that was proposed by the AMA last year?

A. The new system incorporates Eldercare, which was a proposal to benefit the medically needy aged by liberalizing Kerr-Mills. And although the revised program offers many of Eldercare's benefits, it also has many of Eldercare's handicaps. For instance, a Medicaid program cannot materialize without affirmative action by the states. You know how long states took to adopt the original law; some haven't done so yet. Fortunately, the new law builds in so many incentives that I believe all the states will participate.

Q. Then what do you feel may be the biggest potential danger to doctors in Medicaid?

A. Medicaid is a welfare system. And the danger in a welfare system is that we might lose control of the program's spread: The money comes from general taxation—and there's no relationship between benefits and contributions. Thus there are no built-in restraints on demands for expansion to more and more people. I believe that the soundest way to protect people against medical costs is through insurance—private wherever possible. A welfare program like Medicaid should be confined to patients who cannot be covered through a self-supporting insurance mechanism.

Selection 28

National Health Insurance: Story with a Past, Present, and Future*

While the late 1960s and early 1970s were explosive with controversy on health care legislation and proposals of all varieties, at the center of public attention, cutting across all other health policy debates, was a revival of interest in national health insurance (NHI).

The general issue has been on the American political scene for over 50 years. Public discussion of compulsory health insurance started around 1912 when President Theodore Roosevelt's Progressive Party made national health insurance one of the major planks in its platform. In the following decade, health insurance bills were debated in several state legislatures including New York, Massachusetts, and California, and passed one house of the New York

---
*Prepared for this volume by the authors, July 1976.

legislature with a substantial majority. In 1916 Congress held hearings on a federal plan that included invalidity and sickness benefits.

For several years, it appeared that the American Medical Association would endorse such a program and take the opportunity to influence the legislation. Its social insurance committee helped draft the New York and Massachusetts bills and, in 1917, the Association adopted a resolution submitted by this committee which said, in part:

> ... the time is present when the profession should study earnestly to solve the questions of medical care that will arise under various forms of social insurance. Blind opposition, indignant repudiation, bitter denunciation of these laws is worse than useless; it leads nowhere and it leaves the profession in a position of helplessness as the rising tide of social development sweeps over it.[1]

A prophetic statement—and the last of its kind for years to come. In 1920 the House of Delegates reversed its policy in a strong resolution opposing any form of "compulsory contributory insurance against illness,"[2] a statement that more or less expressed its position for the next 50 years.

NHI reemerged as an issue during the Great Depression, as part of President Franklin Roosevelt's New Deal, which brought the federal government for the first time into economic security programs on a broad front. The historic report of the Committee on Economic Security, which led to the Social Security Act of 1935, confined itself to endorsing the principle of national health insurance. In submitting the report to Congress, however, President Roosevelt made it clear that legislation was on the agenda for the future. In 1944, his State of the Union Message and the Social Security Board's Annual Report to Congress indicated that the Administration thought the time had come.

Roosevelt died before he could take further action. But the following year, in a special message to Congress, President Harry Truman proposed a comprehensive NHI Program, through the Social Security system, a plan that became the basis of the second Wagner-Murray-Dingell bill. From 1946 to 1950, NHI was bitterly debated between its proponents, led by the Committee on the Nation's Health, an *ad hoc* group of prominent liberals and union leaders, and its opponents, led by the AMA. The AMA won.

However, Congress took a significant step in amending the Social Security Act to provide federal matching grants to states for "vendor payments" to physicians, nurses, hospitals, and other providers for treatment of individuals on public assistance. This development was important for it created a precedent and a framework for our federal-state public assistance medical programs—an approach that has continued to compete with social insurance as a basis for national health care financing policy.

During the next 15 years advocates of public health insurance concentrated on adding health care protection to Social Security benefits for the aged. Oscar Ewing, then head of the Federal Security Agency, first proposed legislation in

1951 to provide hospital benefits for all Social Security beneficiaries. This was followed by a strong endorsement in the 1953 Report of the President's Commission on the Health Needs of the Nation (the Magnuson Report).

The next year President Dwight Eisenhower proposed legislation to enable private insurers to broaden their health coverage by federal reinsurance against heavy losses. In 1956 he requested legislation to permit small carriers and voluntary health groups to pool resources for this purpose. Neither proposal was adopted.

About the same time several new bills were introduced to provide hospital insurance for the aged. Extensive public hearings went on from 1958 to 1960, with many counterproposals. A temporary compromise was reached with passage of the Kerr-Mills bill in 1960, establishing Medical Assistance for the Aged through extension of the earlier "vendor payment program." This created the important precedent of public financing for the elderly "medically indigent" *not* on public assistance.

Health insurance for the aged was a prominent issue in the presidential elections of 1960 and 1964. After years of acrimonious controversy and as much public debate as any proposal could have, Medicare was finally passed in 1965 (Selection 25). The United States had its first compulsory national health insurance program, for 10 percent of the population.

Within a few years a broad movement for some form of health insurance for the whole population was under way. This time, however, almost all interests decided to get into the act in an affirmative posture. As early as 1968 the AMA, in a dramatic reversion to its 1917 position, sponsored the introduction of its "Medicredit" version of NHI. The following year the American Hospital Association set up its Special Committee on Provision of Health Services (Perloff Committee), whose report was to lead, in a few years, to a bill sponsored by Representative Al Ullman, later to become chairman of the House Ways and Means Committee.

In 1970, Senator Edward Kennedy introduced his "Health Securtiy Program," strongly backed by the AFL-CIO and the Committee for National Health Insurance. With introduction of the Health Insurance Association of America's "National Healthcare Act," in 1971, all the major private interest groups were actively on stage, with the exception of Blue Cross, which chose to play a "behind-the-scenes" role.

This time, also, government was far more heavily involved at both state and federal levels. Prodded by New York Governor Nelson Rockefeller and their own growing Medicaid problems, the National Governors' Conference has been on record favoring the principle of NHI since 1969. The Secretary's (HEW) Task Force on Medicaid and Related Problems, which reported in 1970, took no specific position on NHI but did call for federalization of Medicaid. The Republican Administration's first health insurance bill was introduced in 1971; a revised version was submitted in 1974.

Altogether, dozens of NHI bills have been proposed in Congress during the past few years. Old bills are revised and reintroduced. In the 94th Congress alone (1975-76), 18 separate measures had been introduced by February 1976;[3] more were expected before the end of the session.

MAJOR ISSUES, CIRCA 1976

It is easy to be misled by the apparent consensus. While almost everyone appears to agree that government action of some sort is required to assure access to necessary health services for the entire population, the wide array of proposals under the rubric "national health insurance" has stretched the term into considerable ambiguity. Within the apparent general agreement are a multitude of highly controversial issues, practical and philosophical, and a host of divergent interests seeking to be served.

The major debating points, as they have been filtered over the years, now revolve around the following issues:

1. the degree and character of private health insurance involvement in the public program;
2. the extent, if any, of cost sharing by consumers through direct charges over and above any premiums they may pay;
3. the extent and character of cost and quality controls to be built into the program;
4. whether the insurance program should undertake to reform the health care delivery system.

There are, of course, numerous other questions over which protagonists can and do argue. Some are subsumed within those listed, for example, universality of coverage, administration, and methods of financing. Others, such as coverage of preventive services and long term care, have only recently emerged as major issues. However, it is the four above that have excited the most attention and emotion during the past few years.

The Public-Private Mix

Public-private participation is perhaps the core issue which, directly or indirectly, affects most other major decisions and where the stakes of various interest groups are conspicuously high. The public-private spectrum has many gradations. They include:

1. tax-credit plans, which simply offer a subsidy to purchasers of private insurance by allowing tax credits for premiums paid for insurance meeting established standards;
2. a government mandate requiring the provision by employers of an approved level of private insurance for full time employees and their dependents, supplemented by government subsidy of premiums for the poor and unemployed;

3. a national government-financed and operated plan using private health insurance carriers as fiscal or administrative agents or intermediaries; and

4. a national government-financed and fully operated plan with no role for private carriers.

There are, of course, other gradations and mixes, including the one recommended in Selection 29. Of the four here listed, the tax credit plan, which received a great deal of early attention because of initial endorsement by the AMA, is no longer receiving serious consideration.

The Nixon and Ford Administration bills followed the "mandated" approach. The technique thus received prominent attention, and the principle was incorporated in other bills from other sources. This method has both ideological and pragmatic attraction to many groups. It promises less enlargement of federal responsibilities and expenditures than other methods. It seeks to avoid further strain on the tax tolerance of the population. It is more acceptable to providers of health care because it has less potential for direct federal controls than the other methods. It is attractive to insurance carriers because it does not threaten their underwriting functions. These are significant considerations.

However, as the Administration discovered after many months of labor by a talented staff, there is no way a mandated program can offer universal coverage without imposition of means tests and a fragmented set of programs. It thus cannot meet a fundamental criterion for effective national health insurance. The 1974 bill actually provided a patchwork of four different programs, with people having to shift from one to another with changing circumstances, millions falling between the stools with no coverage, and enormous administrative complexity. Elimination of means tests, to many people a paramount point of NHI, was not achieved.

Moreover, the financing inherent in mandated plans does not result in equitable sharing of cost burdens. Unlike general revenue financing or Social Security payroll taxes, private premiums are set in dollar amounts and related to the actual health care cost experience of individual firms or groups of firms. They are not related to earnings levels. They are thus more regressive than existing Social Security taxes, often criticized on this score.

Many Administration spokesmen conceded the shortcomings, but felt these were necessary to protect their more basic concerns: minimal enlargement of government activities and minimization of additions to the federal budget. The question thus arises: When does an accumulation of shortcomings become so preponderant that one must conclude that they outweigh the advantages and that the important objectives of the program are vitiated? Our own conclusion is that a mandated insurance program does not furnish sufficient net gains to be worth the expense.

Categories 3 and 4, although also beset by shortcomings, can achieve universal coverage through a single program financed by a combination of different federal taxes. The use of private carriers as intermediaries is similar to the arrangement under Medicare. Such a program enlists the skills and support of the private sector and avoids some of the rigidities of an enlarged federal bureaucracy. However, the intermediaries would work under the rule-making authority of the federal administrators, have little leeway of their own, and little incentive for efficiencies of operation. It is questionable whether such arrangements would continue to be desirable for the carriers under NHI.

Under Medicare the "nonprofit" administrative costs that intermediaries are paid help to meet some of the overhead in their own business; and involvement in Medicare has other advantages. But, if they are pushed out of the health insurance business altogether, it would certainly diminish, if not eliminate, the attraction of the job, for commercial carriers at least, although nonprofit enterprises like Blue Cross-Blue Shield might be in a different position. This question is further explored in Selection 29.

Both the proponents of mandated programs and other plans, based on private collection of premiums, and sponsors of the single federally financed plans have, in the enthusiastic promotion of their own schemes, advanced the impression that there is no reconciliation possible between the extremes—that the advantages of a federal revenue-raising system cannot be combined with the advantages of pluralistic risk-taking enterprise. We do not believe this is the case. Section 29 proposes an illustrative plan that demonstrates that a balanced pluralism is feasible.

The Cost Sharing Issue

Cost sharing was controversial even during the debates over Medicare. It has become more emotion-laden since. For many the symbolism is as important as the substance.

Cost sharing can take many forms, most commonly *deductibles, coinsurance,* and *copay,* or a combination of these. The terms are sometimes used interchangeably. As most commonly defined, a deductible requires that the consumer pay directly the initial costs of services for a given period up to a specified dollar amount. Coinsurance requires the consumer to pay some fixed percentage of the costs of services received. Copayment requires a fixed dollar payment—usually small—for each use of a specified service, such as a doctor visit or a drug prescription.

A large body of opinion (those who support the Kennedy-Corman bill, for example) opposes all cost sharing, claiming it establishes discriminatory impediments to use of services, particularly by the poor, and discourages use of preventive care and early diagnosis by all. If the amount is small enough not to inhibit needed care, they say, it is just an administrative nuisance; if the amount is large, it becomes necessary to introduce subsidies and means tests for the poor.

For many supporters, cost sharing represents a relatively painless way of reducing high premium costs since even low cost sharing amounts can be cumulatively large. The more articulate supporters, however, place primary reliance on the argument that "free" coverage encourages excessive and unnecessary utilization of services, thus overburdening the available supply; encourages inflation by removing consumer cost resistance; and results in unnecessarily high total costs.

There is statistical evidence that full coverage, as compared with high cost sharing, does increase demand. But such data can be used to support both positions since they do not indicate whether the additional demand is "necessary" or "unnecessary" (elusive terms in health care, in any case) or whether its denial would have proved damaging. And, of course, the inhibitions fall mainly on low-income groups (although not necessarily welfare cases).[4]

Proponents of cost sharing acknowledge the latter problem by usually proposing that cost sharing be income-related. This is unsatisfactory to opponents on several grounds. It again introduces means tests under another name which, despite good intentions to the contrary, have always resulted in invasions of privacy, indignities, and discrimination. Moreover, all plans for income-related schedules are complex, cumbersome, and costly to administer. Income relatedness would also appear to vitiate the major objective of the "cost consciousness" advocates. If the payments are zero for the very poor, equity demands that they be graduated so as not to represent financial obstacles for the middle classes as well. But, as a practical matter, experience indicates that most people, who can afford it, will buy "first dollar" protection elsewhere, if available, even though economists preach that it is a "poor buy."

The argument that full coverage would place excessive strain upon available facilities appears now to apply largely to ambulatory services. About 90 percent of inpatient hospital bills are already paid by third parties, and additional insurance is not likely to have substantial effect upon demand. Whatever additional demand may be reasonably anticipated could, in most areas, easily be absorbed by the present supply of hospital beds and facilities. In respect to ambulatory services, the objections to cost sharing barriers are: (1) Whatever supply is currently available should be equitably shared; financial ability should not be the determinant of who will have easier access. (2) NHI is inherently inflationary unless measures for direct price control and other regulatory restraints are imposed; these will have to be imposed in any case. (3) Cost sharing barriers will continue emphasis on crisis-oriented medicine and away from preventive care and health education, which are the largest areas of neglect. (4) It is unrealistic to expect equitable control over use and price by imposing high deductibles and coinsurance on the patient, the wrong target.

The argument for cost sharing presupposes a conventional marketplace wherein the consumer can control his expenditures through comparative shopping among doctors, drugs, and hospitals; by avoidance of unnecessary hospital procedures; and similar rational medical-economic judgments. It has often been pointed out that in health services, the physician is the primary decision maker. Particularly in serious or hospitalized illness, which accounts for the great bulk of health care expenditures, the patient is not the real buyer. The doctor, who admits, discharges, and orders all the procedures, is the effective buyer.

Except for the initial contact, the patient generally is the passive recipient of services—usually uninformed as to what is taking place, much less what it costs (sometimes even unwillingly). If he tries to reduce costs or otherwise influence the course of events by taking issue with his doctor's orders, by trying to discharge himself from the hospital, by refusing certain procedures or even, in the case of terminal illness, by pleading against heroic and costly measures that might add a few pain-wracked weeks to his life, he will be accused of being everything from a "noncooperative patient" to a criminal. To say to such an individual or his family that he should assume responsibility for holding down utilization and costs by exercising "consumer sovereignty" is futile. Equitable and rational control, if it comes, will require some system of restraints primarily on providers.

It is not necessary to assume an extreme position on either side of cost sharing. Experience indicates that a system of modest copayment (rather than deductibles or coinsurance) can discourage frivolous utilization, not be an unreasonable strain on anybody, and cumulatively can be helpful in meeting program costs. Flat sum copayments are now used, for example, in the Swedish national health system and for certain services under the British National Health Service (where it is a perennial source of controversy), and in some of the more successful American prepayment plans such as the Kaiser Health Plan. Percentage coinsurance can accelerate to prohibitive sums. Attempts to contain them by establishing maximums become very complex to administer, especially if they are income-related.

Frequently overlooked is the fact that virtually all proposals have provisions that permit invisible forms of cost sharing, which are not labeled as such. For example, many would permit a physician to set his effective fee to the patient at a figure exceeding the amount that the program will pay (aside from coinsurance). The consumer is liable for the difference. This is particularly mischievous because it is concealed cost sharing, it is uncontrollable, and it is a potential inducement for busy practitioners to discriminate among patients in favor of the affluent. In addition, under all proposals, certain services remain uninsured (or uncovered), and the consumer is responsible for all the costs. Such factors make it certain that the average consumer will be paying for a very substantial portion of his health services under NHI, with or without formal cost sharing.

Catastrophic Insurance

This can be considered a more elaborate form of cost sharing. It is health insurance with a very high deductible, usually set at a level where it is assumed expenditures beyond that amount would represent great economic hardship to a family. For example, the most prominent of the catastrophic insurance proposals, the Long-Ribicoff bill, would have hospitalization benefits commence only after 60 days of previous hospitalization for the individual. Outpatient benefits would begin after expenditures of $2,000 for a family had been incurred for that purpose. Catastrophic insurance generally requires additional coinsurance. The original Long-Ribicoff bill included 20 to 25 percent coinsurance with a family maximum of $1,000. The 1976 version eliminated coinsurance.

Such a program is attractive to people who beleive that "routine" health care costs are not now a significant problem for most people and do not justify enactment of a massive full coverage system; it is only with very large costs that most people need help and where present arrangements are inadequate. It also has the attraction of appearing to offer universal protection at low cost because catastrophies are not common. It has some of the same appeal as other forms of cost sharing: lower utilization and alleged consumer price resistance.

Catastrophic insurance from the same liabilities as other cost sharing, only in more extreme form. It is, as cost sharing generally, an old issue about which we wrote in 1961:

> It is impossible to determine a line or even a zone of 'catastrophic' expenses by a monetary definition.... One family's routine expenses are another's catastrophe.... We do not know whether the family with a $1,000 medical bill is finding it, on the average, a heavier burden than the $300 bill family. It is also unclear whether the smaller bill may not often result from the relative financial barrier rather than relative medical need and that a health loss as well as financial loss may not be indicated.[5]

If we attempt to correct that difficulty by defining the point of catastrophe in relation to income, we come right back to means tests and all their undesirable administrative, psychological, and health implications.

Catastrophic insurance can best be defended not as an ultimate self-contained program, but as a step in an evolutionary development of a comprehensive NHI system. Long-Ribicoff, in fact, appears to have that end in view. The sponsors have made the hospital and medical deductibles more apparent than real for most people. Both can be met in part or in total through expenditures covered by any other public or private programs. It is expected that out-of-pocket payments for deductibles would be minimized in practice.

There are, of course, other possible incremental approahces to NHI. As we have noted elsewhere:

> ... the only difference between the catastrophic plans and the comprehensive plans is the deductibles. If, over time, the deductibles are gradually reduced to a very low acceptable level or eventually eliminated, the result is total national health insurance. Another possible path is to gradually cover discrete identifiable groups. We seem to be on that road now. In 1965 we covered the age group 65 and over. The 1972 amendments added two smaller groups, the disabled and victims of renal failure. The next step could be the age group eligible for social security, which now starts at 62 and even 60 in some cases. Or it could be children under 12, for example.... these general roads to NHI... are, of course, not necessarily mutually exclusive.[6]

The approach suggested appears to be gathering interest. In 1976 bills were introduced by Senator Jacob Javits and Representative James Scheuer to provide comprehensive health care for all children under age 18 and a program of maternity benefits for all women.

Controls

There is a great deal of discussion of cost and quality controls, but in the main the interest centers on costs. Even when quality controls are introduced, as in the PSRO (Professional Standards Review Organization) amendments to Medicare, they are advanced primarily as means to contain costs. In fact, many proponents of national health plans emphasize mainly the potential of a national program to apply cost control mechanisms.

This is a matter of grave concern to hospitals, physicians, and other providers of care. It is a powerful factor explaining their almost uniform opposition to a federally financed and administered plan. They believe price regulation and other restrictions are likely to be far more extensive under federal auspices than under plans primarily privately financed and administered.

This seems to us, at most, an interim issue. Whether initially included in the legislation or not, no NHI scheme can long operate without some cost controls, difficult though they may be to administer effectively. All industrial nations have learned that health care financing can be a bottomless pit; some type of cost containment is simply inescapable. Medicare started optimistically with almost no cost controls. These have been gradually added as experience demonstrated the endless drives to price and cost inflation. The inevitable movement to stronger controls is well underway. The Social Security Amendments of 1972 (P.L. 92-603) provide a set of wide-ranging controls over Medicare, Medicaid, and Title V reimbursement, whose full implications are still being tested through Administration regulations and court battles. By 1975, about half the states had adopted certificate-of-need laws (Selection 38). The National Health Planning and Resources Development Act of 1974 requires all states to create such a mechanism. A few have also legislated rate regulation for health care institutions. An increasing number of NHI bills provide for some kind of cost regulation, most often "prospective" rate setting for hospitals instead of retrospective cost reimbursement. There remains great uncertainty regarding the kind of controls that could be implemented effectively and that would prove equitable, but the need becomes less of a question with each day's experience under present arrangements.

Reforming the Delivery System

A recast financing system will inevitably have an effect on the delivery system. To some, this is a primary reason for supporting NHI; to others for opposition. Regardless of one's judgment on the need for such reform, there is an important strategic question as to whether the same piece of legislation should simultaneously attempt both undertakings. We discuss this in Selection 29.

Other Issues

With respect to long term care, the challenge is to bring it, including geriatric, psychiatric, and the management of long term chronic disability, into the mainstream of professional interest and third party financing and to do this without an inordinate rise in the overall costs. This will almost certainly require coverage of home care and some types of residential and day care facilities (Selections 48-51).

Preventive care, including health education, is currently being redefined in a recent rebirth of interest—a rebirth that stems both from considerations of health and of economy (Selections 42-46). Such a redefinition is essential as a prerequisite to any meaningful third party coverage. One significant effort was made by Representatiave Tim Lee Carter, a physician and ranking Republican member of the House Ways and Means Committee, in the 94th Congress. In reintroducing the NHI bill, sponsored by the Administration in the previous Congress, he added coverage, without any cost sharing, for an array of preventive services [H.R. 4747, Sec. 184 (a) (2)]. Selection 46 presents a more detailed effort in the same general direction, including both periodic screening and health counseling.

A LOOK AHEAD

The issues we have enumerated are not entirely technical questions that can be resolved by further research and scientific findings. Every possible resolution affects different interests in different ways, and none is equally favorable to all. Each answer is related to certain value judgments, strongly felt and generally not universally shared. The academic assumption that additional knowledge will bring us closer to agreement is not necessarily valid when dealing with divergent ideologies and where the stakes are high for contending parties. The accommodations required in this field will be slow in coming and probably can only be achieved in a step-by-step progression or a gradual phasing-in of programs.

It thus appears improbable that any comprehensive NHI program can be enacted in the near future. It would require some unprecedented legislative acrobatics, or a social disruption like a major depression, for Congress to resolve so many deep disagreements in one act. But that does not diminish the importance of the current debate. Only an understanding of NHI, viewed as a whole, can enable us to comprehend the significance and appropriateness of steps taken along the way. A view of the demands and objectives of the many contending interests is needed to appreciate the nature and necessity of the accommodations that are made, and why the process is so laborious.

It is also essential to view the issues and arguments in their American context. Many people appear to believe that the programs being considered here are imitations of European practices because most Western societies have long had some type of general government health scheme. The fact is that European programs vary widely from one another; there is no "European-type" of NHI.

Neither of the two European systems best known in this country, the British and the Swedish, can be considered prototypes for any of the major proposals being debated in the United States. Neither is called or operated as "national health insurance." The British is designated a National Health Service, and the Swedish system also operates primarily as a direct service. Both are financed mainly from general revenues, and coverage for all citizens or residents is automatic. Nearly all hospitals are publicly owned in both countries; "reimbursement rates" are not an issue. Primary care physicians are compensated on a capitation basis in England; they are generally on salary in Sweden. These few characteristics should indicate how little the American proposals have in common with the more prominent European plans.

The question does arise, however, as to why there has been so little discussion of the possibility of a health service, rather than insurance, in this country, since many who know such systems regard the former as far less complicated to operate than either private or social insurance. The most relevant answer appears to be that developments in each country must be seen in the light of its own historical background. The Swedes, for example, are quick to remind a visitor that government has always had primary responsibility for health services there; the present system is simply an extension and evolutionary adaptation of the traditional design.

In England, the government took over ownership of hospitals during World War II. Health insurance for workers had been in effect since 1911, but it was a government scheme operated together with local "friendly societies," and no tradition of private health insurance had been established. Moreover, the Health Service was enacted in 1946 immediately following the great social upheavals of a long harsh war and on the basis of promises made by all political parties in the midst of that war.

Our history is, of course, very different. Unlike the other countries, we have developed a large private health insurance industry that plays a major role in the financing of care. Hospitals are, in the main, private institutions. Our medical profession has a more "independent" tradition. The nation has an historical suspicion of direct governmental enterprise. We have generally chosen government regulation of private enterprise rather than government ownership or operation.

However, there is a body of informed opinion that believes that after we live with the type of NHI that is indicated by the areas of commonality in current proposals, the country will inevitably find that it is unnecessarily and burdensomely complex. The structure may totter from the weight of administrative complexity, mountainous paper work, and proliferating bureaucracies. We will then move on to the logic of a more simply framed health service.

Whether that will, in fact, occur is in the realm of long range prognostication, at which nobody has evidenced great success. But even these forecasters do not generally claim that we can, as a practical matter, skip the NHI experience in their scenario. We learn and persuade by cumulative experience. We cannot leapfrog historical development. This is not to say that the process always works itself out in a rational manner or that it yields the best results, only that it is one of the ecological realities. In any case it seems safe to say that for the next decade, at least, we will be wrestling with the problems of creating NHI and then trying to work out its bugs. That is a large enough task to look forward to without further projections.

Finally, we must again note that while NHI legislation is undoubtedly needed, we should not entertain unreasonable expectations. A new financing system, no matter how much better than we now have, is not a cure for all other health care problems. Most of the array of anomalies and needed reforms dealt with in this book will remain difficult and important issues to be resolved with or without NHI. Moreover, the arrival of NHI may force on the nation a host of complicated new decisions, such as setting limits on investment in health services and consequent allocation of health resources, and rationing or denial of some types of service, so sensitive in their implications that thus far we have, for the most part, been unwilling to acknowledge, let alone face, them.

NOTES

1. J.G. Barrow, *AMA: Voice of American Medicine* (Baltimore: Johns Hopkins Press, 1963), p. 144.
2. *Journal of the American Medical Association,* May 1, 1920, p. 1319.
3. U.S. Department of Health, Education, and Welfare, Social Security Administration, *National Health Insurance Proposals,* HEW Publ. (SSA) 76-11920, June 1976.
4. See, for example, A.A. Scitovsky and N.M. Snyder, "Effect of Coinsurance on Use of Physician Services," *Social Security Bulletin,* June 1972, pp. 3-19. This study found that, after introduction of 25 percent coinsurance on all physicians' visits to a prepaid group practice clinic, the average number of per capita visits dropped 24 percent. The drop was particularly striking for lower income females and children. In the year after coinsurance was imposed, 30 percent of lower income males did not see a doctor even once. The per capita number of annual physicals fell 19 percent; for lower income males and females, 51 and 57 percent respectively.

Similar, although less detailed, findings were reported in a study of the impact of cost-sharing on the use of ambulatory services under Medicare in 1969:

> "The impact of SMI cost-sharing... is seen in the relatively larger proportion of enrollees with low-to-moderate family incomes who do not use medical services and who do not incur sufficient charges to meet the deductible. There apparently is a differential impact of the deductible in the use of covered SMI services for persons in this group compared with those of higher family incomes or with private out-of-hospital medical insurance complementary to Medicare." U.S.

Department of Health, Education, and Welfare, Social Security Administration, *Health Insurance Statistics*, HEW Publ. (SSA) 74-11702, October 10, 1973, p. 2.

5. H.M. and A.R. Somers, *Doctors, Patients, and Health Insurance*, (Washington, D.C.: The Brookings Institution, 1961), p. 401.

6. H.M. Somers, "Interview," *Hospitals: Journal of the American Hospital Association*, August 16, 1974, p. 90.

Selection 29

National Health Insurance: Criteria for an Effective Program and a Proposal*

Before undertaking an evaluation of proposed programs and different approaches to national health insurance it is necessary to establish some guidelines or criteria against which the programs may be measured. So large and important a public undertaking should measure up to a demanding set of standards to be acceptable and effective. It should meet the following requirements:

1. *Universal coverage of the resident population without distinction as to income or premium contributions.* The undertaking of national health insurance is justified by the recognition that access to medical care is a necessity, not a luxury, and that universality of protection is required. Universality cannot be achieved by voluntarism, even when supported by incentives. Publicly imposed means tests are destructive to universality and, when accompanied by a separate program for means test eligibles, almost always lead to a double standard and a "two-class" quality of care. One of the objectives of a national system must be to end such discrimination.

2. *Equitable financing, with multiple sources of funds funneled through a single mechanism.* Only in this way can universal coverage of the population be assured. Sources of funds should include a balanced array of employer and employee payroll taxes (including taxes on self-employment income and other individual nonwage income) and general revenues, all centrally collected through one instrumentality and intended for all beneficiaries. This does not mean centralized administration of insurance or of program benefits; we refer only to tax collection and provision of an overall fund.

---

*Excerpt from H.M. Somers and A.R. Somers, "Major Issues in National Health Insurance," presented to Sun Valley Health Forum, 1971; published in *Milbank Memorial Fund Quarterly* L (April 1972): Part 1, pp. 177-210.

3. *Comprehensive and balanced benefit structure.* Comprehensive protection is a relative term in medical care. Nobody believes it is possible or desirable that the program furnish 100 percent of all legitimate health services and goods. The goal is to eliminate, within practicable limits, financial barriers to needed health care without resort to means tests. At the present time, therefore, comprehensive benefits are considered to mean approximately 75-80 percent of the average family's health care expenditures. If furnished in an appropriate mix, this will rarely result in an impossible burden upon families.

4. *Incentives to maximize efficiency and effective use of resources and to discourage health care price inflation.* All insurance is threatened by lack of restraint on the part of both providers and consumers because the necessary money appears forthcoming without immediate visible strain on individuals. Coping with this danger is one of the most important and difficult challenges for a successful national scheme. The primary difficulty is in dealing with providers, who are the major determinants of cost and utilization.

Similarly, hospitals must be induced to make more productive use of personnel and to avoid unnecessary facilities and services. The Medicare experience has made it abundantly clear that open-ended cost reimbursement to hospitals and other institutions establishes disincentives for efficiency and economy. Substitute devices, such as prospective negotiated rates, are being experimented with; and others can be developed. However, any "one correct method" of paying either physicians or providers should be avoided. Frozen universal legislative prescriptions can be self-defeating.

Incentives should also be directed at consumers, including small nondeterrent copayments and identifiable tax-related benefits, as in the Social Security system.

5. *Pluralistic and regulated competition in underwriting and administration.* Monolithic government operation of a field so sensitive, complex, and rapidly changing, for a diverse continent of 206 million persons, is likely to bog down in bureaucratic rigidities or to become excessively vulnerable to political caprice and manipulation. Too little is yet known about "best ways" of delivering care to permit completely centralized decision making with its inevitable demands for universal conformity.

All possible resources and experience will need to be harnessed to make the system operable. Competitive underwriting by a limited number, but wide variety, of private carriers, regulated by controlled centralized funding and standards—along the lines of the Federal Employees Health Benefits Program (FEP)—could provide decentralization, reduction of political vulnerability, and incentives for competitive innovation in both quality and cost controls. (More will be said on this point further on.) It may also be desirable to have a government agency as one of the carriers.

6. *Consumer options in respect to carriers, providers, and delivery systems, as far as geographically feasible, on an informed, meaningful basis.* A sense of choice is necessary not only to promote satisfaction and acceptance but also to develop a responsible attitude toward the use and abuse of the services offered.

The best of the prepaid group practice plans insist that enrollees have at least a dual choice, between joining them or some other type of insurance plan, both initially and at periodic intervals. But so-called "free choice" can be fictitious, unless fortified by information. The uninformed "free choice" available to the middle class in some communities is often less meaningful than the informed choice available, for example, to members of FEP, which undertakes responsibility for informing them on details of each of the available options.

Moreover, government should not become a "Big Brother" deciding for individual consumers which option is "best." Prepaid group practice, for example, has admirable advantages; but it is not necessarily everybody's dish and should not be imposed. It is enough for government to confine the options to a limited number of approved and accountable carriers and delivery systems on the basis of quality and responsibility.

7. *Administrative simplicity.* This is, of course, a relative matter. No national scheme for the United States in a field so diffuse and intensely personal as health care can be easy to administer. But the relative degree of complexity is important. A reading of the array of legislative proposals and published discussions demonstrates that administrative considerations generally get short shrift. They have little popular appeal. Everybody is concerned about "policy," but the problem of how to effectuate policy is assumed to be something to be left to the dull fellows, mechanics. It is little appreciated that administrative structure is itself a major policy question, and often determines the practical outcome of many other policy decisions.

Most important, perhaps, is the necessity for establishing the relationship of program content to administrative capacities. If, for example, a program's organization is fragmented into many separate pieces requiring delicate dovetailing, the administrative process may have to be so complex as to become a major impediment to effective implementation. On the other hand, the attempt to establish a single monolithic structure to control everything will result in cumbersomeness, rigidity, and unresponsiveness.

8. *Flexibility for adaptation to changing circumstances and public preferences.* Health care technologies are advancing at unprecedented exponential rates. Supply and demand structures are shifting rapidly, and the only predictable is change. The financing system must not only be readily adaptive to differing regional conditions, it must be able to shift easily in time. This requires wide administrative discretion, plural approaches, and a relatively loose system. Delivery system preferences, for example, should not be firmly rooted in basic law. Freedom of carriers to innovate and experiment should be assured.

The appropriate portion of national income to be devoted to health care cannot be firmly fixed. Worthwhile alternative uses of national income, including education and housing, will always be available; and public preferences may change. Moreover, health services do not alone bring health, and presumably it is better health that is the objective. Relative investment emphasis may need to be altered to meet that objective most effectively. A point of diminishing returns from health services may be reached as compared with similar investment in the quality of the living environment—pollution, housing, recreation, food and so forth. In the ever-present problem of rational allocation of resources we must be prepared for the possible conclusion that marginal increments to health services, in preference to other social needs, are counterproductive. The way must be left open for the public to change its priorities.

9. *General acceptability to providers and consumers.* In a free society any large public system must have a reasonable degree of general acceptance by providers of care and consumers. A system that is widely resented will be seriously hampered and could become inoperable. It could result in long term deterioration and inadequacy of resources—manpower, investment capital, and philanthropy. It could produce serious stresses that are incompatible with effective delivery of personal services. Successful innovation requires a reasonably congenial climate.

Consumers must see the system as financially equitable, administratively responsive, and consistent with the cultural norms of the community. For providers, it must assure continuation of accepted professional standards of practice and reasonable freedom within them, and also reasonable levels and stability of compensation. It would be rash and counterproductive to attempt to attain economy by taking it out of the providers' hides. Of course, this is all a matter of degree, because what is "fair" and "reasonable" is not scientifically determinable. A controlled system of competition or regulation will not and should not elicit hosannas from either providers or carriers; this would indicate imbalance. On the other hand, so would rebellion. The point is that decisions cannot be arbitrary, punitive, or unilaterally made. The process requires negotiation, bargaining, accommodation, and wide participation.

Other relevant criteria could be added, but these are central.

NATIONAL HEALTH INSURANCE AND THE DELIVERY SYSTEM

Some may feel that this list places insufficient emphasis on restructuring the delivery system. If our assignment dealt with the total problem of health services in this country, we would surely place heavy emphasis on this issue, as we have done in many previous publications.

But here we are dealing only with the development of an insurance system, a technique for financing universal coverage. We believe not only that reordering the delivery system is a necessity, but also that the insurance scheme will be most effective if accompanied by substantial changes in organization.

Remedies for all health care problems cannot be expected from changes in the financing system alone. The range of functions and issues is too numerous, varied, and complex. Other instrumentalities, private and public, and other legislation must be looked to. If an insurance system alone gets too grandiose in its undertakings, too diffuse in its functions and objectives, it will be frustrated.

The financing scheme does have responsibilities that relate to and affect the delivery system, and these are reflected in the list of criteria. The insurance system must encourage efficiency, exert cost controls, and assure responsible fiscal behavior. Cost efficiency and service delivery efficiency are interdependent. The financing system can and should stimulate and encourage innovation, experimentation, and diversity in delivery systems. But the actual decisions on how care will be organized and delivered must be left to others, including physicians, hospitals, the community and appropriate government agencies.

It is hazardous to employ a financial system to mandate or even to regulate delivery of care. For some 25 years we have witnessed distortions in the delivery system, at least partly as a result of health insurance. It downgraded primary care, drove people into the hospital, and favored fee-for-service as the method for paying providers. The faultiness of that bias has become evident and pressures are generating to emphasize primary care, ambulatory service, and capitation payment. Twenty-five years ago it seemed most efficient to concentrate most of the health care resources in the hospital. The shortcomings of that approach are now apparent. Now many feel it most efficient to ignore the hospital and concentrate resources in primary care units. Will the new biases prove less unbalancing in their effects than the old? Will the opposite mistakes be made? Will their harmful imbalances prove less difficult to correct?

Financial systems, including government programs, tend to be dominated by considerations of dollar savings, not an irrelevant consideration, of course. But the financial mechanism ought not be given exclusive or primary authority to recast delivery systems through monetary manipulation. Clearly, no financial machinery can be completely neutral in its impact on the delivery system. The larger the program the greater the impact. In a national program the danger is great that conformity to the contemporary conventional wisdom might be irresistible and change difficult to effect. By minimizing the responsibilities of the financing system for the nature of delivery systems and allowing for strong countervailing forces, we are more likely to achieve necessary balance and flexibility. [There followed a detailed critique of each of the major congressional proposals as of June 1971.]

COSTS

It is beyond the province of this paper to present cost estimates for the various proposals, but a few words about the problem may be appropriate. Each of the proposals, if enacted, would generate significant additional expenditures for health services. This is consistent with one of the major purposes of the legislation, to remove present financial barriers. It is extremely doubtful that the attempted improvements in efficiency of the delivery system will be sufficient to counterbalance the increased demand and prices. In any case, the factors affecting increased costs will take effect promptly; factors designed to improve efficiency can only move slowly.

As might be expected, the figures publicized by proponents of different plans are usually substantial understatements of probable costs, just as figures advanced by opponents often tend to be exaggerations. More important, the advertised figures are rarely comparable, because they often use different definitions of costs and may relate to differing time periods. Some of the cost figures undertake to state the total cost of the program to the federal government; some express only the net, or additional, cost to government, taking into account that some existing programs will be curtailed or abandoned; others describe the overall net additional cost to both public and private sectors, recognizing that part of the new governmental cost represents a transfer of expenditures from the private to public sectors. There are other variations.

These varying portrayals of costs do indicate that a useful analysis of program costs, individual or comparative, must provide more than a global figure. In addition to an estimate of prospective direct program costs to the government, meaningful data would also show, among other things, how much represents additional cost to the federal government (whether in tax losses or in appropriations), how much is a transfer from state and local government expenditures, how much is a transfer from expenditures in the private sector (perhaps broken down between insurance and direct consumer expenditures), how much represents new costs generated by the program itself, and the global cost to the economy. Most often overlooked are the new costs, in terms of additional utilizaton and price effects, that any program undertaken to improve or alter access patterns will generate, offset by any savings from operational economies.

Preliminary examination suggests that the total financial costs to the economy under the various proposals are not likely to vary as greatly as protagonists assert. But the differing incidence of costs, the economic and social effects of transfers and the relative effectiveness of the use of differing channels for expenditure, are all very important.

Programs wherein government contributions take the form of tax credits or deductions tend to conceal the real costs to government; they may also conceal the cost to the economy generated by the legislation. Programs requiring specific appropriations and operating budgets make costs more visible, and visibility is socially desirable. When earmarked taxes are employed to finance a program, it is obviously essential to relate the tax rates to the cost obligations of the program. A tentative analysis of the various plans suggests not only that current estimates tend to be understatements, as has already been indicated, but also that the earmarked tax programs are probably underfunded.

Monetary costs, important as they are, should not, however, be the major criterion for program judgment. A cost is high or low in relation to the desirability and value of what it purchases, and possible alternative use of the funds.

DANGERS OF POLARIZATION AND NEED FOR BALANCE

In varying degrees all the proposals examined, and many others, call for appreciable alteration in financing of health services and reflect a widespread public desire for change. Inevitable and legitimate disagreement centers on the nature of desirable change. Public debate is needed. Unfortunately, indications are that with the passage of time and the consolidation of positions, the controversy may be degenerating into a conflict based on ideology more than pragmatic considerations of workability and practicality. The issue is increasingly being presented in terms of government versus private sector. In an era when demarcations between "public" and "private" have in practice become progressively blurred, the symbolism of old ideologies remains strong. Thus doctrinaire position-taking may interfere with pursuit of the most effective pragmatic blend.

In some quarters disenchantment with the shortcomings of private insurance has apparently led to the conclusion that we must now make a complete reversal and turn the entire problem over to government. Increasingly, such advocates blame all the ills in the financing and organization of health services upon the omissions and commissions of private health insurance. This not only vastly exaggerates the powers that the industry has, or should have, but also ignores the social climate. What is now generally demanded in this field was neither acceptable nor even possible only a few years ago. The social milieu of 1971 cannot sensibly be set as a standard to evaluate behavior in an earlier and different context.

These critics tend to forget that the same errors and omissions they attribute to private health insurance were also made by government. The failure to develop effective controls over costs or to restructure the delivery system is just as true of government programs—Medicare, Medicaid, Champus—as it is of private health insurance, and for the same social reasons. The effect of fragmented insurance policies upon fragmentation of health services is as true of Medicare as it is of Blue Cross-Blue Shield. The unhappy consequences of ineffective state regulation of insurance are certainly in large part attributable to the federal McCarran Act. No automatic solutions are to be found in doctrinaire formulas regarding the preferability of public versus private operations.

It has long been known that monolithism contains the seeds of stagnation. Large bureaucracies, in or out of government, tend to become routinized and tradition-bound in method and outlook unless challenged by the enterprise of other forces. Historically, government has been most effective at picking up and advancing ideas and programs that have started elsewhere and won support, or that need assistance against sluggish or inadequate responses in the private sector. The cutting edge of a new movement is usually in the venturesomeness of relatively small and often new organizations. These stimulate government action, just as government stimulates private institutions to change by inducing fear of government retribution.

Too little is yet known about "right" ways of organizing health care to chance the freezing of any particular patterns. Right now the most significant organizational reform being advocated is the nationwide development of prepaid group practice, based largely on the success of the Kaiser Foundation Health Plan. We fully share the enthusiasm for the Kaiser-type program (although the Kaiser people themselves protest that more is being claimed for it than can yet be validated). It should be recalled, however, that Kaiser emerged from small beginnings in the private sector and persisted against the impediments of governmentally-created legal restrictions as well as the stubborn opposition of organized medicine. Had a unitary system existed in the 1940s, it seems doubtful that a Kaiser scheme could have gotten off the ground. Good as the Kaiser plan is, it will undoubtedly not prove to be the final word in health organization for the distant future. From whence will the next generation's innovators, like Kaiser, get their launching leverage?

We do not have to abandon all the assets of private initiative to obtain the advantages of governmental financial strength, social equity, or democratic control. Nor is it necessary to bind the hands of government to harness the capacities of the private sector in the public interest. We can assimilate both to mutual advantage.

Government undoubtedly must assume resonsibility for financing health care if universal and equitable access are to be assured. The doctrinaires at the other extreme, whose traditional fear of direct government involvement causes them to fabricate patchwork schemes to avoid all government control, end up with programs that are grossly flawed and, if adopted, would likely backfire upon them.

We doubt that there exists in the United States the managerial competence to administer a unitary all-inclusive system of continental dimensions dealing with such sensitive personal servies. We doubt that the political system could withstand the strains of the inevitable multitude of complaints, dissatisfactions, demands, and misfortunes of the entire health system heaped on it alone. To achieve its objectives, government needs help from the private sector.

- It needs the managerial expertise and experience of the private sector, if only for purposes of effective decentralization and exposure to varieties of administrative alternatives.

- It needs the diversity and competitiveness that capacity for risktaking, innovation, and experimentation make possible. Rationalization of the system will require such attributes.

- It needs the political protection of a spread of responsibility and blame for mishaps.

- It needs the involvement of large portions of the private sector to make possible broader understanding and tolerance of the immense difficulties of running such a system.

- It needs the support of such groups as a counterforce to the tendency of governmental budgets for human services to become unduly restrictive.

It is equally true that the private sector needs government to provide the necessary financial strength and stability and to assure universal and equitable coverage.

Rigid attempts at categorization of private and public sectors are obsolete. The challenge is to work out mixed structures that can effectively take advantage of the potentials for cooperative action and competitive initiatives. These are not incompatible; at their best they are complementary. Perhaps it might be called a system of "complementary abrasiveness." Progress does not come in neat fully harmonious packages, but more often from the clash of conflicting ideas, approaches, and needs. Necessary and flexible "trade-offs" in response to differing needs and desires will prove feasible only if room is permitted for diversity, plurality, and private drives in competition for government funds and approbation.

With polarization both sides tend to see less and less merit in the position of the other, and each becomes persuaded that no acceptable accommodation is possible. In a discussion of his and the Administration's plans, Senator Edward Kennedy was quoted as saying, "The most basic difference is that the Administration relies on the private health insurance industry while we rely on the Social Security approach. I don't see how there can be compromise on that issue." Probably private insurance spokesmen would utter similar sentiments.

The fact is that the Social Security approach *can* be reconciled with use of private insurance instrumentalities, although obviously some accommodation will be required on all sides. In fact, with good will, an approach can be developed that borrows significant elements from all the major proposals. The following section will undertake to delineate the broad outlines of one such possibility. The plan is built upon the general approach of the Federal Employees Health Benefits Program (FEP), which now covers over eight million people and has been operating for over a decade—a significant practical experience with a vital public-private mix.

We do not attempt to spell out details because it is not our purpose to peddle a particular plan, but rather to suggest a practical avenue of reconciliation that is workable and effective in its own right. It adheres as closely as possible to the principles enunciated in the above list of criteria.

A NEW PROPOSAL

A national health insurance program would be established to cover the entire civilian population without distinction as to income or contributions. Such universal coverage would be supported by a single national fund, financed by a combination of (1) taxes on employment and self-employment earnings and individual nonemployment income; (2) employer payroll taxes; and (3) federal general revenue. The program would be adminsitered by a federal national health insurance board or agency.

A national minimum standard of benefits, by scope and amount, would be established based on an expansion of benefits now covered under Medicare. The initial expansion would aim to cover about 60 percent of an average family's health care expenditures and move, in easy stages, toward 75 percent. Physicians' and dentists' visits and most prescription drugs would be subject to limited flat-sum copayments.

As in the FEP, a limited number of insurance carriers would participate as underwriters and operators of their own plans. Such carriers could include Blue Cross-Blue Shield, prepaid group practice plans, consortia of insurance companies, medical society foundations, and others. Participating carriers would have to be approved by the board on the basis of standards of operation, and participation would be subject to periodic review.

It is probably desirable that among the approved carriers should also be one federal program available to all. Among other advantages, such a program would serve as a yardstick. Each carrier's plan would be required to meet the minimum benefit standards established by the board or by law.

All persons would be free to choose any approved carrier, available in his area, for his insurance coverage. Opportunity to change would be available at specified enrollment periods. The board would have responsibility for supplying all persons with complete and understandable information regarding their options, presenting each available choice in uniform and nonpreferential style. Carriers could not advertise or engage in direct selling. They could, of course, sell additional protection.

The board would allocate, from the central budget for which it would have responsibility, to each carrier an annual sum based on the number of persons (or families) who had selected it. These sums would represent the "premium" payments for all its enrollees. No additional premium charges would be made. This total premium would be related to the demographic and socioeconomic composition of each carrier's enrolled population. The aim would be to provide each carrier with actuarially equivalent capitation payments. The rates would be negotiated between the board and the carriers.

Each carrier would be free to experiment with reimbursement methods to providers and to develop its own controls. It could, if it wished, contract with medical groups, hospitals, foundations, or other plans for delivery of services. Inasmuch as each carrier would be operating with a controlled total budget, from which it might derive a profit, or loss, or break even, it should have a strong incentive to promote maximum efficiency and economy in its own operations as well as among providers. The carriers would also be permitted to join together to negotiate uniform reimbursement rates with health plans or institutions without violation of antitrust laws.

The carriers would be relieved in good part of their former heavy jobs of direct selling and premium collection and, therefore, could concentrate on service functions and provider relations. They could use any surplus to enrich the minimum benefit package and thus provide a competitive incentive for attracting additional enrollees in the next registration period.

The board's administrative responsibilities would include approval of participating carriers, determination that benefit standards are met, conduct of enrollment elections, determination of the annual national health insurance budget, allocation of annual payments to carriers, and provision of an appeals procedure for consumers and providers. It would not operate any specific insurance plans, nor handle claims, nor itself undertake to determine or impose changes in health services delivery. It would, however, in its regulations have to cooperate with the decisions of the appropriate government health agencies regarding the quality, organization, and delivery of health services.

Even though the program would be financed from earmarked funds, segregated in a health insurance trust fund, the amounts to be turned over to the board for its budget would be subject to a biennial appropriations act of Congress. (The precedent for this is in the Social Security and unemployment insurance laws.) This will avoid freezing the national commitment for health services or tying the nation to a level of expenditures predetermined by established tax rates. It will require keeping Congress informed, permit Congress to evaluate costs in relation to other social needs, and facilitate expression of changes in public preferences.

These are the plan's essentials. As can be seen, it incorporates important elements from most of the major legislative proposals. We do not anticiapte that most protagonists of other plans will promptly cry "hurray;" none will get precisely what he is asking for now. Yet it is a design that all the vital parties at interest can live with.

Labor, the major constituency for the Kennedy proposal, gets a program based on Social Security financing principles, nondiscriminatory universal coverage, and controlled budgets—all among its top priority considerations. The private insurance industry remains in competitive business with its overall volume significantly increased. The small, fly-by-night, and dubious enterprises that are among the thousand or more current carriers will be virtually eliminated, but that would probably be true under any national program with standards and could prove a boon to the better companies.

Physicians and other providers remain free of direct government control or having to deal directly with government as their payer—one of their major concerns. Organizational change is not imposed on the delivery system through a government insurance fund. Employers are not faced with a mandatory obligation for 75 percent of premiums, (as required by the Administration plan), potentially prohibitive to small or marginal employers. Most consumers are assured enlarged and more meaningful free choice.

Equally important, such a plan reserves maximum flexibility for future change. If underwriting and operation by private insurors should not work out satisfactorily, it would not require any cataclysmic change in design to eliminate that feature and use government instrumentalities exclusively. On the other hand, if the private carriers' role proved salutary under the new conditions, their functions could be broadened. Except for the central financing feature, which is inescapable for any plan that aims at universal coverage without a means test, this design gives no irretrievable hostages to fortune.

The overhead economies in administration should be substantial. Centralized collection of tax contributions, reduction in sales promotion, commissions, and also in problems of determining benefit entitlement could result in savings of many millions. Yet this can be achieved without building a new massive federal bureaucracy.

In the important years before such a program takes effect, while its specific provisions are being debated and during its administrative lead-time after passage of the law, anticipation of such a pluralistic competitive program should be conducive to greater experimentation with improved methods of delivery as well as better insurance techniques. On the other hand, anticipation of a monolithic program would discourage new undertakings and lead to a mood of simply waiting for word on what the government wants, a mood unfortunately already visible in some quarters. Anticipation of a government "cop-out," leaving things as they are with a subsidy added, could have similar effects.

It is useful to recall that spokesmen for the Kaiser Foundation Health Plan, the model that many of the leading reformers and NHI advocates seek to emulate, advocated a general FEP approach for the Medicare law when it was being debated. Its president, Dr. Clifford Keene, in urging Congress to revise the proposed bill along FEP lines, said:

> From the viewpoint of promoting sound public policy, the advantages of this approach are substantial. It will effectively implement the concept of significant choices which are fundamental in our society. It will preserve the opportunity for variation and experimentation on which continuing improvements in the organization of health care services depend. It will permit different kinds of health plans to continue covering aged members, and it will permit direct service plans to continue doing this in a manner which stresses quality medical care under a system with built-in incentives for controlling costs.

The general point is even more valid today for effective national health insurance. ...

Chapter Six

Rationalizing the Delivery System: Approaches to Comprehensive Care

In the drive to remove financial barriers to access to health care, most advocates denied, until the late 1960s, any intention to influence methods of delivery. Many did not recognize the inevitable relationship between financing and organization. Some who did felt that organization was of secondary importance; in any case it would be impolitic to stress any such issues because it would jeopardize chances of obtaining financing legislation. Thus, the Medicare law contains a specific statutory injunction against "any supervision or control over the practice of medicine or the manner in which medical services are provided." The only general exception was provided by leaders of prepaid group practice who argued and demonstrated that financing and organization were, and should be, linked.

In fact, the influence of health insurance on health care was visible long before Medicare (Selection 17). The billions of new money, produced by Medicare and Medicaid, and government-guaranteed full reimbursement to providers, vastly magnified such influence. Medicare forced a desirable upgrading of quality among inferior hospitals, nursing homes, and home health services. But almost all were affected by the heady atmosphere of easy money. New institutions multiplied. Old ones were enlarged and subdivided into new departments, services, and programs. Most doctors strove to become specialists, and ordinary hospitals strove to become tertiary care centers. All wanted to be self-sufficient. Primary care and family practice seemed on the verge of disappearing.

Fragmentation was not a new problem. The advent of new programs and monies intensified a process that had long been developing as a result of expanded knowledge and proliferation of specialism (Selection 9). However, the additional resources made it easier to allow the scientists, specialists, researchers, medical centers, and others, each to "do his own thing." By the end of the 1960s, patients were complaining that their care was more "fragmented" and more complicated to obtain than ever. It was also clear that the fragmentation was contributing to the cost spiral.

But even after such splintering is recognized and deplored, it is extremely difficult to assemble or reassemble the pieces. Aside from the intellectual problem of what needs to be done and how, there is the practical problem that nobody is in charge, nobody with the responsibility or authority to rearrange the pattern. Neither the specialists nor hospitals believe in or advocate fragmentation; but, like most other people and institutions, they fervently fight any loss of their own autonomy.

No informed approach to this problem would urge a self-defeating retreat from technological progress or abolition of specialization. Yet it is widely recognized that if the advantages of specialism and high scientific competence are to be made practically available to the patient in some coherent fashion, and if some modicum of control on costs is to be exercised, the pieces of the jigsaw have to be organized and responsibly coordinated. This objective has come to be known as "comprehensive care." The concept implies far-reaching adjustments in both organization and financing, systemization, and an effective coordinating force—one reason it is so controversial. In the late 1960s this goal was primarily the mission of "voluntary planning" and a subject of lively debate.

Selections 30 (1971) and 31 (1972) describe and illustrate one concept for such a system using the *de facto* center of medical care, the hospital, as the responsible coordinating force. Selection 32 (1971) discusses and compares three prominent alternative models. Selection 33 (1974) describes one medical center which successfully embodies the hospital-based model. It goes on, however, to report that the promise of progress in that direction was not materializing, the movement apparently deflected by a multitude of obstacles, including the apparent inability of most hospitals to contain costs and to adapt to the needs of primary care. Selection 34 (1976) narrates some other salient developments in the struggle for rationalization and control that marked the late 1960s and early 1970s.

Selection 30

The Hospital as Center of Community Health Services: A Proposed Model*

In a country with the size and diversity of the United States it is not surprising that no one method for the delivery of health services has won universal approbation. The particular form that is dominant in any given community depends on many local factors, including the socioeconomic status of the patient population; the number, quality, and organization of physicians; the presence or absence of a medical school; the organization and outreach of the community hospital; the presence or absence of neighborhood health centers, nursing homes, and other health facilities; methods of financing; and the relative role of public and private institutions.

---

*Excerpt from A.R. Somers, *Health Care in Transition: Directions for the Future* (Chicago: Hospital Research and Educational Trust, 1971), pp. 99-108.

THE ULTIMATE AIM: COMPREHENSIVE CARE FOR ALL

Despite this diversity, there is a growing consensus among providers and consumers alike that both the organization and financing of health care should be so ordered as to assure to all Americans something called "comprehensive care." It is not possible to define "comprehensive care" to the satisfaction of everyone, any more than we can define precisely what we mean by "democracy" or "freedom." It is possible to identify a number of essential conditions without which comprehensive care cannot be provided. Here are four:

   1. Every individual must have access, as needed, without financial or other barriers, to the whole spectrum of health services—preventive, advisory, rehabilitative, and long term care, as well as diagnostic and therapeutic—through organized referral channels that do not break the primary personal relationship, do not require unnecessary duplication of diagnostic tests or other services, and provide complete and continuous records of all medical and other health-related information.

   2. Every individual must have access to a meaningful personal relationship with at least one health professional, preferably a primary physician or a specialist who can provide the necessary general coordination and continuity. Where this is not possible, he should have access to a professional physician-surrogate who would be responsible for his health records and for coordinating the various specialty services.

   3. There must be enough doctors, nurses, and other health personnel to effect points 1 and 2.

   4. Every physician and other health professional should be subject to an organized system of professional discipline or peer review involving the quality, quantity, and price of services rendered. Every health institution must be subject to some form of price discipline—through market competition, public regulation, or a combination of both.

Not everyone will agree with this approach to the definition of comprehensive care. Some may say it is too broad to be meaningful; others may find it too rigid. With a concept such as this it is neither possible nor necessary to achieve complete agreement. What is essential is enough consensus to enable us to move from the philosophical to the practical plane so we can begin to determine the necessary modifications in the present delivery system or "nonsystem."

We here suggest a redefinition of the role of the hospital as center of community health services, which could go a long way toward facilitating fulfillment of the four prerequisites and thus the achievement of communitywide comprehensive care.

THE CENTRAL ROLE OF THE HOSPITAL

An essential point must be emphasized from the outset: In referring to the hospital, we are not talking about a physical plant but about a complex social organization, including trustees, medical staff, administration, nursing service, and so forth. In Ray E. Brown's words, the hospital should now be viewed primarily as an "organizational arrangement." But what makes it different from "other organizational arrangements," for example, the Garfield system (Selection 32), is that it is not just an abstraction. The hospital is a living, dynamic embodiment of centuries of scientific and humanitarian efforts, an amalgam of often conflicting, but basically complementary, community and professional pressures.

It is proposed that this unique institution, which has emerged as the principal workshop for most of the health professions and could become the community health center, should now actively seek and be officially assigned the role of organizational catalyst, referral center, and professional monitor of the quality and quantity of care rendered not only on its own premises but also throughout its community.

The proposal that it play the central role does not mean that all community health services actually would be provided within its four walls. On the contrary, the community health system of the future not only will call for fewer acute beds per capita than at present but also will stress physical decentralization for all services except those that actually require sophisticated technical equipment and highly specialized personnel. There will be increasing emphasis on neighborhood health centers, which will be located in affluent as well as underprivileged neighborhoods, on private group practice clinics, on first aid stations in isolated localities, on good long term care facilities, and on home health programs.

But the hospital, as the broadest-based source of authority in terms of professional, technical, and financial resources, the site where professional needs and values and community needs and values meet and can be reconciled, will be assigned responsibility for assuring the essential functional and organizational relationships—through satellite units, affiliation agreements, interinstitutional contracts, etc.—to make the complex and interrelated system work for the entire community on a predominantly voluntary (nongovernmental) basis.

This means that the hospital will become both the primary operational center for community health services and the primary center for comprehensive health planning at the community level. Combining of operational and planning responsibility is essential if comprehensive health planning is to be meaningful at the point of actual delivery.

It is true that many hospitals, perhaps most, are not yet prepared—in terms of experience, skills, financing, or even philosophy—to meet such a challenge. But many others, including some of the large, pace-setting institutions, are clearly moving in this direction. So are the American Hospital Association, the Catholic Hospital Association, and many state associations. Given adequate encouragement, moral and political as well as financial, most of the industry would probably be prepared to follow suit.

Moreover, this proposal is not as revolutionary as it may first sound. Increasingly, public opinion and the law are holding the hospital responsible, even legally liable, for the quality and quantity of care rendered within it. This responsibility is increasingly being assumed and, with varying degrees of effectiveness, discharged by a network of hospital-based professional review and audit committees. Thus far, this responsibility and the system of professional review have been limited to care actually rendered on the hospital premises. It is now proposed that this responsibility be extended to care throughout the hospital's entire service area, including care rendered in satellite clinics and neighborhood health centers, mental health clinics and rehabilitation centers, nursing homes, home health programs, by visiting nurses, and even that rendered by affiliated physicians in their private offices.

The concept of grouping community health facilities around the community hospital and the latter's affiliation with a regional teaching hospital or medical center has been advocated by health care authorities for three or four decades. Such a development was implicit in the report and legislation that led to the Regional Medical Program in 1965. It was explicitly recommended by the National Commission on Community Health Services in 1967 and many of the nation's leading hospital and health care authorities.

ILLUSTRATIVE PROJECTIONS

What do the words "organizational catalyst," "referral center," and "professional monitor" mean in practice? In a country of this size, with wide regional and cultural variations, they will mean different things in different places. At the risk of oversimplification, here are two illustrations—two imaginary hospitals operating in the context of the proposed model a few years from now. In projecting these examples, an evolutionary development has been assumed, with all this means in terms of some continuing irrationalities, rather than a drastic revolutionary overhauling of our present nonsystem—an overhauling that might well lose more than it would gain.

Mercy Community Hospital

Mercy is a community hospital, one of six serving a highly urbanized city of about 500,000. Urbanton does not really need six hospitals. Three would probably be enough and more in line with the national trend to fewer, larger institutions. However, until recently, there were seven separate hospitals in this community and the reduction to six, by merger of two, represents progress.

Mercy has about 350 beds, a first-class surgical service, an intensive care unit, a coronary care unit, and a renal dialysis unit. The department of ambulatory services includes most of the usual specialty clinics, a physical rehabilitation service, a geriatric clinic emphasizing psychiatric services, a well-developed social service, an excellent emergency department, and a first-class primary care unit. There are no inpatient pediatric or maternity services.

In addition to these central facilities, Mercy operates a 200-bed extended care facility (ECF) a few blocks away; two neighborhood health centers one mile and three miles from the hospital, respectively; and an extensive home health service. It has referral agreements with two additional ECFs, several nursing homes, and a community mental health center. Most of its nonprofessional services—laundry, dietary, housekeeping, business operations—and most of the routine laboratory work are provided through a multihospital corporation contracting with the six hospitals.

The medical staff consists of approximately 150 physicians, about 50 of whom are full time. These include the medical director, director of professional education, director of community medicine, and chiefs of all the major services; radiology, pathology, anesthesiology, physical medicine, and psychiatry departments *in toto;* and the staffs of the emergency department, primary care unit, and the two satellite neighborhood health centers.

Most of the doctors have their offices in the medical arts building situated next door to the hospital and owned by it. The largest suite is occupied by the Mercy Medical Group—a separate organization of 35 physicians. The rest of the building is occupied by doctors in varying degrees of combination, mostly two- or three-man partnerships. Nearly all—except for the obstetricians and pediatricians—have their primary affiliation with Mercy, although many have joint appointments in other hospitals as well.

Mercy's primary concern is patient care, but it has also become an important clinical teaching center. It is affiliated with Metropolitan University Hospital, about 50 miles away. Thanks to this affiliation, Mercy has an organized referral system for the superspecialties, easy consultation with the staff of University Hospital, close working relations with respect to its residency programs, and even an undergraduate program for fourth-year medical students interested in community medicine. This affiliation, plus the hospital's vastly increased interest in community medicine, have enabled it to obtain a majority of U.S.-trained house staff for the past few years, a situation that never prevailed in the 1960s.

Mercy's diploma school of nursing was discontinued several years ago; but it cooperates closely with a nearby community college in providing the clinical experience for a new three-year nursing school, and it also conducts numerous additional courses for LPNs, nursing aides, and various specialized technicians. The director of professional education, who presides over these extensive educational activities, is one of the busiest men on the staff.

Mercy's patient population is still not defined as precisely as some planners would like. Nevertheless, a pretty clear *de facto* service or target area has gradually emerged, particularly as a result of clearer identification of the community's primary care doctors with a single institution. Since not all the hospitals provide all services, however, there is necessarily some crossing of geographical boundaries.

The policy of institutional specialization was hotly debated for several years. There were community leaders as well as doctors who felt that every hospital should have a maternity and pediatric service, a cobalt unit, a dialysis unit, an emergency department—in effect, the whole gamut of hospital services. Eventually those who favored partial specialization prevailed. Mercy reluctantly gave up its inpatient pediatric and maternity services in return for recognized preeminence in geriatrics and the only dialysis unit in Urbanton. It continues to provide ambulatory pediatric and maternity care through its department of community health, but patients with serious illnesses requiring hospital admission are referred to the Good Neighbor Hospital, only a few miles away, whose facilities and staff have specialized in these services. As *quid pro quo,* Mercy's dialysis unit and geriatric clinic serve the entire community.

Today, several years after the somewhat traumatic realignment of programs, both physicians and community appear generally pleased with the results. Better services are being provided at less cost than would otherwise have been the case. In the late 1960s, Mercy's OB service was running an occupancy of about one-third, Good Neighbor's about one-half. Today, the latter's OB rate averages close to 80 percent—about as high as a maternity service can be expected to operate effectively.

Costs at Mercy are not low. Hospital costs have continued to rise. Fortunately, however, methods of financing care have also continued to develop, so that this high price is rarely borne by an individual patient at the time of illness. The more affluent of Mercy's patients continue to rely on traditional types of insurance, especially the combination of basic hospital coverage and major medical. Under these plans, physicians are still paid on a fee-for-service basis. The majority of patients, however, are now covered by a new type of prepayment plan, modeled somewhat after the Kaiser Foundation Health Plan and also being sold by a number of other carriers and Health Maintenance Organizations. Under its HMO contracts, Mercy Hospital agrees to provide subscribers with all necessary hospital and medical services for a flat monthly fee. As far as medical services are involved, some, for example those in neighborhood health centers, are provided by salaried doctors. For others, the hospital subcontracts with the Mercy Medical Group. Inpatient maternity and pediatric services and highly specialized services such as open heart or brain surgery are purchased by Mercy on behalf of these patients from other institutions with which it has referral agreements.

The financial arrangements are complicated and probably more expensive than if provided under a single national plan. The institution of a capitation or a flat fee-per-person payment for hospital and medical costs and their integration into a single program have helped considerably to make doctors more cost conscious, to force hospitals to greater managerial efficiency, and generally to restrain the rise in costs to bearable dimensions.

Metropolitan University Hospital

Metropolitan University Hospital is one of the nation's best and largest teaching hospitals, the primary teaching arm of a first rate medical school. With 800 beds it has virtually every major specialty and superspecialty. It also has a large and active department of community and family medicine, which is largely responsible for administering the network of affiliations with community hospitals and other community health facilities and programs.

Like Mercy, it also has an active ambulatory service and several neighborhood health centers. Unlike at Mercy, however, these are operated primarily as research, teaching, and demonstration units. They are relatively small and deliberately focused on the most difficult patient populations within reasonable access. For example, one center is located in a skid-row area, where drug addiction and alcoholism, combined with multiple socioeconomic problems, present University's department of community medicine and department of drug and alcohol studies with abundant "teaching material" while providing the inhabitants of this area with as good care as can be found anywhere in the country. Patient care for this grossly atypical population is heavily subsidized by the federal government.

The ambulatory center in University Hospital itself seeks to present students and faculty with a typical cross section of the population. The number it serves, however, is restricted to a number that can be dealt with at the inevitably slower pace required for patient care in an academic setting. This also helps to minimize any town-gown conflict. The costs are paid in the same way as at Mercy—partly by traditional insurance, partly by capitation plans, but in all cases with an educational subsidy. Thus the carriers and subscribers are not charged the extra cost of academic care. The patient population is largely self-selected and comes from a relatively large area of the metropolis.

University's residents and interns, as well as graduate students in public health and hospital administration and even a substantial number of undergraduates, are rotated among several of the affiliated community hospitals, like Mercy. This is particularly true of those who are specializing in community or family medicine. Conversely, residents from the community hospitals come into University at frequent intervals for conferences, grand rounds, and for a two-week residency each year. The interchange between house staff and faculty in the two types of institutions has been enriching to both and has improved the quality of patient care available in the entire area.

Primary Care Facilities

To complete the picture, one would have to give similar vignettes illustrating the organization and work of institutions that are smaller and less sophisticated professionally than Mercy Hospital. Depending on the cultural and physical geography of the area and region, these might include a small rural hospital, a neighborhood health center in a large urban area, a private group practice clinic, an emergency first aid station in a sparsely populated region or in a seasonal resort area, whose primary facility might be a helicopter or a Piper Cub, a college infirmary, a small industrial hospital in the mining or lumbering fields, or any number of other types of primary care units where emergency services must be provided on a standby basis but where the chief requirement in any serious situation is quick transfer to a fully equipped hospital.

The diversity of such institutions precludes doing justice to this echelon of the developing health care system. [More will be said about the neighborhood health center in Selection 32.] It should be clear, however, that such primary care institutions are vitally important links in the total delivery picture if all Americans are to be provided with comprehensive health care. The time for wishful thinking that we can persuade good young doctors to move into such areas on a solo basis is already long past. All efforts should be concentrated on linking these primary outposts of care to our urban hospital system. Simultaneously, the urban hospitals must rise to the challenge of assuming responsibility for these units by developing mutually beneficial satellite arrangements.

THE COMMUNITY HOSPITAL AS AN EDUCATIONAL INSTITUTION

One aspect of the proposed model deserves special consideration—the use of the community hospital as an educational resource in achieving the quantity and quality of personnel needed to assure good personalized care. The following discussion comes from Dr. Ward Darley, former executive director, Association of American Medical Colleges:

> I cannot conceive of an organization of community health services that could get along without the hospital at its core. The hospital medical staff is the community's principal guarantor of good patient care. If these staffs function as they should (perhaps it would be better to say as they could), there is no reason why the peer judgments of the quality of patient care could not be extended from the hospital itself into the community, doctors' offices, etc.
>
> Even if such extension is not in the direct line of staff authority it could come about indirectly, provided the staff took part in the proper kinds of continuing education. By "continuing education," I mean educational programs based upon the peer identification of gaps in the quality of patient care and then the development of educational programs directly aimed at correcting these gaps. Depending upon the circumstances, these programs would be aimed at the whole staff, part of the staff, or even a single individual. The continuation of staff membership should depend upon participation in this educational activity and also upon demonstration that said education has corrected the difficulty....

Of basic relevance is the development of hospital records that can be used for teaching and learning as well as the evaluation of patient care. Dr. Lawrence L. Weed of the University of Vermont is well along with this development, and he and people he has trained are now available to help any hospital staff learn how to do this.

The standard format of these records could be used by all hospitals in a given community and by physicians in their offices. The result would be records that would mean the same thing to different people and pave the way for allied health personnel to fill identified areas of responsibility, as members of a patient-care team headed by physicians, and making proper entries on the chart so that the doctor or anyone else can quickly ascertain the patient's situation at any given time.

The implications of this type of continuing education and record-keeping go far beyond the medical staff. If the staff can really learn something about teaching and learning, it is then in a position to play an effective role in the education of nurses (all kinds, at all levels) and other health personnel. In the expansion of such educational efforts, teaming up with junior colleges (even high schools) and liberal arts colleges would be a natural. Also, the hospital could expect to qualify for internships and residencies and even clerkships for medical students. The student could be assigned to a qualified member of the staff as preceptor and given a great experience in the continuing care of patients, following the patient from office to hospital to home, thus developing an understanding of the natural history of disease—and of health.

The involvement of students (medical, nursing, and others) in home care would be greatly facilitated—particularly if patients who need such care could be discharged from the hospital to their homes but kept on the hospital census. The hospital could then send whatever equipment might be necessary to the patient's home, instruct the family how to care for the patient, and have its personnel (interns, residents, nurses) follow the patient in his home. Then if rehospitalization is needed, a second admission and the setting up of a new record would not be necessary.

I would also make a plea that extended care facilities and nursing homes be placed under the administrative and professional arm of the hospital—upon a nonprofit basis—and that hospital-based personnel render care much on the same basis as I have suggested for home care.

Coming back to the hospital as an educational institution, I see great possibilities in the area of public education. It could be the "schoolhouse" for part of a national program of consumer health education, an important local terminal in any national network that might be established. But a good part of the program should be "homemade" so that the "student group" will feel that it has personal and community relevance.

Given the proper space, equipment, and personnel—physicians, nurses, social workers, dietitians, etc.—the hospital could provide public lectures or courses on how to use the community's health and medical care facilities, accident prevention, dietary management, etc. This kind of activity would easily provide a bridge to patient care by having physicians assign selected patients to classes in weight control, management of diabetes, ulcer, etc. The activity could go further in that doctors could assign selected patients to group therapy for emotional problems, drug addiction, alcoholism, etc.

The community hospital could well serve as the usual point of entry into a community's system of medical care.... The principal innovation here would be the multiphasic screening clinic. The staff physician could tell new patients (except in real emergencies) to come to him after they have gone through this clinic. After the doctor receives the screening report, he would contact the patient for a thorough review of the findings, also a history and physical examination of his own. Multiphasic screening operated by the hospital would carry great implications for extending health and medical care into the area of discovery, evaluation, and management of asymptomatic disease; also into programs of health protection as well as health education.

The hospital could also play a key role as a place where the data necessary to the evaluation of patient care can be concentrated, analyzed, interpreted, and used to develop periodic environmental inventories and morbidity profiles. The input would come from patient records, multiphasic screening records, the doctors' offices, community health and welfare agencies, etc. ...

There are, naturally, debatable details in Dr. Darley's proposal. Perhaps the most exciting thing about it is that it effectively meshes the two important concepts of systemization and personalization. Such a rationalization of regional and community patient care and educational facilities and programs not only assures better patient care but also the opportunity to educate the next generation of health personnel in the personal aspects of patient care. Thus, the "system"—far from destroying personal care—provides the essential "organizational infrastructure" upon which such care can be based.

Selection 31

The Franchised Hospital*

The challenge is to develop an effective regulatory mechanism based on shared authority between federal and state governments, the health professions, and the hospital that will make limited use of essential federal power but will preserve a large degree of professional, institutional, and state responsibility. The following may suggest a viable approach.

1. Enfranchise most general hospitals as public utilities or public service corporations. Unlike the traditional utility, however, they would not only be regulated but would become key elements in the regulatory apparatus, responsible either for providing or assuring provision of the whole spectrum of comprehensive health services, at reasonable cost, to all persons in a defined community or service area. In multihospital communities, overlapping franchises would probably be necessary.
2. A hospital that chose not to take on the burden of the franchise could become a nursing home or some other type of health care facility or could continue to operate as a hospital but without certain financial advantages—for example, participation in Medicare and Medicaid—that could be reserved for the franchised institution. If necessary, tax-exempt status could be limited to the latter.
3. Require all essential health care providers, both individual and institutional, to affiliate with a franchised hospital. Physical decentralization would be encouraged. All would share a single, computerized, hospital-based patient record system. This would not only promote continuity of care but would enable the hospital's professional staff to extend its present inpatient utilization and quality controls to all community health services.
4. Unlike most of the proposals debated in Washington today, state governments would play an important role. Minimal conditions for the franchise and for state administration would be specified in federal law. But each state would administer its own program and could set additional conditions as it sees fit. Existing comprehensive health planning agencies could be utilized.

The emphasis on state and regional participation is in line with current developments. About a third of the states have already enacted hospital rate review laws and/or "certificate of need" programs for approval of new facilities. Several are considering moving to full utility regulation. The hospital industry is generally cooperating. What is missing and is badly needed is some sign of

---

*Excerpt from A.R. Somers, "Remedy for Hospitals," New York *Times*, November 24, 1972, Op-Ed Page.

federal interest—an interest directed toward helping the industry and the states assume effective responsibility. Now there is only an erosion of such responsibility.

Selection 32

Alternative Models*

The franchised hospital is not the only possible model for achieving comprehensive care. Others have been proposed, with impressive sponsorship, and should be carefully studied. On close analysis, however, it appears that there are not many serious alternatives.

Two theoretical possibilities may be dismissed forthwith. At one time, it appeared that the central role in community health care—at least the planning and coordinating role, if not the actual provision of services—could be assumed by the local health department. Large portions of the country simply lack a municipal or county health department. Where such departments do exist, they have, with a few notable exceptions, limited themselves to public health matters, ignoring the much larger area of nongovernmental services.

In New York City and several other large urban centers, municipal hospitals still provide most of the health care available to large segments of the poor. Inadequately financed, inadequately staffed, almost totally lacking in amenities, these hospitals have been increasingly criticized by professionals and consumers alike. Many are now in a real state of crisis. Efforts are being made to upgrade them, through such devices as the Health and Hospitals Corporation of New York. Significantly, however, such efforts usually draw the institutions away from city hall and toward the voluntary sector. In the end, it is the hospital, *as a hospital*, that is a rallying point for both professionals and consumers, not the hospital as an outpost of the city health department.

A few ardent supporters of organized medicine appear to believe that the county medical societies could play this role. This is equally unrealistic. Most of the societies have shown as little interest or competence in community health affairs as the health departments have shown in the problems of the voluntary sector. Both types of organization have disqualified themselves by the narrowness of their interests and their failure to realize that the delivery system of the future must be an amalgam of public and private enterprise, of provider and consumer interests.

---

*Excerpt from A.R. Somers, *Health Care in Transition: Directions for the Future* (Chicago: Hospital Research and Educational Trust), pp. 109-113.

THE GARFIELD "SYSTEM"

Another model, which has attracted a good deal of attention, turns out to be not alternative but complementary. This is Dr. Sidney R. Garfield's carefully charted patient care "system" set forth in the April 1970 issue of *Scientific American*. Drawing on the Kaiser experience, of which he was one of the founding fathers, but going far beyond it, Garfield proposes an ambitious model with heavy emphasis on prevention and the use of paramedical personnel.

His first concern is to find an effective regulator of patient entry into the health care system to substitute for the physician's fee, which he considers a serious barrier to early entry and preventive care. The proposed new regulator would be a computerized health-testing service. After health testing, the patient would be referred, as appropriate, to one of three types of program and facility—health care (health education and prevention, counseling, and so forth), sick care (diagnosis and treatment of the acutely ill), or preventive maintenance (care of the chronically ill who require routine treatment, monitoring, and follow-up).

Three of the four modalities—health testing, health care, and preventive maintenance—could, according to Garfield, be provided entirely by paramedical staff under medical supervision. Only one modality—sick care—would require primarily medical staff; and it, too, would be assisted by paramedical personnel. Garfield claims the system would be much more economical to operate, not only in terms of dollars but also in terms of even scarcer medical manpower.

As thus described and depicted in the charts, the Garfield model is an abstraction, a "system" of interrelated care modalities apart from any specific institutional setting and totally lacking any human or managerial motivating force, financial, political, or other. In his text, however, Dr. Garfield is more concrete:

> In the system being proposed a central medical center, well staffed and equipped, would provide sick care. It could have four or five "outreach" neighborhood clinics, each providing the three primarily paramedical services: health testing, health care, and preventive maintenance.

In practice, therefore, it turns out that the "central medical center" or "hospital" would be the institutional and organizational focus of his system with the testing, preventive, and maintenance activities provided in satellite clinics. Thus there is no inherent conflict between this proposal and the hospital-based model [presented in Selection 30].

There is, however, overemphasis in the Garfield proposal on structural formality and some unnecessary rigidities. Real-life patients will not be willing or able to "flow" as neatly as Garfield would like. Neither will real-life doctors be willing to work exclusively within the confines of his neatly drawn compartments. The personal element in health care is simply ignored. Nevertheless, his systems approach with its emphasis on "patient flow," has contributed an important new conception to our evolving delivery system. In a modified and humanized form, it could be assimilated into the hospital-based model and help to strengthen the preventive and maintenance aspects.

THE NEIGHBORHOOD HEALTH CENTER MODEL

In April 1970, Governor Francis W. Sargent of Massachusetts announced the launching of a new health care program for Boston's poor, under the direction of Dr. Leonard Cronkhite, director of Children's Hospital Medical Center of Boston, and supported by a number of leading Boston businessmen and hospitals. The governor described the plan as follows:

> The target population size for our proposed system would be approximately 300,000 people. They would be served by their own comprehensive program which would include neighborhood health centers, hospitals, nursing homes, and a home care plan, all under a single management. The cornerstone of this system is the primary or family care center, established where people need them—in neighborhoods and communities.... We are designing the typical neighborhood center to serve 15,000-20,000 people.
>
> These centers will accept total responsibility for providing comprehensive, personal, health services for the men, women, and children within their service areas, on a 24-hour-a-day basis. They will have the ability to select the method of care needed by the sick patient, not whatever type of care happens to be covered by an insurance policy as now exists. The care will be offered in such a way that one physician or medical team takes full responsibility for the total care of the patient and his family. The centers will focus on health education and *preventive* medical care, in order to keep people from becoming ill in the first place. They will provide first aid and dispensary services, thus answering many of the needs for those citizens who have been obliged to seek care in our already overcrowded and much higher-priced hospital emergency rooms. They will also provide a wide range of diagnostic and therapeutic services, including dental care, and—when necessary—will refer patients requiring more complex treatment to the appropriate hospital facilities.

Sargent then stated that he was appointing a special committee "to define precisely the management vehicle needed to accomplish this program. This vehicle should not be government itself but something akin to a nonprofit corporation."

Despite all the publicity, the Massachusetts plan is a modest one, limited to some 300,000 of Boston's poor. Cronkhite himself has made no claim to a national model, although some admirers have. It appears to represent a refined formulation of the basic neighborhood health center concept developed by the Office of Economic Opportunity (OEO). With 49 such centers now funded, and 29 additional centers funded by HEW with Section 314(e) money but along lines similar to the OEO centers, it is clear that this model has already become a significant factor in health care delivery.

Its most important features may be identified as follows:

1. It is directed at a disadvantaged population living in a defined geographic area.

2. The programmatic focus is on primary care, and the organizational or institutional focus is a primary care unit—neighborhood health center, family health center, etc.

3. Funding, at least in the early years, is almost entirely through government. Although some plans, such as those in Massachusetts, hope for eventual prepayment, all have started on the basis of free care to recipients, with revenue derived primarily from government grants, secondarily from Medicaid and Medicare.

4. Heavy emphasis is placed on the development and use of nonprofessional, indigenous personnel, and on involvement of "the community" in program planning and operation.

5. The hospital is not generally viewed as part of the system. While its essentiality for acute care is acknowledged, it is generally assumed that this can be provided in emergencies on a "backup basis," without the necessity for close organizational or financial ties.

6. Physicians, in most instances, are salaried. Institutions are paid—or subsidized—on the basis of costs.

7. No one is forced to come to a center. For the target population, however, "free choice" is not, at the moment, of paramount importance. Within the center, patients or sometimes whole families are usually assigned to a health care team—doctor, nurse, social worker, home health aide, etc.

The advantages of this model may be readily identified. For millions of poor Americans, who have traditionally had to rely on indigent clinics or the nearest GP willing to take them on a more or less charity basis, the health center obviously represents a big step forward—in access, quality, and, equally important, in a sense of participation in health care decisions affecting their lives and welfare.

There is another advantage. Since middle class consumers and "mainstream" providers are generally not involved, or only peripherally so, they feel less threatened by this development than by one that touches the entire community. Thus, it may prove easier to establish a totally new neighborhood health center than it would be to improve the ambulatory services in the community hospital or to alter the board of governors of the hospital.

In evaluating the general direction for the future, however, the drawbacks to this approach must also be clearly faced. While the advantages are mostly short term, the disadvantages are mostly long term. First, assuming that the goal is true comprehensive care, calling for fulfillment of the four prerequisites set forth earlier (Selection 30), it is highly doubtful that the neighborhood center model can meet this test.

There is a clear break in continuity between the primary health center services and those required when the patient must be hospitalized, even in maternity cases. In many instances, this break would be as complete as that which usually occurs when a patient from an indigent clinic is admitted as an inpatient, and is also suggestive of the traditional British dichotomy between general practice and hospital care, a historical anachronism which the British themselves are now trying to correct. As European experience indicates, the effort to play down or ignore the hospital simply will not work. It remains the *de facto* center of community health care and must be dealt with as such. To attempt to build two competing systems—one for primary care, the other for hospital care—will result in higher costs and lower quality for both.

The fourth prerequisite also appears inadequately met. Peer review of a sort is provided in many of the neighborhood health centers by their own staffs. In the beginning, idealism and the appeal of novelty and competitive salaries are likely to attract a number of excellent young doctors and other health professionals. But in time, separation from the mainstream, especially the hospital's review mechanisms, and financing difficulties will almost surely lead to second-rate care. This was the history of the union health center movement in the 1940s and 1950s.

It is not easy to reconcile these short run gains and long run dangers in such proposals. As short run therapy for a major crisis, they have clearly played a valuable role. To continue with large doses of the same therapy could be counterproductive. The answer appears to lie in reconciliation of the many positive aspects of this model with the hospital-based model. As one element in a communitywide health care system, an element uniquely appropriate for disadvantaged populations but increasingly applicable to the affluent as well, the neighborhood health center could and should emerge as an important component of U.S. medical care.

PREPAID GROUP PRACTICE*

Prepaid group practice, in the view of many, perhaps most, health care experts, is an idea whose time has come. On February 18, 1971, President Nixon singled out prepaid group practice organizations—in modified form now renamed health maintenance organizations or HMOs—as the Administration's

---

*Excerpt from A.R. Somers, ed., *The Kaiser-Permanente Medical Care Program: A Symposium* (New York: The Commonwealth Fund, 1971), pp. v-vi.

chosen instrument for effecting a rational reorganization in the delivery of health serivce.

The current official popularity represents a remarkable change from the preceding four decades when both organized medicine and government fought the fledgling organizations with numerous potent weapons: state laws outlawing "lay controlled" medical care plans, invocation of the common law rule against "the corporate practice of medicine," professional boycotts, and expulsion of affiliated doctors from medical societies, refusal to extend hospital privileges to these doctors, refusal to make available Hill-Burton funds and other aids to facilities construction, etc.

Despite the overwhelming obstacles that faced prepaid group practice in those days, a handful of sturdy plans survived. Gradually the basic principle upon which prepaid group practice is based—an organized system of care which accepts the responsibility to provide or otherwise assure comprehensive care to a defined population for a fixed periodic payment per person or per family—has won increasing acceptance, especially among providers and within government.

Landmarks in this evolutionary development include a series of United States and state supreme court decisions finding the medical societies guilty of restraint of trade and ordering them to stop boycotting the maverick organizations; a New York state law specifically prohibiting denial of hospital privileges to doctors because of affiliation with a group practice plan; the Report of the AMA Commission on Medical Care Plans (Larson Commission) adopted by the House of Delegates in 1959, affirming the patient's right to free choice of medical plan as well as individual doctor; passage of the Federal Employees Health Benefits Program (FEP) in 1960; and the laudatory endorsement of prepaid group practice by the National Advisory Commission on Health Manpower in 1967.

Under the FEP, for the first time a government agency—other than the courts—adopted a policy of benevolent neutrality vis-à-vis prepaid group practice and enabled the consumer freely to choose such coverage, if he wished and if available in his locality.

As a result of these and related developments, prepaid group practice gradually shook off its professional stigma. Over the years additional plans were started, and the membership gradually increased to several millions. The exact figure varies depending on the definition. If the count is restricted to plans open to the general community and providing comprehensive care, there are only about 20 (25 if Kaiser is counted as six) with less than four million members. If, on the other hand, all the plans serving special union or employee groups are counted, the number is about 125 with a total membership on the order of eight million.

The reasons for this less-than-dramatic rise in enrollment have been widely debated. Opponents claim that the majority of both providers and consumers still find this type of care too restrictive. Proponents point to the continued existence—in over a third of the states—of laws prohibiting formation of consumer-sponsored plans, the difficulty of raising adequate start-up funds, and of launching any innovative method of delivery in the current tight labor market for physicians. Organized labor, the principal advocate of prepaid group practice among consumer groups, has long claimed that this method of delivery provides impressive efficiencies and economies which could be translated into lower health insurance premiums and a smaller transfer of wages into employee fringe benefits.

As health care costs have continued their spectacular rise, especially during the five years since Medicare, the cost-effectiveness argument has impressed more and more economists, journalists, and third party payers. The Nixon Administration, in particular, facing the unanticipated rises in Medicare and Medicaid costs, has officially adopted this view. This appears to be the principal motive behind the new push for HMOs.

Throughout this period—the long years of embattled isolation followed by the recent surge of popularity—one organization has stood out clearly not only for its size but for its dedicated physician corps, its businesslike management, its financial self-reliance, and its quiet (one might almost say old-fashioned) avoidance of publicity or any suggestion of proselytizing. The 25-year growth of the Kaiser-Permanente Medical Care Program to the world's largest private, direct-service health care plan, with 2.2 million members, over 2,000 doctors, 21 hospitals, and assets of about $250 million has not been easy and took place totally independent of government funding or government cheer-leading. It is a record that inspires confidence in the essential validity of the concept of prepaid group practice. But it is also one that should inspire caution in any group considering a similar undertaking and restraint in any government agency or planning body that considers prepaid group practice a panacea for the health care crisis.

THE KAISER MODEL*

Widely acclaimed by health care planners, economists, and informed journalists, Kaiser represents the most original and important contribution to the delivery of health services made by this nation during the past 25 years.

Comparing its major features with those of the neighborhood health center model, the following contrasts emerge:
1. It is directed at a cross section of the population living in a geographic area, but without the rigid geographic or income limits required for neighborhood centers.
2. Something approaching the whole spectrum of comprehensive care is provided (although specific elements such as dental care or extended mental health benefits are not available) under coordinated management and funding. There is no special emphasis on primary care, but neither is it discouraged as under the fee-for-service system.

*A.R. Somers, *Health Care in Transition: Directions for the Future* (Chicago: Hospital Research and Educational Trust, 1971), pp. 113-116.

3. Funding is almost entirely private, with respect both to capital and operating costs. Unlike most other nonprofit hospitals in the United States, Kaiser hospitals have been financed out of operating surplus.

4. Paramedical personnel are used more than in conventional practice, but probably less than in the OEO centers. There is little community involvement. Only in the past year or two have a few public or community representatives been elected to the governing board.

5. The hospital is clearly viewed as the center of the delivery system. Physicians' offices and clinics are either in a hospital or a satellite clinic. However, the real heart of the Kaiser system is the insurance plan. Both hospitals and medical groups depend on the plan for their income and for capital expansion.

6. Physicians are organized in a separate legal entity, a group, and contract with the plan to provide services for a fixed fee per enrollee per year, regardless of the amount of services provided. The amount available for payment to physicians is related to the amount required to pay hospitals. Hence, there is the much publicized incentive to hold down use, especially hospital use.

7. All enrollees are given a periodic choice of joining, or remaining in, the Kaiser plan or some more conventional alternative, such as Blue Cross-Blue Shield. Within the plan, members may choose their own personal doctor, who refers them to specialists as needed.

With its broad, communitywide orientation, a substantial degree of consumer free choice, effective integration of most major hospital and ambulatory services, effective managerial controls combined with considerable provider freedom, and the well-documented lesser use of expensive hospital care and lesser costs, many now advocate the Kaiser model as the ideal for the United States as a whole.

There are, however, other considerations. First, there is the basic fact that less than 4 percent of the population now belongs to a Kaiser-type plan. Kaiser itself, the giant of the group, has less than 1 percent. While it is true that state laws, medical society regulations and prejudices, and hospital discrimination were, historically, very important in inhibiting the growth of prepaid group practice, it is also a fact that the gradual, although still incomplete, erosion of these restrictions and considerable positive encouragement from the federal government and informed public opinion have not been accompanied by any great expansion.

Major causes for the continuing poor showing in this regard probably include the sellers market for physicians' services—resulting in high earnings, no matter how inefficient the practice, and discouraging organizational innovation; the lack of enough managerial talent and start-up money for those interested in emulating the Kaiser example; the existence of some plans of this type which have not been as efficient or successful as Kaiser; and the fear of many consumers of becoming locked into a health care system about whose quality they are doubtful.

In any case, it is clear that not all patients or all doctors would be happy in this type of setting. This means that there is no democratic way that the Kaiser model could be imposed on the entire country. To impose it in any other way would be unthinkable and would clearly defeat its purpose.

One of the prime secrets of Kaiser's success has been its insistence on a large degree of free choice on the part of its members, through the provision for periodic renewal or withdrawal from membership. If no alternative were available, however, and if the entire population were simply divided up among a series of Kaiser-type plans, such choice would not be available; and consumers would be effectively locked in.

In the projection of Mercy Community Hospital, it was suggested that prepaid group practice might well become the majority pattern for the future. But it was also stressed that minority patterns could, and even should, be encouraged to coexist with prepaid group practice, thus providing the discipline of competition on all types. Such competitive coexistence could be reconciled with cost and quality controls, however, only if some universally acceptable institution assumes responsibility for general coordination. This institution, it was suggested, should be the franchised hospital.

Selection 33

The Hospital Model in Action: A Lonely Experiment*

THE HUNTERDON SUCCESS STORY

To indicate that the hospital model is a real-world possibility, we can briefly examine the experience of the Hunterdon Medical Center at Flemington, New Jersey. Hunterdon is the only hospital in a large rural county (population about 70,000) in the western part of the state, half way between New York City and Philadelphia. The hospital considers the entire county as its "community" or service area. It has 195 beds, including 14 for the mentally ill and 30 for long term or continuing care, plus 22 bassinets.

The medical staff consists of 34 fulltime salaried specialists with offices in the hospital and 25 family practitioners in offices scattered throughout the county. Most of these FPs and GPs are in independent practice. But to make sure that adequate primary care is available to the entire population, the hospital initi-

---

*Excerpt from A.R. Somers, "The Hospital as a Management System," Harvey H. Weiss Memorial Lecture, Maryland-Delware-Virginia-D.C. Hospital Association, Thirty-third Annual Conference, January 7, 1974, Washington, D.C.

ated and built three satellite family health centers which operate under varying affiliation agreements.

The hospital also operates a continuing care facility, a community mental health center, a home care program, child evaluation center, methadone and alcoholism clinics, and numerous other outreach services. From its inception, it has maintained affiliation with one or more medical schools, for both graduate and undergraduate education, and tertiary care referrals. Today it is a major teaching hospital for the College of Medicine and Dentistry of New Jersey-Rutgers Medical School.

It has long been a pioneer in the development of the family practice residency. This program has been so successful that most of the FPs practicing in the county today are Hunterdon graduates.

Hunterdon's emphasis on ambulatory care has clearly paid off in terms of reduced hospital utilization. Although the population of the country has doubled during the past two decades, the hospital has increased its acute beds by less than half. By contrast, the number of full-time specialists grew from eight to 34. The hospital's average length of stay—5.7 days in 1973 (first nine months) for Blue Cross members under 65—is considerably below the average for the state (weighted for comparable mix)—7.1.

By current standards, the cost of care at the Hunterdon facilities is relatively low. The standard charge for an ambulatory visit at the Lambertville Family Health Center was $7 as late as 1973, and an emergency room visit at the hospital, $14.

Hunterdon's total budget for 1973 (exclusive of full-time physicians) was $7.7 million, including $468,000 for depreciation. Two years earlier the budget was only $5.4 million; but during the past two years Hunterdon added its mental health unit and continuing care facility. Although there was a sizable deficit in 1973 it was considerably less than the amount set aside for depreciation and was met in large part through community contributions.

In short, the hospital-health center model has not only proved acceptable to the great majority of providers and consumers in Hunterdon County, it is also financially viable. Good comprehensive health care is available to the residents of this county at lower costs than the state or national averages.

Three Basic Requirements

As one reviews the Hunterdon experience and explores the possibility for general diffusion of the concept, three requirements emerge as the *sine qua non* for success.

First, the hospital must be willing to commit a substantial portion of its professional, administrative, financial, and other resources to health care modalities other than traditional inpatient services. Many such services can be better provided in other locations and by other institutions. But all such institutions and all professionals involved in the process should be affiliated or associated with the core hospital in such a way that the patient can be referred from one level of care to another without duplication of tests, records, or costs, and with the assurance of overall quality and cost controls.

For the average community hospital this would probably mean provision of most secondary and some primary care on its own premises, affiliation with a medical school or major teaching hospital for most tertiary care, and supervision of additional primary and long term care through affiliated institutions and professionals.

Second, to develop and to operate the network of community health services contemplated in the first point, the core hospital must gradually transform itself into a communitywide "management system" with authority commensurate with its responsibility.

The definition of "community" may be on the basis of geographical or socioeconomic considerations or through explicit membership. At Hunterdon the definition is *de facto* related to county lines. As the only hospital in the county, the problem is far simpler than it would be in a multihospital community. It would probably be undesirable as well as unrealistic to expect explicit definition in terms of "districting" or some similar statutory device, immediately. However, if the concept of the hospital as an accountable management system is to have real meaning, it must push in the direction of responsibility for a defined popualtion.

Third, to acquire the authority and develop the "management system" contemplated in the second point, the leadership of the core hospital must be strong, cohesive, and acceptable to—preferably representative of—all major provider and consumer elements within the institution and within the community. The leadership must be able to unite these diverse elements in agreement on a common institutional goal: the assurance of high quality comprehensive health care to the defined population at a feasible price.

Sobering Reality: The Trend Is Contrary

In this day of growing concern over the rising costs of health care, the fragmentation of care, and the alleged irresponsibility of many health professionals and institutions, the hospital-health center model would appear to offer an increasingly attractice alternative direction to pursue. Has this been the case? How widely has the concept of hospital responsibility for a broad spectrum of health care been accepted and implemented?

In New Jersey, some eight or ten of the stronger hospitals are moving—at varying rates of speed and with varying success—in this general direction. On the national scene, one can identify individual institutions—for example, Massachusetts General in Boston, Johns Hopkins in Baltimore, Rush-Presbyterian-St. Luke's in Chicago, Mt. Zion in San Francisco, and a few others that have struggled mightily to establish good ambulatory services, neighborhood health centers, community mental health centers, nursing homes, etc.

Throughout the country one hears much talk about the hospital as a "community health center." Many institutions have changed their name to reflect this new orientation.

The American Hospital Association is concerned with its "leadership role" in the entire health care field. The 1970 report of the Perloff Committee, with its recommendation for establishment of health care corporations (HCC), was a quantum leap forward in AHA thinking in this area. The HCC concept—at least partly based on the Hunterdon experience—was brought to the attention of Congress and the general public through incorporation into the national health insurance bill sponsored by the AHA.

However, it is easy to be misled by individual citations and by general rhetoric. What *is* actually happening throughout the country? *Is* the average community hospital moving in this direction?

There is no definitive answer to these questions. The data are incomplete, sometimes inconsistent, and often ambiguous. Nevertheless, an indication of trends can be obtained through analysis of the AHA annual statistical reports with respect to the various hospital facilities and services. I recently studied these data for the decade 1962 to 1972. The results are discouraging.

For example, as late as 1972, only 6 percent of all community hospitals in the United States had a home care department or a family planning service. Only 12 percent had a rehabilitation unit. The proportion with an organized outpatient department (OPD) fell from 41 percent in 1962 to 28 percent in 1972.

By contrast, the proportion with radioactive isotope facilities and electroencephalography—illustrative of the highly specialized, technologically sophisticated, and capital-intensive services—increased from 25 percent to 66 percent and from 17 percent to 36 percent, respectively.

The decline in OPDs may come as a surprise to those who have been watching the historic rise in outpatient visits. Those hospitals with OPDs are obviously experiencing a continuing dramatic rise in utilization. This may be precisely the reason that some hospitals closed these units while others are reluctant to take them on.

The general heavy emphasis on technological services and relatively poor showing for ambulatory and outreach programs is a nationwide phenomenon. However, there are some significant regional variations. For example, hospitals in the mid-Atlantic region (New York, New Jersey, and Pennsylvania) are consistently stronger with respect to the outreach services, especially when contrasted with the south. Nearly 80 percent of the mid-Atlantic group have social service departments; only 24 percent in the west south central area. Nearly half of the mid-Atlantic group have OPDs; only about 20 percent in the two southern regions. Home care units range from 15 percent in the mid-Atlantic down to 1 percent in the west south central.

Too much should not be made of these examples. But, they are of such an order of magnitude that it is impossible not to conclude that the average U.S. hospital of the early 1970s remains pretty much what it was a decade ago—a citadel of specialized, technologically-oriented, inpatient care—probably more so. Efforts to broaden the spectrum to include ambulatory care, preventive care, psychiatric care, rehabilitation, social services, and extended care have made some impact, especially in the larger voluntary and public hospitals in the mid-Atlantic states. In most of the country, however, such services are few and far between.

Why should this be so? If the idea of the hosital as "community health center" is so attractive, has been advocated for four decades, its financial viability demonstrated, and a number of our most progressive hospitals are moving in this direction, why has there been so little overall movement and, in some respects, even retrogression?

The complete answer of course is highly complex and beyond the scope of this discussion. It may be worthwhile, however, to list a few of the major factors, without any order of priority.

1. Medical staff opposition, or at least indifference, to hospital involvement in primary and long term care.
2. The financial bias toward inpatient care that still prevails in most health insurance.
3. Resistance to giving up or reducing individual autonomy by professionals and institutions.
4. The influence of the "technological imperative" on both professionals and consumers.
5. The financial cost bind in which hospitals find themselves.

Selection 34

Redesigning the Delivery System: Unresolved Controversy*

The conflicts, uncertainties, and discontents regarding delivery of health services, indicated in previous selections, have not been resolved, probably exacerbated. The increased dimensions of the industry, continued acceleration of costs, the heavier involvement of government, and the debates over national health insurance all served to call more public attention to the incongruities, inefficiencies, and even obsolescence in traditional modes of delivering care. Threats of unionization, professional and nonprofessional, and divisive movements within professional societies were harassing the industry internally. Externally, there were rising calls for controls and reform. The industry felt it was unfairly being made the target of blame for all that was wrong with U.S. health

---
*Prepared for this volume by the authors, 1976.

care and grew defensive, but it was now generally agreed that substantial change of some sort was needed.

For a time, most forces appeared to be moving in the direction of a restructured community hospital tied into a regional network (Selections 30 and 31). This approach seemed compatible with the medical profession's increasing commitment to a three-level system of patient care—primary, secondary, and tertiary—and with technological advances in transportation, communications, and quality monitoring systems, such as the Problem-Oriented Medical Information System.[1] Generously funded public programs, including Hill-Burton, the Regional Medical Program, Comprehensive Health Planning agencies, and the availability of federally supported full-time hospital and health planning personnel could have facilitated progress toward an apparently widely accepted goal.

The American Hospital Association contributed its concept of the Health Care Corporation (HCC), a concept clearly in the above tradition but unfortunately tied to a particular form of national health insurance for activation.[2] The HCC attracted little support for either providers or consumers.

On the contrary, as indicated in Selection 33, the entire movement was derailed. Progress toward regionalization, particularly the hospital-based model, came to a near halt in the early 1970s. New voices, responding to different drummers, propounded other solutions—many, various, and discordant.

The reasons were apparent. Continuous inflation and the disappointingly slow progress of both voluntary and public health planning not only aggravated impatience with the current delivery system but generated cynicism about reforms proposed by institutions and individuals identified with the existing system. A central role for the hospital in the regional design was particularly vulnerable. As the most expensive segment, with rapidly rising costs, and the stronghold of highly specialized inpatient care, the hospital was often viewed as antithetical both to managerial efficiency and to the needed emphasis on ambulatory and primary care, in addition to the negative influences cited in Selection 33.

Many of the new critics, attracted by the growing size and importance of the industry, had little familiarity with the special historical and structural characteristics of health care. Theoretically attractice nostrums, derived from conventional and noncomparable types of economic activity, were publicized. For a time, considerable emphasis was placed on the "competitive model" as an alternative to the "regional model." There was a call for greater competition and more reliance on the profit motive as a stimulus to efficiency and competitive pricing (Selection 37), a proposal that did not elicit general public support.

The new climate did help to advance a striking, albeit probably temporary, growth of for-profit hospitals, mainly chains operated by large management corporations. To the extent that such new enterprises demonstrated the possibility of greater efficiency and flexibility in an industry burdened with "guildism" and other rigidities, it was a constructive force. Generally, however, the new chains have slowed their buying and constructing of hospitals and are now concentrating their new business on managerial contracts and consultantships with voluntary institutions.

Most of the hospital industry continued to condemn the "profit motive" in health. But even those most vocal in defense of "voluntarism" showed little practical enthusiasm for regional planning or capacity for internal reform. By and large, the hospital industry was heavily preoccupied during the 1970s with fighting off public regulation, cost controls, and the growing threat of unionization.

In part, regionalization may thus have become the victim of the backlash against hospitals. Ironically, this may have been a tacit acknowledgment that, without the hospital as its lever, regionalization could not be achieved. The backlash also ignored the fact that proponents of regionalization and the hospital-based model were simultaneously calling for a restructuring of the organization, functions, and obligations of the hospital. It could not be done away with; we could not do without it; but it might be reformed to meet new needs.

Among the earliest to challenge the coordinating role of the hospital were the advocates of neighborhood health centers (Selection 32), especially those identified with the Office of Economic Opportunity. However, the most prominent challenge came from advocates of health maintenance organizations (HMOs). This model drew support from a variety of different groups ranging the entire ideological spectrum and for diverse and often conflicting reasons—supporters of prepaid group and individual practice plans; economists who envisaged it as a means of introducing competition and avoiding public regulation; elements of the insurance industry who saw it as a way of widening policy offerings and holding down premiums in an increasingly antagonistic environment; the Nixon Administration, which saw it as a way of containing costs and governmental expenditures; and health care progressives who saw it as a vehicle for preventive medicine.

In 1970, with considerable fanfare, the Nixon Administration began to promote the HMO as the "centerpiece" of its new health care strategy; and the Department of Health, Education, and Welfare started a program of limited financial support. Near the close of 1973, Congress enacted a long-debated Health Maintenance Organization Act authorizing $375 million over a five-year period for feasibility studies, planning, and development grants and loans. To qualify, an HMO had to meet specified statutory standards with respect to range of benefits, enrollment policies, quality assurance, grievance procedures, reporting, and other requirements. An added stimulus was the requirement that all employers of 25 or more covered by the Fair Labor Standards Act must offer an HMO option (wherever such an organization exists) in their employee health insurance plans. Restrictive state laws were by-passed, and for-profit HMOs made eligible for limited support.

Controversy developed immediately over the array of mandatory standards, which were so restrictive that many were convinced that they would erode whatever stimulative effect the law might otherwise have by putting HMOs at a competitive disadvantage against conventional carriers, not subject to such requirements. It was claimed that probably no existing HMO in the country could qualify. Several of the most successful prototypes, such as Kaiser and San Joaquin, indicated that they might not even try. Within weeks after passage of the law, there was talk of amendments. A partial accomodation was made in the administrative regulations which permitted a three-year phasing-in period before all standards must be met. But in January 1976, despite almost six years and many millions of federal dollars, there were a total of 166 plans in operation, including those that predated the new drive. Only ten had been "qualified" under federal regulations, although the General Accounting Office attributed part of the slow pace to HEW's own sluggish operations.

After two years of debate over the character of necessary amendments, Congress revised the law in the fall of 1976, substantially relaxing the rigid requirements in order to improve the HMO's competitive position. No one could be sure what the effects would be. By the time Congress acted, HEW had qualified 20 plans and was clearly accelerating its pace.[3] But only some six million people, 3 percent of the population, were yet enrolled, although in local markets, where an HMO was actually available, the proportion was probably closer to 10 percent. Congress's action renewed optimism, but no longer was anybody talking of spotting the country with enough HMOs to be available to 90 percent of the population.[4]

Moreover, in 1974 the Administration's primary attention had shifted to Professional Standards Review Organizations (PSROs) (Selections 39 and 40). Despite PSRO's limited mandate—monitoring the necessity, appropriateness, and quality of institutional services to Medicare, Medicaid, and Title V (Maternal and Child Health) patients—some of its advocates, as well as many of its opponents, saw it as yet another device for reorganizing and controlling the delivery system. Their fears were unfounded. By 1976 it was clear the PSROs would have difficulty fulfilling their limited Congressional mandate.

Each of these concepts—the neighborhood health center, the HMO, the PSRO—has a useful and meritorious purpose, leaving aside the question of the effectiveness of the particular laws which attempt to give them expressions. The neighborhood health center created an organized and dignified channel of medical care for many thousands of poor who never had access to such services. The HMO is a commendable method of delivering and paying for health care which, at least in the form of its original prototypes, the authors have frequently praised (Selections 19, 20, 32). Peer review is indispensable if quality of care is to be monitored at all on an ongoing basis. Malpractice suits, however effective they may be as a warning to incompetent physicians or negligent institutions, can never substitute for continuous professional surveillance (Selection 41).

None of these models, however, can adequately serve as the central coordinating force for a comprehensive health care system. None is committed to regionalizing health care facilities and services. Neither the neighborhood health center nor the HMO can be universalized. The PSRO has limited jurisdiction and no institutional base. Moreover, these conceptions, especially the extravagant claims advanced for each, have succeeded in fractionating both the intellectual and practical movements toward rationalizing the delivery system. As of mid-1976 there is virtually no agreement on a desirable model, probably less than at any time since the beginning of real concern with the problem.

However, the underlying technological and economic necessities continue to dictate movement in the direction of regionalization with defined and related levels of primary, secondary, and tertiary care. An important recent example is the regional network system developed by HEW for the care of patients with chronic kidney disease, under the 1972 amendments to Medicare (Selection 38). Announcing the new program in April 1974, Assistant Secretary Charles Edwards said,

> To facilitate this proper balance of resources, we will certify only those networks that have the proper mix of resources. Reimbursement will be limited only to providers that are associated with a certified network.[5]

Then, looking ahead to some form of national health insurance, Dr. Edwards continued,

> If we are going to be able to assure quality heatlh care, not just for kidney-disease patients but for everyone, and if we are going to make such care available universally at a cost that the American people can afford, then we are going to have to develop the kind of rational balanced systems such as the one we have put together for the kidney program.

The debate is likely to continue indefinitely into the future, as indeed similar debates go on in nations that already have some form of national health service or insurance. This is probably healthy, as such controversy does stimulate innovation and receptivity to change. Even more likely, each of these concepts and practices and many more, including fee-for-service solo practice, will continue to live side by side—although emphasis and forms will shift and change. None will universally prevail. This, too, is probably healthy and inescapable in so large and diversified a nation.

However, this pluralistic scheme of things will have to be embraced by increased public regulation, broad enough and flexible enough to accomodate and tolerate a wide spectrum of differing structures, but effective enough to assure reasonable accountability and some control over costs—a subject to which we return in the next chapter. By 1976, P.L. 93-641—the National Health Planning and Resources Development Act of 1974—had become the nation's chief instrument for trying to bring some order into the fragmented delivery system.

NOTES

1. L.L. Weed, M.D., *Medical Records, Medical Education, and Patient Care: The Problem-Oriented Record as a Basic Tool* (Cleveland: The Press of Case-Western Reserve University, 1969); H.K. Walker, M.D., J.W. Hurst, M.D. and M.F. Woody, eds., *Applying the Problem-Oriented System* (New York: Medcom Press, 1973).

2. American Hospital Association, *Ameriplan, Report of a Special Committee on the Provision of Health Services* (Chicago: 1970); 93rd Cong., H.R. 1, Introduced by Rep. Al Ullman, January 1973.

3. *Congressional Quarterly Weekly Report,* September 18, 1976, p. 2547.

4. Department of Health, Education, and Welfare, *Towards a Comprehensive Health Policy for the 1970's—A White Paper,* May 1971, p. 37.

5. C.C. Edwards, M.D., "Remarks," Regional Communications Seminar, New York, April 17, 1974, pp. 4-5 (processed).

Part III

Inflation, Frustration, and the Search for New Policies

Part II

PART III

Inflation, Frustration, and the Search for New Policies

... our present health non-system, whose goals are to hustle money wherever it can be found by finagling the reimbursement formulae; where the senior doctors do as they please, and the housestaff can run amok with empty order pages in the medical charts; where the goal is to do something for any patient who asks for it, and to ignore those who don't ask. The non-system thrives where most managers are entirely ignorant about production decisions, the placebo effect is maximized, and resource allocation is defined by organizational power politics. The measurement of benefits doesn't matter; costs have to be justified, rather than contained. Today's health care managers have invested years in learning to play these games. It is the system we all know and love and is, therefore, the best of all possible worlds. What could be more obvious?

Duncan Neuhauser (1976)

Acute, curative, technology-dependent medicine reached its apogée in the 1960's—and, as expectations rose, so did the cost.... The next major advances in the health of the American people will result from the assumption of individual responsibility for one's own health. This will require a change in lifestyle for the majority of Americans. The cost of sloth, gluttony, alcoholic overuse, reckless driving, sexual intemperance and smoking [are] ... justified on the ground of individual freedom, but one man's freedom in health is another's shackle in taxes and insurance premiums.

John H. Knowles, M.D. (1976)

From 1950 to 1975 total health care expenditures increased from $12 billion to $118.5 billion, or 88 percent, an annual average of 9.6 percent (Table XI). The rise was almost 14 percent in 1975, with a similar estimate for 1976. In the same 25 years the proportion of GNP spent on health climed 80 percent, reaching 8.3 percent in 1975. The growth of per capita expenditures was equally dramatic, over 10.2 percent per year, equaling $547 per person in 1975.

Total costs are a product of unit prices of goods and services, size of population, per capita utilization, and the changing quality of inputs including the cost of new technology. Since 1950, unit prices have been far the most important factor in the cost rise. As the following table indicates, prices have played proportionately an even greater role since 1965 than before.[1]

Source of Increase	Percentage Distribution		
	1950-75	1950-65	1965-75
Total	100.0	100.0	100.0
Price rise	48.4	44.3	53.0
Population growth	15.0	21.5	8.7
Utilization increase, product change, and technonogy	36.6	34.2	38.3

Other data show that, contrary to common impression, utilization increases played a minor role in cost rises after 1965, and technology advances were more important.[2] American Hospital Association statistics support the Social Security Administration data above. In recent years, more than 50 percent of hospital cost increases are attributable to price rise, less than 10 percent to increased utilization, about 25 percent to growth of "nonpayroll" costs, the remainder to population and payroll change.[3]

Hospital prices have gone up more rapidly than all others. While medical services as a whole increased 39 percent faster than all other services from 1965 to 1976, hospital daily room charges rose 182 percent more sharply (Table XIV). Throughout the pre-Economic Stabilization Program period, hospital prices were increasing three times as fast as other services. When ESP controls were lifted, they took flight again. In the most recent year, 1975-1976, room rates climbed almost 15 percent. Total community hospital expenditures had their largest single-year advance in more than a decade in 1975—19.5 percent (Table VI).

The widely held view that this is primarily attributable to higher labor costs is untrue. Hospitals have indeed been increasing their personnel—from 224 employees per 100 adjusted daily census in 1965 to 298 in 1975, or 33 percent—and salaries—average annual salary per employee went from $4,072 to $8,649 in that decade—which makes all the more striking the fact that payroll actually represents a steadily declining portion of hospital expenses. From 62 percent in 1965, it dropped to 53 percent in 1975, dwarfed by the sharp acceleration in nonpayroll expenditures, especially for new technologies, contracted services, and the cost of financing capital expansion. The nonpayroll category rose an average of 18 percent a year during the decade; over 23 percent in 1975. The new technologies also account for much of the additional personnel.

The increased third party assumption of costs (Tables VIII to X, XIII) made the rises tolerable for most individuals and dampened general public complaint but compounded problems of public finance. The rapid increase in proportion of costs paid through government contributed to the budgetary crises of the mid-1970s, especially at state and municipal levels. Taxpayers grew balky. During New York City's widely publicized fiscal crisis, the mayor pointed out that $2.5 billion, over one-fifth of the city's budget, was being spent for health care.[4]

Moreover, the rise in public expenditures did not result in any decline in the private sector. While government health expenditures went up nearly 12 percent a year, 1950-1975, private-sector expenditures also went up nearly 9 percent. Medicare beneficiaries were paying out-of-pocket 65 percent more for health care in 1975 than they did in 1966, the year Medicare and Medicaid went into effect.[5] Large employers, the backbone of private health insurance, became increasingly critical. A high official of General Motors, for example, said,"there is nothing new about this concern, but never in the 22 years I've been involved in health care have I encountered such an intensity of feeling about it."[6] He pointed out that, in its 1976 model year, GM was spending over $1,700 a year on health care for every employee on its payroll, and it was announced that about $175 of the cost of the average automobile was attributable to the health care bill.

The apparent intractability of the increases in costs and prices has undoubtedly contributed more to the rising public frustration than any other aspect of health care. Gradually, the wishful thinking of an earlier period—the assumption that the industry was merely "catching up" or making up for earlier underpayment of hospital workers and relative public neglect—has been abandoned. Periodically, new culprits are named—malpractice premiums or higher quality or general inflation—but these are now met with increased scepticism.

The statistics might suggest that the providers of care should have been happy. Employment was booming. Earnings of both professional and nonprofessional workers increased steadily. Doctors' incomes rose dramatically, reaching a 1975 median of $58,440 net for physicians in private practice.[7] Hospitals, nursing homes, and other health care institutions expanded in virtually every dimension, including revenue and net operating margins.[8] The drug and appliance industries enjoyed phenomenal prosperity.

Yet, affluence brought neither satisfaction nor serenity. Providers were subjected to public protest and felt they were being unfairly blamed for developments beyond their control. There was rising anxiety over growing dependence on government financing, increased government regulation, the rise in malpractice insurance, and the enlarged role of private health insurers. These and similar disturbing uncertainties led to a widespread feeling of loss of control over their own destinies, culminating in physician strikes in several cities.

The spiraling costs and their sequelae might also have been easier to take were it not for the growing awareness that the vast additional expenditures had not contributed commensurately to improved national health. As the death rates for the 1960s became apparent, it was clear that little, if any, overall improvement was registered during that expansionist decade (Tables I and II). In some age and disease categories there was retrogression. Although there was real improvement in the early 1970s, the net effect on opinion leaders was one of disappointment.

A search for new policies was inevitable. It took many forms. Cost containment was the most frequent demand—with few expressing very clear notions of how it was to be achieved. A growing number saw government itself and public regulation as the principal villains and protested that federal controls had already gone too far, were singularly unproductive, and were at the source of the difficulties. Many still claimed that lack of adequate access remained the major problem and emphasized the unfinished business of national health insurance. Others looked to the delivery system as the major deficiency and advocated reorganization and stronger planning. For some, improvement of quality was the prime consideration; while others saw quality and cost-efficiency as inextricably interrelated.

A small but growing number began to question the heretofore taken-for-granted positive relationship between more health care and better health. They started to look elsewhere—to the environment and particularly to individual life styles—as the more significant determinants of health and more productive per dollar invested. Within the health care field itself there was a heightened groping for forms of health care that were less technology-dependent and more humanistic. More Americans began to look overseas, not to copy but to learn from foreign experience. The selections in Part III reflect this wide-ranging exploration and the diversity of approaches.

NOTES

1. M.S. Mueller and R.M. Gibson, "National Health Expenditures, Fiscal Year 1975," *Social Security Bulletin,* February 1976, p. 13.

2. Marian Gornick, "Ten Years of Medicare: Impact on the Covered Population," *Social Bulletin,* July 1976, pp. 3, 7-11.

3. Derived from American Hospital Association, *Hospital Statistics, 1976 Edition* (Chicago: 1976), p. xiv.

4. Editorial, *New York Times,* February 13, 1976.

5. Gornick, *op. cit.,* p. 18.

6. V.M. Zink, "An Employer Looks at Health Care Costs," *Trustee,* April 1976, p. 17.

7. *Medical Economics,* May 16, 1977, p. 84.

8. J. Pettengill, "The Financial Position of Private Community Hospitals, 1961-71," *Social Security Bulletin,* November 1973, pp. 3-19.

Chapter Seven

Regulation of Facilities: Moving Reluctantly Toward the Inevitable

The merits of public regulation of the health care industry, especially hospitals and nursing homes, have been hotly debated in recent years. Advocates point to the constantly rising costs (Tables VI, X to XIV) and the failure of both third party reimbursement and self-regulation via "voluntary" planning as effective instruments of control. Opponents point to the alleged failure of public utility regulation of other industries and claim the public interest would be better served through competition.

Advocates of regulation generally concede the unimpressive utility record but insist there is no effective free market in the health care industry and that price competition is impractical. Whatever the merits of this debate, a wide variety of public controls over hospitals and other facilities have been exercised in this country for years. Conflicting ideologies aside, health care regulation is now a rapidly expanding fact of life.

The transition from self-regulation and voluntary planning has been gradual but continuous, pushed by the relentless cost spiral. It took only five or six years to move from the "areawide" hospital (later health facilities) planning movement, which started in the early 1960s and was supported by Hill-Burton funds, to the Regional Medical Program (RMP) and Comprehensive Health Planning (CHP) laws of the mid-1960s. Both were well motivated but suffered from lack of defined priorities and authority. Both were still confined to voluntary planning.

Despite some limited achievements, it soon became evident that neither RMP nor CHP was equipped to take effective action against the rising costs. At about the same time, it also became clear that the hope that the enormous increase in supply of health manpower and facilities, which some economists had counted on to create more competition and slow down the inflation, was illusory. Faced with the totally unexpected magnitude of Medicare and Medicaid costs, government at both federal and state levels began to show increasing impatience with the shortcomings of voluntary planning and to search for acceptable ways of adding "teeth," or regulatory authority, to the planning process.

The states acted first, beginning with New York. Through a gradual accretion of state authority from the late 1940s through the mid 1960s, New York established a state review and approval mechanism for all new hospital and nursing home construction or significant expansion of existing facilities. Following this lead, the "certificate-of-need" concept, as it came to be known, was gradually emulated by other states and gradually other elements of a "public utility" approach—including rate regulation—were adopted in a few. However, the historic influence of voluntary planning continued to be reflected in the administrative structures of the newer regulatory machinery—a preponderant reliance on layers of committees composed of interest group representatives.

The federal government, prodded especially by the Senate Finance Committee, also became more critical and more active. In 1968, the Secretary's (HEW) Advisory Committee on Hospital Effectiveness (Barr Committee), on which the "establishment" was well represented, called for state review and approval of all new facilities and physical changes in existing facilities as a condition of federal funding. In 1969 the House Ways and Means Committee embarked on the long and tortuous legislative process which finally culminated, three years later, in the 1972 Social Security Amendment (P.L. 92-603), providing a significant array of statutory controls to be imposed as conditions of Medicare and Medicaid reimbursement. Among these was mandatory state review of construction programs (Sec. 1122), a limitation on payment for institutional costs found by the Secretary to be "unnecessary in the efficient delivery of needed health services" (Sec. 223), and limits on "prevailing" charge levels by practitioners (Sec. 224).

These amendments reflected increasing consensus that voluntarism would not work and that stronger actions would have to follow. Except for the brief interval of national wage and price controls under the Economic Stabilization Program, 1971-1974, costs showed no signs of moderating; and the fragmentation of the industry grew more conspicuous. The question as to whether this was the fault of the planners or other forces over which planners had no control had become academic.

By 1974 Congress had decided to phase out not only RMP and CHP, but Hill-Burton as well. The successor National Health Planning and Resources Development Act (P.L. 93-641) was built on precedents established in the states and in previous federal legislation but went considerably further down the regulatory road. It called for a national network of Health Systems Agencies (HSAs)—independent bodies not part of existing political entities—and endowed them with considerable potential enforcement authority. Not only review, but approval, of new and expanded facilities and services would become mandatory.

Two omissions were conspicuous. First, the law does not provide for rate review, although any state could adopt such a program on its own. (It does provide for experimental demonstration projects in six states to test alternative forms of reimbursement.) Second, the controls are confined to institutional providers; physicians and other practitioners are not dealt with directly.

Selection 35 describes and defines the major forms of health cost regulation as practiced in the states, *circa* 1975. Selection 36 is a case study of the problems and options facing one major metropolitan community at about this time. The situation has its analogues in other metropolitan centers. Selection 37 represents a specific rebuttal to the claim that increasing the number of health care institutions will create effective competition and obviate the need for regulation. Selection 38 relates the experience of one state with its certificate-of-need program.

Selection 35

Development of State Regulation*

The rapidly growing overlay of federal law dealing with health care delivery generally provides for continuation of state responsibility within a framework of federal standards and guidelines. This pattern of federal-state administration was established in the Maternal and Child Health and Crippled Children's Program of 1935 (Title V of the Social Security Act) and the Hill-Burton Act of 1946 and was followed in most subsequent relevant federal health legislation, including Medicaid, the Comprehensive Health Planning Act, the federal "certificate-of-need" provision of the Social Security Amendments of 1972 (Sec. 1122) and, most recently, in the National Health Planning and Resources Development Act of 1974 (P.L. 93-641).

By contrast, Medicare regulations provide primarily for federal administration. Similarly, the short-lived Economic Stabilization Program (ESP) of 1971-1974 attempted to assert federal regulation over all health providers. After the emergency impact of Phases I and II had worn off, however, subsequent phases of ESP were bitterly and successfully opposed by the health care industry. With the demise of the ESP, Congress reverted to the traditional pattern of federal-state participation in enacting P.L. 93-641, with the federal government assuming a greater role than in the earlier programs noted above.

It seems reasonable to expect that future health care regulatory activities will evolve primarily from existing and developing state programs, coordinated and probably increasingly homogenized through federal funding and its accompanying requirements. In anticipation of this development, the Department of Health, Education, and Welfare initiated a comprehensive study of state health regulation in June 1973. The results of this study, conducted by one of the authors, became available in late 1974.[1] This article is based primarily on those findings.

Although often overlooked, structural issues are fundamental. At the heart of all regulatory systems are the two crucial questions: Who will make the key

---

*Excerpt from L.S. Lewin, A.R. Somers, and H.M. Somers, "State Health Cost Regulation: Structure and Administration," *The University of Toledo Law Review* 6 (Spring 1975): 648-653.

decisions? How will they be made? These issues are especially critical in the health field, where basic concepts such as measurement of need, quality, and effectiveness are ill-defined and disputed, thus leaving wide latitutde and discretion to the regulatory bodies.

RATIONALE OF HEALTH CARE REGULATION

Health care regulation has traditionally been aimed primarily at ensuring that services are of adequate quality. These efforts include licensure of professional practitioners and health care institutions. With the passage of the federal Medicare and Medicaid programs in 1965, the rate of increase in health care expenditures sharply accelerated, and both public and private third party payers became increasingly interested in cost controls.

The twin problems of price inflation and possible overutilization of health care services spring from a system of incentives within an industry that has been shaped by a unique combination of influences. Foremost among these is the imprecise and subjective definition of the product itself. Equally imprecise is the definition of "quality" as applied to health care. The inability of the consumer to control hospital use, to "comparison shop" among providers, or to evaluate the reasonableness of costs are all factors peculiar to the health field. The frequent insulation of the consumer from the immediate financial consequences of rising costs by virtue of extensive third party coverage of hospital services plus the general public commitment to care for all—regardless of price—provides little incentive for consumers to resist rising prices and costs.

On the supply side, the freedom of health care providers, seldom at risk financially, to decide on the nature and quantity of care provided to consumers, together with the tradition of fee-for-service payments to individual practitioners whose fees are not demonstrably related to cost, provide minimal incentives toward efficient use of resources. Similarly, the system of retrospective cost reimbursement by third parties for institutional providers is totally devoid of cost containment incentives. Excess hospital bed capacity in many areas results in higher unit costs and incentives to increase utilization of services beyond needed levels in order to recover the fixed costs of underutilized facilities and services. Alternative delivery mechanisms which might reduce overutilization and associated costs by means of positive financial incentives are generally lacking.

[More recent factors inexorably pressing prices upward include: the rapid rise in cost of malpractice insurance (Selection 41), repeal of the voluntary hospitals' exemption from the National Labor Relations Act resulting in greater union activity and higher salaries and wages; sharp increases in construction costs; and more reliance on borrowing and debt financing.]

The interaction of these factors results in a market where the basic supply, demand, and resource decisions are made by health professionals who have few positive incentives, and many disincentives, to provide health care in an economically efficient manner. Recognition of the inherent inability of the health delivery system to contain costs adequately and to allocate health resources efficiently has given rise to numerous government attempts at "cost containment."

FORMS OF STATE REGULATION

Cost containment efforts have taken varied forms. The most common is *disallowance of specified cost items from third party reimbursement formulas*, e.g., expenditures for research and personnel education unrelated to patient care, excessive interest expense, and bad debt costs. This approach has become virtually standardized through Blue Cross and Medicare provisions and is generally based on eliminating cost items judged inappropriate or unreasonable to a specific patient class. It has been used by Blue Cross plans in 16 states as a means of discouraging unnecessary expansion of facilities and services. In these cases the Blue Cross hospital contract disallows reimbursement for the interest and depreciation expenses of facilities deemed unnecessary by designated planning bodies.

This strategy has its limits for a variety of reasons. First, as implemented, it controls classes of costs rather than the appropriate level of expense within cost centers. It is often regarded as inequitable and punitive to disallow expenditures after they are made. Insofar as it depends on Blue Cross, the plans in most states lack adequate penetration to influence hospitals significantly. In such cases, Blue Cross sanctions are without significant effect. Because of the limits inherent in this approach, increasing interest has focused on three other mechanisms for cost containment.

One such is *rate review*. This approach requires that changes in reimbursement rates be established by, or with the concurrence of, agencies external to the health care provider. There are a number of methods by which this approach may be pursued.

Most prominent are systems that set prospective rates for a health care provider to apply over a specified time period. These systems permit the provider to retain funds if efficiencies can be realized and if costs are below projections. The method also places providers at risk if costs exceed projections and is, therefore, regarded as creating incentives for more cost-conscious behavior. Of course, techniques for establishing the prospective rate, the timing and basis of payment, and the extent to which the provider is truly at risk will influence the degree of cost-consciousness induced.

A second approach is the *regulation of capital expenditures and services*. This approach is designed to discourage and prevent the creation of facilities, equipment, and new services in excess of community needs. Mechanisms of this type include direct controls, such as certificate-of-need laws, which can prevent construction or operation of new facilities or services deemed unnecessary or not financially feasible. Approaches to such regulation can also be indirect, as for example, where Blue Cross plans and governmental purchasers do not prohibit the operation of new facilities or services but penalize operators through non-reimbursement of the capital cost of such facilities.

A third method of cost containment aims at reducing overutilization of services by providers and consumers through *utilization controls and claims review*. The federal Professional Standards Review Organization (PSRO) program and Medicaid utilization review requirements are examples. In some states, Blue Cross and Blue Shield plans and medical foundations are experimenting with preadmission or concurrent certification and recertification methods in addition to the more common after-the-fact utilization reviews. . . .

NOTE

1. Lewin and Associates, Inc., *Nationwide Survey of State Health Regulations*, NTIS Accession Number, PB 236660/AS (1974). Lewin and Associates, Inc., *An Analysis of State and Regional Health Regulations, Feb. 1975: Executive Summary* (1975). See, also, Lewin and Associates, Inc., *Summary of Nationwide Survey of State Health Regulations*, DHEW Publ. (HRA) 75-611 (1974).

Selection 36

The Philadelphia Medical Commons: The Choices Ahead*

Once in a long while, an inspired writer or spiritual or political leader will capture in a simple human story or parable one of the great moral or political dilemmas of the day. Aesop's fables, the parables of Jesus, President Lincoln's homely anecdotes, and the fairy tales of Hans Christian Anderson and the Brothers Grimm are all part of the priceless legacy of the human race. Seven years ago, Garrett Hardin, a biologist, published in *Science* (December 13, 1968) an article entitled "The Tragedy of the Commons" and thereby enriched the English language and the American political debate with a significant new parable.

Hardin's concern is directed at a category of broad social problems that defy technological or individual solutions. The concept of "the tragedy of the com-

---

*A.R. Somers, excerpt from paper presented to Philadelphia Health Management Corporation, Special Meeting, October 15, 1975 Philadelphia; published by Blue Cross of Philadelphia, February, 1976.

mons" grows out of the old English practice of permitting each herdsman in the village to graze his cows freely on the village common. The practice worked well as long as both man and beast remained below the carrying capacity of the land. Once this point is passed, however, "the inherent logic of the commons remorselessly generates tragedy."

Each herdsman knows that there is a limit to the capacity of the commons to sustain the increasing number of cattle. But as a rational being, he calculates that his immediate personal gain from adding to his herd outweighs the damage to the community as a whole. The cumulative effect of many such seemingly insignificant individual decisions destroys the value of the commons for all. In Hardin's words:

> Each man is locked into a system that compels him to increase his herd without limit—in a world that is limited. Ruin is the destination toward which all men rush, each pursuing his own best interest in a society that believes in the freedom of the commons.

Salvation, according to Hardin, lies in the development of "social responsibility" which, in turn, is "the product of definite social arrangements," i.e., "arrangements that create coercion of some sort."

> To many, the word coercion implies arbitrary decisions of distant and irresponsible bureaucrats; but this is not a necessary part of its meaning. The only kind of coercion I recommend is mutual coercion mutually agreed upon by the majority of the people affected.

That is to say: regulation by an accountable public authority.

Hardin was not the first scientist, natural or social, to project such a scenario; but rarely has it been done so persuasively. The thesis has, of course, been challenged both by those who disagree that we are anywhere near finite limits on our national resources or "commons" and by those who fear government regulation more than they fear depletion of resources. Within a year, the same journal, *Science* (November 28, 1969) published a strong rebuttal, "The Tragedy of the Commons Revisited." Written by a political scientist, Beryl Crowe, the second article was far more pessimistic than the first.

According to Crowe, there are problems to which there are neither technical nor political solutions. He gives three reasons for his lack of faith in the ability of the American political process to cope with such difficult social problems: (1) the loss of a common value system, (2) the consequent inability of the state to enforce decisions even on minorities if they are strongly opposed, and (3) the corruption of the public regulators through capture by those they are supposed to regulate.

Many social scientists agree with Crowe's third point regarding the alleged ineffectiveness of public utility regulation. For different reasons, many health care leaders oppose regulation; and, in general, public officials have been loath to assume the added responsibility. Since the expiration of the Economic Stabilization Program and the brief period of relative price stability which it produced, however, health care costs are again spiraling upward; and a new sense of national urgency is emerging.

Under these circumstances, it has proved impossible for health insurance, even with the frequent premium rises of recent years, to keep up with the unending cost spiral. The proportion of health care costs that must be met out-of-pocket by publicly and privately insured individuals is again on the rise after years of decline. Contrary to our experience in the 1950s and 1960s, we appear to be into a "revolution of thwarted expectations."

Nor is the sense of disillusionment confined to costs. Consider just one fact: the average life expectancy for a Swedish man, age 40, is more than three years longer than for an American of the same age. Do not blame this on the health care system. Blame it primarily on environmental problems and the typical American life style. What is becoming increasingly clear is the irrelevance of large portions of the expensive health care we are dispensing today.

Many distinguished health authorities and economists have been emphasizing this. Such views are still confined to a minority. But, as they spread and no corrective action is taken, they become more extreme. Witness Ivan Illich's book, *Medical Nemesis,* which opens, "The medical establishment has become a major threat to health." The potential for development of a real medical nihilism on the part of opinion makers and public officials is growing. If this attitude should become dominant, it could be disastrous for providers and consumers alike.

It was inevitable in this atmosphere that someone would relate the "tragedy of the commons" directly to the medical care economy. In the July 1975 issue of the *New England Journal of Medicine,* Dr. Howard Hiatt, dean of the Harvard School of Public Health, published an article, "Protecting the Medical Commons: Who is Responsible?" which did just that. With example after example, he points out three basic weaknesses in the traditional way the medical commons has been used: (1) the assumption that one should do everything possible for, or to, the patient, even to the point that marginal benefits for the individual threaten our ability to provide adequate services for the population as a whole; (2) the utilization of scarce resources for practices that have not been clinically evaluated and may in fact benefit neither the individual nor society; and (3) the narrow interpretation of health as exclusively a medical concern, as opposed to the need for more emphasis on prevention.

Dr. Hiatt joins with Dr. Hardin in pointing out the inadequacy of *laissez-faire* as a monitor of socioeconomic priorities. But he does not propose turning the responsibility entirely over to government. Nor does he think that physicians alone should be asked to make these crucial and often excruciatingly difficult decisions. Rather, he calls for a working partnership between the physician and the public "in the creation of control mechanisms in a manner that reflects both enlightened self-interest and the public interest."

This is the only view that seems to be tenable. If, as now seems likely, the tragedy of the "medical commons" cannot be averted through technology alone and if, as also seems likely, it cannot be averted through political action alone, the one remaining hope is a creative mix of public and private enterprise, individual professional and entrepreneural initiative combined within a context of effective public responsibility, public accountability and, to the extent necessary, public regulation—"mutual coercion mutually arrived at."

One need not adopt Dr. Crowe's extreme pessimism, but it is essential to view this whole undertaking with a strong sense of realism. The chances for success are now perhaps 50-50. But the odds are not foreordained. They can be changed, for better or worse, depending on our ability to handle four major variables: (1) the extent of public and professional understanding of the nature of the problem; (2) the sense of urgency with which the problem is viewed; (3) the quality of leadership that emerges; and (4) the adequacy of the institutional and organizational structures through which the leadership will have to work.

I will try to address two of these four issues through: (1) a brief look at the Philadelphia "medical commons" and some of its major problems; and (2) a brief discussion of P.L. 93-641, the new Health Planning and Resources Development Act, the major instrument now available for averting a tragedy of the Philadelphia commons.

THE PHILADELPHIA MEDICAL COMMONS

According to a recent publication of the Philadelphia Health Management Corporation, Philadelphia is "the health capital of the nation." Several other cities would dispute that claim. Nevertheless, both historically and currently, the health and health care (it is essential to remember that these are not the same) resources of this community are truly impressive. This is a community that takes rightful pride in its historic legacy.

It is of more than historical significance that the Pennsylvania Hospital—the nation's first, founded in 1751, and described by one of our leading medical historians as "a surviving example of the best in 18th century hospital planning"—is still recognized as one of the best in America. Among your other "firsts" are the first medical school in the U.S., the first medical association—the Philadelphia College of Physicians—the first pediatric hospital, and the first and only women's medical college, now coed, of course.

The genealogy of your medical profession is one of the nation's most interesting. Your five medical schools plus the College of Osteopathy make Philadelphia one of the nation's two largest concentrations of academic medicine. When surveyed a few years ago, about 9 percent of all U.S.-trained physicians were produced in Philadelphia. The 9,000 or more physicians in the five counties of southeast Pennsylvania constitute one of the highest physican/population ratios in the nation—a precious and preciously expensive resource that neither you nor the nation can afford to squander.

Your hospital industry, with over a hundred institutions of all types in the five counties and some 26,000 beds, gave you a 1974 bed/population ratio of 6.8/1000. With some 65,000 employees, the hospitals are now reported to constitute the largest single employment group in the area. Your 73 acute care hospitals, with 18,700 beds, produce a 1974 ratio in this category of 4.9/1000 population. Your 200 nursing homes, with an estimated 17,500 beds, result in 4.6/1000.

Home care, traditionally one of the most neglected aspects of health care, received earlier and more sustained attention—both from Blue Cross and the city government—in Philadelphia than in most parts of the country. Eleven hospitals, including the Philadelphia General Hospital (PGH), have organized home care programs. The Community Nursing Services of Philadelphia with 430 employees—community health nurses, home health aides, physical, speech, and occupational therapists, social workers, and outreach workers—and its pragmatic mix of public and private fundings is one of the nation's largest and most respected home care programs.

Another way of measuring the size of the Philadelphia Medical Commons is in dollars. According to the Philadelphia Health Managment Corporation, some $2.4 billion was spent for health care in 1973 in the five Pennsylvania counties. Of this, an estimated $2 billion went for personal health services, including $100 million spent in Philadelphia by citizens of New Jersey. On a per capita basis, this works out to about $630 for every man, woman, and child during that year, 43 percent higher than the $442 national average for 1973. While most of these huge sums flow through Blue Cross and other private sources, the role of government is substantial and ever-growing.

After such figures, it is hardly necessary to add that the Philadelphia Medical Commons involves more than the providers of care. It has to be backed up and underpinned by a first-rate, high level planning and resource development capability and a set of financing institutions with the skill (some would say wizardry) necessary to translate the new and terribly expensive medical science and technology into affordable patient care.

In the five brief years of its life, PHMC has helped to develop an areawide health management information system which, together with the Hospital Survey Committee, the Regional Comprehensive Health Planning Council, the Greater Delaware Valley Regional Medical Program, the Philadelphia College of Physicians, the Delaware Valley Hospital Council, and the city Health Department, should now be in a position to provide this community with one of the best area wide health data bases in the country.

These, then, are some of your many achievements, your many assets. But achievements are generally accompanied by new problems, assets by liabilities. As I understand it, your major health care problems can be summed up in one word: superabundance, a superfluity of good things.

It is commonly accepted that you have too many open-heart and cardiac catheterization units, too many renal transplant facilities, too many operating rooms. It is no news that you have too many OB and pediatric inpatient beds.

Altogether, according to the Hospital Survey Committee, there are 900-1,000 excess acute care beds. Add to this a considerable surplus of long term psychiatric beds, and the current excess has been estimated as high as 2,000.

At the same time, about half of your nursing home beds are rated unsafe from fire and, even with these unsafe beds, there is a shortage in the city. There is a need for more alcohol and drug abuse programs and either a shortage or poor distribution of short term mental health facilities. I am not aware of any organized consumer health education programs.

Are there enough good home care programs and residential homes for the dependent elderly? There are no reliable data, but it would be surprising if there were. How could there be when most of the financial and professional incentives are weighted toward expensive institutional care? The higher-than-average physician/population ratio and the comparatively large number of doctors of osteopathy probably mean that primary care needs are met here more adequately than in many places. But it would be surprising if there were not a serious lack of coordination between the various levels of care—pimary, secondary, tertiary, and long term—and between the city and the suburbs.

There is one particularly disturbing fact: the infant mortality rate for nonwhite babies in the low income areas of Philadelphia is one of the highest in the nation. The 1969-1971 average was 36.9 per 1,000 live births, compared with an average of 33.4 for low income areas in 19 of the largest cities.

Turning to the financial side, you may soon lose your reputation for better-than-average hospital productivity as the personnel/patient ratio continues to rise. Hospital employees are, of course, just as entitled to join unions as any other employees; and I was one of the first to testify to Congress to this effect. Still, it must be recognized that the impact of unionization on a largely unprepared hospital management and the unions' failure to take more responsibility for helping to improve productivity to balance the higher wages are important factors in the ever-rising hospital costs. So, of course, is the continuing rise in the cost of fuel, malpractice insurance, and perhaps most dramatic of all, the amount of debt servicing now loaded onto many hospital per diems.

As a result of these and other problems, Philadelphia has now achieved two new distinctions:

1. One of the highest current rates of increase in health care costs in the country. A total cost rise of 23.5 percent is anticipated for the period July 1975-July 1976.
2. One of the largest premium rises for any Blue Cross plan in 1975—37 percent—with a request for an equal amount scheduled for 1977.

Many of these disturbing financial problems came to a head in the 1975 Blue Cross rate hearings. The dilemma which the commissioner of insurance faced must have been excruciatingly difficult. In his decision, Commissioner Sheppard cited "the deteriorating financial condition of the plan, saying that, without rate relief, it would exhaust its reserves by December 1 and face eventual bankruptcy." You know what that would mean not just to the 2.5 million subscribers but to the hospitals and other health care institutions that depend on Blue Cross to transform those millions of dollars of employer and employee monthly contributions into hospital reimbursement payments.

The new premium rise comes to $10.45 a month for families dependent on small group coverage, bringing their total premium to over $40 a month. This could spell disaster for some small employers as well as their employees, coming on top of the recession and general inflation. The problem is complicated by the fact that 29 hospitals have been operating for over a year without Blue Cross contracts—a situation that responsible authorities obviously could not allow to go on indefinitely.

To complicate matters even further, the area is losing population. The Census Bureau estimates that the population of the five counties went down by 1.9 percent between 1970 and 1974. Philadelphia County alone fell by nearly 6 percent. Already, inpatient utilization has been falling for four straight years as the average length-of-stay comes more into line with the national average. (It is still one day longer than the average.) The Hospital Survey Committee has projected a further substantial decline in bed needs.

There are two overriding priorities facing Philadelphians as you look to the preservation of your historic medical commons:

1. The deliberate adoption of an areawide policy aimed both at better cost containment and a better balance between primary and tertiary care, between prevention and health education on the one hand and curative treatment on the other. This should include an immediate moratorium on all additional inpatient beds and other facilities, more and better interinstitutional arrangements for shared services—for patient care as well as laundries—and a gradual transfer of substantial resources from subspecialty tertiary care to primary care, prevention, and long term care.

2. The immediate establishment, by means of P.L. 93-641 and other instrumentalities, of an effective areawide decision-making process to enable you to make these difficult decisions as objectively and democratically as possible, with due regard to the legitimate needs and values of the providers as well as the consumers, with adequate protection for the quality of care at all levels, and with respect for the fact that the Philadelphia medical commons is a state and national, as well as a local and regional, resource. What all this adds up to is the necessity for a first-rate capability with respect both to techniques of resource management and political negotiation.

THE NEW PLANNING INSTRUMENT

There are various ways of looking at P.L. 93-641. You can take a ho-hum view that it is just another in a long list of fumbling and ineffective federal efforts, over nearly three decades, to persuade the health care providers and consumers to behave more responsibly and rationally in relation to the medical commons. Or you can conclude that it provides a new and significant opportunity that has to be taken more seriously.

It will be some time before we know which of these views prevails. The official regulations have not yet been published; the national guidelines not even written. My basis for very cautious optimism depends on two assumptions: (1) the changed economic and political environment; and (2) some differences in this law compared to Hill-Burton planning, CHP, and RMP. Here are four such differences:

Authority

Unlike previous efforts, the new law has potential teeth. State regulatory functions under certificate-of-need laws and Section 1122 of the Social Security Act, the so-called federal certificate-of-need, are strengthened. States that do not have such programs are given until 1979 to participate or lose all forms of assistance under the Public Health Service Act.

Once fully operative, any application for a federal grant or loan for health facilities construction and modernization must be approved or disapproved—not just reviewed as was the case with CHP bodies—by the Health Systems Agency (HSA) in which the facility is located. Apparently this even includes the NIH and professional education funds insofar as they are intended for use in the delivery system. Moreover, all such applications have to conform to state plans and the state certificate-of-need process.

The precise nature of the relations between federal, state, and area bodies is still far from clear and will probably emerge only gradually as a result of experience over time. But one generalization seems predictable: power and authority will remain at the area level vis-à-vis the state, and at the state level vis-à-vis the federal, only to the extent that the lower level is equipped and prepared to exercise such authority effectively.

Comprehensiveness

In theory, the new law appears less broad than the old CHP program: The jurisdiction is limited to personal health services, deemphasizing environmental issues. Since the CHPs were never able to deal effectively with the latter, the specific focus on health services combined with enlarged functions, authority, and funding, provide the first serious possibility for a comprehensive approach to the entire "health care system."

Title XVI, with its $610 million three-year authorization for health resources development, replaces Title VI, the old Hill-Burton program, and is intended to provide substantial funds for carefully allocated health resources development. The actual appropriations are likely to fall far short of the authorization. The point, however, is that, whatever the total amount finally available, all applications will have to be approved by area and state bodies and will be expected to conform to comprehensive plans. The result should be substantially less fragmentation than in the past. It is also worth noting that Title XVI emphasizes ambulatory facilities far more than any previous federal planning law.

One of the most interesting aspects of the new law is the provision for establishment of a National Council on Health Planning and Development and a set of national guidelines for health planning. The latter are expected to include a statement of national health planning goals. The Secretary of HEW has until July 1976 to issue such guidelines, and no one has any idea at this point what they will contain or how useful they will be. It is significant, however, that for the first time in our history Congress has mandated an overall statement of goals. Whether this effort will, in fact, help to reduce the actual fragmentation that has been proliferating for years remains to be seen.

Involvement of Both Providers and Consumers

Previous planning efforts have been directed primarily at one or the other. The Hill-Burton areawide planning bodies were dominated by provider interests. The Comprehensive Health Planning agencies were consumer-oriented. The Regional Medical Program was oriented to academic medicine. The new law has gone to great lengths to try to assure maximum participation by both providers and consumers and by both public and private interests in the governance of the new planning bodies at both the area and state levels.

The result is an HSA representation formula that calls for 51 to 60 percent representation for consumers (the term is very restrictively defined), the remainder to be providers, with the latter spelled out in five categories—physicians and other professionals, health care institutions, insurers, professional schools, and the allied health professions. It even distinguishes between "direct" and "indirect" providers. There are also further requirements to assure representation for government, both elected and appointed officials.

The complexity of this formula is obvious. It will usually end with a governing board considerably larger than the suggested 10 to 30, with an executive committee of 25 which must also meet the consumer-provider requirements, i.e., 13 to 15 consumers; 10 to 12 providers. Even a committee of 25 seems too large for real effectiveness. The problem here—and its solution will call for real statesmanship—is to reconcile the law's legitimate concern for maximum representational equity and local participation with the managerial strength and flexibility needed to get anything done.

Regionalization

Regionalization implies two components: (1) horizontal relations, based on rational geographic distribution of facilities and programs within a given area or region, and (2) vertical relations, based on affiliation agreements and referral patterns between institutions and practitioners providing different levels of care—primary, secondary, tertiary, and long term care.

The concept has received lip service from both providers and planners for nearly half a century. Thus far, however, very little progress has been made with respect to either component. The problem has always been that regionalization involves some surrender of autonomy on the part of the institutions and individuals involved. Rarely, indeed, does this ever take place on a voluntary basis, as the history of the Regional Medical Program amply demonstrates.

The new law seeks to advance the concept in several ways: (1) There is the obvious three-level geographic structure: health service areas, states, and the country as a whole. (2) There is the effort to establish Health Service Areas that are meaningful in terms both of population and resources. The basic population guidelines—500,000 to 3 million with exceptions for metropolitan areas—appear generally reasonable.

So does the requirement that "to the extent practicable, the area shall include at least one center for the provision of highly specialized services." The meaning of the phrase "to the extent practicable" will require careful study, however.

Some services are more "highly specialized" than others. We certainly do not need over 200 centers for open heart surgery. I doubt if we need even 50. The role and identification of the true national subspecialty centers is largely ignored in the law, a gap that the new National Council on Health Planning and Development and the national guidelines will have to address.

Nevertheless, P.L. 93-641 represents considerable progress in the direction of potential regionalization, especially geographic, but with the opportunity for developing meaningful vertical or programmatic relations as well. Under what circumstances is a favorable outcome likely? These will obviously vary from area to area but in general three conditions seem essential:

1. The area must be large enough and inclusive of a broad enough range of facilities and programs to permit provision of a full range of primary and secondary services and long term care, i.e., all necessary services, including prevention and health education, short of the subspecialties, and, "to the extent practicable," one subspecialty or tertiary care center. For some purposes, the area might well be broken down into subareas, as provided in the law. But if meaningful planning is to be carried out for hospitals and other major secondary and tertiary institutions, a broad base is essential.

2. The area must be large enough to permit the recruitment and employment of a first-rate set of officers and staff, men and women capable of commanding the respect of providers, consumers, and government officials.

3. Areas that encompass major tertiary care centers will be faced with special problems. On the one hand, the HSA will have to take special pains to make sure that primary and long term care are not neglected, as has been the case too often in the past. On the other hand, it will require particularly sophisticated staff to make sure that the area's tertiary role—possibly a national one—is not lost in the new, more egalitarian planning effort. Again, a larger area, permitting greater human and financial resources, appears desirable.

In brief, P.L. 93-641 may provide the Philadelphia area with its last chance at meaningful local control or self-government in the health field. The best way for an area to retain a considerable degree of autonomy is to consolidate its strength internally, to assume responsibility for reconciling internal differences as fully as possible, to make sure that it can command the leadership, the expertise, the technical and financial resources, and the population base to make its voice felt, strong and clear, throughout the state and in Washington.

The argument is essentially the same as that advanced, nearly 200 years ago, by Alexander Hamilton on behalf of the U.S. Constitution, in opposition to those who opposed the federal union and wished to maintain autonomous states. Writing in the sixth *Federalist* paper, he said:

> The three last numbers of this paper have been dedicated to an enumeration of the dangers to which we should be exposed in a state of disunion, from the arms and arts of foreign nations. I shall now proceed to delineate dangers of a different and, perhaps, still more alarming kind—those which will in all probability flow from dissensions between the States themselves, and from domestic factions and convulsions....
>
> It has from long observation of the progress of society become a sort of axiom in politics, that vicinity, or a nearness of situation, constitutes nations as natural enemies ... 'unless their common weakness enforces them to league in a CONFEDERATIVE REPUBLIC and their constitution prevents the differences that neighborhood occasions, extinguishing that secret jealousy which disposes all states to aggrandize themselves at the expense of their neighbors.'

Selection 37

"Certificate-of-Need" versus the "Market" as Regulator*

As I understand the major thrusts of the preceding papers, they are:

1. Competition and market incentives in health care should be fostered, encouraged, and maximized to the extent practicable. As my wife and I, in our writings and public lectures, have for many years been extolling the attractions of pluralism, my agreement is not likely to surprise anyone. I would, however, give more emphasis to the limitations on the practicability of significant competition in major sectors of this field. Moreover, I doubt that competition is the only conceivable way of maintaining quality of services or to contain costs, as has been alleged. If it is, large sections of the country appear doomed to grave difficulty.

2. Health maintenance organizations are a highly desirable vehicle for creating and augmenting competition. My support goes even further. I regard the HMO—particularly in its prepaid group practice form—as a meritorious structure for health care delivery even when the assets of competition are absent. However, I do not believe there is any substantial evidence to support the view that either legislation or administrative regulation has been the major restriction upon the emergence or growth of such organizations.

3. Legal restraints on free market entry (of hospitals, HMOs, or other health institutions) are unjustified and damaging when the motivation is simply restriction of competition. This, I would add, is particularly true when the form of restraint results in the curbing of innovation.

4. Adding a significant consumer input into the decision-making apparatus has my enthusiastic support, although the difficulties are multifold.

I find the principles underlying these main themes relatively unassailable. But, as indicated, I am puzzled by some of the supporting statements, some that appear to misrepresent important facts, and some blithe assumptions about the problems associated with building competition into this monopolistic field that tend to reduce complex issues to simplistic levels.

I dislike picking on allegations that seem to me quite unnecessary to support the basic themes. But I do think it is important that we be accurate about our facts and that we understand what the real problems are.

---

*Excerpt from H.M. Somers, "Commentary" on three papers presented to American Enterprise Institute for Public Policy Research and Committee on Legal Issues in Health Care, Duke University School of Law, Conference, June 1972, Washington, D.C.; published in C.C. Havighurst,ed., *Regulating Health Facilities Construction* (Washington, D.C.: American Institute for Public Policy Research, 1974), pp. 293-299.

Let me illustrate with the argument about "certificate-of-need," because that phenomenon has been a central concern of these meetings. The notion and the allegations that "cream-skimming" (or "protectionism" as some call it) is a major, if not the major, justification advanced for certificates-of-need has been pervasive. That is an unfair and inaccurate representation of the position taken by certificate-of-need advocates. The skimming argument has been a rather minor one, even if it is periodically blurted out by frustrated hospital administrators. Its attraction to debating economists is that it is the easiest argument to demolish—thus we get an apparent magnification of a small point and the beclouding of issues.

Since the authors feel that certificate-of-need legislation is dangerous, it would seem that they ought to confront the real arguments of its advocates, whether correct or incorrect. Such arguments, therefore, seem to me worth listing, without necessarily taking sides. Such a recital may also throw some light on aspects of the industry that have been neglected in the discussions thus far.

First, the impression has been given in several papers that certificate-of-need legislation has been aimed primarily, if not exclusively, at keeping out new institutions. This has not been the case in the states with whose legislative history I am acquainted. The recent laws have been aimed primarily at containing the expansion of existing hospitals. The tendency of existing hospitals to expand is ever present, and that is where the big threat of overbedding is. That threat should not be brushed aside by conventional economic arguments that oversupply will correct itself by bringing down prices and shutting down beds, arguments which have little empirical validity in this atypical industry.

Second, in contrast to the assumptions made in several of the papers, the advocates of certificates-of-need argue that overbedding or underoccupancy is very expensive for the entire community, not just for the hospitals directly affected. The paper by Judith and Lester Laves, for example, argues that in the event of substantial underoccupancy in hospitals, such facilities will go broke and out of business. I would argue that it would be desirable for some hospitals to go broke and out of business; but, unfortunately, for the most part that is unlikely. They will not go out of business because the community, or their special constituency, will not permit it. There are a great many one-hospital areas, where the market is so limited that competition is highly improbable—by the politics of the situation if not the economics—and the community will not let its hospital die even if it is losing money (sometimes an imprecise concept in hospital accounting).

More important, hospitals are not ordinary business enterprises. They go beyond the business of rendering medical care for a price. Very often they are symbols for constituent groups—religious symbols, fraternal symbols, prestige and status symbols for a community. For the Catholic church, Jewish communities, and Protestant denominations, their hospitals are matters with high institutional and emotional attributes that go far beyond the question of balancing the books. They symbolize the cohesion, the devotion, and the status of the constituent groups. This is also true of many small communities. They will find the money to keep "their" hospital solvent. (Parenthetically, such hospitals also answer a deep psychic need for many individuals; rendering free volunteer services is a way of getting a posthumous foot into the door of heaven.)

Third, the certificate-of-need advocates deny the assumption that excess supply is automatically self-eliminating—that is, that demand remains independent of supply. Empty beds will in fact be filled at great cost to the community. Hospitals and their medical staffs have impressive and demonstrated means of expanding or contracting so-called "demand," within broad limits, almost at will. By and large, people are not invited into hospitals; they are ordered. And they are not often asked to select their hospital, even if a choice were available, which frequently it is not. This is not necessarily due to "irresponsibility" by the medical staff. The twilight zone of those who need and those who do not need hospitalization is very broad. The availability of beds is inevitably a powerful determinant in physician decision making. Moreover, the hospital is the natural workshop of the doctor; he has a professional interest in keeping it solvent.

Fourth, and probably most important to many proponents, and to most of the legislators to whom I have talked, is the issue of quality. As Clark Havighurst stated, proprietary institutions have somehow achieved a bad reputation on quality. The medical profession, by and large, is suspicious of them. The Laves correctly pointed out that this is really a licensing problem. True, the authority to reject poor quality already exists in the licensing body of some states, and could be added in the others. But the existence of formal authority and the political power to make it effective are not the same. (We may well have the same experience with certificates-of-need. Lawyers and economists have a tendency to confuse formal authority with real practice. The certificate-of-need may turn out to be a paper tiger because of the realities of political power.)

A second aspect of the quality argument is the conviction that excess, or underutilized, facilities result in poor quality, quite aside from costs. The most common example is the superfluity of cardiac surgery facilities in many areas where few institutions have sufficient cases per month to maintain the relevant skills of the surgeons and other personnel. In short, slackness is not just an economic issue but also a quality problem.

A third feature of the quality concern is the widely held belief that, wherever possible, small institutions should be discouraged, that institutions with less than 200 beds (the precise number varies) cannot offer optimum care.

I do not claim that these arguments of the advocates, either individually or collectively, justify certificates-of-need. I suppose my mere recital of their case may cause you to assume that I am one of the advocates. In fact, I have considerable skepticism about certificates-of-need. I believe there is a persuasive case that can be made against them. But such a case should confront the real arguments, and "protectionism" is not prominent among them.

There appears to be in some of the certificate-of-need discussion an implicit assumption that we have been suffering a supply scarcity. It is, of course, quite natural for economists to assume that a rapid rise in prices is virtually synonymous with scarcity, and that theoretical assumption seems sturdy enough to withstand any amount of empirical evidence to the contrary. But most American communities have more beds than they can use effectively. Occupancy rates are, on average, low; in some places, very low. Most metropolitan areas have more technologically advanced equipment than they can keep in reasonably active use. Restrictions do not appear to have had much impact yet. Of course, surplus supply does not necessarily imply effective competition, and that is not what I am claiming. But it is useful to be straight on whether we are suffering from shortages.

A related point: The Joseph Newhouse-Jan Acton (Rand Corporation) paper places considerable emphasis on the allegation that "reimbursement insurance" has been a major cause (perhaps *the* major cause) of increased utilization and thus the increase of total expenditures to an unacceptable level. According to data recently published by the Social Security Administration (SSA)—and also the House Ways and Means Committee—this common impression may need some modification or at least further examination, particularly in the case of hospitals. The data indicate that increased utilization has been a relatively minor factor in the growth of total expenditures.

The studies by Dorothy Rice and her associates show that during the period 1950-1970, 47 percent of the rise in personal health care expenditures was attributable to price increases, another 17 percent resulted from population growth, and the remaining 36 percent was due to "increased use of services and the introduction of new medical techniques." Since increased utilization is not separated from product change, we can only say roughly that the former probably represented substantially less than one-third of causal influences, perhaps not more than 25 percent. The differential in the roles of prices and utilization in the cost of hospital care is even greater.

All of which underlines the precaution that conventional demand-supply analysis is not very rewarding when applied to the idiosyncratic health care industry.

I was surprised to hear so much sharp criticism of Medicare and health insurance for causing increases in utilization. I should have thought that to remove financial barriers to access was one of their major purposes. Certainly Medicare was legislated on the justification that it would enable people, who could not otherwise afford it, to use more health services. Yes, seems to be the reply; but now they are using too much. How much is too much? In his monumental Michigan study some years ago, Walter McNerney showed that if you took the degree of overutilization and matched it against underutilization, insofar as these could be identified, you would emerge with a pretty close balance. The only convincing data we have indicate that utilization has, in fact, increased; but we have no evidence as to whether the increase is more or less than the amount medically necessary.

The central thesis of Havighurst's paper is, I believe, that HMOs would change the cost and utilization picture without regulation if they are allowed to enter the market freely. He seems to believe that if they were only allowed to enter the market freely, they would rapidly proliferate through the nation. This seems an odd assumption in the light of history. The HMO idea (at least in its pure form as prepaid group practice) is an old one, having achieved wide national attention and discussion through the classic reports of the Committee on the Costs of Medical Care in the early 1930s. We have had considerable experience with such plans for some 25 years. They have not been growing or spreading proportionately. Why?

What have been the barriers? Surely, certificate-of-need laws had nothing to do with the situation. They are a very recent development, and HMOs were showing no signs of national expansion before certificates-of-need were even thought of. True, there is legislation restrictive of HMOs in some 22 states, but these laws long antedate certificates-of-need and are based on an entirely different principle, generally of the antiquated "corporate practice of medicine" vintage. Such laws ought to be abolished. But the point here is that HMOs have not been developing rapidly in other states either.

Good HMOs are very expensive in capital costs and start-up costs. It has proven difficult to attract physicians to prepaid group practice for a variety of professional, ideological, and economic reasons. It has proven even more difficult to attract patients to enroll. Ordinarily, some 30,000 enrollees are required for a sound and viable plan. Those of us who have been close to many attempts to inaugurate HMOs know this is a formidable task, with failure far more common than success. In New Jersey, for example, groups of intelligent and dedicated men and women have been struggling for six years to get at least one HMO under way, and success has not yet crowned their efforts.

I see nothing on the horizon now to offer any confidence that we could, within the next ten years, do any better than double the proportion of the population cared for by *bona fide* HMOs. At best we might reach 10 percent! How we might change that is the question that ought to concern us.

Competition and economic incentives are highly desirable. They should be built into the health services economy wherever possible. But careful examination of health care institutions and behavior (devoid of the conventional "reasonable assumptions" that economists like to make when they are uncertain of the facts) will show that there are inherent limitations upon effective competition and that normal incentives have limited efficacy. Health care *is* a unique market, as I and other writers have demonstrated in many publications. With or without the augmentation of HMOs, we will have to face up to the unpleasant necessity of regulation. We will be moving more rapidly toward rate regulation and quality controls. Any increase in effective competition may reduce the range of such regulations, but it seems quite improbable that they can be avoided altogether.

Such talk leads to ready accusation of an antimarket bias. As it happens, I have a rather strong promarket bias in economics. But neither bias nor rhetoric can create effective competition where special factors militate to the contrary. The movement toward regulation did not develop from bias or ideology. It has emerged because of failure of the marketplace to operate according to the competitive model, with the resultant waste, injury, and public dismay that cause meetings like this to be held. Some of that failure was avoidable and is correctable. But a large part of the difficulty lies in the special technological and behavioral aspects of health care, about which economists must take the time and trouble to learn more before their very useful skills and tools can make their maximum contribution to curing the ills in this field.

Selection 38

The New Jersey Certificate-of-Need Experience*

As of October 1, 1975, 27 states had enacted certificate-of-need (C/N) laws, and similar legislation was pending in seven others. Although there are variations among the states, the general pattern calls for mandatory state review and approval, in the form of a "certificate-of-need," of new health facility construction and program expansion above a stated dollar limit. Failure to obtain such a certificate, which, as the name implies, involves primarily proof of "need," usually results in prohibition to proceed with the contemplated project, denial of an operating license, state funds, and/or a substantial fine.

The ambitious objectives of such legislation are illustrated by the New Jersey law:

> It is hereby declared to be public policy of the State that hospital and related health care services of the highest quality, of demonstrated need, efficiently provided and properly utilized, at a reasonable cost are of vital concern to the public health.

The rationale was the apparent inability of the market economy to meet these objectives. The primary stimulus was the spectacular rise in health care costs, particularly in hospitals, over the past two decades.

The C/N development is very recent. Prior to 1971, there were only four states with such laws. Ten more were added that year. Additional impetus came with passage of the Social Security Amendments of 1972. Section 1122 of that law stopped short of mandating C/N; but, in states that have such laws, it required review of all health facility capital expenditures over $100,000 as a condition of payment for depreciation and interest costs under Medicare, Medicaid, and Maternal and Child Health reimbursement. It also provided additional federal funds to participating states for the operation of their programs. As of late 1975,

---

*Excerpt from A.R. and H.M. Somers, "Certificate-of-Need Regulation: The Case of New Jersey," written early in 1976 for Eli Ginzberg, ed., *Regionalization and Health Policy* (Washington, D.C.: U.S. Government Printing Office—in press).

41 were participating in the 1122 program; all but one of the remainder had their own C/N laws. The National Health Planning and Resources Development Act of 1974 (P.L. 93-641) goes further and requires C/N legislation by each participating state.

Since nearly half of the state laws have been on the books for less than four years, some less than one, it is much too soon for definitive appraisal of their effectiveness. Nevertheless, certain trends, problems, and issues can be identified and should be the object of careful study as the nation moves, tentatively and uncertainly, toward the next stage in health care regulation and regionalization, mandated by the new planning act.

NEW JERSEY HEALTH CARE FACILITIES PLANNING ACT

The New Jersey law (NJSA 26:2H-1, *et seq.*), approved May 1971 and effective August of the same year, is one of the broadest such statutes in the nation. In addition to the C/N authority, which was debated for several years and had the support of both providers and consumers, the law also included strengthened licensing authority and a controversial rate-control provision, thus encompassing three of the main instrumentalities widely considered essential to an effective regulatory program.

The definition of a "health care facility" is unusally comprehensive, including not only general hospitals but 18 other categories. The definition of "health care services" is equally broad, matching services with the kinds of facilities in the preceding definition. It excludes only "services provided by a physician in his private practice or by practitioners of healing solely by prayer." Existing facilities and services, including those applying for a license before the effective date, were "grandfathered," i.e., exempt from the C/N requirement—a continuing source of difficulty for the Department of Health, the responsible agency.

During the first four years, 84 percent of C/N applications, representing 760 separate projects and estimated expenditures of nearly $600 million were approved. Sixteen percent, representing $193 million, were disapproved. Over the years, the ratio of approvals to disapprovals has increased. During the first year, 65 percent of the applications, representing 73 percent of the dollar value, were approved; during the last year, 90 percent of applications, representing 88 percent of the dollar value.

Differing interpretations of this trend, as well as the overall high rate of approvals, are possible. It could mean considerable and increasing leniency on the part of the state, possibly under heavy political pressures from many sources. It could mean that most applications have become more reasonable. Awareness that a proposal must run the gauntlet of a multiple review process and is given considerable public exposure has undoubtedly introduced a substantial factor of caution and self-selection. Moreover, some denied applications have been amended and presumably improved, thus gaining final approval.

These simple facts do not tell us much, however. Loopholes, especially the "grandfather" provision, continue to be exploited nearly five years after passage of the law. Approved projects are rarely contested, but the contested cases are obviously the most important in terms of establishing policy and precedent. The proportionate number of appeals has been rising recently.

Moreover, there are reports of numerous violations without any enforcement action being taken. Most of these relate to small projects, which are difficult to monitor. A fair number are said to be unintentional, resulting from ambiguities in coverage. Others involve exploitation of loopholes, which results in violation of the spirit, if not the letter, of the law. For example, some facilities may have abused the emergency exemption for new equipment necessary to replace old equipment deemed "hazardous to the patient."

SOME ILLUSTRATIVE CASES

Three recent cases have been selected to illustrate the interrelationship between C/N and regionalization.

Perth Amboy Hospital

In November 1975 Perth Amboy Hospital received approval from the state Commissioner of Health to construct a satellite hospital with 80 beds in Madison Township, lower Middlesex County, about ten miles from the parent institution, and to modernize and renovate the latter. The application was submitted in October 1973 and experienced an unusual degree of bureaucratic exchanges and delays in the intervening 25 months.

Perth Amboy is an old hospital, badly in need of repairs and modernization, in a relatively low income Puerto Rican community. However, it has a reputation for good management and its occupancy rate has been exceptionally high—87 percent in 1974. The hospital planned to eliminate 107 medical-surgical beds and thereby make room for modernized psychiatric beds, and a number of new programs including a regional trauma center, intermediate renal dialysis center, and an ambulatory surgical facility.

The beds would be, in part, replaced by construction of the new satellite in a middle class suburban area. The satellite would offer only short term inpatient and minimal emergency services. Complicated cases would continue to be handled at the major facility. Overall there would be a net reduction of 17 beds. The total project cost was originally set at $13 million, of which only 30 percent was attributable to the satellite. But it was that portion of the proposal that generated most of the protracted controversy.

The commissioner had officially rejected the application in August 1974, conforming to the recommendation of the State Health Planning Council (SHPC). The commissioner cited the negative impact on nearby hospitals as a major concern. Several hospitals within commuting distance had raised objections, feeling threatened by a new facility in an area from which they had been drawing patients.

The commissioner did express support of the planned renovation work and the ambulatory program and urged Perth Amboy to revise the application. The hospital refused and announced that it planned to appeal to the Health Care Administration Board (HCAB) and to the courts if necessary. It claimed both procedural and substantive errors.

The commissioner reopened the case. A new series of studies of bed needs and financial feasibility were undertaken by the newly activated Region III "B" agency as well as the SHPC ("A" agency). Surrounding hospitals again entered strong protests that the satellite would adversely affect their operations. After a long period of surveys, meetings, and movement of the application up and down between administrative levels, including an unsuccessful effort to promote a merger between Perth Amboy and a small hospital in nearby South Amboy, both the "B" and "A" agencies joined in recommending approval. The commissioner issued a certificate on November 6, 1975.

In so doing, the commissioner conceded that the satellite might have negative financial effects on most of the objecting hospitals, but she considered the amounts insubstantial and of lesser weight than the advantageous effects of the proposal—including the needed ambulatory and specialized services at Perth Amboy and the comparatively low costs anticipated at the satellite.

Five of the neighboring hospitals decided they could not accept that decision. Since none was itself a rejected applicant, they could not appeal to the Health Care Administration Board (HCAB), the highest administrative appeal forum. That recourse is available only in case of an application that has been disapproved by the commissioner. On December 19, the five institutions brought a notice of appeal to the appellate division, asking for "special relief." They asked that the commissioner's decision be upset on grounds of underestimated deleterious financial effects on them, alleged failure to follow rules and regulations, and allegations that the regulations were not reasonably developed to deal with this kind of situation.

Twenty-six months after the original application the final outcome remains uncertain. Meantime the projected costs have escalated substantially, reopening questions of financial feasibility. In any case, construction and related problems would put the satellite at least three years in the future.

We are not here concerned with the specific merits of the case, which would require a far more detailed recital of facts, figures, and guesstimates. But this much of the story is sufficient to illustrate that regulation can rarely be a simple, clean-cut process in a democratic society. Affected interests are often numerous and diverse. In this case, although the "third party" interests—the objecting hospitals—were informally consulted and heard on several occasions, they had no formal "rights" for getting into the system at administrative levels, through hearings or otherwise. Thus, the early, and perhaps otherwise unnecessary, resort to the courts.

The case also raises basic questions about the appropriate and feasible functions of a C/N program and its role in promoting regionalization. Is the satellite relationship one that should be encouraged? Does the program have an obligation to protect the interests of existing institutions against competition? Or should it seek to encourage innovation, even when this means risk for established institutions?

Does it have any special responsibility to institutions and patients in low-income areas? Should it, and can it, seek to correct inequities in health care resources resulting from inadequate financing mechanisms such as Medicaid or the absence of universal entitlement to health care? The issue is complicated by the fact that none of the existing institutions is likely to close down any beds. Most likely they will raise prices or take aggressive measures to increase occupancy. In such cases, how does one measure equity or the "public interest?"

St. Joseph's Cardiac Surgery Unit

In June 1975 St. Joseph's Hospital and Medical Center, Paterson, in Area I, applied for a C/N for a cardiac surgery unit at an estimated cost of $47,000. The justification includes the claim that this is simply the logical next step in a planned development of cardiology services, going back to 1969, which had hitherto received the department's approval, including a certificate for an enlarged catheterization capacity in 1974; the large number of catheterizations currently being performed; the alleged need for an additional surgical unit in New Jersey; the fact that St. Joseph's medical staff is currently referring many cases to St. Luke's Hospital in New York City; and plans by the Department of Surgery to expand through recruitment of a surgical specialist from St. Luke's. The application was approved by a local autonomous planning body, the Passaic Valley Health Facilities Council.

Both the SHPC Committee on Regionalization and the Northern New Jersey "B" agency made strong recommendations against approval. In arriving at this decision, they applied the Guidelines for Cardiovascular Surgical Units, adopted by the New Jersey RMP and the State Department of Health in 1970 and based on national guidelines developed by the Inter-Society Commission for Heart Disease Resources. All the guidelines agreed that such a unit should perform at least 200 procedures a year to assure safety and quality, as well as reasonable costs. Both bodies agreed that there was no evidence of need for any additional cardiac surgical units in New Jersey at the present time. Nine units had received "grandfather" authorization at the time the C/N law was passed, and almost everyone agreed there was already excess capacity. According to the Area I Planning Council, the two hospitals in that area now performing open heart surgery performed 17 and 19 cases, respectively, in 1974. The case against the application was further strengthened by the report of an independent consultant, a heart surgeon from Harvard Medical School, who visited the hospital at the request of RMP and found its relevant capabilities weak in several respects.

Following these reviews, the SHPC recommended denial; and the commissioner acted accordingly on October 8, 1975. The hospital has already appealed to the HCAB, and a hearing has been set for February 1976. The hospital has also announced that, if it loses, it will go to court.

Obviously, the issue is, first, the familiar conflict between the "haves" and the "have nots." While the "grandfathered" "haves" point to the underutilization of currently approved units, the "have nots"—St. Joseph's and its surgical staff—claim that the existing units are not doing a good job and should not be allowed to stand in the way of a new, high quality operation. St. Joseph's long range planning, its aggressive recruitment of a surgeon from New York, and its high rate of catheterizations suggests that it might well generate a higher case load than several of the existing units.

The case for granting St. Joseph a certificate would be greatly strengthened if it were clear that the commissioner could couple it with revocation of the licenses of some underutilized units. The department apparently has the legal authority to do this; but it has never been tested in court, and there is little disposition to force such a test.

Underlying the question as to whether Hospital X or Hospital Y should be licensed for cardiac surgery is the basic issue of general overutilization. Good institutional planning, aggressive marketing, and a change of "franchise" could create more demand and possibly lower the unit cost of production. But would this improve the health of the people of New Jersey? Or is it likely to result in overdiagnosis and more unnecessary surgery?

Underlying hospital rivalries to become "regional centers" for the various high cost subspecialty programs is the basic issue of the role of technology in modern medical care and the extent to which the "technological imperative"—the dynamism inherent in recent technological developments—will be permitted to dominate the health care system. More important than the problem of duplicate facilities and financial waste is the possibility of unnecessary procedures. In a situation where supply creates demand and where demand is met primarily through third party payments, the possibility becomes a probability, and the challenge to health care planning extremely difficult.

Renal Disease Program

The Social Security Amendments of 1972 extended Medicare coverage to most persons with end-stage renal disease (ESRD) requiring dialysis or transplantation, and authorized the Secretary of HEW to limit reimbursement to facilities meeting departmental regulations, including minimal utilization rates and procedures for assuring the appropriateness of treatment. These regulations, issued July 1975, provided the first mandatory nationwide regional system, albeit for a single disease.

Twenty-nine ESRD networks were designated, each serving a minimum population base of 3.5 million, each expected to have at least two transplant centers to serve approximately 2 million, and with enough dialysis centers to serve a population of about 500,000 each. Under the original regulations, all

New Jersey except Bergen County was assigned to Network 24, along with most of Pennsylvania and all Delaware. Philadelphia was to be the center of this network. Bergen County was assigned to the metropolitan New York network.

Unlike most states, however, New Jersey was already operating its own controls and developing a statewide kidney disease treatment network. New Jersey had originally emphasized home, as distinguished from institutional, dialysis due to a combination of private and public initiatives in the 1960s. At the time ESRD was started, approximately 70 percent of the state's patients were on, or being trained for, home dialysis, compared with a national average of 40 percent. When the Medicare program eliminated most of the financial barriers to use of a hospital-based facility, it removed the incentive for patients to dialyze at home—often a difficult undertaking, especially for low income families. The home program has dropped sharply to 15 to 20 percent of the state's caseload.

In 1971 the New Jersey RMP, through its Subcommittee on Hypertension and Renal Disease and in cooperation with the Department of Health, undertook to encourage the planned development of more adequate hemodialysis facilities. It developed guidelines, published in 1972, suggesting the requisite population base, beds and other equipment, and personnel for all types of kidney disease centers.

Almost concurrently, the state C/N law came into being. All renal disease facilities then required state approval. The RMP guidelines were not binding on the health department but were adopted as its points of reference. Their significance was underlined in 1973 when SHPC's Committee for Regionalization of Health Services requested RMP, in collaboration with the Chronic Renal Disease Program, to update the guidelines, focusing on C/N procedures. The department then issued these guidelines to assist "B" agencies in their reviews.

For C/N, the state has defined three levels of care: (1) acute hemodialysis on an inpatient basis; (2) maintenance, or chronic, dialysis, either hospital or non-hospital-based; and (3) transplantation. The utilization standards developed by RMP were adopted for approval of new facilities (e.g., for a transplant center, a minimum of ten transplants in the first year and 25 for each succeeding year).

With the passage of the federal law and its generous payment for renal care, providers anticipated a burst of new demand and the threat of inadequately equipped and randomly located excess facilities was real. The C/N procedure was the only available means of constraint. It resulted in denial of applications for ten dialysis facilities, while 20 have been approved. Four transplant centers have been approved, compared with seven in Philadelphia alone.

In light of this history, the consternation that met the original HEW plans is not surprising. The fragmentation of the state's own network of controlled treatment centers and their assignment to federally determined networks centered in other states probably had some justification from the remote perspective of Washington because of the interstate SMSAs, as well as the outstanding medical centers in New York and Philadelphia.

To New Jersey, however, such a plan appeared to disregard important state developments, especially its own long standing efforts toward regionalization in kidney disease and the emergence of its own tertiary care centers sparked by development of the new medical schools, including a campus in the Camden area. The HEW plan was also seen as ignoring political realities. It could damage the state's sense of identity and thus the public motivation to support the difficult requirements of regionalization.

The HEW plan would have also damaged the credibility of the state's C/N program. A case in point arose in 1974. Our Lady of Lourdes Hospital in Camden was operating a renal dialysis and transplant center for which it had received a New Jersey C/N. The HEW authorities initially determined that the transplanting, at least, should be performed in a Philadelphia center. They were preparing to deny reimbursement to Our Lady of Lourdes under the Medicare program. A vigorous battle ensued with the hospital and its nephrologists mobilizing all the state's political resources to halt that decision. They succeeded.

As of this writing, it appears that New Jersey will be recognized as a single state network under the federal program. The state's professional leaders have moved ahead on their own, without waiting for publication of the final federal regulations. It now appears that there will be an effort to consolidate the planning functions of the ESRD program with those of the new health systems agencies (HSAs) and the professional review functions of PSROs. If successful this should help to strengthen all three programs.

SUMMARY AND MAJOR ISSUES

Whether government regulation of the health care industry is wise or necessary has long been a provocative subject for dispute. For our purposes it is sufficient to say that the political decision has been made and is unlikely to be reversed. The further extension of regulation is a fact of political life. When Congress and state legislatures wrote the principle, "the right to health care," into law, they sounded the death knell to further realistic expectation of a "free market" as an alternative to regulation.

But there are, of course, many types and methods of regulation. There is a school of thought that alleges that control of operating revenues, through rate or price regulation, would be more effective than control over capital expenditures to achieve regionalization as well as cost containment. Such advocates are discouraged by the complexity and cumbersomeness of the C/N and believe that rate control is both simpler and more effective.

Rate control in New Jersey has had much too brief a history to be instructive. However, it may be summarily observed that rate control is no less cumbersome and complex than C/N controls. And it is even more prickly politically since there is no terminal point to disputes over rates. The issue remains open indefinitely as rates must be periodically redetermined. This may be one reason so few states have thus far elected to try rate regulation as compared with C/N.

We do not here undertake to evaluate which method may be better in the absence of empirical evidence. However, it is important to note that the two are not mutually exclusive. In fact, it is reasonable to expect that before the health regulatory process becomes stabilized, the two will be joined in some fashion to be mutually supportive. For example, the ability to deny payments—in whole or in part—to violators of C/N regulations (as the federal government may do under Section 1122) might give C/N administration more credibility by increasing the range, flexibility, and practicality of its sanctions.

Despite its limitations, the New Jersey C/N program has to be considered an important step forward. While it may not have greatly altered the course of events in New Jersey health care history, it has proved to be a catalyst for progressive health care planning in both public and private sectors. The problems facing the program are be coming increasingly difficult, however, as the demands of regulation multiply and the department's inadequate internal resources are further overtaxed. The issues are procedural and substantive, frequently a combination of both. [There followed a discussion of six issues; three are summarized here.]

What Is a "Health Care Facility?"

As noted, the statutory definitions of "health care facility" and "health care service" under the New Jersey Health Facilities Planning Act are exceptionally broad. Since its jurisdiction is still less than universal, however, there have been many questions of interpretation as to who, or what, is intended to be covered. Thus far, the problem of drawing a tenable line between the exempt "physician in his private practice" and the covered "service" or "facility" has defied solution. As a practical matter, the problem involves primarily free-standing radiology, pathology, and physical medicine facilities, usually owned and operated by physicians as part of their "private practice" but performing essentially the same services or using the same equipment as a hospital.

What is "a physician in his private practice"? What of a partnership of four doctors, with well-equipped, shared offices? What of a group of, say, ten doctors whose office constitutes a clinic? Such "private practice" may involve expensive equipment and facilities which are essentially the same as those for which a hospital would require a C/N. The problem of duplication of resources can as readily arise between an office partnership and a hospital as between two hospitals. This is apparent in a situation where a group of radiologists establishes a fully equipped laboratory in their "private practice" in their "private office." Even a solo radiologist might do that.

Early in 1976, for example, applications were received from three independent radiologists for computerized brain scanners, which normally cost in the order of $250,000-$450,000. Moreover, any hospital can evade the C/N requirement for any of the RAPP (radiology, anesthesiology, pathology, and psychiatry) services by putting the specialist on a "concession" basis, thus converting him to "private practice."

Both the Commissioner of Health and the Health Care Administration Board have repeatedly tried to clarify the issue by explicit inclusion of free-standing radiology, pathology, and physical medicine facilities in departmental regulations. The medical profession, led by the radiologists, has bitterly opposed these efforts.

The definitional difficulty is related to the minimum monetary level at which a C/N is required. Theoretically it might be argued that the threshold should be very low because, otherwise, an applicant could circumvent the intent of the law by a series of small, seemingly discrete but actually interrelated proposals. But, as a practical matter, it is clear that administrative resources are not, and will not be, available to handle a multitude of small applications with any degree of efficiency.

But if we are to require review and approval of particular types of equipment costing more than a set amount, what justification remains for excluding them under one label rather than another? (Actually, are not the services rendered by an attending physician in a hospital "private practice?") Some delicate problems of administrative judgment as to legal coverage (and ensuing court tests) could be avoided, and the purposes of regionalization better served, if the criteria for coverage related solely to the nature of the equipment sought and its cost, irrespective of whether the owner or user is an institution, a group of physicians, or a single physician.

Governing and Advisory Boards

The organization for planning and administration of C/N is a system of government-by-committee. The normal organizational structure of an agency headed by a responsible administrator is largely absent. Numerous boards and councils predominate. This was in part propelled by the provisions of the national CHP law, in part by the consumerism movement, and contributed to by the uncertainties and anxieties that accompany a new venture with high stakes.

It is, of course, customary in American government that regulatory agencies are multiheaded, but normally they are relatively small, rarely exceeding seven members. In recent years, recognition that such bodies are administratively cumbersome has resulted in giving full administrative responsibility to the chairman with the other members retaining primarily judicial functions. The health planning and C/N boards are different. They are typically very large, often resembling a parliamentary assembly, and their composition, in terms of the interests they represent—consumers versus providers—is partially mandated by law.

The relative size of the New Jersey SHPC and the area councils is often excused by the claim that they only have an advisory role. This is only technically true; their role is in fact much larger. These bodies are integral parts of the formal administrative process. Neither the commissioner nor HCAB can legally act on a C/N until recommendations are received from the "B" agency and SHPC. What is offered by SHPC is more than "advice" because the law says "no decision shall be made contrary to the recommendations of the State Health Planning Council unless the council and the applicant shall have been granted opportunity for hearing" by the HCAB. Moreover, the law gives SHPC an explicit administrative function; it "shall act as the coordinating agency for the comprehensive area-wide health planning agencies and area planning councils in all matters."

In describing to the authors how one area council had reached a membership of 75, an official explained, "They started by inviting representatives of medical societies, specialty societies, various types of hospitals, nursing homes, nurses, insurance carriers, and every type of legitimately involved group in health care that might otherwise howl if it was excluded. When they were through, they found that they had 37, but they are required to have a majority of consumer representatives, so they had to dig up at least 38 consumers. The irony is, of course, that the larger the membership, the tougher it is to assemble a quorum for a meeting. So, despite the requirement that consumers hold majority membership, an actual quorum at any given meeting is just as likely to show a majority of providers among those present and voting." It is interesting to note that those who complain most loudly about special interest dominance in government were among the leading advocates of this type of council structure.

Among the major issues regarding these bodies is the definition of a "consumer." The national CHP law defined a consumer, in effect, as a nonprovider. P.L. 93-641 does the same, but it has elaborated the definition of providers to encompass virtually everyone with a direct or indirect relationship to provision of health care, including medical school personnel, public members of boards of HMOs, hospitals, insurance carriers, *and their families*. Presumably, the assumption was that only "pure" consumers would adopt a "public interest" perspective, or perhaps an analogy was being made to labor-management collective bargaining. The experience in New Jersey, as elsewhere, casts considerable doubt on the premises of such arrangements. Consumers are no less enthusiastic about the prospect of more and better facilities than providers—especially when told by providers that it will improve access or quality. Generally they perceive no direct costs to themselves; the money appears to derive from remote sources like government, philanthropy, or insurance carriers.

The conflicts in the reviewing bodies are more likely to arise between competing provider interests—one hospital against another, or a free-standing laboratory versus a hospital interest. Ironically, even those interest groups with an immediate and visible stake in containing capital and operating expenditures, such as Blue Cross and some other carriers, have been classified among providers.

Consumer representatives generally participate less actively than other members. Their attendance is not as regular, partially because of a less direct interest and because the work is less likely to be related to their normal employment responsibilities. Their relative lack of technical knowledge, compared with experts from the industry, places them at a disadvantage. The severe limitations on who may legally qualify as a "consumer" diminishes the opportunity to obtain well-informed public representation. Anyone public-spirited enough to volunteer his time on an unpaid hospital, Blue Cross, or HMO board is automatically disqualified from representing the public or "consumers."

Although such anomalies and ambiguities can be viewed as the inescapable birth pains in an evolutionary process, it is, of course, possible that with passage of time they can become frozen into the structure, as part of the traditional conventions. More optimistically, it may be hoped that this is a transitional phase; that as the regulatory process becomes more fully established and accepted, when standards have become less controversial, we may be able to move to a structure that permits appointment of persons as meritorious and knowledgeable individuals rather than interest-group spokesmen, and to avoid the invidious and divisive practices that label some members as having more of a public interest concern than others—as long as clear conflicts of interest are avoided.

Taking the Long View—And Its Difficulties

A C/N program is in constant danger of concentrating on current crises and short term situations. This is what brings forth proper fears that it will tend to freeze the status quo and inhibit innovation. Difficult as it is, administration of such a program must be future-oriented, developing a sensitivity to, and research capacity for, long terms trends. Many of the most difficult decisions facing the Department of Health today could have been anticipated years ago and possibly avoided if the necessary educational and negotiating activities had been pursued in the interim.

The C/N administration cannot be held responsible for "grandfathering" the nine cardiac surgical units when the C/N law was passed in 1971, but it was responsible for granting St. Joseph's a certificate to enlarge its catheterization capacity in 1974; and, as a result, it will now be harder to sustain a denial of the surgical unit. The department's inability or unwillingness to mandate closing of underutilized units is also a serious handicap to long range planning.

Both New Jersey and the Congress have mandated institutional planning by hospitals. If public authorities at both levels do not provide the consistent guidelines and leadership essential to intelligent regional planning, they are in no position to complain if the institutions establish their own priorities.

Among the trends that were anticipatible in New Jersey, at least for several years, but continue to produce "crises" for the C/N program, several stand out. On the demand side, these include: (1) the leveling off in population and economic growth; (2) the middle class exodus from most older cities; (3) the southward movement of industry and people, resulting in a substantial population decline in several northern and central counties; (4) the increasing need for long term care facilities, associated with a gradually aging population; and (5) significant changes in health care purchasing power, in total amount and among different population groups.

On the supply side we note: (1) the overproduction and continuous narrowing of medical specialists; (2) the related burst of increasingly sophisticated and specialized technologies; (3) related organizational and institutional changes; (4) changing patterns of institutional affiliations and patient referrals associated with the development of a statewide system of medical education; and (5) the increasing importance of the health care industry as a major employer and income producer in many communities already hurt by severe unemployment. The New Jersey experience indicates the importance of such considerations in designing effective regulatory strategies.

The shift from a rapidly growing population with rising incomes to the current static situation caught both the regulated and the regulators unprepared. The middle class "flight to the suburbs" and the relative decline of the industrial northern counties have left many good urban hospitals stranded with an inordinate proportion of Medicaid or medically indigent patients. As these hospitals struggle to survive, they have employed various strategems. Several, including St. Barnabas (formerly of Newark) and Hamilton (formerly in Trenton) moved to the suburbs, over the objection of planning agencies, before a C/N was required. They are now thriving.

Others, including St. Joseph's and Cooper Hospital in Camden, whose application for a $42 million C/N is currently pending on the commissioner's desk, are seeking to adjust by becoming tertiary care centers and thus attracting patients from outside their immediate service areas. Perth Amboy Hospital is trying to straddle both worlds, by developing a number of tertiary or regional facilities in its central city hospital, while constructing a suburban satellite.

In each case, the efforts of these institutions to survive have been opposed by other hospitals that feel themselves threatened. If regionalization is not to be permitted to become the bureaucratic dead hand of the past, some such adjustments have to be made, even encouraged. This inevitably means that some institutions will have to be closed or converted to long term or ambulatory facilities, a development that would probably be useful for other reasons, as the need for long term care facilities continues to rise. Needless to say, a regulatory agency must actively promote broad understanding of its purposes to make such decisions politically viable. Indeed, the most desirable course is for the agency to negotiate such adjustments with the parties involved without having to resort to formal regulatory action.

Constructive adjustments of this sort, however, are vastly handicapped by the inequities and inconsistencies in health care financing programs. Many of the difficulties of the New Jersey program, especially its inability to control the proliferation of tertiary care services and the rising costs thereof, are part of a national phenomenon which includes a conflict of goals between financing programs designed to increase access, such as Medicare and Medicaid, and regulatory programs designed to control costs and quality, plus continued inconsistency within the federally mandated planning and regulatory programs themselves.

There would probably be incentives for hospitals and their staffs to move to the suburbs, even if all patients enjoyed the same health insurance coverage. But under existing discriminatory conditions (particularly bad in New Jersey, where Medicaid covers only those on categorical assistance and even these programs are being cut back due to lack of state funds), the incentive is particularly strong. There would probably remain incentives for many physicians and institutions to focus on the acutely ill rather than the "chronics," but under most existing third party programs only the truly dedicated or the second-rate opt for the latter. Lack of universal health insurance is not a C/N responsibility, but it severely complicates its regulatory responsibilities.

The ominous supply trends were also foreseeable. As medical education focused increasingly on specialist and superspecialist training, as the proportion of physicians in primary care declined, and as generous open-ended funding became increasingly available for acute inpatient care, it was inevitable that increasingly specialized diagnostic and treatment technology would proliferate, with no relation to cost-benefit considerations. As the state-supported medical schools expanded their tertiary facilities and affiliation agreements, conflicts with prior referral patterns were inevitable. All problems have been exacerbated by the persistent unemployment, which makes it harder than ever to close or reduce an existing health care facility. As in the case of many military bases, "need" now relates as much, or more, to jobs as to the stated purpose of the facility.

Such unanticipated factors contributed to what is now generally regarded as a bad skewing of resources and the spectacular cost rise, even during periods of expanding utilization when it might have been anticipated that greater institutionalization and greater use of mechanical diagnostic aids and paramedical personnel should help to reduce or contain costs. This did not happen, of course, because medical prices do not operate in a free market, nor do they respond to economies of scale. The whole-body scanner makes the head-scanner obsolete within about a year after it is introduced and threatens to consign much of the hospital's radiological diagnostic equipment to the dustbin—and every hospital wants one! Each hospital wants to be *the* "regional center." The pressures for excess capacity are tremendous.

Even where the medical profession fully supports the concept of regionalization, it is viewed primarily in terms that call for increased technological equipment and more specialist care. In one of the health department's most ambitious efforts, SHPC's Advisory Committee on Maternal and Infant Services recommended, following a year's study, a system of regional networks for maternal and neonatal services, geographically contiguous and based on three progressively more sophisticated levels of care. Although approved without question by SHPC, the report has twice been referred back to the council by the Health Care Administration Board on grounds of unwarranted cost in both additional equipment and personnel.

The difficult issue raised by HCAB—"Cadillac care" for the few neonates with severe congenital problems versus "Volkswagen care" for hundreds of thousands of normal birth infants—is not easily answered. Withholding authorization for the former will not necessarily result in making the latter available. Moreover, the positive results of advanced technologies sometimes obviate the need for subsequent routine care, as experience with the polio and rubella vaccines have proved.

But the opposite is also true. Advanced technology does not always redound to the benefit of the patient, as the Karen Quinlan case makes clear. Many of the nation's leading medical specialists as well as health planners now recognize the need for limiting and regionalizing specialty services. But such cost-benefit considerations are not likely to be foremost in the list of priorities of a hospital, preoccupied with access to the Medicare and private health insurance dollar and dependent for survival as an acute care institution on certification as a subspecialty or tertiary care "center."

THE LIMITS OF A C/N PROGRAM

Just as private enterprise is having to learn that it must operate within a context of public accountability and even a fair degree of public regulation, government also has to realize that there are important limits to its effective authority. Health care is, and will continue to be, a "mix" of private enterprise (profit and nonprofit), public enterprise, and public regulation. The difficult objective is to strike an optimal balance. In the dynamic health care economy, that is a moving target, not likely to be squarely hit.

If regulation is to succeed, its mission should not be too large or unrealistic. The New Jersey C/N experience makes clear that regulation is suffused with inherent difficulties. It runs against the grain of a free society, and the formal or legal authority cannot be confused with real or effective authority. That must be won, over and above the legislative mandate.

The first task is to make clear that the regulatory system is not responsible for all aspects of health policy. Health care is not the chief determinant of health, and the two should not be confused. Other aspects of health policy require other strategies.

Most of New Jersey's positive public health programs—environmental protection, occupational health, school health, education for the health professions, mental health—are now outside the jurisdiction of the Department of Health. Even in areas where it has clear responsibility, such as health education and community health services, the effort has been restricted both by lack of resources and a low priority at the leadership level. The result is not only undue emphasis on regulation, but it also handicaps the latter effort since it forecloses avenues to constructive relations with the providers.

The limits of regulation are also emphasized by its dependence on planning. The state of the planning art is still primitive. Much of the relevant data are hard to come by. "Need" has never been satisfactorily defined. "Health status" indicators are incomplete. The relation of health care to health status remains ambiguous.

The nature and rate of technological change cannot be precisely predicted. Even population projections have proven unreliable in recent decades. That does not reduce the necessity to try to anticipate future needs and problems. But the public and the regulators must be conscious of the limits of our knowledge and not mistake the formal print in which planning documents appear as endowing them with enduring "truths" or rigid "mandates."

The New Jersey experience with C/N demonstrates that no wonders are likely to be achieved, but progress can be made. Our fragmentary data do suggest that this state has, on the whole, fared better with facility utilization and health care costs than those without regulation. Most important, it has shown that a C/N program can win public acceptance and that provider cooperation can be obtained, within limits. For individual institutions, these limits tend to be rather narrowly identified with their own interests. For prominent physicians and other influentials in the industry—many of whom have a history of declared commitment to planning, regionalization, and even regulation where necessary—the limits are rather broad and tend to be identified primarily with degree of respect for the public capability.

Chapter Eight

PSRO and Malpractice: Two Aspects of the Quality Quandry

Some pre-Medicare efforts to protect the quality of health care through state licensure, specialty certification, and the development of voluntary performance standards were noted in Selections 5 and 6. Steadily growing concern, spurred in part by related cost pressures, culminated in the 1972 PSRO law, Sec. 249F of P.L. 92-603. This represented a compromise with the medical profession in that it called for mandatory "professional standards review" in federally funded programs but provided that such review would be performed by the profession itself. The pattern that emerged was based in good part on the San Joaquin Medical Foundation model (Selection 20).

Every area of the country encompassing a minimum of 300 physicians is required to have a Professional Standards Review Organization, comprised entirely of local physicians, to monitor the necessity, appropriateness, and quality of inpatient services to Medicare, Medicaid, and Title V (Maternal and Child Health) patients. Local PSROs are accountable to the Secretary of HEW, who is advised by a National Professional Standards Review Council, also made up entirely of doctors.

In general, the AMA leadership reluctantly accepted the program. Most specialty organizations and the medical care foundations have also supported PSROs. But a substantial minority of the profession, especially in the south and midwest, has continued to fight the entire undertaking, politically and legally. Federal leadership has also vacillated. Emphasis has shifted over time between utilization controls, designed to measure necessity and appropriateness, and quality, although the two factors do overlap. Financial support has fluctuated inconsistently.

Implementation has been disappointingly slow. Only about half the designated PSRO areas were actually operative by early 1977. Obviously, it is too soon to attempt evaluation. The department is officially optimistic, stressing greater physician acceptance and improvement in the state of the art of peer review. On the latter score, three related components are being developed: concurrent review of the medical necessity and appropriateness of admissions and continued stays, short term retrospective evaluation studies of procedures and outcomes, and profile analyses of institutions, physicians, and patients.

Given its broad mandate, it has never been entirely clear which function would assume priority: utilization or quality controls. Although it is intended that both receive the necessary attention, as long as the costs of Medicaid and Medicare continue their astronomical rise, it is likely that the government will increasingly stress the utilization aspects.

Sensing this development, several of the major specialty societies, which provided much of the initial professional enthusiasm, including the American Society of Internal Medicine and the American College of Physicians, now appear more interested in developing quality standards through their own organizations and/or through the hospitals, which, of course, is what they should have been doing all along—with or without PSROs.

The original PSRO proposal provided that all physicians' services be reviewed, not just institutional care. As passed, the law was limited to inpatient care. In effect, this has meant inpatient hospital care only, although procedures for review of long term care are being developed and the department hopes to move on a voluntary basis, to review of ambulatory care and care provided under nonfederal financing.

Selection 39 indicates our reservations about PSRO as an ideal approach, but states our endorsement as the best, realistic, available option. Selection 40 urges that, whatever form quality review may eventually assume, it must be performed in a context of public accountability if it is to achieve credibility as well as effectiveness. Selection 41 probes a different but related issue, the controversy over sharply rising malpractice costs. Generally viewed primarily as a set of legal and insurance problems, here it is examined as a symptom of the character of doctor-patient relationships and the quality of care.

Selection 39

PSRO: Friend or Foe?*

I was among those who opposed PSRO (Professional Standards Review Organization) throughout the Congressional debate. I believed that the objective—effective professional review of the quality and quantity of health care within a context of public accountability—could be achieved more easily for more patients, at less cost, and with less danger of political manipulation, by strengthening existing hospital-based peer review, extending it to noninstitutional services in the area, and making its accountability more explicit.

This would mean fixing responsibility on the hospital professional staff and clarifying its accountability to the public via the board of trustees, in line with the dominant theme of recent court decisions.[1] Conversely, I feared that rechanneling the flow of accountability from the hospital staff to an outside PSRO and thence to state and federal government would lead to an erosion of the trustees'

---

*A.R. Somers, "PSRO: Friend or Foe?" Editorial, *New England Journal of Medicine*, 289 (August 9, 1973): pp. 321-322.

still inadequate, but increasing, accountability and a general decline in responsibility at the community level on the part of both providers and consumers.

Among the other advantages I saw for the hospital-based model, it would permit involvement, as appropriate, of nurses and other health professionals in the review process. This, in addition to the buffer role of the trustees, would mean that the physician would not have to assume sole responsibility for the care rendered by the entire health care team. Under PSRO he will have to bear this responsibility in virtual isolation—a situation that is understandably attractive in terms of freedom from interdisciplinary committee work, "lay interference," etc.—but also means that the medical profession's prestige is more vulnerable than ever before.

Neither Congress nor the medical profession accepted this view. The result is a law that will be difficult to administer, expensive, and highly susceptible to political manipulation. For those of us who have lived through the ebb and flow of federal enthusiasm for RMPs, CHPs, OEO health centers, and other acronymic nostrums, the current excitement over PSRO also conjures up a sense of *déjà vu*.

Nevertheless, at this point, I am constrained to agree with Dr. C.E. Welch in his excellent special article in this issue of the *Journal*[2] that there is now no viable alternative. It is probably too late to return to the hospital-based model. As he points out, if the medical profession now refuses to accept this responsibility, "other organizations are waiting in the wings to assume direction of the profession." These "other organizations" are almost sure to be governmental or government-surrogates.

The AMA apparently understands this warning. How long will it take some other sections of the profession to realize that the issue is no longer "controls" versus "no controls," but simply "what kind of controls?"

Moreover, there are, as Dr. Welch points out, positive aspects to the PSRO program. Among the more promising are the possibility of establishing review of noninstitutional care, a possible stimulus to medical education, and increasing cost-consciousness on the part of doctors.

What are the chances that PSRO will work any better than RMP or voluntary hospital utilization review? Dr. Welch presents an admirably objective discussion of the problems and prospects. He ends on an optimistic note. But neither optimism nor resigned acceptance is enough. For highly motivated physicians who want to see the PSRO experiment work, I ask their indulgence in submitting three practical suggestions:

1. Concentrate on the immediate task—surveillance of the quality and quantity of care in hospitals and other institutions—and work within the existing system as much as possible. Rather than dismantle the existing hospital review mechanisms, try to strengthen them and delegate as much as possible to them. Although there is a logical relation between PSROs and health care planning, and although some realignment of power within the health care establishment is inherent in the PSRO concept, as Dr. Welch suggests, restructuring the system is not the primary objective. The more grandiose the

aims that any specific PSRO sets for itself, the more likely it is to run into serious trouble, and the less likely to accomplish the primary objective.

2. In the effort to arrive at the required norms of care and criteria for evaluation, do not ignore your own experience and the common sense of your colleagues for the theoretically superior wisdom inherent in regression equations and computer printouts. I am not arguing for intellectual sloppiness or sanctification of conventional wisdom. I am not downgrading quantitative analysis and technology as an aid in such analysis. I do say that, in this amorphous area, the consumer-patient and taxpayer—on whose behalf you will be acting—would prefer to have you get going with somewhat crude norms, based on the experience of the best doctors in the area, that can be modified as the program progresses, rather than postpone corrective action for months, or even years, while engaged in pursuit of some statistical magic formula. The highly inconsistent and questionable results that emerged from a recent comparison of five different peer review methods of assessing quality indicate the lack of precision in even sophisticated techniques.[3] In this atmosphere of pseudoscience, and with money available for almost anything that calls itself "evaluation," it would be easy to end up doing more harm than good.

3. Prepare carefully for the first disciplinary showdowns. It will not help the prestige of a PSRO to be overruled by the Secretary of Health, Education, and Welfare or the courts. A new PSRO would be well advised to consolidate its own position and to exhaust all educational possibilities before beginning to throw its weight around. On the other hand, if it shies away too long from corrective action, when required, this will be the beginning of the end. PSRO will go the way of voluntary planning and voluntary peer review, and the medical profession will have forfeited an unprecedented opportunity to make good on its historic claim to be "the guardian of the nation's health."

NOTES

1. *Darling vs. Charleston Community Memorial Hospital,* 211 N.E. 2d 253 (1965); *cert. denied,* 383 U.S. 946 (1966); also *Moore vs. Board of Trustees of Carson-Tahoe Hospital et al.,* 495 P. 2d 605 (1972).

2. C.E. Welch, M.D., "Professional Standards Review Organizations—Problems and Prospects," *New England Journal of Medicine* 289 (August 9, 1973): 291-295.

3. R.H. Brook and F.A. Appel, "Quality-of-Care Assessment: Choosing a Method for Peer Review," *New England Journal of Medicine* 288 (1973): 1323-1329.

Selection 40

Public Accountability and Quality Protection in Ambulatory Care*

Two hundred years ago the founding fathers wrote into the U.S. Constitution civilian control of the military, anticipating by more than a century the famous aphorism attributed to the French statesman Georges Clemenceau, "War is too important to leave to the generals."

Today, more and more Americans seem to be saying, "Medicine is too important to leave entirely to the doctors." Note that I say "medicine," not "health." To say "Health is too important to leave to the doctors" would be equivalent to saying "Peace is too important to leave to the generals." The real meaning would be lost. "Peace" and "health" are universal goals that everyone can agree on—as "motherhood" used to be. But "war" and "medicine" are instrumentalities involving vast resources and the power of life and death. These are the provinces of the experts, the professionals, where laymen are rarely welcome, and where real-life policies evolve more in relation to immediate professional needs and prerogatives than to long run public goals.

On June 3, 1976, *The Evening Times* of Trenton, N.J., carried as a first page, six-column headline (an honor usually reserved for presidential elections or declarations of war) the following banner, "Estrogen linked to uterine cancer increase." The Associated Press story that followed was based on two articles that had appeared in the *New England Journal of Medicine* of the same date. Presumably the story was carried in hundreds of papers throughout the country.

The reason for this tremendous public interest in a highly technical medical subject is obvious: millions of American women are, or have been, taking postmenopausal estrogen and thus feel their lives threatened. The impact of such public interest and public concern on the practice of medicine is very great, especially in ambulatory care, where consumers feel a little more confident or, perhaps, less intimidated than they do once admitted to a hospital bed.

This development should be welcomed as a sign of increasing public knowledge or at least the desire for knowledge. It is symbolic of what is happening to medicine generally; the public is beginning to demand "accountability," not only in terms of professional integrity and fiscal responsibility but also in the quality of care it is receiving.

---

*Excerpt from A.R. Somers, Keynote Address, American Society of Internal Medicine, Conference on "Assessing Physician Performance in Ambulatory Care," June 18, 1976, San Francisco, Calif.: published in ASIM, *Conference Proceedings* (San Francisco: 1976), pp. 4-15.

To a profession long accustomed to operating in a context of professional privilege and almost unquestioned authority, adjustment to the frequently harsh and, sometimes, unfair glare of the public limelight is bound to be difficult and, at times, traumatic. The results, as the current malpractice controversy indicates, are not always positive, either for the profession or the public. Nevertheless, this is a development implicit in our historic commitments to universal education and universal suffrage, and the final results can be both significant and constructive if the leadership of both the profession and the public is willing to work hard enough and make the necessary adjustments.

PUBLIC ACCOUNTABILITY IN THE HEALTH FIELD

The concept of public accountability is especially appropriate to the health field. It is not the same thing as public operation, public utility, or any other conventional type of public regulation. On the contrary, it not only presupposes continued existence of a substantial private sector but also a large degree of professional independence. The opposite side of the coin is that such private institutions and professions are expected to act in a fiduciary or stewardship role, accepting publicly-defined goals, objectives, and procedures for "accounting" to the public with respect to such stewardship. In effect, the private institutions may expect to retain their private status only as long as they act as if they were public.

This is a very important distinction. If we, in America, can achieve the benefits of public accountability, without the evils of overcentralization and overbureaucratization implicit in too much government ownership or too detailed government control, we will have made a major contribution to the development of democratic self-government.

The concept might be likened to the "categorical imperative" propounded some 200 years ago by Immanuel Kant. At a time when philosophers were hotly debating the existence of God and the relevance of competing ethical principles, Kant concluded that, while His existence could not be proved, it behooved the individual to conduct himself *"als ob"* or "as if" the universe were ordered in accordance with universally binding moral law.

For various reasons, public accountability has been slower in emerging in the health field than in some others. Among these are the atypical role of the health care consumer, the persistence of the "medical mystique," and the traditional sharp distinction between the public and private sectors in the health care economy, with public involvement and surveillance almost exclusively concentrated in the public sector. Most of these conditions are changing, and pressures for "public" (or "consumer" or "patient") involvement are building up rapidly. Despite lingering resistance—some of it very strong—many health care institutions and agencies are trying to respond to these pressures in a positive fashion.

One of the first examples of what we now call public accountability was the program of the American College of Surgeons, which eventually led to the Joint Commission on Hospital Accreditation. More recently, the commitments and activities of a number of foundations for medical care and prepaid group practice plans fall under this rubric.

I would so classify the efforts on the part of many Blue Cross and Blue Shield plans to increase public or consumer representation on their boards. And the move on the part of some hospitals to set up "ombudsmen," "patient representatives," or "consumer advisory committees." And the American Hospital Association's effort—not highly successful but still significant—to develop a uniform Patient's Bill of Rights. Indeed, this movement has reached the point that a Society of Patient Representatives has been established within the AHA.

PSRO is, of course, the most far-reaching example to date. It is still far from clear what direction PSROs will take in the future—whether government will move in with too heavy a hand and turn public accountability into public regulation; whether the profession will try to convert PSROs into "fig leaves" for nonaccountability; or whether a real cooperative effort on the part of government and the profession will permit them to achieve their full potential as instruments of public accountability. But the potential is there and should be welcomed by all who cherish the continued independence of the medical profession.

With U.S. health care costs now running about $135 billion a year (more than the entire gross national product of all but a handful of nations) and again in the vanguard of national inflation, in the absence of competitive pricing and other attributes of the "free market," and with continuing pressures for ever-tighter government controls, the future of the private sector may well depend on its willingness and ability to observe this new "categorical imperative." That is, to act "as if" it were a public, rather than a private, enterprise and to accept the public's own definition of the "public interest."

At this point, however, public accountability becomes more than an idealistic slogan. It has to be given substantive content and definition. And so, for the sake of discussion and debate, I suggest the following summary statement: *Meaningful public accountability in the health field involves a set of commitments, institutions, and procedures which will promote the reconciliation of private ownership, private operation, and professional independence with public goals and public standards of integrity, quality, and financial responsibility.*

Here, I will be concerned with quality only. But it must be kept in mind that it is impossible completely to separate quality from either professional integrity or costs.

AMBULATORY CARE

Application of this concept of public accountability to the ambulatory setting is far more difficult than in the case of inpatient care. There are two major differences. First is the general absence of an institutional setting and the aggregation of patients, physicians, and records, which greatly simplifies the technical problem of quality assessment. In the case of hospitals, there is also an existing tradition of public accountability via the trustees, and varying degrees of experience with peer review.

Equally important, but less obvious perhaps, is the fact that the goals of ambulatory care are more difficult to define; as a result, so are the standards or criteria against which performance can be judged. Some physicians insist that it is literally impossible to define the goals of ambulatory care. In their view it is purely and simply an art, not a science; and real art does not commit itself to external goals.

There is some validity to this view. With most acute hospital care, where peer review has achieved its greatest success, the goal is comparatively clear: to cure the patient of a specific disease or, if cure is impossible as in the case of most chronic illness, to achieve manageable stability. In other words, the patient's own goals—and, by extension, those of the public at large—can be stated in professionally meaningful terms. (There is, of course, one increasingly important area of acute care where the public itself has been unable to achieve agreement as to goals—the management of terminal illness—and hence standards and criteria for professional performance are under great strain.)

In the ambulatory setting, however, the patient's goals are increasingly expressed not in terms of "medical cure" but of "health maintenance." And despite the widespread popularization, of the concept of health maintenance, it remains extremely complex, not to be fulfilled by applying a series of protocols dealing with specific complaints any more than by some single financial or organizational formula.

What is involved is the meaning of "health," and no one has been able to come up with a fully satisfactory definition of that elusive concept, despite all the efforts of such eminent bodies as the World Health Organization. The best definition I have heard recently puts it this way, "Health is feeling well enough to do whatever it is you want and expect to do." This means, of course, that health means something quite different to the 20-year-old professional athlete than it does to the 75-year-old retired accountant. So does "health maintenance." And so does quality ambulatory care with such very different patients.

Despite the obvious difficulties, however, the problem is not insuperable. In the first place, we know that numerous health care programs which provide, or finance, ambulatory benefits have been able to establish and maintain standards that have proved acceptable both to the consumer-patients and to the professional providers. Secondly, it was not so long ago that the same objections were being made to hospital-based peer review. (In some quarters they still are!)

Third, the problem of goal-setting for ambulatory care can be approached in a fairly practical way, at least definite enough to permit agreement on standards and criteria. Even accepting the highly flexible definition of health quoted above, we know that, for the vast majority of patients, their expectations are realistic; indeed, a substantial portion are unnecessarily fatalistic. For every hypochondriac or middle-aged fanatic in search of the fountain of youth, there are probably hundreds whose health goals and self-image are lower than necessary.

Thanks to the intelligent and patient work and voluminous records of the National Center for Health Statistics, we now know a great deal about the health and health behavior of Americans, as well as about their illnesses and disabilities. Some of us would like to know even more, but we now have more information available on this score than we begin to make use of in the everyday practice of medicine.

As an approach to professional "health maintenance" standards and criteria, I suggest a combination of effective management of chronic illness and minor acute illness combined with a schedule of age- and sex-specific preventive procedures designed to avoid as much illness as possible. (See, for example, Selection 46.) In other words, a distillate of clinical medicine at the primary care level, epidemiology, and what used to be called "public health."

QUALITY PROTECTION

Up to this point, you have been asked to accept a definition of public accountability which calls for the development of professional values and expertise within a context of publicly defined goals. It has been suggested that the goals of ambulatory care can be distilled, through a process of public-professional exchange, out of a mixture of epidemiological information, presenting complaints to primary care physicians, and direct consumer-patient input.

At this point, it becomes the responsibility of the profession to spell out the services and procedures needed to meet or try to meet these goals, standards of performance for each service or procedure, and to establish institutions and methods for monitoring and enforcement of such standards.

Parenthetically, may I call your attention to the small change in the title from "quality assurance" to "quality protection." This is more than just a literary nicety. I now deliberately try to avoid use of either "quality assurance" or "quality control." "Control" suggests too mechanical an approach; "assurance" promises too much. If quality assurance is related to outcome, not only process, as it should be, no one can guarantee or assure the results. "Quality protection" comes closer to expressing realistic commitments and procedures.

Under this heading, there are four separate aspects of "quality protection" which I believe the public at large and individual consumer-patients are beginning to expect from the medical profession. First is *technical competence.* This, of course, is the *sine qua non.* It is what makes a doctor a doctor. It is the characteristic which the public would simply like to take for granted. It is prepared, even anxious, to leave the education and training of physicians to the profession itself and is prepared to support such education and training generously. It only asks that you do a competent and conscientious job.

Has the profession met the public's expectations with respect to technical competence? Obviously, not in all cases; but I would think that, on balance, the answer has to be "yes." American medical education in the technical sense, both undergraduate and graduate, is almost certainly better than it has ever been, despite the pressures for rapid expansion and for a student body more representative of the total population. Certifying examinations for medical specialists are more rigorous than ever before. Continuing education has also helped, despite its shortcomings, and is now a requirement for membership in several specialty organizations and the medical societies of several states.

The two big issues in this area involve: (a) the qualifications of the foreign medical graduate now that about half of all new licentiates each year are foreign-educated; and (b) the question of relicensure and/or recertification. It is a pleasure to be able to congratulate the American Society of Internal Medicine, the American College of Physicians, and the American Board of Internal Medicine for their stand on recertification, just as I have long congratulated the American Academy and the American Board of Family Practice for their pioneer stand on this question. Both of these are issues that deserve serious and prompt attention to round out the profession's generally good record with respect to technical competence.

The second factor is *a good doctor-patient relationship*. I placed technical competence before the doctor-patient relationship because if I, as a patient, had to make a choice, this would be my order of priority. Millions of Americans feel differently, however; and, when forced to choose, select the doctor who, they feel, takes a personal interest in them. Without question, the public believes that this is an essential aspect of quality medical care. And this is an aspect where, it is also widely believed, the profession is seriously deficient.

The reasons for this deficiency are, in part, overloaded practices; in part, the same as those that have led to the increase in technical competence: as emphasis on specialization and the "science of medicine" has increased, there has been less attention, both at the undergraduate and graduate level, to the "art of medicine."

To some extent this has been compensated for by increasing emphasis on the behavioral sciences in medical school curricula. But a more scientific approach to the neurotic housewife, the middle-aged alcoholic, or the general field of behavior modification—important as these new professional concerns may be—is not what the public is talking about. What it *is* talking about is a doctor who really cares about his patients, who sees them as individual human beings, and is prepared to take time to help them achieve their own health goals.

Whether this is too much to expect of a doctor, today, is perhaps debatable; but the fact that the public wants it is not. And if the medical profession has decided that it cannot provide this kind of care to 215 million people, then it should say so and help to develop alternative sources for this human relationship that most people both want and need so badly.

Dr. Edmund Pellegrino, Chairman, Yale-New Haven Medical Center, a student of this subject, has suggested that primary or ambulatory care should be delivered by primary care teams, including a physician, a nurse clinician, and a nurse educator or "health practitioner." The latter, working under the supervision of the doctor, would presumably have more time to relate personally to the patient. In one way or another, this question will have to be addressed if the public is ever to be satisfied with its ambulatory care. If, as I suspect, the answer does involve some sort of team approach, then this fact should begin to be reflected in medical education, in quality criteria, and in review procedures.

The third consideration includes *institutions and procedures for monitoring care*. Recognition of the desirability of some sort of peer review or professional self-discipline goes back at least half a century to the time, already noted, when the American College of Surgeons first began to call for review of hospital surgery. We have moved a long way since those days, through the era dominated by the Joint Commission on Hospital Accreditation, to the present PSRO period. We still have quite a way to go, however, before either the profession or the public can be satisfied that incompetence has been reduced to the absolute minimum.

Probably it never will be completely eliminated. Doctors are human beings, and human beings get older, get tired, get distracted, and make mistakes. Most patients are prepared to accept some degree of honest error, even from their own doctors and involving their own bodies. Here again the degree of tolerance has a lot to do with the nature of the doctor-patient relationship.

But beyond this zone of tolerance, there is now a rapidly growing conviction that the profession, both academic and practitioners, should match the constant talk of "quality medicine" and its inevitably high cost with more effective institutions and procedures to make sure that such quality medicine is actually getting to all patients.

At the moment, there is less pressure for monitoring at the ambulatory level than in the hospital. The primary care physician is less likely to make an irreversible "goof" than his colleague in the operating room. But when we consider that most chronic illness is cared for on an ambulatory basis, that most initial diagnoses are made on this basis, and that most medications are prescribed, rightly or wrongly, on this basis, the opportunity for error and the need for monitoring become obvious.

As you consider the methodology of peer review, I hope you will not lose sight of the equally important problem that might be identified as the "politics of peer review." Who will do the monitoring? What institution(s) will be responsible?

If these questions were difficult in the hospital setting, they will be even more so in ambulatory care. The institutions that stand at the interface of public goals and professional expertise are inevitably caught in a current no-man's land, the target of criticism from traditionalists in both camps. But it is also an important, perhaps history-making, opportunity, with far-reaching implications, not just for health but for American society as a whole.

The final factor is *corrective action when necessary*. This is the ultimate test of the profession's seriousness in assuming stewardship for quality care on behalf of the public. It has been said that with all physicians well trained, periodically reexamined and recertified, operating under a system of peer review or collegial monitoring, there should be very little incompetent care. Perhaps this will be the case. The effectiveness of the monitoring, however, and to some extent continued improvement in medical education may depend on the seriousness with which the profession undertakes corrective action when necessary. . . .

Selection 41

The Malpractice Controversy and the Quality of Patient Care*

The year 1975 was a landmark of sorts. In that year America was treated to its first exhibition of real and threatened doctor strikes, most conspicuously in California and New York, where doctors withheld their services except for emergency cases, and hospitals were forced either to close their doors or to contract services sharply. These actions were mainly triggered by disputes over malpractice insurance: extraordinary increases in premium rates demanded by insurance carriers and, in some areas, real or threatened withdrawal of carriers from the malpractice business creating the possibility of no available coverage. The actions and the great publicity—much of it in the form of paid newspaper advertisements—were designed to press state legislatures into prompt remedial action as perceived by the medical organizations. They were, on the whole, successful.

State legislatures moved with great haste to mitigate what was represented as a genuine health care crisis. The great outpouring of legislation was mainly aimed at strengthening the defense of physicians and hospitals against claims, reducing potential legal liability, and, most important, assuring the availability of insurance coverage to health care providers. There was, and still is, much to be corrected along these and related aspects of the wide-ranging and complex issues. But, useful as such immediate steps are, they do not penetrate to the more fundamental causes of the problem. Many legislatures acknowledged the short term nature of the new laws (including dubious constitutionality in some cases) and established study commissions to weigh more considered and effective actions for the future.

*Excerpt from H.M. Somers, "The Malpractice Insurance Controversy and Patient Care," *Milbank Memorial Fund Quarterly/Health and Society*, 55 (Spring 1977): 193-232.

It must be recognized that the legal and cost problems of malpractice will probably never be eliminated so long as torts and tort liability remain facts of normal life. (Nor can they be eliminated by "no fault" programs.) But it is my thesis that such problems will not be satisfactorily or equitably alleviated until malpractice is effectively related to problems of quality of care and the doctor-patient relationship in modern society. It is this aspect of the subject which is primarily addressed here.

Commenting on the legislation passed in 1975, William J. Curran, professor of legal medicine at Harvard, noted that on the whole it "seems reasonably well designed to deal with the immediate crisis," but the atmosphere was "mainly technical... not involving the general public or most of the consumer-oriented medical-care groups [who] have taken little notice of these issues, considering them of much lower priority than increased medical benefits as such. This attitude may not continue in the future if the impact of these laws becomes overprotective of providers and insurance companies and forgets the patient in the bargain. I believe there is a danger in this eventuality, which must be watched for and avoided."[1]

Crises often have value. They eventually force real problems to the surface and offer unusual opportunities for constructive remedy. Encouragingly, there are increasing signs that, out of a variety of motives, such opportunities are beginning to be grasped. Fear, illumination, and dismay have already prodded many legislators and health care providers into activities focused on alleviation of the causes of the malpractice crisis rather than their expensive symptoms alone. History may yet record that out of all the travail a substantial net gain for the patient emerged.

INSURANCE TRENDS

Until 1974, with the exception of 1969 and 1970, when premiums jumped a total of 198 percent, the rise in malpractice insurance premiums was reasonably consistent with the rise in national health care expenditures and increases in annual malpractice claims and payments. The fragmentary available data suggest a fairly steady rate of increase of about 10 to 12 percent in number of claims closed annually and about 10 to 20 percent in the value of the average settlement.[2]

But for 1974 and 1975, the Insurance Services Office (ISO), which acts as actuarial advisor for insurors who underwrite about 75 to 80 percent of the nation's short term hospitals and about half the country's doctors, recommended increases of 50 and 170 percent for hospitals and 53 and 170 percent for physicians and surgeons. What explains the wildly erratic movement of premium rates? For example, a recommended 1.4 percent increase in hospital premiums in 1973, and 50 percent and 170 percent in 1974 and 1975, respectively?

The industry explanation was essentially the same as for the spurt in 1969 and 1970: actuarial miscalculation of future losses to be covered by present premiums. The exceptionally long drag in disposition of malpractice cases, what actuaries call "the tail," makes the setting of rates primarily a game of intuition. The commission* reported that in 1971 only about one-third of claims were settled within three years after occurrence of the "accident"; the average case in about five years; and even at the end of eight years some 12 percent remained unsettled.[3] So, in 1975, worried insurance carriers instituted new claims frequency and severity projection techniques, which they believed would correct what they perceived to be serious underprediction of future trends. It is these alterations that were responsible for the bulk of the great rate increases requested in 1974 and 1975.[4]

The resulting variations in actuarial projections and rate setting are enormous. In New York state, for example, where Argonaut Insurance Company was carrying most of the malpractice insurance, the doctor rebellion was triggered when the company requested a 197 percent increase in premiums in 1975 which it said it needed in order to break even. (It had asked for 274 percent in California.) The Joint Underwriters Association[5] said a 100 percent increase would be sufficient. The state Insurance Department cut the request to 20 percent. The consulting actuary of the new doctor-owned mutual company, established by the state medical society, claimed that Argonaut had been working with a "cushion" in 1974, and he recommended to the company an increase of only 10 percent for 1975 over the previous year's rates, despite an estimated 20 percent rise in malpractice settlement costs. The medical society company cautiously decided on 20 percent, later reduced to 15. Many other states found the apparent lack of relationship between requested premium increases and actual claims experience a mystery apparently intelligible only to the insurors.

It is now widely believed that the insurers' troubles were primarily due to investment losses in their securities portfolios. The carriers were conspicuously reluctant to furnish information to investigative bodies. Doctors began to compile evidence claiming that some companies that were demanding large rate increases had been making good profits on malpractice insurance.[6] In California, a study by the Auditor General presented a mixed report—that the seven major insurers had paid out more than they collected from 1960 through 1974, but at the same time it concluded that their potential insolvency "has been brought about primarily by common and preferred stock investments."[7]

Doctors and hospitals had been reluctant to establish their own insurance companies but now felt forced to do so. As the movement spread, they began to find they had uncovered a real means for containing premiums. The New Jersey Hospital Association, the first to establish a hospital-owned insurance company, found that for an earlier year that Argonaut had projected a loss of

---

*The Secretary's (HEW) Commission on Medical Malpractice published in 1973 the most comprehensive and authoritative survey yet made of malpractice insurance. All statements and data attributed to the commission in this article can be found in *Report on the Secretary's Commission on Medical Malpractice,* January 16, 1972, HEW Publication (OS) 73-88, and the *Appendix,* HEW Publication (OS) 73-89.

$2,503,091; its own consulting actuaries, using the same data, came up with earnings of $1,525,989, a difference of over $4 million! The main reasons were that Argonaut had not considered the investment income that could be earned on "available funds" not used to pay claims, and that Argonaut had consistently overestimated its "claim reserves 2.68 times greater than necessary."

It seems clear that the explosion of premium rate increases in the "year of the doctors' strikes" was caused less by any sudden or dramatic increase in actual malpractice claims and payments than by new pessimistic anticipations by insurance carriers of reserves needed to meet future claims and by bad experience in the securities markets. Additionally, many companies were signaling their interest in getting out of the malpractice business or sharply reducing their volume, mainly because of the exceptional volatility and uncertainties of the business.[8] It was, in short, primarily a malpractice *insurance* crisis.

PREMIUM COSTS

Estimates of total premiums paid by all health providers differ widely, but are generally believed to be somewhat above $1 billion in 1975. This would represent less than 1 percent of all personal health care expenditures. It is a great deal of money, but hardly enough to upset the stability of the health care industry, as some have been led to believe.

Premiums vary greatly, of course, by geography and type of practice. A recent survey, based on reports from physicians, showed that the median premium in 1976 was $3,000, representing no more than 3 percent of gross receipts and about 8 percent of tax deductible professional expenses.[9] The highest risk categories, such as surgical specialties, in the highest risk states paid much more. In California, the top risk class was charged $19,000 for a claims-made policy. In New York, premiums ranged from $470 (lowest risk category in upstate New York) to $19,880 (highest risk category in a metropolitan area) with the physician-owned company, now the dominant carrier.[10] In the lowest rate states, such as New Hampshire and South Carolina, premiums may run to about 10 percent of those levels. Some individual physicians pay more, due to penalty premiums resulting from a record of claims filed against them. But there is no parallel rate reduction for years of practice without claims.

Premium rates for hospitals differ greatly. They are usually "experience rated." Estimates of total premiums paid by private hospitals in 1975 range from $200 million to $700 million. Assuming a figure of $500 million, it would represent slightly more than 1 percent of hospital costs in that year. Hospitals pay for the coverage of their salaried physicians, as do other institutions like health maintenance organizations. Increasingly, however, hospitals are also paying or sharing the costs for attending physicians. There are indications that hospital premiums are rising more rapidly than physicians'. Hospitals are complaining that, for the most part, the increases have no relation to actual malpractice experience.

CLAIMS, AWARDS, AND SETTLEMENTS

Contrary to impressions one might get from the press, most people who experience some injury in the course of medical treatment do not make malpractice claims; and most doctors rarely, if ever, experience a malpractice case. In 1975, Dr. Roger Egeberg, special assistant to the Secretary of Health, Education, and Welfare, with responsibility for malpractice problems, publicly estimated that there are about two million medical injuries annually, of which some 700,000 appear to involve some form of negligent conduct. But the number of malpractice claims is estimated at about 20,000.

A survey prepared for the commission showed that lawyers refused the majority of potential malpractice cases brought to them, usually because they saw no adequate basis for liability or because the potential award was too small. Among all lawyers the rejection rate was 88 percent; among a select sample of experienced trial attorneys the rate was 71 percent. This should not be surprising. Since most cases are handled on a contingency basis, lawyers cannot make a living from cases they are unlikely to win or which yield trivial awards. Defendants usually are represented by competent counsel, generally from law firms which on average are twice the size of those of plaintiffs' attorneys. A case that is not won may represent a substantial financial loss for the plaintiff attorney. Thus the contingency fee system, much maligned as a major cause of unwarranted claims, may actually serve as a screen to inhibit cases that lawyers do not perceive as strong and substantial.

Similarly, the frequent allegation that cases are proliferating because patients have too high expectations of medical procedures, or merely because treatment achieves an unfortunate end result, overlooks the fact that a favorable verdict requires evidence of negligence on the part of the defendant and establishment of a causal relation between the negligence and the injury to the patient. The commission found that 99 percent of plaintiffs' lawyers reported that they would not proceed with a case unless a medical evaluation from a consulted physician was supportive of both negligence and causal relation.

According to commission studies, most claim actions are resolved out of court, i.e., settled by mutual agreement or dropped. Fewer than 10 percent reach trial stage. Thus a jury is not usually involved—although anticipations of what juries are likely to decide undoubtedly influence the out-of-court resolutions. In fact, jury verdicts are far more frequently in favor of the defendant than the plaintiff. Of all claims filed, about 45 percent resulted in some payment to the plaintiff; of those which actually went to trial, only 20 percent resulted in payment.

A 1975-76 study of the National Association of Insurance Commissioners (NAIC), indicates that plaintiffs are doing even more poorly than in the past. It showed that, in 56 percent of all claims, the claimant received no indemnity. Of all cases settled by trial, the doctor won 80 percent of the time.[11] Plaintiff lawyers do not appear to be nearly as powerful or persuasive as physicians seem to believe, and considering that more than half their cases result in no payment, their "cut" in winning cases—usually one-third—takes on a different dimension.

The commission studies showed that among those who did receive payments in 1970, three-fourths of the incidents were closed with less than $10,000 paid, and about half with less than $2,000. Awards in six figures were extremely rare, only 3 percent exceeded $100,000. The commission concluded that less than one out of every 1,000 claims paid was for $1 million or more, "and there are probably not more than seven such payments each year."

Considering the general economic inflation following 1970, it is striking that more recent data from the Insurance Services Office render so similar a general picture. In 1974, 43 percent of the claims paid were for less than $5,000, and over 56 percent received less than $10,000. Only 1 percent of all awards exceeded $500,000. The large awards are, of course, a proportionately larger share of the dollar total than their ratio of the number of cases. The over $500,000 awards represented about 23 percent of money paid out.[12] Since such cases are extremely rare, serious, and costly to pursue, they cannot be consigned to any category of frivolous undertakings of irresponsible lawyers.

The available data do not support the view that the proportion of claims successfully pursued to an award has been going up. They indicate that the average size of awards has been increasing about 10 to 15 percent per year, generally consistent with the inflation of costs in the health care system as a whole. It is still fair to say that the bulk of malpractice compensation remains a small claims business.

The commission's comprehensive survey of the insurance industry showed that most doctors had never had a malpractice suit filed against them. It cautiously advanced the hypothesis that some physicians, as well as hospitals, may be suit-prone—a view widely shared by students of the subject as well as insurance carriers.

RECENT STATE LEGISLATION

The volume of malpractice legislation in 1975-1976 was torrential, probably unmatched in legislative history—a tribute to the political influence of medicine. Virtually all states passed some type of new law by the end of 1976. The new laws were mainly designed to "get over the hump." It appears dubious that most will contribute much to longer term solutions, and questions of equity and constitutionality leave doubts as to how much of the new legislation will survive. Some were labeled temporary and set an expiration date. A large majority of states provided for special study commissions to make recommendations for future action.

The preponderant emphasis of the new laws has been to assure the availability of insurance and to contain costs.[13] There have been relatively few attempts to control or mitigate the actual occurrences of malpractice, or the medical environment which may generate suits. In general, this is more true of the states that acted earliest in greatest haste; the later laws tend to show increasing concern with prevention, attempting to associate tort reform with quality control and professional discipline.

Two devices have been most commonly employed to make sure that insurance is available. The more frequent is the legislating of joint underwriting pools among all companies offering personal injury liability insurance in the state. They would share the risks for total liability or, in most cases, only for "umbrella" policies which cover losses above some large amount, say, $100,000. The latter are generally referred to as patient compensation or excess liability funds. They are generally self-financed by a surcharge on the premiums for basic coverage, usually 10 percent. In three states (Nevada, Rhode Island, and South Carolina), the joint underwriting association has become the sole source for purchase of new insurance. More than half the states enacted authorization for some type of pooling arrangement.

A second device is legalizing the establishment of physician-owned and/or hospital-owned mutual insurance associations, through state medical societies or state hospital associations. At least 15 states have such legislation, including some of the largest like California, New York, and Ohio. The movement appears likely to spread as the associations report significant savings compared with commercial insurance. The American Hospital Association has officially authorized a "captive" reinsurance company for all member hospitals. The American Medical Association established an independent, but sponsored, company to aid with capital financing of state plans.

A variety of related devices toward the same end are exemplified by Oklahoma's authorization to its State Insurance Fund, which writes workmen's compensation insurance, to offer medical malpractice insurance to health care providers, and New Jersey's requirement that every firm that sells personal liability insurance in the state shall provide basic malpractice coverage.

The other most prominent group of state actions deals with "legal-system," mainly tort, reforms designed to reduce the number of claims, lessen liability, expedite settlements, and to improve the defendant's relative position in contested suits. The most common device intended to reduce the number of claims as well as to shorten the "long tail" was to curtail statutes of limitation. Most states enacted such a change. Most common are specific limitations on the time within which delayed discovery injuries could be brought for action. The amendments differ substantially in their severity. At one extreme of contraction is the Indiana statute, which sets a two-year limit from the date of *occurrence* of the incident, irrespective of the time of *discovery* of the damage. Children under six years of age have until age eight to file a claim. The Maryland statute is among the least restrictive, although tighter than in the past. Suit must be brought within five years from date of occurrence or three years from date of discovery, whichever is shorter. Minors are still able to sue until they attain the age of majority, now 18.

The most radical attempt to limit liability was the setting of arbitrary ceilings in a half dozen states on the amount of recovery that is permitted irrespective of the severity or extent of damages suffered by the patient. Indiana adopted an absolute recovery limit of $500,000. (Interestingly, the highest award ever achieved in Indiana to that time was $212,000.) Each health care provider must assume (via his insurance, as a rule) responsibility for awards up to $100,000 and a special state fund is created to finance larger awards, financed by a surcharge on all malpractice insurance premiums. Idaho is even more restrictive. It limits liability in malpractice cases to $150,000 for an injury to any one person and, where more than one person is injured, to $300,000. In multiple person injuries involving hospital liability the limit is either $300,000 or $10,000 times the number of beds, whichever is greater.

The constitutionality of such restrictions is doubted by most authorities and is being challenged. That portion of the Illinois law (together with some other features) which had a $500,000 limit, similar to Indiana, has been declared unconstitutional by the state's supreme court on the grounds that it was arbitrary and conferred a special privilege; it established a classification for which there was no substantive basis and, thus, violated equal protection and due process clauses of the state constitution. The Idaho law suffered a similar fate in a state district court. However, the state supreme court has tentatively reversed that decision, stating that constitutionality would depend on the severity of the "medical malpractice insurance crisis" at the time the law was enacted, a matter that it has asked the lower court to determine.

Another device to limit liability, which a dozen or more states have adopted, is some modification of the "collateral source" rule. In varying degrees, these changes would reduce recovery from the defendant by the amount of compensation from insurance or other sources to which the plaintiff was entitled. Since the courts have been gradually moving away from the "locality rule," as the standard for medical care, attempts were made to get legislative sanction for a return to the old rule, but few legislatures responded.

Apparently to assuage the bitter feeling of physicians about contingent fee practices of lawyers—to which doctors often attribute the increase in claims—some states passed limiting laws. While it is doubtful whether any of these laws will have any effect on either the number of suits or the size of recoveries, they may in some cases result in larger net payouts to claimants. A host of other legal process changes have been adopted.

One type of liability limitation that has a high priority in the American Medical Association's list of objectives was not enacted by any state: a "no-fault" system of recovery for all medical injuries, or what the AMA chose to call "workmen's compensation-type" legislation. Most legislators apparently failed to see any substantial parallel between the medical liability proposals and workmen's compensation. They also have been disappointed by experience with the alleged cost savings and reductions in litigation that were supposed to be obtained from no-fault automobile insurance. Many perceived great inequities against patients in the specific proposals. But the AMA has indicated it will keep trying. In the meantime, several important studies have been initiated by organizations including the American Bar Association and the National

Academy of Sciences' Institute of Medicine, which will examine a variety of "automatic" compensation formulas.

About half the states have provided "screening panels" and/or arbitration procedures of various sorts to expedite claims handling and to try to settle them before they get to the trial stage. Where screening panels are established, the submission of the case to the panel is generally compulsory, but findings or recommendations are not binding on either party. In most cases the findings of the panel are admissable as evidence in court.

Generally, the panel is representative of various perspectives. For example, in New York, it will consist of one judge, one lawyer, and one member of the defendant's profession. The panel's determination of whether liability exists is submissible as evidence to the court only in such cases where the determination is unanimous. The panel is not empowered to decide the level of damages to be awarded. Quite different is Indiana's medical review panel. It consists only of three physicians who make the determination, plus one nonvoting lawyer. Its findings on both liability and amount can, in all cases, be submitted as evidence in court. In Massachusetts and Arizona, an appeal to the courts from the findings of the panel requires the appellant to place a $2,000 bond for court costs. Other states include various measures to encourage acceptance of panel findings.

Arbitration provisions generally permit parties, either before or after a claim, to enter voluntarily into agreement to accept binding arbitration. The tribunal is usually mutually selected or agreed to by the parties. Arbitration arrangements of various kinds have been operating on a small scale in various communities for a long time. A majority of states have recognized an award made under voluntary arbitration based on prior agreement as enforceable, and all states accepted arbitration based on post-injury agreements, even before various 1975-1976 amendments. Under its new law, Michigan has gone farther than other states to promote arbitration. In order to qualify for any malpractice insurance, hospitals and doctors must offer each patient a voluntary arbitration agreement. By signing, a patient agrees to submit to arbitration any potential malpractice dispute; but he has 60 days after discharge from the hospital to cancel the agreement. An agreement with a physician is also cancellable. Other states will be watching the Michigan experience carefully.

STEPS TOWARD PREVENTION AND CONTROL

Some states have taken modest steps that indicate awareness that the malpractice problem did not derive entirely from shortcomings in the legal system or insurance practices, that there remained the fact of malpractice itself, and the medical environment which might induce malpractice claims. Mainly these fall into three general categories: (1) mandatory reporting of claims and/or financial recoveries to insurance companies and/or to a state medical licensing or review board for investigation (the latter are designated by an astonishing variety of names); (2) strengthening and/or enlarging the disciplinary powers and mechanisms of existing or newly created boards; and (3) requiring periodic relicensing and/or continuing medical education. A few states have mandatory imposition of insurance surcharges on "repeater" physicians.

An example of the first category is Indiana, where all successful claims against health care providers must be reported to the state insurance commissioner who, in turn, must submit the particulars of the cases to the appropriate board of professional registration and examination for review of the fitness of the health care provider. The Rhode Island statute is broader. It requires the insurance companies to submit annual reports in-depth to the Board of Medical Review and the state insurance commissioner. The board is also charged with investigating all complaints against physicians in the state. At least five additional states have given their boards similar investigatory responsibilities. Georgia requires notification to the licensing authority when a physician's hospital privileges are revoked.

In the second category, the disciplinary powers of licensing boards were in some cases expanded to include professional incompetence as a new ground for suspension or revocation, and a stronger range of sanctions including limits on scope of practice. About 20 states passed some revision of the power or scope of health care licensing agencies. New York provided some rather complicated arrangements. It removed from the State Board of Medicine in the Department of Education responsibility for discipline, although it retains licensing authority. A state Board for Professional Medical Conduct is created consisting of not less than 18 physicians and seven lay members. Two or more committees, consisting of four physicians and one lay member each, are to be appointed from among members of the board. A committee is to investigate each complaint received and also conduct self-initiated investigations of suspected misconduct. After investigation and hearings, the committee's recommendations are to be transmitted to the Commissioner of Health, who shall make recommendations as to the committee's findings and its recommendations. The commissioner must then transfer the entire record to the Board of Regents, which must make a final decision after 60 days.

Oregon amended its Medical Practice Act and defined unprofessional and dishonorable conduct. It requires physicians and medical societies to report to the Board of Medical Examiners suspected malpractice and authorizes competency examination by the board. It permits temporary suspension of a physician's license where the board finds continuation in practice would constitute immediate danger to the public. California, in its statute, indicated a concern with the relationship of malpractice to quality. It changed the title of the licensing agency from the Board of Medical Examiners to the Board of Medical Quality Assurance. Its work was functionally divided into medical quality, licensing, and allied health professions.

In addition, states took various measures to facilitate the work of these bodies. Almost every state now provides immunity in all good faith actions to members of peer review committees and boards. Kansas, Maine, Maryland, and

Montana provide civil immunity to persons reporting information to review or disciplinary bodies. Oklahoma gave patients increased access to their medical records.

In the third category, some 15 states have provisions for continuing professional education either on a mandatory basis or as a disciplinary action. Kansas and Ohio require triennial renewal of medical licenses, including 150 hours of continuing medical education during the three years. Wisconsin requires 15 hours every year. Florida and New York permit their boards to require retraining or continuing education as disciplinary measures. In addition, a number of laws provide for revocation of license, limiting practices, or rehabilitation of "impaired" physicians.

Most legislators recognized that there are limits to what legislatures alone could achieve. Encouragingly, it did begin to appear that the crisis itself, its costs, and the fear of additional legislative disciplinary acts, might have the salutary effect of energizing health care institutions and professions into aggressive activities directed at risk control and prevention. Ultimately, results will depend more on professional responsibility than on any other force.

PROFESSIONAL RESPONSES

It frequently takes a "crisis," or the appearance of one, to galvanize action. Recent years, particularly since the surge of malpractice publicity, have witnessed significant and salutary increases in willingness of the profession to acknowledge and face up to unnecessary shortcomings in the quality of care and in doctor-patient relationships. Severe admonitions from leaders of the profession are now almost commonplace in the literature and at such ceremonies as medical school commencement exercises.

About a dozen state medical societies have voted to require members to participate in continuing education or be removed from the society. Moreover, medical societies supported, or did not oppose, the state laws that permit boards of medical examiners to compel all doctors to continue their education or lose their licenses or have them suspended. We are still a long way from the hopeful forecast of Dr. Robert Derbyshire, a leader in this movement, "The days of the lifelong license are coming to an end." But acknowledgment of the problem is an important step.

There has also been a reaction against the inability or unwillingness of licensing authorities to revoke licenses for demonstrated incompetence and a reluctance of medical societies to censure members, and this is reflected in some of the new laws as well as within the profession.[14] Against considerable resistance, some doctors are demanding professional self-policing to deal with those who are disabled by drug addiction, alcoholism, mental illness, and the like,[15] as well as those who refuse to retire long after advanced age has caused them to lose their effectiveness.

Refusal to testify for plaintiffs and failure to report the observed malfeasance of other physicians—the so-called "conspiracy of silence"—are diminishing and are no longer quietly accepted as appropriate professional conduct. Specialty boards are displaying increased sensitivity to their responsibilities for quality performance.

As the initial anger at the sudden spurt in premium costs subsided, leaders of the medical profession and of hospitals began to urge that the providers of care examine their own contributions to the problem. Addressing the American College of Surgeons, Dr. H. William Scott, Jr., its president, stated that the "gut issue of medical professional liability is far more than an insurance program." He soberly noted that the first element of malpractice is injury to a patient as a result of care administered, and called upon physicians and hospitals to determine the kind of injuries taking place and why, how to prevent as many as possible, and to place blame on the shoulders of those truly responsible. "If the frequency of claims and suits is to be reduced, it is vital to obtain facts concerning the medical injuries that initiate them," he said.

The American College of Hospital Administrators has moved to impress on its members the relationship of the conduct and care of hospitals to malpractice vulnerability. For example, it is distributing a cassette whose purpose, it describes, is "to demonstrate how the quality of medical care delivery can be improved by identifying and correcting specific and potential sources of hospital malpractice common to the various medical specialties and to the hospital."

In 1976 medical magazines increasingly featured articles which departed from the earlier mode of berating lawyers and juries and concentrated on advising doctors on elements of their own behavior, their relations and communications with patients that might stimulate malpractice suits. Traditional public postures were being abandoned, and it was no longer "it just isn't done" for professional organizations to acknowledge publicly the reality of incompetence and negligence and even to urge public officials to assume more disciplinary authority over the profession. For example, in a remarkable official statement, which probably could not have happened even five years earlier, the American Surgical Association proclaimed,

> Physicians who have been found incompetent, negligent or careless should be appropriately identified and disciplined. Findings arising within the system of professional liability claims should be reported to the appropriate state licensing board, local hospital authorities, and regional or national professional organizations. Discipline should involve the withdrawal of the license to practice in some cases, withdrawal of specialty credentials or staff privileges in others. In still others, psychiatric or medical care is needed. For some, upon re-engaging in practice, there should be the requirement of continuing education with mandatory supervision.[16]

CONCLUDING OBSERVATIONS

It seems probable that the net effect of the volley of legislative and private activity will be a subsiding of insurance pressures. In the past, legislatures and insurance commissioners have lacked reliable data. Commissioners are now being pressed to exercise powers they have long held nominally, to regulate rates, and review the procedures of insurance companies in arriving at rates. They will now have better tools for effective regulation as well as more public support.

The widespread experimentation with "screening panels" and with arbitration are positive and hopeful trends. The panels should reduce the number of cases that are filed and might otherwise reach trial stage, thus reducing the duration of time consumed and expenses on all sides. However, screening could also cause protraction because of the two-stage requirement. Screening must be accepted as *bona fide*, not as a hurdle before trial, to be effective. The effectiveness of the panels will, in part, depend upon their credibility as fair and impartial tribunals. Thus the one-sided structure of the type of panels prescribed in Indiana and Nebraska—with only physicians as voting members—offers less promise than those which represent a diversity of interests and skills. The experience of screening panels will require careful evaluation.

Arbitration, in lieu of court cases, is growing and appears to be gaining acceptance rapidly. The American Arbitration Association has become actively engaged in keeping track of all types of arbitration and is conducting experimental projects to help design the best instruments for resolving health conflicts. It provides expert guidance around the country. The preliminary signs are that arbitration reduces the "tail" as well as costs and avoids the glare of sensational publicity that often accompanies a court case. The informality of the process, compared to court trials, appears to offer more equity. Even the existence of the arbitration option appears to raise sensitivity and reduce claims.

On the insurance side, potentially the most significant development is the emergence, with legislative sanction, of doctor-owned and hospital-owned malpractice insurance carriers. In a very brief time several of these mutual companies have demonstrated that they can provide coverage at lower premium rates than commercial carriers were asking, and there are good reasons why they should. Such companies are spreading rapidly. They could quite possibly become the dominant medical liability insurors. In addition to cost saving, there are other heartening prospects in this development. Such companies will give health care providers a more immediate and palpable stake in prevention, and they will be in a better position to exercise controls. All malpractice claims will automatically come to their attention and be known to fellow professionals. The financial burdens will be more readily traceable to their source. These companies will be less inhibited about intervening in the medical practice arena, where insurance companies feared to tread. They are likely to find it profitable to cooperate with and help underpin the disciplinary powers of state licensing authorities and medical societies. A movement toward self-insurance among health care institutions has also begun.

Such developments furnish cause for optimism that the insurance crisis will pass. Whether that will be enduring depends more upon whether all involved continue to take alert and active advantage of the new climate for containing the causes of malpractice suits within the health care system itself, now that malpractice is "out in the open."

Reformed insurance practices can establish better and more direct incentives to prevention. In this respect, the hospital obviously warrants primary attention—not only because the large majority of malpractice events originate within its walls (and also the most expensive ones), but also because systematic preventive and policing programs are more readily feasible in an institutional setting. Since the vast majority of physicians are hospital-affiliated, the institution's principles and practices can have substantial effect upon physician behavior in their own offices as well.

Despite continued resistance from medical staff, who cherish and protect their independence, hospitals are being forced by court decisions to assume larger responsibility for all care rendered in the institution whether by its own employees or by private attending physicians. Ever since the historic *Darling* case was decided by the Illinois Supreme Court in 1965, courts have increasingly enlarged the accountability of the hospital itself. In the notorious *Nork* case, the Superior Court of California ruled that if a hospital knows, or should have known, that one of its patients is liable to be a victim of malpractice by a physician on its staff, whether that physician is an employee or an independent practitioner, "it is liable on the basis of corporate liability." It is not immune from liability merely because it conformed to the standards of the industry and because it is required to function under a self-governing medical staff. The fact that the medical staff is theoretically independent and that its audit and disciplining procedures are inadequate offers no excuse for the hospital.[17]

Such legal trends strengthen the case for tying differential premium rates to the development of preventive and prompt-remedy programs. A hospital which, in addition to meeting standards of accreditation and certification for participation in government programs and the requirements of the Professional Standards Review Organization, has effected an approved preventive program would be given a substantial discount on its basic insurance rates. The program should combine standards of care with patient education, formal patient rights, preventive methods for overcoming misunderstanding and disagreement, and accessible prompt means for settling unresolved claims and differences, involving the participation of those served as well as those who serve.

Even now, some of the more progressive hospitals have begun to develop risk control programs with consistent reports of success, not only in financial aspects but also in terms of patient relations. An organization called Hospital Association of Risk Managers has recently been established. One of the hospitals that has been using a patient grievance mechanism, which includes several of the elements listed above, the 500-bed Halifax Medical Center in Daytona Beach, Florida, saved, according to outside analysts, an estimated $750,000 to $1 million in the three-year period 1972-1975.

Another positive action process that insurance can foster is to set aside a small fraction of premiums, say 2 percent, for a fund to be employed for development, dissemination, and technical assistance in preventive and risk control measures. At least one prominent carrier has begun to provide such a service. The better workmen's compensation carriers have been doing this for years in their "safety" programs and found it profitable. It is the type of activity especially appropriate for the doctor- and hospital-owned insurance companies. [Here followed a proposal for a positive insurance program for self-employed physicians.]

One of the most frequent arguments against greater or more direct penalties on doctors is that they cause indulgence in extravagant "defensive medicine"—unnecessary x rays, laboratory tests, hospital days, etc. Nobody really knows how much defensive medicine is really being practiced; monetary guesses range very widely. In the muddy definitional waters of medical practice, it is not even clear what defensive medicine is. It is often subdivided into "negative defensive medicine" and "positive defensive medicine"—the latter being procedures that *should* have been undertaken in any case—and these concepts are not entirely clear either. It is not known how much of the unnecessary procedures are attributable to malpractice fears and how much to the fact that the victimized patient's bills are covered by health insurance, or how much to the "technological imperative" that characterizes modern medical care, or to other causes.[18] Before the malpractice crisis we heard almost as many complaints about excessive medical procedures, but then they were being wholly blamed on health insurance.[19] Insofar as "defensive medicine" causes deliberate wasteful practices, it should, of course, be deplored. But insofar as it stimulates appropriate caution and care, it is a plus.

These foregoing suggestions are of less consequence than the spirit behind them, a primary concern for the health aspects of the malpractice problem. As indicated, the situation is complex and multidimensional. I have been able to discuss only a few of its many aspects. But I have tried to emphasize that among its many significations is the often neglected fact that it signals something amiss in health care itself and in the relationships between the providers and receivers of care. While there is much to be remedied in many elements of this complicated problem, the most urgent needs and the most promising paths lie in seizing the malpractice crisis as an opportunity for dealing more effectively with the quality of care and introducing counterinfluences against the technological depersonalization of the health care process. If such actions are taken, whatever effects they may have on malpractice costs—and I believe they will be highly salutary—we will have gained much as a society.

NOTES

1. W.J. Curran, "Law-Medicine Notes," *New England Journal of Medicine* (December 4, 1975): 1183.

2. These are based on preliminary data from a comprehensive study being performed by Walter Cooper, vice president and actuary of Chubb and Son Insurance Company. The figures are similar to those reported by Congressman James Hastings in a background paper prepared for the National Conference on Medical Malpractice in 1975: an average annual increase of 11 percent in claims between 1970 and 1975 and of 18 percent in size of awards between 1970 and 1973. According to an article in *American Medical News*, November 4, 1974, claims filed had been increasing about 8 to 9 percent per year.

3. If the commission's estimates were accurate, the situation has improved. The Natonal Association of Insurance Commissioners' comprehensive survey covering the year ending June 30, 1976, showed that the time between an incident's occurrence and its reporting to the insuror, in cases in which the claimant was eventually paid, averaged 20 months for minors and 15 for adults. Disposing of such cases took an average of 22 months after they were reported. "Latest Findings on All U.S. Claims," *Medical World News*, November 15, 1976, p. 37.

4. It should be noted that settlement inflation, caused by passage of time, is at least in part balanced by the earnings of reserves held by the insurance carriers. A prudent investment return of 7 percent would increase the value of the original premiums by 40 percent in five years and by 72 percent in eight years. Such company earnings are not taken into account when premium rates are calculated. When this question was raised at New York state hearings, an industry spokesman replied that investments are too speculative to be considered in advance and would be only a small percent of the whole.

5. A mandated consortium of all personal liability carriers in the state, legally required to provide a market for malpractice insurance.

6. The Detroit-based Physicians Crisis Committee claimed to have turned up evidence that one of the country's major carriers, Medical Protective Company of Fort Wayne, Indiana, had grossly overcharged doctors for insurance. The committee claimed the company had exploited the crisis to increase its after-tax profit from 11 percent in 1965 to nearly 32 percent in 1975. The company's officials refused to comment on the charges. "MDs Say Carrier Makes 32% After-Tax Profits," *Medical World News*, May 3, 1976, pp. 21-22. In another study, the consulting actuary to the New York State Medical Society found that malpractice coverage over the last several years had not been unprofitable for the two private companies underwriting the coverage, as had been claimed. "State Malpractice Insurers Found to Be Profit-Making," *N.Y. Times*, June 11, 1975.

7. *Medical World News*, December 22, 1975, p. 12. At a hearing in California, former Argonaut officials attributed the financial plight of the company to a withdrawal of tax credits by its parent company, Teledyne, a conglomerate. Without this act of dubious propriety, Argonaut might have shown a profit on its old rates. It was also testified that the California Insurance Commissioner had not examined the affairs of the company nor inquired into the precise method used for establishing its reserves. *Medical World News*, July 14, 1975, pp. 23-25.

8. To meet this problem some carriers have recently introduced "claims-made," pay-as-you-go policies. Only claims reported within the policy year are covered by that year's policy. Next year's claims will be covered by next year's policy, and so forth. The conventional "occurrence" policy premium is paid in advance for the risk of a claim, which occurred in the policy year, reported anytime in the future. The device will, of course, not reduce the long term actual costs of malpractice, but it does help to alleviate pricing problems. One major company, St. Paul Fire and Marine Insurance Co., has discontinued all marketing of occurrence coverage in favor of claims-made, although some states do not authorize such policies.

9. A. Owens, "How Much Have Malpractice Premiums Gone Up?" *Medical Economics,* December 27, 1976, pp. 101-108. Only one doctor in 70 paid as much as $25,000. See, also, *Medical Economics,* October 18, 1976, pp. 146-148, and November 1, 1976, pp. 81-91.

10. American Medical Association, *State By State Report on the Professional Liability Issue,* October 1976. Of the New York State Medical Society's approximately 28,000 doctors only 384 pay the top rates. "Malpractice Claims: Many Are Filed, but Few Are Paid," *New York Times,* June 1, 1975.

11. National Association of Insurance Commissioners, *Medical Professional Liability Survey,* Vol. 1, No. 3 (Milwaukee, Wis.: September 1976), pp. 58, 59.

12. Insurance Services Office, *All-Industry Committee Special Malpractice Review: 1974 Closed Claim Survey: Condensed Analysis* (November 1976), p. 25. These figures are higher than actual figures reported to ISO. Since cases closed in 1974 included occurrences spread over many preceeding years, the dollar amounts associated with each claim were, for purposes of comparability, adjusted to a common occurrence year, 1974, by a percentage amount equivalent to the average increase in claims costs over the period. The NAIC 1975-1976 survey showed that these large awards equaled only 17 percent of the money paid out.

13. Brief summaries of the laws of every state have been assembled by the American Insurance Association, "Medical Malpractice Insurance Reports, Revised 10/1/76," (December 1, 1976) (processed).

14. According to Dr. Derbyshire, in the five years 1968-1972, 20 states had taken no disciplinary action against any physician. "Medical Society Faces Discipline Issue," *New York Times,* February 25, 1973. But in the year ending in mid-1975, six Maryland physicians had their medical licenses revoked by the Maryland Commission of Medical Discipline, the most revocations in any 12-month period since the board began in 1969. *American Medical News,* August 2, 1976, p. 2.

15. See " 'Disabled' Doctors: Ignored by Peers," *Medical World News,* June 2, 1975, p. 43. The AMA recently announced that 20 state medical societies have started programs to identify and rehabilitate physicians who are mentally ill or who have alcohol or drug dependence. At least four states—Utah, New Mexico, Nebraska, and Kansas—enacted "disabled physician" laws patterned after the AMA's model statute, which responded to a House of Delegates resolution in December 1975 urging legislative action on rehabilitation of disabled physicians. *American Medical News,* May 31, 1976.

16. "American Surgical Association Statement on Professional Liability, September, 1976," *New England Journal of Medicine* 295 (December 2, 1976): 1294.

17. Although admittedly an extreme instance, the *Nork* case offers no comfort to those who argue that all apparent malpractice derives from unfortunate accidents rather than misconduct. Dr. Nork, who admitted guilt, was involved in at least 50 unnecessary and damaging operations in what the court called "a systematic scheme of fraud by the physician [who] for nine years made a practice of performing unnecessary surgery and performing it badly simply to line his pockets." During all these years of malfeasances his medical staff colleagues did and said nothing. At the time the decision was handed down, Dr. Nork was still in the practice of medicine. His license was finally withdrawn three months later. For an excellent summary of the legal aspects of the case, see Marsha L. Jahns, "Court Decision Would Extend Liability," *Hospitals,* January 16, 1974, pp. 31-34.

18. West Germany, for example, has been experiencing at least as large an increase in "defensive medicine"—defined as additional diagnostic procedures per medical en-

counter—without the impetus of any malpractice crisis. See, U.E. Reinhardt, "Health Manpower Policy in the U.S.," paper presented to Bicentennial Conference on Health Policy, University of Pennsylvania, November 11-12, 1976, Philadelphia (processed), pp. 39-40.

19. There is a new tendency to make malpractice and "defensive medicine" convenient explanations for all increases in medical prices and costs. Total costs have been rising at a compounded rate of over 11 percent a year, and health service prices at about 8 percent for a decade. But hospitals and physicians, in statements to the press, were attributing their 1975 increases to malpractice premiums. See, for example, L.K. Altman "Malpractice Rates Drive Up Doctor Fees," *New York Times*, July 27, 1975. Similarly, hospitals have been increasing required tests of patients for many years. But in 1975, such inflation of care was being attributed to "defensive medicine." As one hospital in a community adds two routine tests upon admission—and such tests represent the more profitable features of a hospital's business—others follow, and then that becomes the accepted "community standard of care." See, for example, *Medical Economics*, July 21, 1975, pp. 11-12.

Chapter Nine

Consumer Health Education: Revitalizing an Old Idea

The rudimentary idea of health education is probably as old as recorded history. Even primitive tribes prescribed instruction of the young in various procedures and tabus related to personal and tribal health. Personal responsibility for health maintenance was a cardinal principle of the ancient Greeks. Throughout history, most of the great doctors regarded themselves as educators as well as healers. The very title derives from the latin, *docere,* to teach.

However, as better knowledge of the human body and disease mechanisms was acquired and medical practice became more scientific, society came to place increasing dependence on medical intervention, together with required public health measures. Concomitantly, individual behavior and individual responsibility were neglected. The patient accepted the authoritarian curative role of the physician as the appropriate avenue to health, while most doctors encouraged that view.

The limitations on the effectiveness of this approach, especially in relation to chronic and psychosomatic illness, were discussed in Selection 10, originally published in 1961. We pointed to the need to reestablish the physician's role as educator, as an essential aspect in the management of disease and disability and the maintenance of health.

In Selection 11, also 1961, we suggested another reason for the importance of health education: the virtually boundless potential of health care demand, including substantial elements of irrationality. We urged doctors, patients, and third parties to recognize the necessity for seeking effective ways to promote rational and responsible consumer health behavior.

During the 1960s, however, amid the growing concern with increased access to health services, very little attention was given to health education. Prevention was generally narrowly perceived in terms of the annual "check-up" or early visit to the doctor. Most health professionals, preoccupied with the pursuit of ever more precise scientific knowledge and the development of dramatic interventions, and burdened with rapidly increasing demands for care, had neither time nor interest in helping the consumer-patient to understand his own health problems, to cope with them himself, or how to avoid or minimize them. The physician, even when acknowledging the importance of such patient knowledge and behavior, generally took the position that this was not his responsibility; he was a healer. The patient, in turn, increasingly acclimated to the magic of cure—the surgeon's knife or the new miracle drug—assumed he could effectively assign responsibility for his health to the professionals, underpinned by third party payers, including government.

People spoke of medical treatment as if it were synonymous with cure, and of health services as if that meant health itself. The profession of health education, once a respected speciality within public health, appeared to lose its sense of mission and its credibility.

Medical science, new technologies, and improved services have indeed produced dramatic breakthroughs and contributed historically to better health status for the American people. But the billions of dollars channeled into additional health care during the 1960s had a relatively small influence on the nation's health (Table I and Selection 43).

By the early 1970s a few concerned health care leaders began to say that the time had come to develop a new thrust in American health policy: one directed primarily at the consumer-patient, with emphasis on his own behavior and responsibility, and at giving him the tools to exercise this responsibility effectively. This would require some reorientation of the health professions and redefinition of health policy. It would also require redefining the traditional approaches and methodology of health education.

Some progress has been made. In 1971 the President's Committee on Health Education was appointed and its report published in 1973.[1] In 1974 a small Bureau of Health Education was established in the Center for Disease Control in Atlanta, Georgia. Later that year, the American College of Preventive Medicine and the National Institutes of Health's Fogarty International Center appointed a Task Force on Consumer Health Education, of which one of the authors was chairman. Its report was made public at the National Conference on Preventive Medicine in 1975.[2] Many of the recommendations from this report were incorporated into the National Health Information and Health Promotion Act of 1976 (Title I of P.L. 94-317).

The following selections reflect these developments: In Selection 42, published in 1971 prior to establishment of the President's Committee, we call for a national program of consumer health education; Selection 43 (1972) makes two specific proposals; Selections 44 and 45 (1973) report progress in carrying out one of these proposals and raise some important questions as to the validity of current efforts.

NOTES

1. The President's Committee on Health Education, *Report* (Washington, D.C.: Department of Health, Education, and Welfare, 1973).
2. A.R. Somers, ed., *Promoting Health: Consumer Education and National Policy* (Germantown, Md.: Aspen Systems Corp., 1976).

Selection 42

A National Program of Consumer Health Education*

Many of the nation's major health problems, including motor vehicle accidents, alcoholism, drug addiction, venereal disease, obesity, premature birth, certain cancers, and much heart disease, are primarily attributable not to shortcomings on the part of the providers of care but to ignorance or irresponsibility of the individual consumer or the community as a whole. This has always been true. But in the past, when ignorance and poor health were so often associated with poverty, there was a tendency to believe that reduction in poverty, along with better access to medical care, would almost automatically bring better health. The health-threatening aspects of affluence were not understood.

Today, however, there is little excuse for continued blindness on this point. Findings such as those reported in the 1969 Auster-Leveson-Saracheck study make two points clear: (1) environmental variables, especially education, are far more important than medical care in determining death rates, and (2) high income is associated with high mortality unless offset by education and medical care.[1] Both conclusions point to the essentiality of education.

The teenage child of wealthy parents who turns to drugs for everything from weight control to complexion control, to constipation, to birth control, to keeping awake to study for an exam, to going to sleep after the exam is over, and to finding togetherness, peace, and happiness in an alien world, is looking for trouble just as surely as the middle-aged businessman who eats too much, drinks too much, smokes too much, takes no exercise, and spends most of his free time sitting in front of television.

THE UNINFORMED CONSUMER: A THREAT TO ANY HEALTH CARE SYSTEM

Given the national commitment to "comprehensive health services of high quality for every person"—written into the Comprehensive Health Planning Act of 1966 (P.L. 89-749)—such individuals are not only endangering their own health but are also building up a formidable health care bill for the nation as a whole and are a threat to the future viability of any health care system. The commitment assumes rational individual responsibility for one's own health. Without this ingredient, the commitment cannot be honored.

Moreover, the community or nation that permits its air and water supplies to be poisoned, its food contaminated by harmful additives, the safety of its streets

---

*Excerpt from A.R. Somers, *Health Care in Transition: Directions for the Future* (Chicago: Hospital Research and Educational Trust, 1971), pp. 79-85.

and highways threatened by drug addicts and drunken drivers, the welfare of its children undermined by too many unwanted babies, and the health of its senior citizens eroded through inactivity and a general sense of uselessness: such a community or nation makes a mockery of its professed commitment to health and safety.

The medical profession cannot be held primarily responsible for the individual or collective irresponsibility of millions of American patient-consumers and their poor health. However, the profession and other providers are responsible for abdicating one of their most important roles—that of the health educator. Individual doctors and a few medical societies do the best they can on this score, but the profession as a whole has been either silent or ineffective with respect to many of the major problems such as air and water pollution, cigarette smoking, overuse of drugs, birth control, automobile safety, food additives, and so forth. By failure to assume leadership on such issues, doctors have not only contributed to the patients' own irresponsibility but have helped to build up the formidable demand for medical services that is now threatening the entire health care economy.

For example, a recent study of automobile accidents concluded:

> More and more physicians, as well as nonmedical specialists, are coming to the conclusion that another massive part of the highway accident epidemic is really a problem in public health and preventive medicine and that the medical profession bears a heavy share of the responsibility for its solution. Drug effects are but one of the medical factors.

Even doctors and institutions that specialize in "preventive medicine," such as "executive health examinations," have all too often been so preoccupied with the mechanics of early diagnosis and the measurement of "yield" that they neglect the more important aspect of prevention—education of the asymptomatic patient to maintain his own health.

NEW RESPONSIBILITIES FOR THE PATIENT-CONSUMER

In recent years new dimensions have been added to the problem. It is now necessary for the consumer to learn not only how to prevent illness, to the best of his ability, but how to help in the treatment once he is ill. Dr. Michael Crichton underscored this point:

> It is a fact of medical life, which can be dated quite precisely in terms of origin: it began in 1923, with Banting and Best. The discovery of insulin by these workers led directly to the first chronic therapy of complexity and seriousness, where administration lay in the hands of the patient. Prior to that time, there were indeed chronic medications—such as digitalis for heart failure or colchicine for gout—but a patient taking such medications did not need to be terribly careful about it or

terribly knowledgeable about his disease process. That is to say, if he took his medicines irregularly, he developed medical difficulties fairly slowly, or else he developed difficulties that were not life-threatening.

Insulin was different. A patient had to be careful or he might die in a matter of hours. And since insulin there has come a whole range of chronic therapies that are equally complex and serious, and that require a knowledgeable, responsible patient.

Partly in response to these demands, partly as a consequence of better education, patients are more knowledgeable about medicine than ever before. Only the most insecure and unintelligent physicians wish to keep patients from becoming even more knowledgeable.

Thus, the patient must now become a member of the health care team. Indeeed, unless the professional members of that team become better organized and better oriented—both to each other and to the patient—the latter may end up, by default, as "captain" of the team, the one who has to make the choices, however uninformed, among various specialties and modalities. This is a role that most consumers do not want. However, the consumer must be prepared and educated to play an informed, responsible role in his own treatment and cure— especially in cases of chronic illness.

Now the demand for consumer participation is being advanced still further. It has recently become customary for government to require a majority, or at least a substantial number, of consumers on most health care advisory boards. Third party payers, hospitals, neighborhood health centers are all required or urged to include meaningful consumer representation. The move toward "consumerism," "Naderism," or "consumer participation" in health care, as in other aspects of American life, reflects many diverse factors—political and economic as well as health.

Many health care providers have resisted this trend, which they see as the "politicalization" of health care or as a threat to the quality of care. These are real dangers. There is an inordinate amount of fumbling and wasted time going on in this respect. Neither the new consumer representatives nor the providers, working with them, know quite what is expected of them. But for the long run this is a promising development. It provides a good opportunity to educate key individuals who, in turn, can help to educate their fellow consumers. The union officials who have participated for some years in running their local health and welfare funds have learned something about the limits, as well as the cost, of health care and are now more temperate in their demands and expectations. The black mothers who are serving on advisory committees for neighborhood health centers are going through the same educational process.

For better or worse, the health care "consumer" is here to stay as part of the health care picture. Since he is ultimately footing the bill, he is going to have some say, either directly through the provider institutions, or indirectly through government, or through both. It would appear the wiser course, from the point of view of the providers, to encourage direct participation. It would also appear the course of wisdom to do everything possible to promote effective programs in health education for all citizens, starting in the home and continuing through school, college, and adult life.

FAILURES AND OPPORTUNITIES

The idea of health education is far from radical. Something under this name has been taught in schools of public health for many years. Many elementary and secondary schools have courses officially labeled "health education" or some equivalent. However, as is generally known, they have not been successful in reaching the youngsters. For the most part, these courses have little relation to real-life problems and show no imagination. Start with a lecture on the evils of smoking, either tobacco or marijuana, and the instructor might as well give up immediately. But start with a realistic discussion of drugs, or sex, or weight problems, and a skillful instructor may be able to lay a basis for lifetime understanding of the use and abuse of drugs, nutrition, exercise, healthy marital relations, and general self-control.

The point is frequently made that education alone is inadequate, that knowledge does not necessarily lead to desirable changes of behavior. This is true, but it does not follow that education is useless. The point is to relate education to personal experience, to give meaning to this experience, to help the youngster anticipate future experience, good and bad, and, above all, to avoid hypocrisy and half-truths.

Young people are frequently more concerned about illness and health than adults think they are. As long as the possibility of death or maiming in a distant war, which appears to have neither purpose nor end, hangs like the sword of Damocles over most young males, it is unrealistic to expect them to get too excited over the possible ill effects of marijuana or speeding. Moreover, adults must appreciate the extent to which more or less deliberate self-abuse may be seen as a means of rebuking the older generation for the many negative aspects of the American life style—a life style in which war, violence, racial prejuduce, overpopulation, and environmental pollution play such conspicuous roles.

The fact remains that the majority of young Americans, like the majority of their elders, want to be healthy and appreciate intelligent help in that direction. For example, a recent study by the American Cancer Society reports that a majority of American teenagers oppose smoking, but environmental magnets like advertisements and the habits of parents and peers still draw about 40 percent to smoking.

We desperately need a new approach to curricula, teaching materials, and teaching techniques at the elementary and secondary school levels. Obviously,

this also calls for a redefinition of health education at the teacher-training level
and a whole new approach in the schools of public health and medicine.

HEALTH EDUCATION FOR ALL

The current multimillion dollar business in do-it-yourself health books,
magazines, and articles, the popularity of "health" food stores and their ever-
growing coterie of dedicated diet-conscious customers, the success of Weight
Watchers and other "health clubs" outside the health care Establishment all
testify to the widespread hunger for intelligent, informative health guidance.
This attitude is probably far more widespread than the irresponsibility we have
already noted, although the two are not necessarily incompatible.

The official attitude of the medical profession and of the U.S. Food and Drug
Administration has generally been one of contemptuous opposition to all such
"extra-Establishment" activities. Given the inability of most doctors to find
time to deal with such problems, it would be far more helpful to light a few can-
dles of effective health education than to curse the darkness.

The importance of television in the continuing health education of adults and
young people alike cannot be exaggerated. The negative effects are with us constantly. Even with the new antismoking advertisements, teenagers are exposed
to more than three times as many messages supporting smoking as assailing it.
Heroin and LSD are not sold on television, but the drug habit is. Clearly there is
need for some national policy, guidelines, and leadership with respect to use of
television and other mass media for this purpose.

It might be desirable to require all third parties, public and private, to devote
1 percent of their health care revenue to general health education. All schools of
the health professions and all hospitals could be required to allocate a similar
percentage of their budgets to the same cause.

Of course, the one individual with the greatest potential as a health educator
is the doctor. He is the one who sees the patient when he is most receptive to
health counsel. He is the one who is really listened to. Here is a great "teachable
moment," and there is either a positive or negative educational outcome depending upon the quality of the doctor-patient relationship during the time they
are together. Some doctors are making an earnest effort to incorporate patient
education into their daily patient contacts. But most are too busy to take on this
extra burden. And even if they had time, many lack both the inclination and the
general knowledge to do the job effectively. This is the price of modern
specialization. It is a high price—so high, in terms of frequently ineffective
medical care as well as frequent patient dissatisfaction—that some corrective
action should not be delayed.

Some hospitals also give lip service to the concept of consumer health education. A few, such as Lankenau in Philadelphia, do something about it. In 1964
the American Hospital Association, in cooperation with the Metropolitan Life
Insurance Company, sponsored an interesting conference on the subject. The

net results are almost zero. Most hospitals are totally unprepared for this work. However, with a little imagination, a little money, and the cooperation of the medical staff, patient education could be effectively tied to patient care.

A NATIONAL COUNCIL ON HEALTH EDUCATION

In order to provide a national center for interest, expertise, promotion, and evaluation in all the areas of actual or potential health education noted in this chapter, the establishment of a permanent high level National Council on Health Education is recommended. The council would be responsible for recommending and monitoring national policy in such areas as:
- national goals with respect to health education,
- teacher training for formal health education courses,
- curricula for grade schools and colleges,
- programs for adult education,
- programs for the mass media,
- health education in hospitals and other public or publicly supported institutions,
- health education and third party reimbursement, and
- consumer participation in health care programs as a technique of health education.

Membership should include the leadership of the medical profession, schools of health professions, hospitals, and other provider groups; business, labor, minority, and other consumer groups; third party carriers; and government. The council should be advisory to the Secretary of Health, Education, and Welfare. It should be adequately funded, imaginatively staffed, including experts in audiovisual techniques, and prepared to play a leadership role vis-à-vis the health and education establishments and the mass media.

NOTES

1. R. Auster, I. Leveson, D. Sarachek, "The Production of Health, An Exploratory Study," *Journal of Human Resources* 4, no. 4, (Fall 1969): 411 ff.

Selection 43

Death Rates, Life Style, and National Morale: Two Proposals*

The crude death rate in the United States (that is, the ratio of all deaths to total population in a given year) has been almost stationary for over two decades—fluctuating between 9.4 and 9.6 deaths per 1,000. Obscured by this overall stability, however, are a number of significant changes.

The most disturbing trends emerge when the data are broken down by age as well as by sex. When the 1964-1968 experience of various age groups is compared, we find that mortality rates rose for all ages between 15 and 74. Improvement was registered only for the very young and the very old. The big news is the rising death rates of young and middle-aged American men.

A study of this phenomenon was released in late 1971 by the National Center for Health Statistics.[1] Death rates for young white men, 15 to 19, rose 21 percent from 1963-1968. For nonwhites, the rise was a shocking 35 percent. This does not include battle deaths. Increases, smaller yet still significant, applied to all white males under 45 and to all nonwhites under 65. Additional data suggest that death rates for men under 45 are continuing to rise.

The principal causes of death for the whole population in 1968 were still heart disease, cancer, and stroke—plus accidents, mostly auto. Heart disease accounted for nearly 40 percent of all deaths. During the late 1960s, however, other causes were primarily responsible. Here, according to the National Center for Health Statistics, are the principal offenders:

1. For young men, 15 to 24, of all races, motor vehicle accidents accounted for most of the upturn; suicide and homicide came next. Blacks 20 to 24 had a homicide death rate of 106 per 100,000.

2. For white men 25 to 44, motor vehicles were still the principal cause of the upturn, followed by lung cancer, cirrhosis of the liver, suicide, and homicide. Blacks of this age group were increasingly subject to violent deaths but also to an increase in cancer.

3. For men of all races, 45 to 64, there were substantial increases in the death rate for lung cancer, emphysema, diseases of the heart and circulatory system, bronchitis, cirrhosis. For blacks of this age group, diabetes, cancer of the urinary organs, and homicide were also factors.

Death is, of course, the ultimate in poor health, and also best reported. But it is only the tip of the iceberg. For every youngster killed in an auto accident, how many thousands are injured, even permanently disabled? For every middle-aged man who dies of cirrhosis, how many million alcoholics or near alcoholics

---

*Excerpt from A.R. Somers, paper presented to Protestant Health and Welfare General Assembly, March 8, 1972, Chicago, Illinois; published in *Bulletin of the American Protestant Hospital Association* 36 (Spring 1972): 4-30.

exist? For every death from an overdose of heroin, how many are hooked to a habit that will cause crime and other problems? For the relatively few whom syphilis actually kills, how many are infected by this easily preventable disease? According to *Newsweek,* venereal disease has reached such proportions in Los Angeles that if the present rate of increase continues, "one in five of the city's high schoolers will have contracted gonorrhea or syphilis by the time they graduate."

Implications of these trends are deeply disturbing. This retrogression in the national health (at least for men) has occurred at precisely the period when almost every available input index of health care progress has been rising. By 1968, expenditures for biomedical research had reached $2 billion a year, and total health care expenditures nearly $57 billion. Between 1966 and 1968, the annual rate of increase was nearly 13 percent, far in excess of the increase in gross national product (GNP). Is there, then, no positive relationship between input and output?

Apparently it all depends on the definition of output. What *is* the product of the health services industry? Is it a healthier people? Or is it so many doctor visits? Or so many patient days in the hospital? So many aspirins sold? If it is the first, the industry will complain, and rightly, that health is affected by many factors other than medical care and that it cannot be held responsible for shortcomings in the living conditions, education, and life style of the American male.

But if output is measured purely in terms of health services delivered, then the primary justification for the massive increases in expenditures and the rapidly rising federal subsidies disappears. The welfare of the four million individuals employed in the health services industry is, of course, an important concern for national policy. Nevertheless, any effort to disassociate the ultimate purpose of the health care industry from consumer health cannot long be sustained.

HEALTH AND HEALTH CARE: ARE THEY RELATED?

Carried to its logical conclusion, the effort to disassociate the health care industry from accountability for the nation's health would mean that doctors and hospitals should not attend anyone except those who are definitely ill; that health insurance should be renamed "sickness insurance;" that prepaid group practice organizations should not be permitted to call themselves health maintenance organizations; and that a clear-cut distinction should be made between the "sickness industry" and those programs and activities designed to improve people's health. A doctor from upstate New York, in a recent letter to the *New England Journal of Medicine,* put the issue bluntly:

> The medical profession has a major responsibility to change the American life style.... Or are the doctors too preoccupied with coronary-care units ... to bother with preventive programs?

Consumer Health Educat...

No such distinction can be made in practice. A national commission of heart disease specialists recently pointed out that a major cause of death from heart attacks is the victim's indecision and delay in calling doctor or ambulance. This indecision, the commission continued, is often related to ignorance about the symptoms of heart attacks and how to get medical help rapidly.

We are just now reaching the point at which the concept of "comprehensive care" is beginning to be accepted. The challenge today is to implement this concept and adjust our programs accordingly, rather than to abandon it and cut our institutions back to "sick services."

Yet some will surely ask, "Is this practical?" How can doctors and hospitals influence the homicide rate? Or the rise in motor vehicle deaths? Or cigarette-induced lung cancer and emphysema? More profoundly, is the very concept of health not a mirage, ever beckoning but ever elusive?

The dictionary definition of "health" encompasses a number of meanings, including the absence of disease or infirmity, a state of well-being, and optimal functioning. Until fairly recently, most people accepted the first meaning almost exclusively. The inadequacy of this definition was particularly felt by leaders of the public health movement, whose brilliant achievements in the battle against infectious and deficiency diseases contributed so decisively to the lowering of death rates and raising of life expectancy from about 1850 to 1950.

The often-quoted World Health Organization (WHO) definition—"Health is a state of complete physical, mental, and social well-being, and not merely the absence of disease or infirmity"—was widely hailed for its emphasis on "positive health." In line with the definition, some segments of the medical profession have tried to broaden the boundaries of health care to include psychosocial factors, a welcome development.

Still, something **is** obviously missing. That "something," or rather "someone" is the consumer-patient himself. Of all the many and varied causes of the current "health care crisis," none has been more overlooked than the consumer-patient.

In his brilliant book, *The Mirage of Health,* Dr. René Dubos of the Rockefeller Institute of Medical Research makes a point that is highly relevant in our present dilemma. Health, according to his view, is not the product of a perfect adjustment between man and a static environment. In his words:

> Harmonious equilibrium with nature is an abstract concept with a Platonic beauty but lacking flesh and blood of life. It fails, in particular, to convey the creative emergent quality of human existence.... In the world of reality, places change and man changes also.... Thus, health and happiness cannot be absolute and permanent values.... Biological success in all its manifestations is a measure of fitness, and fitness requires never ending efforts of adaptation to the total environment, which is ever changing.

From this it follows:

1. Health, like happiness, is not a commodity that one individual can bestow on another. Health has to be earned by the individual himself.
2. Health, like happiness, cannot be successfully pursued as an end in itself. It is a byproduct of the individual's striving for some goal larger than physical well-being. It is dependent on the individual's morale and sense of purpose and maintenance of a life style consistent with that purpose.
3. Individual life style and morale are profoundly influenced by those of society. Yet the environment is ever-changing. A way of life that was healthy for our parents may no longer be healthy for our children.

At first glance, this thesis may appear discouraging in its vision of man as an ever-questing Don Quixote in pursuit of the "Impossible Dream," and health as a byproduct of that struggle. In fact, however, it appears to correspond not only to the record of history but also to the evidence of our own lives.

The Protestant Ethic, the Marxist Ethic, the Zionist Ethic: each of these value systems, as well as older Catholic and Islamic religions, has proved a powerful builder of men as well as of nations and of empires. But value systems are related to the socioeconomic conditions which give birth to them, and once conditions change, the old values lose much of their motivating power. In our society, where one computer can do the work of hundreds of human beings, the Work Ethic obviously has limited appeal, especially to youth.

But hedonism is no answer. This attitude toward life has always been inimical to health. The collapse of the Roman Empire, the France of Louis XVI, and virtually all great affluent societies of the past should be lesson enough. Even for those who stick their historical heads in the sand, there are the current statistics on drug abuse, alcoholism, lung cancer, heart attacks, and venereal disease. Contrary to some wishful thinking, these are not primarily the result of poverty or deprivation and cannot be cured by increasing GNP. These diseases (as well as the rise in violent deaths among our young men and in deaths from smoking, drinking, and overeating among the middle aged) are probably related to each other, and are all related to a loss of morale or purpose in our individual and national lives.

A recent review of a new book, *Voices From the Drug Culture,* in the *New England Journal of Medicine,* had this to say:

> Why does the expression 'drug culture' now commonly apply to white youth of the middle and upper classes who have relatively recently begun to experiment with cannabis and the hallucinogens, rather than, for example, to the much larger 'generation' of chronic ethanol, barbiturate, amphetamine and nicotine users who continue to enjoy their drugs and their 'culture'? Or the advertising firms that work to convince television viewers that expensive salicylates are more effective than cheap ones? Or those of us in or about to enter a medical profession that has come to rely on diazepam three times a day more than on a comforting talk with an obviously troubled patient?

For the health care industry, the lesson of all this is a sobering one. For years, we have gone on the assumption that by spending more dollars, turning out more doctors and nurses, building more beds and health centers, inventing new technologies and drugs, we could make people healthier. For perhaps two decades after World War II, the results were positive as we caught up with previously unmet needs. But around the middle 1960s, the net result of this relatively narrow approach began to be negative. Now, it seems additional funds for medical care, unless accompanied by some far-reaching reforms, could actually contribute to further consumer irresponsibility especially with respect to use of drugs, x rays, and some forms of surgery....

Here are two suggestions directed to different groups. The first is aimed primarily at those who already have some concern for health; it seeks to reach them through the community hospital. The second is aimed at the young. It is not a health program in the traditional sense of the word. But, if implemented, it might do more for the health of the nation than any comparable effort.

A NATIONAL PROGRAM OF HOSPITAL-BASED CONSUMER HEALTH EDUCATION

With national awareness of the need for consumer health education growing, perhaps the biggest single inhibiting factor today is uncertainty as to how to proceed. The inadequacy of traditional approaches is widely recognized and gives pause to many who would like to move faster. The great difficulty in changing behavior in the health field discourages many. So does the difficulty of evaluation.

On the other hand, there is a tendency to ignore examples of effective health education now being carried on by such experiments as Weight Watchers, Alcoholics Anonymous, Planned Parenthood, television ads on antismoking, and hundreds of small projects in hospitals, mental health centers, local health departments, neighborhood health centers, prepaid group practice clinics, and so forth.

One of the values of such projects is precisely their small size and experimental nature. The general idea behind many is that ordinary people, with some training, can help each other. This seems to be the secret of success of such disparate programs as the Chinese "barefoot doctors," the indigenous health aides trained by some of the Office of Economic Opportunity health centers, and the "Learning by Teaching" programs now being tried in some of our more experimental schools.[2]

One of the most promising of these local approaches is the hospital-based program. This can in many instances reach the consumer at precisely the point where he is most receptive—the point at which he has begun to feel concern. It is also relevant that the hospital itself, the most expensive of all health care institutions, badly needs consumer support.

Such experiments are already going on. Frequently the impetus has come from individual staff physicians. Internists, obstetricians, pediatricians, specialists in rehabilitation medicine, psychiatrists, and others are seeking ways of providing their own patients with instruction on how to cope with diabetes, high blood pressure, obesity, pregnancy, child care, family planning, and addictions of various types. However, many such experiments remain isolated with no method of objective evaluation or even a clearinghouse for exchange of experience.

I am proposing that the hospital industry as a whole, under leadership of the American Hospital Association, the American Protestant Hospital Association, the Catholic Hospital Association, and the various state organizations, in cooperation with the appropriate professional associations, take the lead in expanding and evaluating such programs on a nationwide basis.

A NATIONAL SERVICE CORPS FOR AMERICAN YOUTH

"Many forms of delinquency among our overfed teenagers probably come from their unspent creative energy." This is another quotation from Dr. Dubos. While he was referring primarily to antisocial activities, he could easily have included antihealth activities. The major health problems of American youth (death and injury from motor vehicle accidents and other forms of violence, venereal disease, drugs) have been noted.

The challenge, however, is not to tranquilize youth or mislead them with refurbished dreams of happiness through material gains, but to find new ways to harness their physical and emotional energy. To this end I suggest the creation of a National Service Corps, involving one or two years of service between high school and college, or at age 18, for all boys and girls. They would be given their choice of military service or a wide range of civilian activities. It would absorb the Peace Corps and Vista as well as the present military draft. The federal government would be primarily responsible for organizing and operating the corps, although private nonprofit organizations with experience could be delegated responsibility for operating subsidiary branches or projects.

The success of any such undertaking would depend largely on the value of the work projects. Any suggestion of "make-work" would discredit the concept. But to suggest that there is not enough real work to occupy four million 18-year-olds is to shut one's eyes to massive problems. With a work force of this size and with moderate wages, undertakings could be started that are now all but impossible.

The advantage to the typical high school graduate of such a transitional work experience before going on to college or deciding on his life's work should be great. It would provide an opportunity for expressing youthful idealism and creativity, for acquiring healthy living and working habits and self-reliance away from the frequent irritants of family life. For those who do decide to go on to college, it would be a maturing experience and probably result in more highly motivated students, as was the case with the World War II GIs. Those who decide to seek advanced vocational training or go straight to work should be better prepared for this decision.

Obviously, there would be problems. It would be essential to guard against exploitation of corpsmen. Or against using them to undermine regular labor standards of the adult population. Institutions of higher education would have to cope with a serious, though temporary, hiatus. Any new program entails problems. But the proposal would have obvious advantages—to distraught parents, to frightened communities, to a nation groping for ways of channeling the energy of its youth, and most of all to the young people themselves who have been crying out for meaningful purpose and usefulness.

Once again, the American conscience and American technology could be joined, and pride in country could be restored. In the typical American way, we seem to have been edging toward such a program, piecemeal, bit by bit. When President Richard Nixon announced his decision to seek a merger of the Peace Corps, Vista, and certain other federal agencies in January 1971, he spoke of it as a new volunteer service corps "that will give young Americans an expanded opportunity" to serve the poor at home and abroad. The merger was effected, but the new agency never received anything like the federal attention, funding, or sense of mission necessary for it to be taken seriously.

A year later, in January 1972, the Commissioner of the Youth Services Department of Massachusetts announced a program to abolish institutions for juvenile offenders and to replace them with community-based work and educational programs. The reasons were not entirely idealistic. The per capita cost of jailing a juvenile for a year is about $10,000, "enough to send a child to Harvard with $100 a week allowance, a summer vacation in Europe, and once-a-week psychotherapy."

In April 1971, in a column devoted primarily to reclaiming the loyalty of youthful war protesters, *New York Times* columnist James Reston endorsed the concept of a volunteer army but insisted that it "must be part of a broader volunteer national service program." "It's absurd," he said, "to think of the military as the only way to serve one's country.... Military recruiters should have to compete, especially in poverty areas, with recruiters from the Peace Corps, the Job Corps, and other youth corps programs. The poor youth, whether in the ghetto or Appalachia, must have an alternative to the military as an escape from his environment."

The proposed federal sponsorship has been questioned, even the whole concept of a compulsory, as opposed to a voluntary, service. A respected friend writes as follows:

> I fear the ideological indoctrination and suppression possible in a monolithic program. My many acquaintances in VISTA and the Peace Corps have some hairy tales about the changes subsequent to 1969.... However, your proposal of a pluralistic set of opportunities within a comprehensive federal program of financing, guidelines, and parameters makes much sense.

I agree as to the preferability of private auspices. But I do not believe it is possible to launch such a program on a sufficient scale without federal sponsorship. Nor do I think it possible to give equal value to military and nonmilitary service unless there is an equal public and Congressional commitment to the importance and conditions of both types of service. Finally, we have to recognize that, like it or not, we live in an era of big government. We simply must work to make government more accountable and more responsive to human needs.

In any case, this is a program of such magnitude and importance that it would require a great deal of study and public debate. These are not easy tasks that I am suggesting. I close with another quotation from Dr. Dubos:

> The earth is not a resting place. Man has elected to fight not necessarily for himself but for a process of emotional, intellectual, and ethical growth which goes on forever. To grow in the midst of danger is a fate of the human race because it is the law of the spirit.

It is also, I believe, the road to individual and national health.

NOTES

1. U.S. Department of Health, Education, and Welfare, National Center for Health Statistics, A. Joan Klebba, *Leading Components of Upturn in Mortality for Men, U.S. 1952-67,* (Washington, D.C.: U.S. Government Printing Office, 1971).
2. A. Gartner, M. Kohler, and F. Riessman, *Children Teach Children: Learning by Teaching,* (New York: Harper and Row, 1971).

Selection 44

Health Education at Monmouth Medical Center: A Case Study*

Samuel Smith, M.D., a Long Branch, New Jersey, internist specializing in diabetes, has a lot of problem patients. When Paul Brown first appeared in Dr. Smith's office, he looked like a prisoner of war. Although he was 16 years old and five feet, 11 inches tall, he weighed only 104 pounds. An adolescent diabetic, Paul had been administering his own insulin for over a year and doing the best he could with diet modification. But he had no idea how to adjust his insulin dosage and was almost literally starving to death.

*Excerpt from A.R. Somers and William Vaun, M.D., "What $34,000 Has Done for Long Branch," *Prism* (December 1973): 36-59.

Paul was the son of a military father. Because of repeated household moves, everyone involved in his case—the various doctors, nurses, his parents—assumed that someone else had given him the necessary instruction. But, in fact, nobody had—even though Paul had been hospitalized when the diagnosis of diabetes was made.

Fortunately, a schoolmate at Long Branch High School, a patient of Dr. Smith's, brought Paul to Smith's office about a year ago. He was admitted to Monmouth Medical Center for a week, during which time he attended his first diabetic education class. After discharge, he went back for three more sessions, completing the eight-hour course. Today, Paul weighs 140, and his diabetes is completely under control.

Mrs. Mary White, age 44, has been a problem diabetic for several years. About five feet, five inches tall, she weighed 235 pounds last December. Menopause aggravated the situation. She telephoned her doctor constantly, always with the same complaints of depression and inability to maintain her diet.

Last January, Dr. Smith sent her to Monmouth Medical Center's diabetes class. Not only did she pick up information that she had missed before; but, more important, she benefited from the informal group encounter and interpersonal support which her classmates generated from their own experience. Within eight months, Mrs. White reduced to 195 pounds, far from ideal, but a real improvement. Her diabetes was under better control, and menopause was less of a problem. Her morale improved, and her family was deeply grateful. Says Dr. Smith, "The health education class took the albatross off my back!"

THE MONMOUTH (N.J.) HEALTH EDUCATION PROGRAM

Dr. Smith, Mrs. White, and Paul Brown have all been involved in Monmouth Medical Center's Community Health Education Program. This program has become so pervasive that a local newspaper said recently, "For many men and women, Monmouth Medical Center is not primarily a hospital but a public school."

Between September 1, 1972 and June 1, 1973, over 3,000 residents of Monmouth and Ocean Counties, with a variety of actual or potential health problems, attended classes, conferences, or other activities sponsored by the Monmouth program. Seventy doctors, nurses, and other health professionals were involved in the planning and teaching (see the table pp. 308-309).

During one week in May, for example, when the program was at a peak activity for the year, the following educational activities were going on. The weekly class for diabetic patients met Monday night. Forty-two couples attended the expectant parents' class. Postnatal instruction for both parents was conducted twice a day on three separate days. A colostomy patient received five hours of individualized instruction (one preoperative, four postoperative). Preoperative instruction via closed-circuit television was presented to all surgical patients every night, Sunday through Thursday. An in-service training

Community Health Education Programs of Monmouth Medical Center
September 1, 1972, to May 31, 1973

Patient and In-Service Training Programs	No. Student Hours per Activity	No. Times Activity Repeated	Total No. Student Hours	No. Participants	No. Professionals (Instructors)
Patient Activities:					
Diabetes	8	7	56	122	8
Prenatal instruction (both expectant parents)	15	6	90	222	12
Postnatal instruction (both parents)	8	8	64	135	3
Colostomy[1]	5	9	45	9	4
General preoperative instruction[2]	5	1	5	40	2
Nurse In-Service Courses:					
Patient education for obstetrical nurses	6	1	6	9	2
Patient education for nurses on teen-age unit[3]	9	1	9	43	3
TOTAL	56	33	275	580	34

[1] Individual instruction.
[2] One-week experimental closed-circuit television program in May 1973. The 40 patients represent number evaluated for impact of telecast that covers both pre- and postoperative procedures. It became a regular hospital program in September, 1973, broadcast five nights a week, Monday through Friday. Available to all surgical inpatients.
[3] Emphasizes prevention and treatment of VD, contraception, and drugs.
[4] Program includes sex education, marriage counseling, and family planning.
[5] Continuous, seven nights a week.

Consumer Health Education

Community Programs	No. Student Hours per Activity	No. Times Activity Repeated	Total No. Student Hours	No. Participants	No. Professionals (Instructors)
VD instruction (high school students)	4	15	60	780	3
Family living (high school students)[4]	4	6	24	172	4
Drug education (high school students and community)	4	3	12	342	1
Emergency childbirth instruction (first-aid squads)	3	5	15	248	1
Cardiopulmonary resuscitation (first-aid squads)	6	3	18	94	5
Lifeguard programs	6	2	12	35	2
VD information hotline[5]	—	—	—	225+	4
Sickle cell screening	—	16	—	428	8
Sickle cell screening[1]	0.5	—	129	258	8
TOTAL	27.5	50	270	2582	36
GRAND TOTAL	83.5	83	545	3162	70

[1] Individual instruction.
[2] One-week experimental closed-circuit television program in May 1973. The 40 patients represent number evaluated for impact of telecast that covers both pre- and postoperative procedures. It became a regular hospital program in September, 1973, broadcast five nights a week, Monday through Friday. Available to all surgical inpatients.
[3] Emphasizes prevention and treatment of VD, contraception, and drugs.
[4] Program includes sex education, marriage counseling, and family planning.
[5] Continuous, seven nights a week.

program for obstetrical nurses, to enable them to carry on patient education, met for two hours; and another in-service course for nurses on the teen-age unit met for three hours.

At the local high school, meanwhile, hospital staff members spent more than 12 hours discussing drug abuse, venereal disease, and "family living" with the students. Three hours were devoted to individual counseling of patients with sickle cell anemia following the screening program for this disease.

For those in need of emergency counseling, the venereal disease information "hotline" was open every night. This service operates from a desk in the emergency room in Monmouth Medical Center. Two needs are served by this arrangement: first, a special telephone for VD counseling relieves normal emergency room telephones from this type of call; second, specially trained personnel can give accurate information and immediate and effective counseling.

During the same week, the hospital conducted emergency childbirth and cardiopulmonary resuscitation classes for the community's first-aid squad and a special program for lifeguards—a key group in this seashore community.

What sort of an institution is Monmouth Medical Center? How did such an extensive educational program develop? Does it pay off in terms of better health for patients and the community at large? Can useful conclusions be drawn from the Monmouth experience?

To begin with, except for its larger-than-usual size and special interest in education, Monmouth is a fairly typical community hospital, serving a population ranging from the very rich to the very poor.

It began its first efforts at consumer health education several years ago. Informal instruction for expectant parents and diabetic patients was given by physicians and nurses without compensation. In September 1971, Monmouth joined with Rutgers Medical School, a division of the College of Medicine and Dentistry of New Jersey, and two other community hospitals in developing a proposal for a pilot program in hospital-based community health education. In due course, the proposal was funded by a modest grant, and a central Office of Community Health Education was established in the Department of Community Medicine at the medical school.

Monmouth started receiving its share of funds in September 1972, and began developing its program under the general supervision of the director of medical education. The first step was to find a project director, a position eventually filled by a young man already working at the hospital as a psychiatric nurse who had considerable experience in education. Aside from his secretary, all other staff members, volunteer or salaried, are part-time. Space, always a problem in a crowded hospital, was secured, and a visible office of Community Health Education was officially established.

Next, the project director established his priorities: (1) identification of every existing program or activity within the hospital that related to patient or community health education; (2) establishment of a method to involve the community and the health professionals in planning and decision making; and (3) organization of an expanded community program ("outreach") using existing personnel and resources as fully and as effectively as possible.

Identification of existing efforts was not difficult. The program for prospective parents, initiated by the Department of Obstetrics and Gynecology, was particularly well organized, well received, and already financially self-sufficient. The experience gained through this program proved valuable to the planning of subsequent programs.

The main tasks before the project director were to coordinate and expand the existing fragmented activities, to fill in the gaps, and to develop meaningful evaluation techniques. He had to put the whole enterprise on a businesslike basis, with visibility and credibility within the hospital hierarchy and the community.

An advisory group to the new program was established at the outset. It included representatives from all the hospital-based health professions, the community, inhospital and ambulatory patients, and selected community health agencies. Together with the director of medical education and the project director, they developed a program relevant both to the needs of the community and to existing hospital resources. Out of these discussions two major aims emerged:

1. To educate individuals who are now, or have been, patients either of a member of the medical staff or one of the hospital clinics, especially those with a chronic illness or disability. The purpose is to enable such patients to cope more effectively with their health problems and to help the doctor achieve more effective management of their problems.

2. To develop outreach programs, open to the general community, designed to meet some of the community's health needs and to prevent, whenever possible, the need for individual hospitalization. [There followed discussion of these illustrative programs—diabetes patient education, VD hotline, and expectant parents classes. Only the second is presented here.]

VD INFORMATION HOTLINE

The venereal disease hotline operates seven nights a week under the aegis of the outpatient department. The telephones are manned by three highly motivated and specially trained young college students associated with Youth Horizons, a Long Branch community group, and one adult licensed practical nurse. They have full-time back-up from physicians in the emergency room and VD clinic.

From January 2, 1973, when the current program was started, through May 31, 1973, over 225 calls were received. The monthly and weekly averages have increased steadily as a result of favorable publicity, including free spot announcements on the local radio station.

It is impossible to evaluate precisely the full impact of this service. There is no way of measuring the total follow-up, since numerous other health care resources are also available to callers. However, the number of visits to the hospital VD clinic and emergency room by patients seeking advice or treatment has increased substantially since the hotline was started. Equally important, the proportion of patients going to the clinic rather than to the emergency room has also increased. This suggests not only that more patients are seeking proper treatment, but that they are seeking it in the proper place—the VD clinic— rather than going to the emergency room with a condition that is not an emergency. [For a follow-up evaluation, see N.H. Bryant et al., "V.D. Hotline: An Evaluation," *Public Health Reports* 91 (May-June 1976): 231-235.]

EDUCATIONAL METHODOLOGY

At Monmouth Medical Center, every type of educational technique is under consideration, investigation, or experimentation. These include closed-circuit television and other audiovisual aids, panel and small group discussions, individual consultation and instruction, and even the "old-fashioned" lecture.

Merely changing traditional classroom methods does not work, neither does instituting new methods solely for the reason of change. Courses must be designed to involve the adult learner actively in the learning process. The total organization of a community health education program must take into consideration the need for maximum freedom and flexibility. At the same time, the program must be so structured as to impose a high degree of self-discipline, especially with respect to evaluation—a characteristic frequently lacking in traditional health education programs. The need for flexibility and self-discipline will affect every aspect of the program, including organizational structure, choice of a director, teachers, and members of the advisory committee.

Staffing is, of course, crucial. The ideal director is one who combines a background in one of the health professions with some knowledge of modern educational techniques, and strong leadership qualities in program development with flexibility in implementation. A frequent misconception is that such programs must be directed by health educators with advanced degrees.

Finally, each course must be evaluated according to its effectiveness in improving the status of the patient's health. The class for expectant parents, for example, although popular and very well attended, placed too little emphasis on physical exercise. Without evaluation of this course, Monmouth might have drifted along, content with the course's popularity, regardless of objective results.

FINANCING THE PROGRAM

The cost of the Monmouth program for the year, Septembe1972 to August 1973, was approximately $34,000, the amount of their grant. This included salaries for a full-time director and secretary, 65 part-time instructors and other personnel, and money for instructional and promotional materials. Space and office equipment were provided by the hospital.

While $34,000 is not a negligible sum, neither is it very large in terms of current hospital financing. It represents less than 0.2 percent of Monmouth's 1973 budget. Spread over 525 beds, this sum represents about $65 per bed for the year. Health education, then, need not be an expensive undertaking. Indeed, depending on the nature and size of a hospital, a simple reorganization and reorientation of individuals already engaged in segments of the total job may be all that is needed to start. Regardless of the size of budget, however, it is essential to fix the overall responsibility on some one individual; and space and resources commensurate to the job are obviously necessary.

With respect to instructors, the Monmouth policy provides that anyone salaried by the hospital may not receive additional remuneration when serving during regular hours, whatever those regular hours are for the individual concerned. After hours, all receive an honorarium.

Smaller hospitals with no previous experience in community health education might be advised to work with neighboring institutions, pooling resources on a regional basis. In any case, the resources of the numerous public and private health agencies—local, regional, and state—should be thoroughly explored. The Monmouth experience indicates that an impressive pool of volunteer talent and teaching materials, as well as potential financial assistance, are available during the development stage. One of the high points of the year was the unsolicited donation of $1,500 to the program from a black professional women's group in Long Branch, which was impressed with the sickle cell anemia screening program.

Monmouth got most of its start-up money from a special grant. From the beginning, however, the hospital understood that this was a short term subsidy and made plans to integrate the program into its regular operating budget. Every effort has been made to make individual programs as self-supporting as possible. It has been our experience that modest registration fees, waived in cases of financial need, are entirely feasible and not resented.

Such a program cannot be supported entirely by patient or student fees, however; and, at the moment, long term financing presents a problem. But within the foreseeable future, it appears that hospital-based patient and community health education may be considered allowable expenses for third party reimbursement. The Department of Health, Education, and Welfare is apparently moving in this direction with respect to Medicare and Medicaid. So is the New Jersey Department of Insurance. A corollary of such reimbursement would be the requirement of more rigorous criteria for health education programs than was formerly true.

We believe that this pilot program has already contributed substantially to the experience necessary to the development of such criteria. As to the hospital itself, there is nearly unanimous opinion that the experience has been valuable. The proof is the commitment to continue the program after the project funds expire. Participation has been an enriching experience for all the professionals. For the physician, in particular, patient education of this sort adds yet another dimension to the art of medicine.

Selection 45

Consumer Health Education:
Some Critical Questions*

In 1972 with the support of Dr. Stanley Bergen, Jr., President of the College of Medicine and Dentistry of New Jersey, and the cooperation of several community hospitals, I established a small experimental program in hospital-based consumer health education. During the past two years, this program has grown into a network of associated programs, involving a dozen New Jersey hospitals and other community institutions, hundreds of physicians, nurses and other professionals, with a documented record of reaching nearly 13,000 patients and other consumers through a variety of classes, seminars, conferences, screenings, individual counseling, etc.

By the usual standards in the health care field—increase in budget, space, personnel, utilization, local and national publicity—the program may be considered a success. In the areas of our principal concentration—the goals, organization, and management of hospital-based programs—we feel that we are beginning to come up with at least some tentative answers. A manual incorporating some of this experience is now available.[1]

Still, the worrisome questions remain: Is this program an accident of circumstances or are we producing a model that can be generally replicated? More basically, do we really know what we are doing? What exactly *is* "health education?" Do we know how to motivate young people and others who are still asymptomatic, to health-maintaining behavior? What success rate can we anticipate for patients with the various forms of chronic illness or disability? Is "behavior modification" a good thing or bad?

What institutions and what professions should be responsible? What, specifically, is the role of the hospital? Can we build health education into the delivery system and assure payment therefore—for ambulatory as well as inpatients? Can this be done on a purely voluntary basis?

How to move toward a more balanced relationship between the minuscule national investment in health education and other aspects of preventive medicine and the overwhelming commitment to tertiary care and other aspects of therapeutic medicine? Can *this* be done on a purely voluntary basis?

How to reconcile national objectives in health protection, for example in respect to nutrition and environmental pollution, with the far stronger national goal of maximizing jobs and income in all areas regardless of effect on individual health?

---

*Excerpt from A.R. Somers, "Consumer Health Edcuation: An Idea Whose Time Has Come?" *Hospital Progress, Journal of the Catholic Hospital Association* 56 (February 1975): 10-11.

Do we know how to define "quality" in this area and how to measure our effectiveness—or the lack of it? The latter question is particularly important, and the way we approach it may be crucial to the future of health education. On the one hand, we must be prepared to subject ourselves to meaningful evaluation and to accept the consequences even when the studies tell us that our programs are not meeting their goals. On the other hand, we cannot be so lacking in the courage of our convictions that we allow ourselves to be scared out of experimentation or subjected to more rigorous evaluation than other elements of the health care system.

After all, it is the almost exclusive concentration on the traditional therapeutic system that has resulted in the current $100 billion U.S. health care bill and the 10 to 15 percent recent annual increases. All preventive programs taken together probably account for less than 3 percent of the total. We will never move toward a more sensible balance between preventive and therapeutic medicine if those who believe in the former accept the existing double standard with respect to evaluation or commit statistical hara-kiri.

These and many other thorny questions are currently being studied by the NIH-ACPM Task Force in Consumer Health Education. If, through the combined efforts of this task force and the many other groups and individuals studying these problems, we can come up with practical answers, the future will be far brighter—not only for the individuals involved but also for the health status of the nation and the health care economy in general. If we cannot, the current explosion of interest in consumer health education may turn out to be just one more passing fad without any real impact either on the delivery of care or the health of the public.

NOTES

1.. *A Guide to the Development of a Hospital-Based Consumer Health Education Program* (Piscataway, N.J.: College of Medicine and Dentistry of New Jersey-Office of Consumer Health Education, 1975).

Chapter Ten

Some Special Problem Areas: Prevention, Violence, The Elderly

Historically, "prevention" was identified almost exclusively with traditional "public health" activities, such as infectious disease controls, school health exams, and food service inspections. More recently, there emerged a concept of "preventive medicine," which many believed should also be practiced by private physicians as part of normal health maintenance routines—although too often this was narrowly perceived to mean simply the "annual checkup." In part this movement was nurtured by the growing recognition that, with the shift in major illness patterns from infectious to chronic diseases, the "risk factors" had become more complex and involved a broad range of environmental influences as well as individual behavior. Many of these were factors in which public health had not been traditionally involved. There was a growing demand that "somebody" assume responsibility.

Selections 46 and 47 represent two original approaches to prevention in this new mood. The first is an effort to define appropriate health goals for specified periods throughout the lifecycle and cost-effective preventive procedures to help individuals attain those goals. The second discusses violence—symbolic as well as actual—as a risk factor in the health of American youth.

The "geriatric problem" was forcefully brought to official and public attention by the rapidly growing numbers, and proportions, of the elderly in the population, and the alarming rise in the cost of providing them with health care. As of 1975, there were 22.3 million persons 65 or over, 10.5 percent of the population.[1] In nine states, they already exceeded 12 percent, including Florida with over 16 percent. By 1985 the figure is expected to reach 26.7 million; by the year 2000, 30.6 million. If the present low birthrate continues, these 31 million will constitute nearly 12 percent of the total population. By 2030, when the post-World War II baby boom cohort passes 65, the elderly may represent 1 in 6.[2]

In 1975 life expectancy at 65 averaged 15 years—13 for men, 18 for women. Only 14 percent of older people, not quite 3 million, were in the labor force, either working or actively seeking work. Nearly 16 percent, 3.3 million, were below the poverty level; most of the remainder would be except for the aid of various public programs.

Over $30 billion was spent for health care of the elderly in fiscal year 1975, accounting for nearly 30 percent of all national health care expenditures.[3] Per capita, this averaged $1,360, of which almost 70 percent went for hospital and nursing home care.

Official dismay is readily understood when we note that the government paid for more than two-thirds of these costs in 1975 and that the figures rise every year, both absolutely and proportionately. The major avenues for these expenditures were Medicare, $13 billion,[4] and Medicaid for elderly patients, $5 billion. Each is rising at an alarming rate. Medicare expenditures doubled between 1969 and 1975. Between fiscal years 1974 and 1975, government spending for elderly health care increased 22 percent; Medicare expenditures rose 29 percent; Medicaid, 31 percent.

Prospects for the future are even more ominous because dependency and disability among the aged are likely to grow more rapidly than the gross "65 and over" data indicate. The numbers in this category are getting so large that distinctions must be made within it. Those 75 and over, as well as those 80 and over, are growing faster than the category as a whole. For example, the Bureau of the Census projects that by the year 2000, while the entire 65-and-over population will have increased 37 percent, those 75-and-over will be up 60 percent, and those 80-and-over 64 percent.[5]

United States policy for the elderly is reaching a critical stage. Increasingly the complaint is heard that an undue proportion of national resources is being expended on the aged at the sacrifice of younger people. The problem, however, is not with the elderly themselves who have little to say about the amount, kind, and price of the care they receive. These decisions are largely determined by physicians and by government programs and policies. It is, for example, not generally the choice of older patients that so many are "warehoused" for years in so-called nursing homes or that so many others, with terminal illness, are kept alive for a few extra days or weeks by inordinately expensive and often extremely painful "heroic" procedures.

The nation is being forced into awareness that new means must be found to meet the needs of the elderly, at less expense and with more respect for their own preferences. Selection 48 examines one relatively inexpensive but neglected modality for such care. Selection 50, which compares geriatric philosophy and practices in the United States and the United Kingdom, is also relevant.

NOTES

1. U.S. Bureau of the Census, *Projections of the Population of the United States, 1975 to 2050,* Series P-25, No. 601, October 1975, pp. 41, 51, 66.
2. "17% of Nation is Expected to be over 65 in Year 2030," *New York Times,* June 1, 1976.
3. M.S. Mueller and R.M. Gibson, "Age Differences in Health Care Spending, FY 1975," *Social Security Bulletin* 39 (June 1976): 19.
4. The balance of Medicare expenditures (Table XIII) went for the disabled under 65.
5. U.S. Bureau of the Census, *op. cit.*

Selection 46

The Lifetime Health Monitoring Program*

Is the periodic physical examination—annual or otherwise—worthwhile? How useful are mass screenings for specific diseases? What about multiphasic screening? Is health education a form of preventive medicine? If so, where and how should it be practiced?

What, exactly, is "preventive medicine?" How does it relate to personal health care? Is it compatible with fee-for-service payment of health professionals? Can it be financed through health insurance? What proportion of the national health care dollar should be spent on prevention?

These and related questions are being asked more and more insistently as responsible policy makers grope for ways to restrain the seemingly endless spiral of rising health care costs, nearly $119 billion in 1975, and to get the most out of the huge expenditure.

They are not easy questions to answer. Despite the obvious "common sense" proposition that preventing illness is not only good for health but also for the pocketbook, we have relegated prevention to a very low rank on the national health priority list. According to one high level estimate, total expenditures for preventive services in the early 1970s amounted to only 2 to 2.5 percent of our total health care bill; for health education, probably less than one-half of 1 percent.

There are many reasons for this neglect; many are beyond the capability of those interested in preventive medicine to do anything about. But there is one important matter that advocates of prevention can and should do something about, i.e., failure to define precisely what is meant by "preventive medicine." The term has been used to encompass all types of activities aimed at the prevention or reduction of disease, including individual preventive services provided by physicians and other health care professionals, environmental and occupational health controls, and consumer health education. This paper is limited to one of these modalities: preventive measures that can be incorporated into personal health services and financed through direct patient payments, health insurance, or other mechanisms normally used to pay for such services.

At an earlier period, when preventive measures were directed primarily to infectious disease, their meaning and methodology were more obvious. More recent efforts to deal with noninfectious chronic diseases have been far less successful. Partisans of the periodic "check-up," multiphasic screening, and health education have too often tended to promote their causes with nonspecific goals and insufficient data. This lack of precision has hurt the entire concept of pre-

---

*Excerpt from Lester Breslow, M.D., and A.R. Somers, "The Lifetime Health Monitoring Program: A Practical Approach to Preventive Medicine," *New England Journal of Medicine* 296 (March 17, 1977): 601-608.

vention. For example, there is the inaccurate but widespread tendency to equate all periodic preventive services with the "annual check-up."

Fortunately, there is evidence that this situation is improving, as leaders of preventive medicine, epidemiologists, health educators, behavioral scientists, and physicians in primary care get away from such broad and ill-defined concepts as the annual check-up or health education in the abstract and approach prevention with more reference to specific chronic illness and with more emphasis on current major risk factors—cigarette smoking, obesity, hyperlipidemia, hypertension, and alcoholism. We must also ask what is relevant and cost-effective for specific populations, at specific age levels.

The growing length and quality of the relevant bibliographies[1] indicate that something along this line is already happening. Tests that have been accepted uncritically for years by some public health personnel and physicians are now being questioned on the basis of controlled studies. At the same time, many clinicians who traditionally discounted the value of preventive procedures are now incorporating them into their regular practice. The time is ripe for a major effort in this respect.

THE LHMP: RECONCILING PUBLIC HEALTH AND PRIVATE PRACTICE GOALS

This paper represents one such effort—an effort to construct a lifetime schedule, or series of "packages" of effective individual preventive procedures, tentatively called the "Lifetime Health Monitoring Program" (LHMP). Most of this program can be incorporated into existing patterns of medical practice and health care financing, although a few components, such as school health education, should continue as public health measures. LHMP is not presented as a finished product. It is an exploratory proposal to be reviewed and refined by health professionals and knowledgeable consumers. Empirical studies will be needed to test and validate the effectiveness and acceptability of the various components.

We have divided the lifespan into ten periods, based on changing life styles, health needs, and problems:

I. Pregnancy and perinatal period
II. Infancy (1st year of life)
III. Preschool child (1-5 years)
IV. School child (6-11)
V. Adolescence (12-17)
VI. Young adulthood (18-24)
VII. Young middle age (25-39)
VIII. Older middle age (40-59)
IX. Elderly (60-74)
X. Old age (75 plus)

For each of these ten periods, we have formulated a brief set of overall health goals and professional services or requirements related to these goals. Some may say that the goals are too general and the range of required services impractical, but the very act of definition helps to get us all—professionals and consumers alike—away from the usual complaint-response medicine toward health maintenance medicine. It forces us to think positively about health and what it means and requires at different ages.

We also present a series of criteria for determining the appropriateness of specific preventive procedures, and suggest "packages" of procedures for two age groups—illustrative of what needs to be done for all ten.

Within the professional community, LHMP seeks to bring together two hitherto separate approaches: one primarily epidemiological; the other, clinical. The former has been summarized in a report prepared for the 1975 National Conference on Preventive Medicine; the latter in a series of articles on periodic health screening by Doctors Frame and Carlson (see Note 1).

Although there are differences in the two approaches—one based primarily on public health, the other on medical practice—the similarities are striking and far more important. For example:

1. Both focus on personal health service, preferably involving a continuing doctor-patient relationship.
2. Both identify specific preventive measures for specific age groups, rather than calling for a vague "check-up."
3. Both call for some rational and varying periodicity, rather than an annual ritual.
4. Both rely heavily on scientific proof of efficacy but, in the absence of 100 percent proof, temper this with a "prudent" interpretation of available evidence concerning potential benefits, costs, and dangers.
5. Both include educational and counseling procedures, designed to influence individual health-related behavior, as well as specified testing procedures designed to ascertain the early onset of disease or the presence of certain risk factors associated with the development of disease.

All five of these points have been incorporated in the Lifetime Health Monitoring Program.

THE TEN AGE GROUPS: GOALS AND PROFESSIONAL SERVICES

The 10 age groups, each with its distinct health goals and professional services are listed below. [Here we have retained only the goals and services for Groups II and VIII.]

II. Infancy (1st year)

Health Goals
1. To establish immunity against specified infectious diseases.
2. To detect and prevent certain other diseases and problems before irreparable damage occurs.
3. To assure growth and development to the infant's maximum potential.
4. To help to provide a basis for lifetime emotional stability, especially through a loving relationship with mother, father, and other family members.

Professional Services
1. Prior to discharge from hospital: tests for inherited metabolic disorders and certain other congenital disorders; parent counseling.
2. Four postdischarge professional visits with the healthy infant during the year for observation, specified immunizations, and parent counseling.

VIII. Older Middle Age (40-59)

Health Goals
1. To prolong the period of maximum physical energy and optimum mental and social activity, including menopausal adjustment.
2. To detect as early as possible any of the major chronic diseases, including hypertension, heart disease, diabetes, and cancer, as well as vision, hearing, and dental impairments.

Professional Services
1. Four professional visits with the healthy individual, once every 5 years—at about 40, 45, 50, 55—with complete physical examination and medical history; tests for specific chronic conditions; appropriate immunizations; and counseling in regard to changing nutritional needs; physical activities; occupational, sex, marital and parental problems; and use of cigarettes, alcohol, and drugs.
2. Tests at annual intervals for hypertension, obesity, and certain cancers.
3. Annual dental prophylaxis....

CRITERIA FOR INCLUDING SPECIFIC PROCEDURES

In deciding which specific procedures to include, eight criteria were applied, derived in part from those adopted by the National Conference on Preventive Medicine, June 1975, and in part from those used by Frame and Carlson.
1. The procedure is appropriate to the health goals of the relevant age group(s) and is acceptable to the relevant population.
2. The procedure is directed to primary or secondary prevention of a clearly identified disease or condition which has a significant effect on the length or quality of life.

3. The natural history of the disease(s) associated with the condition is understood sufficiently to justify the procedure as outweighing any adverse effects of intervention.
4. In the case of screening, the disease or condition has an asymptomatic period during which detection and treatment can significantly reduce morbidity and/or mortality.
5. Acceptable methods of effective treatment are available for conditions discovered.
6. The prevalence and significance of the disease or condition justify the cost.
7. The procedure is relatively easy to administer, preferably by paramedical personnel with guidance and interpretation by physicians, and generally available at reasonable cost.
8. Resources are generally available for follow-up diagnostic or therapeutic intervention if required. . . .

SPECIFIC PROCEDURES FOR TWO AGE GROUPS

Applying these criteria to *infancy* and *older middle age,* we suggest the following list of specific procedures. The first was relatively easy to draw up. The basic criteria for well-baby care are fairly well established in both private practice and public health clinics.

Infancy (1st year)

Specific screening procedures to be carried out before discharge from hospital or during four postdischarge visits:

Suspected or Possible Condition	Procedure
Metabolic disorders	PKU screening
Gonorrheal ophthalmia	Silver nitrate prophylaxis
Diphtheria, tetanus, and pertussis	Immunization
Measles, mumps, rubella	Immunization
Poliomyelitis	Immunization
Hemorrhagic disease	Vitamin K
Anemia	Hematocrit
Growth and development disorders, including congenital dislocation of the hip	Developmental assessment including observation for congenital disorders, height, and weight.

Older Middle Age (40-59)

By contrast with the list for infants, it is impossible at this time to present a list of preventive procedures for this age group which would receive universal professional approval. The spectrum of opinion still varies from those who hold firmly to the need for a complete annual "check-up" to those who claim that nearly all preventive services are wasted.

The following list—featuring one complete professional examination at 40 and subsequent examinations at 5-year intervals, with a few selected tests which could generally be handled by nonphysician personnel at 2 to 3 year intervals, i.e., once between the 5-year intervals—is a compromise. It is based on the criteria set forth above and reflects our judgment of carefully evaluated experience to date.

Note particularly, the absence of x ray of the lungs and tonometry as routine screening procedures. Except for heavy smokers and other high risk groups, the routine chest x ray can no longer be justified at this age. In the case of glaucoma, both the reliability of the existing screening procedures and the value of treatment prior to the onset of visual field loss are now being questioned.

Among other tests where routine application is professionally questioned by some are those for diabetes. The standard tests—fasting blood sugar and abnormal glucose tolerance—are reasonably reliable; but the value of detecting the disease in the asymptomatic stage in this age group, as compared to withholding treatment until symptoms appear, is not clear. The importance of detecting breast cancer as early as possible is generally recognized. However, there is no good evidence, as yet, that mammography contributes to that purpose among women under 50.

On the other hand, there is strong emphasis on self-monitoring. Patient responsibility in this respect, however, can be increased by periodic reports to, and instructions from, a physician or other qualified health professional.

Older Middle Age (40-59) Specific Screening Procedures

Suspected or Possible Condition　　　　*Screening Procedure*

2-3 Year Intervals

Suspected or Possible Condition	Screening Procedure
Malnutrition, including obesity	Weight and height measurements—history of nutrition and activity*
Hypertension and associated conditions	Blood pressure*
Cervical cancer	Pap smear
Intestinal cancer	Stool for blood*
Breast cancer	Professional breast examination, with mammography for those over 50*
Complications from smoking	Smoking history
Endometrial cancer (postmenopausal women)	History of postmenopausal bleeding*

*Once a year over 50.

5-year Intervals

Coronary artery disease	Cholesterol, triglycerides, ECG
Alcoholism	Drinking history
Anemia	Hematocrit
Diabetes	Blood sugar test
Vision defect	Refraction
Hearing defect	Audiogram

High Risk Groups

Add to 5 year intervals:

Tuberculosis	PPD
Syphilis	VDRL

HOW MUCH WOULD LHMP COST?

No one can say precisely. Physician charges for "check-ups" now range from about $60 to $150, depending on number of tests, degree of automation, extent of physician involvement, geographic location, etc. Full scale "executive examinations" go as high as $500.

At the other end of the scale, several organizations provide automated multiphasic testing for $25 to $50 per exam. These are carried out by technicians in fixed locations or on vans; the data are generally computerized and reviewed by physicians who send the results to the examinee's personal physician. Commonly included are ECG and blood pressure; weight and height; hearing and vision tests; urinalysis; pulmonary function; blood tests for cholesterol, hemoglobin, and sugar; and cervical cytology.

The LHMP differs significantly from both the above examples. As a program designed to encourage inclusion of periodic preventive measures in health insurance and prepayment plans, it assumes that the proposed services will be used only at the suggested time intervals. The annual per capita premium should be much less than the average fee-for-service charge now common for annual checkups. This would be true even if the physician and other professional personnel were paid at current rates. High volume and some resulting economies in the testing procedures may also enable the providers to reduce costs and charges. On the other hand, since LHMP requires individual counseling as well as screening and since the former cannot be automated, the cost can never be reduced to the level achieved by some computerized multiphasic programs.

There is reason to hope that such a program of preventive medicine would eventually reduce the amount of expensive curative care now needed, although it would be misleading to claim that any such savings could be achieved in the short run. By definition, the potential savings, if any, from preventive medicine—to the individual and to society—should show up in future years. Even so, the amount is problematical. Those who are saved by good preventive services from heart attacks and cancer in their 40s and 50s will eventually die of something else. It has been rightly said that life itself is the one fatal condition that cannot be avoided. The primary object of preventive care is not to save money but to save lives, to avoid premature death, and to improve the quality of life.

HOW SHOULD WE PAY FOR THE LHMP?

The underfinancing of preventive care in the United States was noted at the outset. Virtually all health insurance (which should be called "sickness insurance") discriminates against preventive services. This is true of both public and private programs. In theory, health maintenance organizations are expected to provide more preventive care, as the name implies. This is true of the better HMOs, but not all.

In recent years there has been a growing conviction that this situation must be changed, that the health insurance carriers and programs, starting with Medicare and looking toward national health insurance, must be persuaded or mandated to provide coverage for at least a substantial portion of preventive services. A number of health insurance leaders have indicated interest in doing this but have demanded more precise definition of the services to be included in the "preventive package" than has hitherto been available. The LHMP is an effort at such a definition.

It might also be wise to phase in the program with a minimum "starter package." It is usually better that a large new program start modestly, perhaps on a multisite demonstration and evaluation basis, enlarging as capability and acceptance increase. Such a "starter package" might include complete physical examinations, along with appropriate tests, medical behavioral histories, and counseling at the following times:

1. Predischarge, for newborn infant
2. Postdischarge, two visits during first year of life
3. Preschool child (school entry)
4. School child (6-11)
5. Adolescence (12-17)
6. On entering college, Armed Forces, first full-time job, or marriage (18-25)
7. At age 40
8. At age 62-65 (pre-Medicare)

In the case of child-bearing women, there should be four additional visits, three prenatal and one postnatal.

What are the chances of persuading Congress, state governments, and the private health insurance industry that something like this should be included in Medicare and private insurance, now, and in national health insurance when it comes? A few years ago, we would have been pessimistic. Today we are hopeful. For example, John Kittredge, Vice-President of Prudential Life Insurance Company, one of the largest, has written:

> I see no real problem with having the benefit included in the group insurance provided by employers. But we cannot unilaterally change our contracts to provide benefits that were not included before.... One way would be to require employers, through revision of state laws, to make such coverage available or to make such benefits available to employees on a self-insured basis. Similarly with individual policies, a state requirement for inclusion in new policies would be necessary....
>
> In the past two or three years, however, I have become disillusioned over the prospect of such extensions through state laws. We already have an appalling lack of uniformity in this type of legislation.... I would rather see this come through national health insurance and, perhaps before that, through adoption in the bargaining patterns of one or more of the trend-setter unions. The United Auto Workers seems to be most influential in this respect.

We agree as to the long run advantages of national health insurance (NHI) coverage. However, the uncertainties respecting adoption of NHI and the fact that NHI benefits are likely to reflect preexisting benefit patterns make it desirable to begin to move as soon as possible. In addition to experimentation by a number of collective bargaining groups, we would urge immediate action by Congress on behalf of Medicare and Medicaid patients and by at least a few of the more active state insurance commissioners.

CONSUMER AND PROFESSIONAL INCENTIVES

Assuming such benefits are made generally available through health insurance, there is still the problem of individual participation. Even where preventive procedures are compulsory, as in the case of childhood immunizations, noncompliance is substantial. Making the entire program compulsory would be neither feasible nor acceptable at the present time. What is needed, most of all, is a more positive view of prevention on the part of the medical profession, which sets the tone for the attitude of other health professionals and consumers as well. In this respect it is distressing to note what appears to be a more than coincidental recent attack on preventive medicine.

In addition, however, various incentives for consumer/patient participation should be considered. Kittredge has suggested:

> Perhaps there is an analogy in some of our dental insurance plans. For preventive types of dentistry, we purposely pay 70 percent of the eligible charges in the first year and progressively increase by 10 percent each year so long as the insured has had a dental examination in the prior year and has obtained the treatment recommended by the dentist. Perhaps it would be possible to impose some sort of financial penalty for failure to participate or reward for doing so.

These are difficult issues that need a great deal of study, along with problems of improving the effectiveness of some of the recommended procedures, such as school health education, determining the most effective organizational settings, and the development of the needed manpower.

The question of manpower for preventive services, not dealt with in this paper, has been ably discussed elsewhere.[2] We cannot conclude, however, without emphasizing the importance of the organizational issue. Some authorities maintain that preventive care is simply not compatible with the predominant U.S. fee-for-service method of payment. For example, Walter McNerney, President, Blue Cross Association, has written:

> It has often proven easier to change the organizational configuration for delivering health services (à la HMOs) to stimulate changes in individual behaviors, rather than skewing individual behaviors though incentives in the financing mechanism, and then expecting the delivery system to respond appropriately. In order to provide for the efficient delivery of the proposed benefit package, stimulating the creation of facilities and services specifically designed to comply with the elements of this program could prove appropriate.

Fee-for-service practice and the health insurance plans built up around it are better adapted to episodic therapeutic medicine than to health maintenance. Some prepaid group practice plans, such as the Kaiser-Permanente Program, have been shown in several studies to provide more preventive services than traditional arrangements for medical care. However, the fee-for-service system has shown itself reasonably flexible and capable of assimilating prevention—at least at the primary care level, where it is most relevant. At the same time, not all capitation systems have shown the devotion to prevention demonstrated by Kaiser. Furthermore, we believe that the general inclusion of a package of professionally approved and reasonably priced preventive health services could be a major stimulus to organizational response. Such has already been the case with Hawaii Blue Shield when confronted with the opportunity of providing "health examinations" to its subscribers.

The LHMP must not be seen as an organizational straitjacket for all preventive medicine. The recommended time intervals as well as the specific procedures are intended primarily as guides to practical scheduling, pricing, and financing. The identification of broad health goals and relevant professional services is far more basic. They can, and probably should, be implemented in different ways under different forms of health care organization.

The United States is unlikely to move, in the foreseeable future, to universal capitation or any other radically different new delivery system. We are likely to continue our existing pluralistic patterns, albeit with increasingly centralized financing as dictated by the high costs, and with increasing capitation or salaried practice at the primary care level. Within this pluralism, it is our hope to promote closer relations (1) between clinical medicine and epidemiology, and (2) between professional care and individual consumer/patient knowledge and responsibility.

LHMP is far from a blueprint. It is, primarily, a call for a philosophical reorientation in personal health care: more emphasis on primary care and, within primary care, more emphasis on prevention, including health education or patient counseling. It is also an attempt to demonstrate that such reorientation can be gradually assimilated into medical practice and ongoing health care institutions without traumatic changes in these institutions or their financing.

As to the important doctor-patient relationship, far from driving a "preventive medicine wedge" between the personal physician and his patient, LHMP seeks to strengthen that relationship by making it financially feasible for the personal physician to incorporate prevention into his day-to-day patient care. And far from depersonalizing care by putting the computer or any other form of technology in control, LHMP seeks to maximize individual professional-patient contact at the point where it really counts: not in carrying out routine tests, which the machine can do as well or better, but in counseling on the basis of individual findings within an epidemiological framework. Such a reorientation of U.S. health care could have a significant long range effect on individual and national health status as well as costs.

NOTES

1. For example, National Institutes of Health—Fogarty International Center and American College of Preventive Medicine, National Conference on Preventive Medicine, Report of Task Force III, Lester Breslow, M.D., Chairman, *Theory and Application of Preventive Medicine in Personal Health Services* (New York: Prodist, 1976), selected bibliography of 97 references. P.S. Frame, M.D. and S.J. Carlson, M.D., "A Critical Review of Periodic Health Screening Using Specific Screening Criteria," *Journal of Family Practice* 2 (1975), four-part series: Part I: "Selected Diseases of Respiratory, Cardiovascular, and Central Nervous Systems," 2:29-36; Part 2: "Selected Endocrine, Metabolic, and Gastrointestinal Diseases," 2:123-29; Part 3: "Selected Diseases of the Genitourinary System," 2:189-94; Part 4: "Selected Miscellaneous Diseases," 2:283-89, 222 references.

W.O. Spitzer, M.D. and B.P. Brown, M.D., "Unanswered Questions About the Periodic Health Examination," *Annals of Internal Medicine* 83 (1975): 257-63. L.C. Robbins, M.D. and J.H. Hall, M.D., *How to Practice Prospective Medicine* (Indianapolis: Health Hazard Appraisal, Methodist Hospital of Indiana, 1970).
2. Edmund D. Pellegrino, M.D., "Preventive Health Care and the Allied Health Professions," in *Review of Allied Health Education I,* Joseph Hamburg, M.D., ed. (Lexington, Ky.: University Press of Kentucky, 1974), pp. 1-18.

Selection 47

Violence, Television, and the Health of American Youth*

For a considerable proportion of American children and youth, violence has become a major health problem. For an alarming number it is a way of life. In 1973, 18,032 young Americans, 15 to 24, died in motor vehcile accidents, 5,182 were murdered, and 4,098 committed suicide.[1] During the same year, 425 children, 5 to 14, and 342, aged 1 to 4, were reported murdered. The actual figures for child murders are assumed to be very much higher. The death rate, for ages 15 to 24, from all causes, was 19 percent higher in 1973-1974 than it had been in 1960-1961. The rise was entirely due to deaths by violence.

As affluence has made automobiles and motorcycles more accessible, the young have increasingly become both victims and agents of traffic accidents. In 1973, motor vehicle accidents for those 15 to 24 accounted for 46.2 deaths per 100,000, a 16 percent rise from 1963. For every youth killed in a car accident, nearly 40 are injured, an estimated total of 700,000.

The rising trend of youthful suicides continues. The rate for ages 15 to 24 more than doubled between 1950 and 1973, to 10.6 per 100,000. In addition, many auto deaths, recorded as accidental, are considered by many experts to be suicides. According to studies at Baylor College of Medicine in Houston, and in Kansas City, 14-15 percent, one in six or seven of auto accident fatalities are suicides, not accidents as reported on death certificates.

Violent crime in the United States continues to accelerate: murder is the fastest growing cause of death in the United States. The annual rate rose over 100 percent from 1960 to 1974. Our homicide rate is roughly ten times that of the Scandinavian countries. More murders are committed yearly in Manhattan (population 1.5 million) than in the entire United Kingdom (population 60 million). The age group most involved, with both the greatest number of victims

*Excerpt from A.R. Somers, "Violence, Television and the Health of American Youth," *New England Journal of Medicine* 294 (April 8, 1976): 811-817.

and persons arrested, is 20 to 24. In 1972, 17.0 percent of all homicide victims and an estimated 23.7 percent of all arrests were in this age group. Teenagers, 15 to 19, accounted for 9 percent of all victims and nearly 19 percent of the arrests.

In 1964 in New York City, 1,279 children under 16 were arrested for robbery, 131 for rape, and 30 for murder. In 1973, the figures were 4,449 for robbery, 181 for rape, and 94 for murder. "It is," wrote the author of a soberly documented account of several such youthful crimes and the law's impotence in dealing with them, "as though our society had bred a new genetic strain, the child-murderer who feels no remorse and is scarcely conscious of his acts."

The big city child murderer is still relatively rare, but youthful skirmishes with the law are becoming almost commonplace. According to a 1966-1970 survey of youngsters, 12 to 17, by the National Center for Health Statistics, almost one youth in five reported having had one or more contacts with the police or juvenile authorities over something he or she had done or was thought to have done. About 44 percent of 17-year-old boys reported such contact.

According to the National Center for Health Statistics, the largest rise in deaths from homicide during the past two decades was at ages 1 to 4. More than a million American children suffer physical abuse or neglect each year, and at least one in five dies from mistreatment, according to a 1975 study released by the Department of Health, Education, and Welfare, which said the figures represented a "social problem" of "epidemic" proportions.

The pediatric profession, which historically played a leadership role in the improvement of child health and welfare, has again demonstrated a combination of scientific and ethical responsibility by mounting, in cooperation with child welfare agencies, the current crusade against child abuse, culminating in the Child Abuse Prevention and Treatment Act of 1974.

Has it any chance of reversing current trends? It is much too soon to say. But the odds seem highly unfavorable unless something can be done to change the moral, as well as socioeconomic, environment in which American children are growing up today. One of the most relevant and urgent areas of concern is that represented by television's massive indoctrination of both children and adults in the "culture of violence."

VIOLENCE ON TV: MIRROR OR MODEL?

The extent and impact of television's massive daily diet of symbolic crime and violence, in so-called "entertainment" programs, is hard for anyone who is not a heavy viewer to comprehend. According to the annual "Violence Profile" maintained at the Annenberg Institute of Communications, University of Pennsylvania, approximately three-fourths of all network dramatic programs during evening prime time (8 p.m. to 11 p.m.) and children's dramatic programs on Saturday and Sunday mornings, 1967-1973, contained violence as standard content. The proportion declined slightly from 80 percent in 1967 to 73 percent in 1973. However, the rate of violent episodes remained virtually unchanged:

about eight per hour. One authority has estimated that "between the ages of five and fifteen, the average American child will view the killing of more than 13,000 persons on television."

Television is not the only entertainment medium to emphasize violence today. Violence, along with sex, pervades the comics, paperback books, and fiction magazines. The film industry is far worse than television in proportion of violence or horror material to total output, and some of the worst violence in television today originates in movies.

The portrayal of murder, mayhem, war, and all kinds of fighting in drama, opera, novels, and painting probably goes back to the beginning of each of these art forms. There are at least two major differences, however, between the usual historical treatment of violence and the typical current situation.

Traditionally, violence was portrayed in a context of high tragedy (the Bible, Greek and Shakespearean tragedy, Tolstoy's *War and Peace*, etc.), fantasy (fairy tales, Wagnerian legends, early cowboy and Indian stories, etc.), or outright slapstick (Marx Brothers, Charlie Chaplin, etc.). It was generally not related to contemporary people or current "real-life" situations. By contrast, much of today's movie and television violence is presented in the context of ordinary life and routine problem-solving. The implications for the viewer are very different; his personal identification, either with the murderer, the murdered, or both, is likely to be much greater.

Television is also distinguished from other entertainment media, even movies, by its pervasive impact on children. Historically, few children had access to theater or other dramatic entertainment. For some decades the Saturday afternoon movie was a ritual for many American children. But with the rising cost of movie admissions and nearly universal free access to television, this is no longer the case. Television has become *the* medium for children. It is difficult to overstate its influence on them.

As of the early 1970s, 96 percent of American homes had one or more television sets. Frequent viewing begins at about age three. A recent Nielsen survey reports that preschoolers watch an average of 54 hours a week. This means seven to eight hours a day! More than 20 million 2 to 17-year-olds are still watching at 9 p.m., 13 million at 10 p.m., and 5.3 million at 11 p.m. For many children, watching television will consume as many hours from age two to six as classroom hours for the next ten years.

Low income children spend even more time in front of the television than others. One study of 15 to 17-year-olds in the late 1960s found that middle class youngsters average four hours on Sundays; low income youngsters "upwards of five to six hours."

It is this almost total immersion in the home setting, combined with the audio-visual impact, that sets television apart from other entertainment media and necessitates special consideration as a risk factor influencing the health of American youth. Television not only offers, it imposes, vicarious experience and psychological conditioning on our children. In the words of the respected movie critic, Joseph Morgenstern,

> It's not enough to say that Shakespeare and Marlow were violent and civilization still survived. Technology has brought a new amplification effect into play. Never before has so much violence been shown so graphically to so many.

In singling out television for special treatment, however, there is no implication that this industry's motivations are any worse than, or generically different from, those of other industries. The difference lies in the nature of the medium and its unique impact on children.

What is this impact? Is the picture of society that children are viewing on television reasonably accurate or distorted? Does the role of violence in television entertainment conform roughly to that in society in general, or is it exaggerated? In other words, is television a mirror or a molder of social values? If the latter, is the net result positive or negative? Does constant exposure to symbolic violence act as a "catharsis" to aggressive tendencies in children and thus provide a sort of antidote or immunization to real violence? Or does it tend to promote insensitivity and/or emulation? [Here followed a summary and discussion of two major federal reports directed at these issues.]

The need for additional research to justify action is questionable. Psychologist Robert Liebert, who had participated in some of the research for the Surgeon General's Committee, and his colleagues at the State University of New York, Stony Brook, summarized the situation as of 1973:

> The quibbling is unwarranted. On the basis of evaluation of many lines of coverging evidence, involving more than 50 studies which have included more than 10,000 normal children and adolescents from every conceivable background, the weight of the evidence is clear: The demonstrated teaching and instigating effects of aggressive television fare upon youth are of sufficient importance to warrant immediate remedial action.

Which brings us back to the point the National Commission had reached in 1969! But no closer to answering the question, "What action?"

VIOLENCE, MONEY, AND FREE SPEECH

The stakes in the "game" of television violence are enormous. On July 9, 1975, Paramount Pictures announced that it had leased to the networks the rights to 42 recent movies, including *The Godfather* and *The Godfather Part II*, for about $76 million. NBC-TV, which paid about $7 million for a single showing of *The Godfather* in 1974, has reportedly paid $15 million for a single run of the two films in television format. According to Michael Rothenberg, a pediatric psychiatrist, 24 percent of the television industry's profits come from the 7 percent of its programming directed at children.

Understandably, the industry is strongly opposed to any new regulation and, at the slightest suspicion of such, invokes the First Amendment and charges critics with impending censorship. This has complicated and confused the issue, especially since many of the same people, most concerned about television violence, are also deeply concerned over civil liberties, and with good reason. The two are closely related. Violence is the enemy of a healthy democratic society as it is the enemy of a healthy body. But the suspicion is growing that the censorship issue is probably a red herring.

A recommendation by a Task Force on Consumer Health Education (see p. 292) that Congress establish some form of "reporting mechanism" on television violence for fact-finding and publicity purposes was opposed by an industry spokesman just as strongly as if it had called for censorship. Dr. Albert Bandura was probably correct when he said,

> In reality, the industry fears the threat of adverse publicity more than the threat of censorship, and Johnson, an outspoken FCC commissioner, was probably accurate in characterizing many of the disputes in this area as more concerned with profitable speech than with free speech.

One of the major arguments of the defenders of television violence is that virtue almost always triumphs in the end. This is no longer true—if it ever was. Who, in *The Godfather,* are the "good guys" and who the "bad guys?" We are very close to the idealization of violence. And, year by year, the real world conforms more and more closely to the world of television violence.

The number of warning voices are increasing daily. For example, Anatole Broyard, reviewing Barbara Geld's 1975 book, *On the Track of Murder,* starts "I had not realized how desensitized I had become to the fact of murder as a result of seeing it so often on television or in the movies...."

The New Yorker, reviewing some of the spectacular crimes of 1975, including the attempts on President Gerald Ford's life, commented,

> Murder of every sort, even as it was universally deplored, was gaining in respectability. An atmosphere of assassination had spread across the country, and in that atmosphere distinctions were blurring and disappearing—distinctions between fame and notoriety, between entertainment and tragedy, between law enforcement and criminality.... The C.I.A., the S.L.A., the F.B.I., and Charles Manson's family were mingling on our television screens, in our thought, and, it seemed, in the real world, and it was getting harder by the minute to tell them apart.

Even so ardent a defender of civil liberties as Walter Lippmann wrote:

> A continual exposure of a generation to the commercial exploitation of the enjoyment of violence and cruelty is one way to corrode the foundations of a civilized society. For my own part, believing as I do in freedom of speech and thought, I see no objection in principle to censorship of the mass entertainment of the young. Until some more refined way is worked out of controlling this evil thing, the risks to our liberties are, I believe, decidedly less than the risks of unmanageable violence.

Douglass Cater and Stephen Strickland conclude their study of television violence:

> Admittedly, probing television's effects raises First Amendment concerns.... But the issue remains. For television programming goes to one of society's most urgent problems—how it educates its youth. From the earliest days of the Republic, education has been the subject of social management. The solution is not to declare a no-man's land in exploring television's effects on the young, but to develop more enlightened ways of exploration.... We cannot avoid "1984" by merely condemning it. Rather our ambition should be to invent an alternative vision of 1984. The first necessity is to expose our communications system to the bright glare of examination and debate....

The time may be fast approaching, however, when Pastore's "Dutch Uncle" pronouncements and even the threat of license forfeiture may be of little avail. Technology—by cable, satellite, cassette, and perhaps ultimately by fiber optics—promises a fissioning of our communication channels. Increased competition could open the way for greater diversity and choice in television viewing. But it could also push program producers to extend ever further the outer limits of audience arousal.

NEED FOR A BROAD EPIDEMIOLOGICAL APPROACH

The problem of youthful violence is obviously highly complex and is challenging an increasing number of eminent jurists, educators, social scientists, journalists, and politicians, as well as a few health professionals. Thus far, the answers have baffled liberals and conservatives alike. The liberal orthodoxy, that crime is due largely to poverty and repression, was widely discredited during the 1960s when affluence, civil liberties, and crime expanded simultaneously. On the other hand, a more conservative national Administration and Supreme Court, the election of tough "law and order" mayors in several major cities, and the serious recession of 1973-1975 did nothing to reverse the rising crime wave, thus undermining the conservative orthodoxy.

The only area where the medical profession has, thus far, played an active leadership role is in child abuse. While it is still too early to know the outcome of such action—epidemiologically rather than ideologically oriented—it could turn out to be the most creative effort of the past decade in this whole area. Otherwise, public policy—stalemated between two discredited ideologies—appears at a loss either to diagnose the situation or to effect any empirical remedy.

And yet something must be done. For as Arnold Barnett, an MIT mathematician, and his colleagues have demonstrated, the linear projection of current increases in murder rates leads to astonishing levels, with murder probabilities "up to 1 in 12 and life expectancies diminished by more than 3 years." The speed with which retrogressive developments can take place in the volatile American climate is also indicated by another Barnett finding: "In the last eight years [1966-1973] the rise in murder rates has more than 'wiped out' the accumulated decline of the previous forty."

Before the Barnett projections could become fact, however, the increasing fear and frustration would, almost certainly, lead to drastic changes in our form of government and in our civil liberties. Thus, the irony that those who invoke civil liberties most loudly in defense of television violence may be paving the way for serious curtailment of such liberties. Violence does not always lead to dictatorship, but violence is always an ingredient of dictatorship; and we entertain ourselves and our children with violence at the peril of our political future. Surely, in this situation, the search for the causes and cures of violence merits the same degree of moral and intellectual commitment on the part of the health professions as we are currently devoting to the war on cancer, or once did to the war on tuberculosis.

An epidemiological approach would also rule out any single factor etiology. In our present state of ignorance, every possible risk factor—physical, demographic, socioeconomic, political, moral, cultural, and, of course, our ineffective system of juvenile criminal justice—should be explored. This paper has concentrated on just one of the many factors—television's indoctrination of children in the "culture of violence"—but it is one where the medical profession may be able to play an important part in remedial action.

WHAT CAN THE PROFESSION DO?

The essential first step is general professional acceptance of the role of television violence as a risk factor threatening the health and welfare of American children and youth and official organizational commitment to remedial action. Recent publication of Dr. Rothenberg's brilliant "call to arms" on this subject[2] was an important beginning.

Next, it is essential that the American Medical Association and other organizational spokesmen for the profession make their views known to the industry—both the networks and local stations, to the FCC, and to federal and state legislators, especially the two responsible committees of Congress. The approach should be twofold: a reduction of violence in general entertaining programming and support for the concept of the "family viewing hour." The primary argument for the latter is not that it will save children from exposure to violence; it will not. But the very existence of such a family hour commits the industry to values other than commercialism and may force them, and the rest of us, to come up with some positive guidelines for realizing television's enormous positive cultural and educational potential.

A few braver-than-average psychiatrists, pediatricians, and physicians interested in preventive medicine, communications, behavior change, and national policy for health promotion may be sufficiently challenged to devote their major efforts in the next few years to help formulate such positive guidelines and to produce some experimental programs of this type.

Perhaps most important of all, individual practitioners, especially those dealing with children, adolescents, and young parents, can try to help them understand and minimize the television risk factor.

To some leaders of the medical profession, as well as individual physicians, the call to involvement in the problem of violence may seem unreasonable. But it is worth recalling the circumstances that led to the birth of pediatrics in this country. In the latter part of the 19th century, in the midst of an epidemic of infant mortality, infanticide, and child abuse, far worse than the present one, it gradually dawned on physicians and public officials alike that a high infant death rate was not an Act of God but evidence of human weakness, ignorance, and cupidity, and could be corrected. There was also the growing recognition that, in the words of the poet Wordsworth, "The child is father of the man."

At the turn of the century, Dr. Abraham Jacobi, founder of the American Pediatric Society, made clear the profession's willingness to assume a heavy burden:

> The young are the future makers and owners of the world. Their physical, intellectual, and moral condition will decide whether the world will be more Cossack or more republican, more criminal or more righteous. For their education and training and capacities the physician, mainly the pediatrist, as the representative of medical science and art, should become responsible.

The dramatic decline in the infant and early childhood death rates and the general improvement in the condition of children after the turn of the century are tributes to a combination of medical science, technological progress, enlightened public policy, and human courage. This same combination is now needed for an attack on this new risk factor—pollution of the mind—which has contributed to an epidemic of youthful violence, an epidemic that seriously threatens the health of American youth.

NOTES

1. Homicide figures reported by the National Center for Health Statistics, based on nationwide reporting from death certificates, are consistently higher than those of the FBI, based on voluntary reporting from local law enforcement agencies.
2. M.B. Rothenberg, M.D., "Effect of Television Violence on Children and Youth," *Journal of the American Medical Association* (Dec. 8, 1975): 1043-46.

Selection 48

Homemaker Services: An Essential Option for the Elderly*

Mrs. L. was admitted to the nursing home on October 2, two days after neighbors learned she had lived for a week on water, a half-loaf of bread, and a box of cereal. Various infirmities kept her from shopping for groceries and even from preparing meals and she had nobody to do it for her.

The kindly neighbors watched as Mrs. L. was helped down the stairs on her way to an institution, and their own taxes were helped up. Her care would cost about $400 a month or about three or four times what it would cost to have a part-time homemaker-home health aide to do her shopping, help with her meals and do her housekeeping. Such help was all Mrs. L. needed and all she wanted.

This story appeared in an American Medical Association news release, March 16, 1973. Three years later, hundreds of thousands of Mrs. L.s are still being sent to nursing homes, when less expensive in-home services are often all that they want or need.

According to the U.S. Senate's Subcommittee on Long Term Care,

If home health services are readily available *prior* to placement in a nursing home there is convincing evidence to conclude that such care may not only postpone but possibly prevent more costly institu-

---

*Excerpt from A.R. Somers and F.M. Moore, in *Public Health Reports* 91 (July-August 1976): 354-359.

tionalization. What is particularly appealing from the standpoint of the elderly is that home health services can enable them to live independently in their own homes, where most of them would prefer to be.[1]

The subcommittee reached this conclusion after 15 years of study of long term care and the testimony of hundreds of witnesses, representing both professionals and consumers. Other studies make the same point. For example, W.G. Bell of Florida State University found that 85 percent of elderly persons—those in nursing homes as well as those at home—preferred to be at home.

In-home services can also lead to faster discharges after hospital or other institutional care. Hospital utilization review committees are under increasing pressure to find safe alternatives for many who no longer need such care. New York State now mandates an "organized discharge planning program... acceptable to the Commissioner [of Health] and in writing to ensure that each patient has a planned program of continuing care which meets the patient's post-discharge needs."[2] Homemaker-home health aide services can be an essential component in such "a planned program of continuing care."

Such services are also often needed by the disabled and families with small children where the mother is incapacitated for one reason or another. In fact, homemaker services began as a substitute mother service in the early part of this century. The hyphenated title, "homemaker-home health aide," results from superimposition of the term "home health aide"—formally introduced in Title 18 of the Social Security Act of 1965 (Medicare)—on the older term "homemaker." In this selection, "homemaker" is generally used in lieu of the longer title. Also, since more homemaker services are now provided to the elderly than to families with children, the focus is on this aspect of their work.

The number of agencies providing homemaker services is growing but not fast enough in relation to need. There were, in 1975, less than 1,800 administrative units providing homemaker services; and less than half of these were among the 2,300 certified home health agencies. The number of homemakers is estimated at about 44,000. The National Council places the need at 300,000, approximately one for every 1,000 Americans under 65, and one to 100 for those 65 and over.

Currently the United States has one for every 5,000 persons, a very low ratio compared with other industrialized nations such as Norway, the Netherlands, Sweden, or the United Kingdom. Sweden has the highest ratio, with approximately one aide for each 121 persons. Norway has 1 to 173; the Netherlands, 1 to 247; and the United Kingdom, 1 to 726. The United Kingdom leads with the greatest absolute number, 67,440. Sweden has 65,700.

TASKS AND QUALIFICATIONS OF HOMEMAKERS

The homemaker, working under supervision of a health professional, helps older people—those with arthritis, heart conditions, terminal cancer, or those who are simply too old or too frail to keep house and care for themselves adequately—with those personal and household activities which they can no longer do for themselves. Included are laundry, shopping, preparing nutritious meals, bathing, shaving, and washing hair.

Under supervision of a therapist, the homemaker may also assist with a physical, speech, or occupational therapy routine. She provides emotional support and observes and reports the condition of those being served to the public health nurse or other supervisor. Both personal and household tasks are included. Most homemaker agencies see no justification—other than the reimbursement requirements of Medicare and other third parties—for separating these closely allied functions.

The formal definition, developed by the National Council for Homemaker-Home Health Aide Services, Inc., the recognized standard-setting body for the field, assumes both types of activity:

> Homemaker-home health aide service helps families to remain together or elderly persons to remain in their own homes when a health and/or social problem occurs or to return to their homes after specialized care. The trained homemaker-home health aide, who works for a community agency [which could be a hospital], carries out assigned tasks in the family's or individual's place of residence, working under the supervision of a professional person who also assesses the need for the service and implements the plan of care.

The tasks of the homemaker should be seen as part of a broad spectrum of in-home services, which include medical care, nursing, physical and speech therapy, social work, nutrition, and a host of paraprofessional or volunteer services, such as telephone reassurance, friendly visiting, meals-on-wheels, and transportation. In a given community all such services should be administered by a single agency or a closely linked group of agencies to assure maximum utility, flexibility, and economy for any one individual or family.

Although the homemaker should always work under supervision of a nurse, social worker, or other professional, she is usually a mature woman. Personal qualifications, such as maturity, warmth, integrity and experience are more important in this work than formal education. Since long term formal training, or even a high school diploma, are not needed, the homemaker job is ideal for many unemployed women, particularly those who have raised families of their own. It offers a useful opportunity for jobs and training under the Comprehensive Training and Employment Act of 1973 (CETA). The latter is being used for this purpose in a number of localities.

If the homemaker field is not to go the way of the nursing home field, proper attention must be given now to standards and adequate monitoring. The goal should be to have each agency's performance monitored by a properly qualified body—either a national voluntary organization such as the National Council for Homemaker-Home Health Aide Services or a department of state government.

COSTS AND FINANCING

The cost-effectiveness and even the cost of home care, including homemaker services, have been debated for some years. Advocates of home care point to the high and still rapidly rising costs of institutional care and contrast these figures with the relatively low hourly or per-visit costs of inhome services. For example, unpublished data reported to the National Council by 74 approved programs, primarily voluntary, nonprofit, but from all sections of the country, indicate a 1974-1975 average cost per hour for homemaker services of $5.28. This includes homemaker salaries and benefits, supervisory and other administrative costs, and some costs of professional assessment. For the 74 programs, the average number of hours per case in that year was 122; and the average cost per case, $644.

Spokesmen for nursing homes as well as objective observers point out that such figures are incomplete and can be misleading. Obviously, all services essential to maintaining people in their homes must be compared with all services essential to maintaining people in institutions. One Maryland nursing home administrator recently put the counterargument this way:

> As for the cost of home care, it costs upwards of $45.00 per shift for private duty care in the home plus ancillary costs such as equipment, nutrition, transportation, etc. In addition, to have a visiting nurse come to the home for one hour would cost approximately $25.00. This does not include the homemaker, physical therapist, or occupational therapist fees if needed.... In reality, home care will cost more than inpatient care both in terms of money and human resources. It may be sociologically acceptable, but we must be ready to pay the price.

Such a view is a useful antidote to too facile or purely ideological acceptance of home care as a universal cost-effective alternative. However, it is also misleading in the opposite direction; the implication is left that home-care requires constant, rather than intermittent, attendance.... Even the visiting nurse will not usually come in every day; sometimes only once in ten or 15 days.

For example, three large approved urban agencies with 1,000 patients 65 years of age and over—in San Francisco and Washington, D.C.—report that for this group, utilization of homemakers averages less than 25 hours a month per case, plus fewer than two professional visits a month. The latter includes all related responsibilities such as assessment, supervision, and coordination with other community resources.

The crucial test is the appropriateness of the care to the needs of the individual patient. One who needs 24-hour-a-day service should usually not be cared for at home; one who needs only intermittent services usually should not be in an institution. The complexity of services also has to be considered. In other words, each type of care can be cost-effective when appropriately used. Among the individuals and groups endorsing this view are the Comptroller

General of the United States, the Health Insurance Benefits Advisory Council (HIBAC) to the Secretary of HEW, the U.S. Senate's Subcommittee on Long Term Care of the Special Committee on Aging, Senators Frank Moss and Frank Church, Chairmen of these two committees, and Representative Edward Koch of New York. According to the Comptroller General:

> Several studies—focusing on savings realized by early transfer of patients from hospitals to home care programs—have pointed out that such care can be less expensive than institutional care....
>
> A study by the Rochester, New York, Home Care Association showed an estimated reduction of 13,713 patient-days and a savings of $1,055,000 in calendar year 1970 and an estimated reduction of 12,579 days and a savings of $1,068,000 in calendar year 1971 as a result of early release of patients from hospitals to home health programs.

In its own cost study, the National Council stresses the potential economy resulting from the greater flexibility inherent in home services:

> Institutional care, which requires that employees be on duty around the clock, cannot easily be varied nor does it allow individuals to do as much for themselves as possible. In-home care, on the other hand, can be custom-fitted to the needs of the individual and families served, while simultaneously making the most of their strengths. For example, the hours a week of care, the duration of care, and the tasks performed by the homemaker-home health aide all can be fitted to the need and can be changed to meet a changing situation.

Despite this agreement on potential cost savings as well as the strong preference of most of the elderly to remain in their own homes, health care in the United States remains heavily institution oriented. A major explanation for this fact, as well as the striking differences between homemaker population ratios in the United States and European countries, is the relatively low level of U.S. government support. A beginning toward federal support was made in the 1962 social services amendments to the Social Security Act, and Titles 18 and 19 of the 1965 law provided some funding for home health services, including "to the extent permitted in regulations, part-time or intermittent services of a home health aide." Medicare permits reimbursement of home health aide services, however, only if skilled nursing, physical therapy, or speech therapy is also required by the patient.

Over the years, the Social Security Administration has interpreted this provision very strictly. Only personal care services for the patient, not housekeeping duties, are reimbursable, unless the housekeeping is incidental and does not increase the time spent by the home health aide. In contrast, the equivalent of many household services such as food preparation, laundry, and cleaning are included in institutional reimbursable expenses.

Although Medicaid is less restrictive, the constant financial pinch felt by that program, and the pervasive influence of the Medicare pattern have resulted in a similar downgrading of home care. It is not surprising that all home health programs account for less than 1 percent of Medicare expenditures and an estimated 0.4 percent of federal-state expenditures under Medicaid—a situation that has been severely criticized by the Comptroller General, HIBAC, and the Senate Special Committee on Aging. One result of such criticism is the establishment of several experimental home care and homemaker projects under Sec. 222 of the Social Security Amendments of 1972 (P.L. 92-603).

A similar struggle over reimbursement is taking place in the private health insurance industry. Blue Cross and commercial carriers are gradually including some aspects of homemaker services as covered benefits, with carefully worked-out limitations. Unfortunately, these developments have generally followed the Medicare model. The overall result is that, while some lower income individuals obtain inhome service through public social service and health programs and some well-to-do persons may purchase service from the rapidly developing proprietary homemaker agencies, the middle income group is generally left without an adequate funding source.

NEED FOR A NATIONAL POLICY

While the reluctance of third party payers, especially Medicare, to reimburse for homemaker services is the most visible obstacle to expansion, it is only the tip of the iceberg. Indeed, the Medicare restrictions are themselves the result of other deep-seated obstacles. Among these are: the overwhelming priority that physicians and most other health professionals give to care for acute illnesses as opposed to the prevention and management of chronic illness; the fact that most "health insurance" is in reality "sickness insurance;" the fear, among both public and private third parties, of abuse of noninstitutional care which, it is widely believed, is more difficult to monitor than institutional care; the tremendous national and institutional investment in acute-care hospital beds, nursing homes, and other institutional facilities, an investment which virtually mandates high occupancy as a measure of acceptable productivity; and changing consumer attitudes, mores, and life styles. The typically small urban apartment, the fewer number of children to share the burden of providing a home for aging parents, crime and the fear it engenders among older people living alone, all militate against home care.

Underlying most of the provider and third party concerns is the virtual impossibility of establishing a neat boundary between health care and other community services. The homemaker-home health aide concept—relatively new and poorly funded—is caught precisely in the middle of these basic philosophical and societal conflicts. The awkward hyphenated name—a product of the effort to link needed social services with reimbursable health services—symbolizes the dilemma. While we Americans continue to give lip service to one set of values—individual autonomy and responsibility, the family, the community, prevention, and health maintenance—all the major incentives—financial, professional, status—are skewed in the opposite direction.

But there is some reason to believe, or at least hope, that these priorities may now be in the process of gradual change. The Senate Subcommittee on Long Term Care is beginning to crystallize and mobilize public and professional opinion:

> A national policy on long-term care—comprehensive, coherent, and attentive to the needs of older Americans—does not exist in the U.S. today. The need for such a policy becomes more evident with each passing day that brings an increasing number of older Americans. The rapid increase in America's over-75 population indicates that (1) a policy is needed immediately, and (2) long-term care should properly be considered within the context of national health insurance plans.[3]

The importance assigned by the subcommittee to home care as an "alternative" to institutionalization is also made clear:

> Home health care receives a very low priority in the U.S..... all the more evident when American health delivery systems are compared with some European systems where home health is a full partner in a genuine continuum of care....
>
> Older Americans, more than any other group. have been adversely affected by the failure. Some 2.5 million seniors are without necessary care, which could postpone or prevent institutionalization if provided in a timely fashion.

Within this "genuine continuum of care," the desirability of appropriate, approved, carefully supervised homemaker services, a key component of long term noninstitutional care, can be related to four separate but reinforcing considerations:

1. Homemaker services provide an essential option to the infirm elderly, the disabled, and to handicapped families who need some assistance with personal and household tasks but do not need institutional care. Such services permit them to remain in their own homes where most prefer to be, and with families as nearly intact as possible.
2. Homemaker services provide needed assistance to overworked health professionals, often permitting them to care for patients in their own homes without the time-consuming strain of unnecessary visits to those homes.

3. Homemaker services provide an opportunity for useful work to mature individuals with homemaking experience without the necessity for much formal education, thus suggesting a major opportunity for public service jobs, as well as private employment, during the years of anticipated high unemployment immediately ahead.
4. Homemaker services often provide an opportunity for substantial savings to third party health insurance carriers and taxpayers. The urgency of this point is underscored by the rapidly rising number of the elderly and their generally low income status.

Although substantial overall savings are possible only if there is a moratorium on the construction of unneeded beds and other institutional facilities, there is some reason to hope that national policy is gradually changing in this respect because (1) there is now less public subsidy of institutional facilities, and (2) planning mechanisms designed to encourage rational allocation of health care resources are gradually coming into existence through the new National Health Planning and Resources Development Act and state certificate-of-need laws.

SOME RECOMMENDATIONS

In the hope that the leadership of the health professions, in cooperation with government and appropriate representatives of the public, will help the homemaker services meet their full potential, we recommend the following immediate steps:

1. Agree on a definition of homemaker service that recognizes the inclusion of both personal care and household tasks, and covers benefits and patient eligibility.
2. Agree on a set of standards to assure appropriate, safe, efficient, and effective services, and on one or more mechanisms for approval or accreditation of programs meeting such standards.
3. Extend, through amendment of the Medicare *Conditions of Participation,* state regulations, or both, the policy contained in the New York State Hospital Code requiring every hospital to maintain an "organized discharge planning program ... which meets the patient's post-discharge needs."
4. Agree on basic recordkeeping and accounting procedures to provide an essential data-base for quality controls and for actuarial estimation of the costs of insurance coverage.
5. Implement the recommendations of the Senate Subcommittee on Long Term Care, the Comptroller General, and the Health Insurance Benefits Advisory Council with respect to benefits for home health services under Medicare and Medicaid.

6. Encourage voluntary coverage of home health benefits, including homemaker services, in Blue Cross and other private health insurance, and explore with all interested parties the desirability of mandatory coverage.
7. Formulate a realistic package of home health, including homemaker, benefits to be included in national health insurance when enacted.
8. Encourage the employment and training of homemakers under the Comprehensive Employment and Training Act of 1973 and other public service employment programs as a means of providing useful jobs and skills to the unemployed, as well as attracting much-needed recruits, especially to work in low income areas.

Finally we urge health professionals, consumers, and governments to recognize that much more is involved in health than just health care, no matter how broadly the latter is defined. Even the most skilled, dedicated, and well-financed professionals in the world cannot stem the tide of environmental and behavioral threats to health inherent in many of the conditions of contemporary American society, particularly the decline of the family and the family homestead, the disintegration of communities, the prevalence of violence and fear, and overreliance on institutionalized care.

Obviously, homemaker services alone cannot stem this tide. They are a symbol, however, of the need for reintegrating health, welfare, and community services as they apply to the individual and to the family.

NOTES

1. U.S. Senate, Subcommittee on Long-Term Care of the Special Committee on Aging, *Nursing Home Care in the United States: Failure in Public Policy, Introductory Report*, 93rd Cong., 2nd Sess. (Washington, D.C.: U.S. Government Printing Office, 1974).
2. New York State Hospital Code, Chap. V, Subchap. C., Sec. 720.7.
3. U.S. Senate, *op. cit.*

Chapter Eleven
Some Relevant Foreign Experience

Despite some much publicized differences in financing, most of the economically advanced nations share a commonality of health problems, a basic philosophy with respect to health care, and similar institutions for providing such care. This is hardly surprising. Middle aged men die of heart attacks and women of breast cancer in communist Russia just as they do in the United States. Old age is no respecter of political ideology. Infants born under "socialized medicine" need the same immunizations and other well-baby care as infants born to an American "Blue Cross" family.

Virtually all these countries—capitalist, socialist, and communist—share the same faith in medical science, medical technology, and professional intervention. The hospital has emerged as the principal site of technological medicine and the most expensive element in the national health care bill. The costs of health care are rising much faster than other necessities of life. Although the proportion of gross national product spent for health care in the United States is now probably the highest in the world, the ratio is increasing rapidly in most advanced nations. In 1973 the proportions among a representative group ranged from 5.3 to 7.7 percent (Figure 1), and all were groping for ways to control these costs. Even in the one area of conspicuous difference—the extent to which the costs of care are borne through taxation as opposed to private health insurance and direct consumer payments—the differences are narrowing as the United States moves, gradually but apparently inexorably, toward increased government participation (Table X).[1]

The primary reason for studying foreign experience is not to promote emulation. Important social institutions are not generally transferable from one country to another. Health care systems are, and should be, the product of demographic, socioeconomic, and cultural differences among nations as well as of common health problems and shared scientific and professional traditions. Still, there is much that each country can learn—both positive and negative—from the experience of others. Thanks to our size, resources, and perhaps some accidents of history, America still enjoys a degree of choice with respect to health and health care policies denied to less fortunate countries. Whether this additional time and latitude will be used wisely, or wasted, can be influenced by the extent to which we seize the opportunity to study the experience of others and learn both from their forward steps and their mistakes.

The selections in this chapter deal with three aspects of national health policy where the United States is also searching for direction. Selection 49 focuses on the effort to overcome the widely deplored fragmentation of services and programs. Selection 50 discusses health care for the universally rising numbers and proportions of the elderly, an area where medical, social, and economic policies are inescapably interrelated. Selection 51 spotlights one nation's effort to reorder its policies in the direction of health promotion.

NOTE

1. A recent Rand Corporation study claims that over 90 percent of the variance in per capita medical expenditures in the developed countries can be explained by variation in per capita gross domestic product and has little relation to differences in prices or methods of paying physicians. Joseph T. Newhouse, *Income and Medical Care Expenditures Across Countries*, (Santa Monica, California: Rand Corporation, 1976).

Selection 49

The Rationalization of Health Services in Britain and Sweden*

The rationalization of health facilities and services—in the interest both of cost controls and better patient care—is emerging as a major public policy issue throughout Western Europe. This is true despite the fact that in most European countries health care is already financed mainly through public funds. As Dr. Arthur Engel of Sweden has observed:

> With the enormously rising costs of hospital building and of hospital operation, carefully rationalized hospital planning inside a comprehensive system of health and social care is of utmost importance.

Similar views were expressed in a 1970 Green Paper on the British National Health Service, and in the "Resolution on Recommendations Concerning Lowering the Cost of Medical Treatment," by the European Public Health Committee of the Council of Europe. Specific recommendations include:

---

*Excerpt from A.R. Somers, "The Rationalization of Health Services: A Universal Priority," *Inquiry* 8 (March 1971): 48-60. Based on visits by the author to England, Sweden, and Denmark in the Spring of 1970.

> Promoting the closest possible integration between preventive and curative medicine, both with regard to medical and ancillary staff, and the use of organizations, establishments, and installations....
>
> Interchange of patients between different levels of hospitals or health services....
>
> Close cooperation between the hospital and family physician....
>
> Coordinated planning between the various authorities responsible for health services....
>
> Coordination of planning between the different hospital authorities within the area... to allow rationalization of the scope of work among the hospitals....
>
> An information system should be set up to cover several hospitals and also community services. This may raise a demand for an automated data processing system.[1]

This is a sobering thought for both proponents and opponents of national compulsory health insurance in the United States. Public financing has not proved a panacea in Europe. It has solved some problems and created or exacerbated others. Clearly, also our health problems and theirs are basically similar, despite certain historical variations and differences in timing.

EUROPEAN HEALTH CARE ECONOMICS

A few background facts are essential. First, the European health care economies are almost completely "socialized." Except in The Netherlands, most of the hospitals are owned and operated by government at one level or another. In Britain, since 1948, they have been the responsibility of the national government, with their operation delegated to 14 regional councils and some 400 hospital management committees, plus a special separate arrangement for the teaching hospitals.

In Sweden most hospitals are the responsibility of local governments. Twenty-five county councils and separate authorities for the three largest cities carry the responsibility. These bodies are autonomous and empowered to impose special taxes for the construction and operation of their hospitals. Ninety percent of the hospitals' revenue comes from local taxes—with the balance coming from the central government, insurance payments, and direct patient payments.

In theory, inpatient ward care is free[2] to all residents without limitation as to time or type of service. In fact, of course, shortages of beds and personnel impose limits, especially in Britain, where there are substantial waiting lists for elective surgery. In Sweden, persons 67 or over are limited to one year in an acute care hospital.

In both countries, physicians' services are free, or nearly so, to all or most of the population. Inpatient medical care, provided in all instances by salaried doctors is completely free. The financing of family doctor (out-of-hospital) services differs rather significantly among the three, chiefly as a result of historical differences in the relation of "family-doctoring" to hospital care.

The Swedish system is most complicated and nearest to ours. About half the ambulatory care is rendered in the outpatient departments of the hospitals by hospital-based doctors. Until January 1970, these doctors billed their patients, who were then partially reimbursed by the national insurance scheme. Starting in 1970, however, all hospital doctors are fully salaried. The patient pays directly to the hospital a small fee—seven kronor (about $1.40)—for each visit regardless of the amount of services required.

About a fourth of ambulatory care is rendered by salaried doctors working out of district health centers. Patients pay the same seven kronor (15 for a home visit) for these services. A final quarter is provided by private practitioners in their own offices who may charge what they wish. The patient is reimbursed, through national health insurance, for three-fourths of the official fee schedule. Dental care is covered in the same way, although there are many limitations. In 1969 per capita sickness insurance contributions averaged about 450 kronor ($90) for the year. Employers pay somewhat more, and government subsidy is about 12 percent of total costs.

In Britain the hospitals are not generally used for primary care. Outpatient services are restricted to diagnostic services or special therapy. Primary care is provided free by the general practitioner service, one of the three major arms of the National Health Service. General practitioners are paid on a modified capitation basis.

Drugs are supplied free to children, the elderly, and to those with certain long standing chronic conditions. For others, there is a flat charge of two shillings, sixpence (about 35¢) per prescription. In Sweden, certain life-sustaining drugs are covered in full. For others there is a discount and a maximum charge of $3.00 per prescription.

GENERAL CONSUMER AND PROVIDER SATISFACTION

The impact of the various forms of health care on national mortality and morbidity has never been effectively measured. Perhaps the most ambitious attempt—by Dr. Osler Peterson working with researchers from England, Sweden, and the United States—concluded that meaningful international comparisons were impossible in the present state of international health data.[3] Despite this caution against relating health statistics to systems of care, Dr. Peterson *et al.* did point out that the United States, with the highest death rates of the three countries at that time, also had the highest levels of utilization—as measured by per capita doctor-patient contacts or hospital admission rates—and the highest per capita expenditures.

In any case, it is evident that the health care systems are overwhelmingly popular with the public in both Britain and Sweden. In neither country is there any serious demand for repeal. They are as fully accepted by the conservative parties as by the labor or socialist parties through which the systems were originally introduced.

In Britain, the Conservatives would like to increase the small private sector, represented primarily by the British United Provident Association (BUPA), a successful nonprofit health insurance organization with about 3.5 percent of the population enrolled. With a handful of private hospitals financed out of its own funds, a flair for innovation, and able management, BUPA enjoys the support of many top leaders in the British health care field; but no one even considers it as a potential substitute for the National Health Service. It has been said that the three most popular items in Britain today are the monarchy, tea, and the NHS.

Alongside the public satisfaction must be placed the general satisfaction of the providers of care. "Socialized medicine" represented much less of a change in Europe than it would in the United States. In the Scandinavian countries the hospitals have been the responsibility of local government for a century or more. In England most of the world famous teaching hospitals were voluntary until 1948, but this was not true in Scotland; and even in England perhaps half the acute beds and nearly all the mental and other long term beds were run by government, even prior to the NHS. The nationalization of all hospitals under the NHS was in accord with the desires of both the hospitals, which, even before World War II, were in disastrous financial condition, and of the hospital-based physicians whose primary concern was to avoid being placed under local government.

With respect to physicians, most of the senior consultants have been pleased from the outset—with good reason. Paid by the NHS for whatever proportion of their time they choose to give to hospital work (much of which they had previously done for nothing), they are permitted to retain whatever private practice they wish to handle. There has been dissatisfaction among junior hospital staff, who have accounted for most of the emigration; but their complaints appear to be directed primarily against hospital staffing patterns rather than against the NHS per se.

The GPs, who originally chose to be paid on a capitation basis rather than salary, found themselves nearly overwhelmed in the first few years. In 1970 however, thanks to a tapering off in this backlog of demand, substantial pay increases, modifications in the capitation system of payment, and more attention from the central government, they appear generally satisfied. The end of the old British tradition of having to buy a practice and increasing government assistance in establishing GP "health centres" appear to be special sources of satisfaction. Dr. William Thompson, editor of *The Practitioner*, probably spoke for most of his constituency when he reported that most British doctors were much better off now than before NHS and were basically pleased with it.

As already noted, the Swedish hospital doctors were recently involved in a basic change of policy—from what we would call "geographic full-time" to "strict full-time." For about 15 percent of the highest paid this resulted in some loss of earnings, and some grumbling is still heard. For some younger doctors it meant an increase. The majority remained at the same level. And in the Swedish welfare state where taxes consume nearly half of the average family income, money wages are less important than shorter hours and a more rational professional life. There is no serious professional opposition to the health service in Sweden.

COSTS RISING RAPIDLY

In terms of costs, two facts stand out most prominently. First, although costs, and the utilization they reflect, still vary from country to country, they are all going up rapidly, especially in the past few years. Second, despite the continuing differences in organization of services, in every country the hospital is consuming an increasing share of national health care expenditures.

Some of the significant differences in use patterns, as of the late 1950s and early 1960s, have been reported by Peterson and his associates. For example, the Swedes averaged only 2.8 physician visits per capita per year, while the English averaged 4.7; and Americans, at a roughly comparable date, 5.3. On the other hand, the Swedes were admitted to short term hospitals at the rate of 127 per 1,000 population; the English, only 82 per 1,000; and Americans 134 per 1,000. Although the English balance their low admission rate with an exceptionally long length of stay, the Swedes have both a high admission rate and a long length of stay. The mean length of stay for the United States, England, and Sweden, as reported by Peterson et al., was 7.7 days, 14.8 days, and 12.5 days, respectively.

Whether there is a sort of balancing trade-off as between physician and hospital services, or for some other reasons, the proportion of gross national product spent for the health services in the various advanced countries of the world remained relatively similar throughout the 1950s and 1960s. An International Labor Office study based on data of the early 1950s reported a range from 3.7 percent in Denmark to 4.5 in Norway and the United States and 4.6 in New Zealand. Using data from the late 1950s, Professor Brian Abel-Smith of England reported a range from 4.9 percent in Sweden to 5.3 percent in the United States.

During the 1960s health care costs increased dramatically in Europe, as in America. In Sweden costs have been rising about 10 percent annually. In England, where expenditures were rigidly held down for the first decade of NHS, they have also begun to escalate, the rise for the year ending March 1968 being 10 percent. A Netherlands study reports a rise of 243 percent in health care costs during the decade 1958-1968, with hospital care rising 339 percent.

The latter phenomenon, the hospitals' increasing share of total health care costs, appears to be the pattern throughout Europe. Fifty-six percent of the NHS budget went for hosptials in 1969-1970, all but six percent for operating expenses. The operating costs alone of Swedish hospitals consume 51 percent of total public expenditures for health. Current investment in new hospitals is very high. Odin Anderson and Duncan Neuhauser compared the rise in hospital costs in Sweden, England and Wales, and the United States for the decade 1955-1965 and found the following: Sweden up 323 percent; England and Wales up 228 percent; United States up 231 percent. Even with the effect of general price increases eliminated, they found these rises: Sweden, 206 percent; England, 179 percent; United States, 191 percent.[4]

The Swedes' growing concern about their out-of-hand hospital costs was clearly stated by Goth Nilsson, Chairman of the Örebro County Council. Citing a study of health costs and gross national income by the City of Stockholm Finance Department, assuming a continuing increase in the former of 10 percent per year, Nilsson pointed out that the health share of gross national income would rise from 5 percent in 1967 to 13 percent in 1987. Under certain assumptions the health share could reach 37 percent by that year.

Nilsson continued: "This would mean a considerable reshuffle of public resources to the benefit of the hospital and health services. Is this realisitic? Is it reasonable? Are the present aims and structure of the health services the right ones? Does not the situation force the leaders in the health services to decide on a structure to suit these possibilities? To what extent can illness be prevented?" He then continues with a long and urgent plea for more preventive services and health education.

THE DRIVE TOWARD RATIONALIZATION

Against this background of general satisfaction accompanied by accelerating cost increases, concerned public officials and health authorities are casting about in many directions for cost restraints. According to Dr. Robert Logan, of the London School of Hygiene and Tropical Medicine, "There is no ceiling to the costs of a perfect comprehensive health service." Or, in the more pungent words of Richard Titmuss of the London School of Economics, "It is a bottomless pit."

Since it is now unthinkable in these countries that demand should be restricted by reimposition of financial barriers, the officials and planners are concentrating on other approaches, principally the administrative manipulation of supply and demand. The recommendations, with respect to lowering the cost of medical treatment advanced by the Council of Europe's Public Health Committee are illustrative. One of these recommendations dealt with greater patient participation in the costs of care (copayment). After considerable debate, the committee adopted a statement saying that such a measure is acceptable provided the contribution is small and that it can be reduced or abolished in cases of special need or where there is no fear of abuse. Sweden's new "seven kronor" system suggests that this recommendation may be heeded.

All the other recommendations dealt with rationalization of supply in one form or another; the integration or coordination of all types of facilities, services, and programs, hopefully with the ultimate aim of redirecting demand to the less expensive programs and facilities as well as the avoidance of duplication, waste, and poor quality care.

The Swedish Regional Hospital System

One of the first to stress this approach to cost controls was Sweden, a country with a smaller than average supply of doctors, a greater than average supply of beds, nurses, and other health personnel, and the financial and technological resources to make possible an imaginative approach to rationalization. In addition, there is in Sweden what Gunnar Myrdal calls "an organizational infrastructure" through which health care planning and other desirable public policies could be undertaken with a minimum of compulsion and national government controls. "In recent times," says Myrdal, "Sweden has become the organizational state." Employers, labor—now organized virtually 100 percent, including hospital workers—a powerful cooperative movement, hospitals, doctors, "even very specific common interests—for instance old-age pensioners and invalids, or those suffering from rheumatism, diabetes, and even less frequent illnesses—have now their own nationwide organizations with district branches." While such an organizational network has its drawbacks and dangers—especially the danger of overbureaucratization, which Myrdal pointed out—it did facilitate the development of hospital planning on an area or regional basis, totally at variance with British policy under the National Health Service.

As already noted, Sweden has long been divided, for purposes of hospital administration, into 25 autonomous counties and three major cities. In the late 1950s, however, Dr. Engel, then Director General, National Board of Health, concluded that a new organizational level was necessary to avoid duplication and irrational use of resources and personnel. In 1960 his proposal was accepted by Parliament. The new level was designated a region, and the country was divided into seven such regions, each with roughly a million people. (The population of the country is now about 8 million.) Each of the five existing teaching hospitals was designated a regional hospital, and two others were named as potential regional hospitals. Collaboration between the counties within each region remains on a voluntary basis with governmental health authorities supervising, guiding, and advising the counties as they move toward greater coordination.

At the national level, supervision is exercised by the National Board of Health through its Planning Department and a semiautonomous body, the Committee for the Construction of Health and Social Welfare Buildings (NSB).

which must approve all new construction. The Institute for the Planning and Rationalization of Health and Welfare Services in Sweden (SPRI), formed in 1968 as a result of an agreement between the national government and the Federation of Swedish County Councils and supported one-third by the former, two-thirds by the latter, now serves an important function as technical advisor to the county councils.

Under the guidance of this voluntary but coordinated effort at rationalization, a four-level model of care is emerging:

1. At the regional level a single regional hospital serves a population of a million or more. The superspecialties are concentrated at this level.
2. The county central hospital serves a population from 250,000 to 300,000. As a rule this hospital has 800 to 1,000 beds, most of the usual specialties, a large outpatient department, rehabilitation facilities, family planning, welfare services, etc.
3. The local district hospital, typically serving 60,000 to 90,000, is still in process of transition. Nearly all authorities agree on the need for merging, closing, or converting many of the formerly small district hospitals into nursing homes, health centers, or a combination of the two. Local resistance is considerable, but the policy remains to eliminate all district hospitals with less than 300 beds.
4. The local health center, serving a population of 10,000 to 20,000 with ambulatory preventive and curative care, is not formally part of the hospital system. However, with 300 such centers in operation today, the goal is to integrate their activities with the nearest district hospital.

Illustrative of the new, rationalized, automated, Swedish hospital is Danderyd, the central hospital for North Stockholm. With some 1,000 beds to which 400 new psychiatric beds will be added by 1972, it was recently described as "a medical-technical industry for human repair, it books by computer, is run by an economist [University of California, M.H.A.], functions through employee participation, is totally free, assigns private rooms for need but not for money, and really cares for and about each patient." One could add that it boasts the record of the lowest infant mortality rate of any hospital in the world—a record won from another Swedish hospital, Karolinska—and despite the fact that all medical care is given by salaried physicians it operates with a personnel/patient ratio of about 1:5 [compared with a 1970 U.S. ratio of 2.7:1 (Table VI)].

The guiding principle of the Swedish planners is that "care should be provided at the lowest acceptable organizational level of the medical care system." The motivation was both economy and higher quality care. In the words of Dr. Engel:

> The main goal is to provide qualified medical treatment for the population of every area of the country.... If we had not launched the regional hospital system we would have witnessed the growth of small specialist services in many places. They would not have had the

capacity to develop the highest quality of care and to keep abreast of scientific progress. That would have meant a bad investment of capital and medical personnel.

It is still too soon to evaluate the results. But it is already obvious that more has been achieved with respect to quality than economy. The rapid rise in overall and hospital costs has been cited.... The fear expressed by Nilsson that too great a proportion of national resources are going into health care is rather widely shared by public officials. Despite planning, the combined pressures of consumers and professionals continue to produce more beds than needed. To control the situation in Stockholm, starting in 1971, the city will be divided into six health care districts with a central hospital in each district and rather strict limitations on patient crossing of district lines.

British Efforts at Coordination

Prior to World War II, the British voluntary hospital, despite recurrent financial crises, defied systematic planning. Even the nationalization of the hospitals in 1948 and establishment of the regional hospital boards and area management committees have been described by one of England's leading health care authorities as, in reality, "no more than reshuffling of the same people who had always run the hospitals—the unpaid volunteers who had attained some expert knowledge and the medical profession."

While this appraisal of the impact of the NHS on British hospitals undoubtedly represents British understatement, the almost total absence of investment capital during the first ten years of the NHS precluded any serious effort at restructuring or rationalization. Starting in the mid 1950s, modest but increasing sums were made available for new construction. Leaders, both in and out of government, began to recognize the need for planning. In 1962 the Ministry of Health presented to Parliament an ambitious program, *A Hospital Plan for England and Wales*. Central to the new plan was the concept of the "district general hospital." Normally 600 to 800 beds, it would serve a population of 100,000 to 150,000 and provide treatment and diagnostic facilities for both inpatients and outpatients, including a short-stay psychiatric unit and geriatric unit. One of its major purposes was the integration of the many existing single-specialty institutions.

By the end of the 1960s the concept of the district general hospital was further expanded to one of 1,000 to 1,500 beds, serving a population of 200,000 to 300,000, with greater emphasis on psychiatric (including mental subnormality) and geriatric treatment; on joint planning of hospital and community health services; and on bridging the gap between hospital and general practitioner services through the introduction of "general practitioner beds" at the district hospital.

Meanwhile governmental leaders became increasingly concerned with the dysfunctions resulting from the tripartite division of the National Health Service. A Ministerial Green Paper, published in 1968, urged integration of the three branches with responsibility for provision of all services allocated to 40 to 50 area boards. The 14 regional hospital boards and the 400 area management committees would be abolished.

Despite widespread agreement as to the desirability of integrating the three branches, a storm of criticism greeted the Green Paper. It was widely alleged that the new area boards would be too remote from the people, would probably be dominated by the hospitals, and would discourage regional planning. Shortly thereafter another report, this one by the Royal Commission on Local Government in England (Maud Commission), recommended that integration be achieved by turning all the services over to strengthened local government. Again a storm of protest, this time from the hospitals and doctors.

The latest proposal, contained in a second Green Paper published early in 1970, seeks to reconcile the opposing positions and recommends integration, not through existing local government, and not through 40 to 50 area authorities, but by some 90 of these bodies designed to correspond to the 90 "unitary authorities" recommended by the Maud Commission. To guarantee local participation (presumably consumers) it was proposed that the new area bodies should consist of only one-third professionals, with one-third persons appointed by local governments, and one-third by the Secretary of State for Health and Social Security. In place of the existing 14 regional hospital boards, the Green Paper recommended 14 advisory regional health councils.

How the emerging district general hospital would fit into the new administrative pattern is unclear. In theory, at least, the integration of hospital, general practitioner, and other health services should make it easier for the district hospital to become the hub and center of all the health services and thus contribute to a general rationalization. On the other hand, opposition to the hospital as the major consumer of scarce NHS financial resources and as the citadel of specialist-dominated curative medicine could prevent it from developing the desirable outreach.

Comparing the British and Swedish scenes, it may seem ironic that the British are moving to erode the power of their new regional hospital boards at the same time that the Swedes are trying to strengthen their regional organization. In fact they are both groping toward some effective balance between centralization and decentralization, between national and local responsibility.

In all cases, this issue is complicated by the overlap of provider versus consumer interests. The historical opposition of English doctors and hospitals to local control—in striking contrast to the Swedish experience—apparently relates both to the relative financial weakness of British local government and to fear that professional interests would not be adequately protected. Although one may anticipate some continuing opposition to the proposed 90 area authorities by hospitals and doctors, especially by the teaching hospitals and their staffs if, as proposed in a separate document, their autonomy is now removed and they are brought into the general health services grid, it seems likely that this compromise will be acceptable to enough of the various interests that it will pass Parliament. [With some modifications, this was the general pattern established by the NHS Reorganization Act of 1973.]

Beyond these broad areas of agreement, there appears to be a growing conviction that real integration of health services will not, and cannot, be achieved simply by juggling administrative units. How, it is now beginning to be asked, can even a fully integrated area authority, with responsibility for all branches of the health services, provide continuity of patient care, and the economies presumed to result therefrom, as long as the traditional dichotomy between hospital care and primary care persists? Undoubtedly those who are asking this question are still in the minority. From Labor Party spokesmen one hears more about the "rationing" of supply as a means of controlling demand than of changes in the fundamental organization of physician services or consumer attitudes.

But occasional voices are being raised to question these generally taken-for-granted "givens" in the growing supply and demand imbalance. Some are beginning to point out that the dramatic increase in hospital use and costs is not the fault of the hospital, but of the GP who determines the hospital caseload; or, more fundamentally, the system which forces the conscientious GP to send his patient to the hospital whenever he suspects anything seriously wrong with his patient.

Dr. Robert Logan recently concluded a penetrating analysis of NHS problems with a renewed attack on "the gap between general practice and hospital practice in Britain."

> This break in contact between care in the hospital ward and in the home existed in England long before 1948 (when the nationalization of all the hospitals merely aggravated and froze it) and now both the public and the profession so accept it that to discharge a semi-ambulant patient to his own well-furnished home a few days after an operation (or even after a normal childbirth) is an experiment if not revolutionary! Yet every patient in England has his own free family doctor backed up by a potential army of nurses and home helps—and each redundant day in hospital consumes at least £6 of limited resources and skills....
>
> Another consequence of the break in continuity... is to be seen in outpatient departments. Here again the hospital doctor is so remote from the family doctor with whom the patient is registered that, six months after the first visit for an outpatient "consultation," some one-fifth of all patients in general medicine, surgery, pediatrics, and gynecology are still retained by the hospital and are not discharged to the care of their own doctor.... No system for the delivery of technical skills can afford such a polarization of medical manpower, particularly in a country like ours which has no alternative routes in our comprehensive, but closed, National Health Service.

To correct this situation and to achieve some meaningful rationalization at the crucial point—where care is actually delivered—Dr. Logan refers hopefully to ideas apparently fermenting in Scotland under the leadership of Dr. John Brotherston, Scotland's Principal Medical Officer.

> The discerning Scottish eye views the isolation as so wide and fundamental that it needs a radically new working vehicle run by a new hybrid doctor, half general and half hospital practitioner. Essentially doctors would not work in groups of less than five and would care for 10,000 population with half their work concerned with "hospital" medicine, much of which would be carried out in a new medical center equipped as for present outpatient's hardware and dealing more appropriately with much of the current outpatient caseload of investigation, follow-up, and care of the chronic ambulatory patient. The new buildings would also incorporate the day centers and day hospitals for the handicapped, the elderly, and the psychiatric, and thus would be nearer to the neighborhood of the homes of such long-term patients than at present. The relatives and the public would be increasingly participating in their care.... To run such a new setup would naturally need a new breed of doctor, but he would be practicing up to the rising level of his professional interests and competence. Such a new kind of doctor would be delivering the modern medicine he has been taught in both the community and in the hospital. Besides providing the most effective use of the educational investment from his long training, it should also satisfy his ambitions and thereby reduce the "brain drain."

OUR COMMON PROBLEMS

For the American observer there appear to be a number of relevant observations in the European experience. First, there is the comforting discovery that we are not alone in our difficulties. Despite differences in financing, not only Britain and Sweden but Western Europe in general share our concern over fragmented care and rising costs and are looking for ways of dealing with these problems.

Second, there is the realization that in all these countries, the hospital is the special target of criticism. Consuming the lion's share of national health care expenditures in all countries, perhaps this mixture of resentment, envy, and distrust of the modern "medi-factory" is understandable, but it is particularly unfortunate just at the time when the need for systemization or rationalization of health services is increasingly recognized. The implication is clear: either the hospital will take the initiative in rationalizing the health services as a whole, including out-of-hospital care, or it will be done by forces hostile to the hospital with resulting downgrading of its role.

Third, there is the conviction that, underneath all the socioeconomic, political, and cultural differences between these nations and ourselves there are a number of common problems regarding the health care system in a modern, affluent, technologically advanced society:

1. How to provide a financial base broad enough and stable enough to sustain the comprehensive and expensive system demanded both by consumers and providers in such a society?
2. How to provide the "organizational infrastructure" necessary to provide something approaching comprehensive care to the entire population?
3. How to revitalize the health professions educational endeavor so as to meet the enlarged needs and demands of such a society, both quantitatively and qualitatively?
4. How to enlist the intelligent participation of the general public and the individual consumer in the national health care endeavor in such a way as to improve individual health while restraining costs to bearable dimensions?

It appears that the public's first concern—an adequate financial base—is perhaps intuitively correct. As Myrdal said, affluence is an absolute prerequisite to the welfare state. But if an adequate financial mechanism is essential it is only one of several essentials, as the experience of the socialized health economies makes clear, and by itself is no guarantor of either adequate cost controls or quality controls.

At the present time both Britain and Sweden are concentrating, each in its own way, on the second issue—the organizational infrastructure. They are making some progress. But at the same time, there is the growing realization that organizational reform cannot solve the problems without going even deeper into reform of professional education (Logan and Brotherston), and consumer education (Nilsson). The overriding fact is that we are growing closer together both in our problems and in our solutions, as well as in the difficulty of our task.

NOTES

1. Council of Europe, European Public Health Committee, "Resolution on Recommendations Concerning Lowering the Cost of Medical Treatment," (Strasbourg: March 1969), pp. 66-67.
2. Strictly speaking, of course, no services are "free." The term is used here, as it is generally in those countries, to indicate services financed either by taxes or health insurance contributions and for which no payment is required at the time of delivery.
3. O.L. Peterson, M.D., et al., "What Is Value for Money in Medical Care?" *The Lancet* (April 8, 1967): 771-776.
4. O.W. Anderson and D. Neuhauser, "Rising Costs Are Incorrect in Modern Health Care Systems," *Hospitals* (Feb. 16, 1969): 50-52.

Selection 50

Geriatric Care in the United Kingdom: An American Perspective*

Geriatric care is probably the most complex, neglected, and challenging aspect of health care facing the developed countries during the last quarter of the twentieth century. In all these countries both the number and proportion of the elderly continue to rise steadily. In the United Kingdom—where the retirement age for women is 60, for men, 65—by 1973 pensioners constituted nearly 17 percent of the population; 13.6 percent were 65 or over.[1]

While few, if any, other countries have reached this extreme (the U.S. ratio for 1973 was 10.1 percent) and the proportions continue to vary considerably, the ratios are now rising throughout the developed world. Particularly dramatic is the rise in numbers and proportion of those over 75 and even over 85.

Only in case of a major war, depression, or some totally unforeseen catastrophe is this trend likely to be reversed. Every advance in the treatment of cancer, heart disease, stroke, diabetes, arthritis, and in the salvage and rehabilitation of victims of trauma will increase the need for geriatric care. Every month added to the life expectancy of those 65 and over means a higher proportion of those in the most dependent age groups—the over-75s and over-85s. At the same time, the sharply reduced birthrates mean smaller cohorts of employed workers to support the elderly.

To compound the problem, relatively few physicians, health planners, and even public health authorities are professionally engaged in, or committed to, long term care of the elderly. In most countries, pressure groups working for health care legislation and appropriations are overwhelmingly oriented to acute care. Nevertheless, the inexorable pressure of growing proportions of the elderly on limited health care resources, is forcing most nations, regardless of political philosophy, to face up to this problem.

This report on geriatric care in the United Kingdom suggests a number of trends and issues that will become increasingly relevant to U.S. experience as our population continues to age, and limits on our national resources become more apparent.

MAJOR CHARACTERISTICS

In 1973 the crude birthrate in the United Kingdom was 13.9 per 1,000 population. The average life expectancy at birth was 69.0 for men; 75.2 for women. The average life expectancy at age 65 was 12.2 for men; 16.1 for women. There were 7.6 million 65 and over. The over-75s numbered 2.7 million and accounted for

---

*Excerpt from A.R. Somers, in *Annals of Internal Medicine* 84 (April 1976): 466-476.

4.8 percent of the population; those over 85, 0.5 million and 0.9 percent. In 1973, there were 27.9 elderly per 100 population of working age compared with only 14.5 in 1931. The projection for 1981 is 28.3.

The differences in health care for the elderly between the United Kingdom and the United States are more striking than in any other aspect of health care. These differences are discussed below.

Financing

The existence of the National Health Service (NHS) providing complete and nearly free (at time of delivery) health and medical care to all ages, for all conditions, and with no limits on duration, means that there are no special problems of financing care for the elderly as opposed to the general population, or long term care as opposed to acute care.

The main source of finance is the central government which, directly or indirectly through grants to local authorities, provided in 1974 about 88 percent of total health and social services costs [including 7 percent from NHS payroll taxes]. In 1975 the central government share was expected to rise by another 10 percentage points. The consolidated NHS budget is thus clearly dominant, providing a more powerful instrument for controlling both overall costs and the allocation of resources within the system than is available in most democratic countries, including the United States.

In practice, it is often alleged that acute hospital services receive a disproportionate share of national health resources, both manpower and financial. The hospitals do receive the lion's share of the health and social services dollar, approximately half in 1973 and 1974. But there are no built-in statutory biases in this direction. Funds are now in seriously short supply for the health service as a whole, but there is a continuing effort to protect and even enlarge somewhat the proportion of resources devoted to geriatric care. When increasing financial stringencies dictated a general cutback in projected capital expenditures for 1974-1975, there was no reduction in the allocation for geriatric services.

General Practice

Britain's more than 25,000 GPs constitute a much higher ratio of all practicing physicians than in the United States. The percentages for 1973 were 45 and 18, respectively. [For primary care potential in the United States, see Table V.]

The heavy emphasis on primary care and the persistence of a strong, officially encouraged GP service within the reorganized NHS permit greater continuity than is usual with specialty services, more attention to social and community factors, and generally provide an important base for the supportive type of care so frequently needed by the elderly.

Moreover, GPs receive small supplements for each elderly person on their patient lists, an amount which may not fully compensate for the extra care needed, but at least helps to reduce any disincentive. GPs who care for residents of old people's homes (residential homes) also receive a title of Visiting Health Officer and an additioanl supplement.

Geriatrics as a Medical Specialty

According to the Royal College of Physicians, geriatrics is "the branch of general medicine concerned with the clinical, preventive, remedial, and social aspects of health and disease in the elderly." However, an increasing number of able and aggressive English and Scottish physicians have succeeded in establishing geriatrics as a separate specialty, officially recognized as one in which hospital consultant appointments are made, and, to an increasing extent, recognized as a specialty in medical education.

The British Geriatric Society (originally called Medical Society for Care of the Elderly) was founded in 1948. By 1974 there were almost 300 geriatric specialists in the United Kingdom. Each serves an average of 250,000 elderly people, deals with more than 100 GPs, and admits to hospital about 700 patients annually. The geriatricians are responsible for about two-fifths of the hospital beds occupied by the elderly, but less than one-fifth of the elderly admitted to hospital.

There is an important distinction between elderly patients in general and geriatric patients. The latter are confined to those who have a combination of physical, mental, and social problems and who require long term care. Hence the need for special training and special interest on the part of the geriatric specialist as opposed to general surgeons, general physicians, or even specialists in internal medicine. So important are the mental problems that a subspecialty of psychogeriatrics has recently emerged—the only division of psychiatry with expanding chronic bed occupancy. Some 25 psychogeriatricians are now employed in British hospitals.

As of 1972, 246 hospital geriatric consultant (specialist) posts were filled plus about 100 registrars (intermediate hospital physicians) and 300 senior house officers (junior physicians). Many positions in all three categories were unfilled, and the great majority of registrars and SHOs were foreign-born, a source of distress to those seeking to strengthen the specialty.

It is not possible to make a precise comparison with American medicine in this respect. The American Geriatric Society has about 8,000 members, the majority internists. According to Dr. Ewald Busse, president, there are about 200 physicians giving full-time clinical practice to care of the elderly. While this is a growing field in the United States, the relatively stronger position of British geriatrics is probably a major factor in both the qualitative and quantitative development of long term care for the elderly in Britain.

Institutional Care

Nursing homes, in the American sense of the term, are virtually nonexistent.[2] Nonacute care for stroke patients and other elderly requiring medical attention is provided in geriatric beds in general hospitals. There were, in 1973, some 70,000 geriatric beds in Great Britain, 14 percent of all hospital beds. Official guidelines call for ten such beds per 1,000 population over 65. Typically they are provided in departments of 100 to 300 in district general hospitals.

The quality of care in the geriatric wards is frequently criticized by health authorities, while the public complains that it is extremely difficult—in some areas nearly impossible—to gain admission. The occupancy rate for 1973 was 93 percent, with a reported waiting list of 9,000. However, with a 1974 average length of stay of only 99 days (down slightly from 102 in 1973), it is clear that these beds have not been permitted to become "warehouses" for the long term "storage" of the ailing and homeless elderly.

Part of the pressure for more institutional services has been relieved by the development of "geriatric day hospitals"—a new concept in hospital outpatient care that emerged in the late 1950s and has grown rapidly in recent years. The day hospital, usually operated by a general hospital, provides facilities for physiotherapy and occupational therapy, medical examination, nursing treatment, dentistry, chiropody, and other health-related activities. Patients spend four to eight hours a day in the center, including lunch and afternoon tea, and are usually brought by special transport. Inpatients also come over from their wards.

In 1959 there were only ten day hospitals in the United Kingdom; by 1971 there were 111. Between 1964 and 1974 the number of new geriatric "day patients" rose from 4,800 to over 28,000. The majority of patients using day hospitals suffer from stroke, arthritis, or "chronic brain syndrome." The principal reasons for attendance are physical maintenance, rehabilitation, and relief of relatives. Although the evidence as to cost-effectiveness of the day hospital is not conclusive, most studies indicate reduced inpatient admissions, shorter inpatient length of stay, lower per diem costs, and/or improved quality of care.

Day hospitals are distinguished from "day centers," which are run by local authorities or voluntary agencies and provide social facilities, a meal, possibly a bath and chiropody, but none of the remedial services found in the day hospital.

Residential accommodations for the elderly, as well as the physically handicapped and mentally disordered, have been required of local government authorities since the National Assistance Act of 1948. Official norms call for 25 places per 1,000 elderly by 1983. They can be provided by the local authority directly or through delegation to voluntary organizations. The present "old people's homes" evolved out of the traditional public assistance or welfare homes. Some 10 to 12 percent of the local authority homes are still of the traditional variety—overlarge, outmoded, and impersonal. The newer type aims for an occupancy of 30 to 60 and a "homelike" atmosphere with numerous physical and social amenities. All meals are eaten communally. At the end of 1974, 108,000 persons 65 and over were in such homes, nearly 90 percent in local authority units. The reported average cost as £30 a week (about $65).

"Sheltered homes," operated by local authority housing divisions, permit a greater degree of independence. Residents frequently have private bed-sitting rooms, bring some of their own furniture and belongings, prepare their own breakfast, and are watched over by a "warden." Apparently there are no national norms for this category, but the Scottish Development Department suggests 25 per 1,000 elderly.

Among the voluntary organizations, Age Concern has played an important leadership role not only in publicizing the need for nonhospital residential facilities but also in establishing and operating model units. The Abbeyfield Society, a smaller group, provides places for some 4,000 in homes of seven to 12 each, at an average cost of £12 a week. The difference may be explained partly by the younger age and better health of Abbeyfield residents, partly by the voluntary or semivoluntary nature of the personnel.

Home Care

The personal social services, especially those available for care of the geriatric patient at home, appear more completely developed, to enjoy higher official status, and are relatively better financed than in the United States. As of 1974 the social service share of the total Department of Health and Social Security (DHSS) budget for health and social services was 15.5 percent.

The roots of Britain's extensive social service system go back several centuries. The modern phase dates from the immediate post-World War II period. Under the National Service Act, local authorities were empowered to provide "home helps" (homemaker services) to the elderly, and, under the National Assistance Act of 1948, meals and recreation.

Starting in the mid-1960s, the social services began to receive increasing attention. Section 45 of the Health Services and Public Health Act of 1968 (implemented 1971) increased the range of personal services which local authorities were required—not just empowered—to provide. Following a much publicized, high level study of the entire social services by the Seebohm Committee, 1965-1968, the Local Authority Social Services Act of 1970 (effective 1971) attempted to consolidate and streamline the administration of the numerous services by the responsible local authorities. Further administrative reorganization was mandated in the NHS Reorganization Act of 1973.

The range of personal services now potentially available to the elderly is virtually limitless. In practice, the principal services consist of: meals, in the home (meals-on-wheels) or elsewhere; home helps; visiting service and social work as needed; and minor physical adaptations of the home for the physically handicapped. District nurse and health visitor services, ambulance and other transport, chiropody, and bathing services are provided by the District Health Service rather than the local authority. All prescription drugs for the elderly are free.

At the end of 1974, nearly 500,000 elderly persons, nearly seven percent of the total, were receiving home help from a service of about 43,000. Eighty-six percent of all home help recipients were over 65. The number receiving meals at home during a sample week in 1973 was reported to be 158,000, about 2 percent of the elderly. About 60 percent as many free meals are also served in clubs and centers of various types. Most meals-on-wheels are delivered by volunteers. However, the planning, preparation, and cost of the food is the responsibility of the local authority.

A related benefit, administered separately through the social security system, is the "attendance allowance." This is a small cash benefit, made available to the severely disabled and those who need continual or frequent personal care attendance, in addition to other domiciliary services. Certification of need is required from an Attendance Allowance Board or a physician with authority delegated by the board. The intent, of course, is to further help the disabled remain at home.

Financial Constraints

The British health services have long operated under far greater financial constraints than those in the United States. The proportion of gross national product (GNP) going for all health care in the United Kingdom—an estimated 5.3 percent in 1973 (Figure 1)—and per capita expenditures in that year, $158—were substantially lower than in most other developed countries; dramatically less than in the United States.

Such figures should not be taken as "absolute truth." Both GNP and health expenditures are estimates, and changes in the ratios obviously reflect changes in GNP as well as in health costs. Both are affected by changes in price as well as quantity and quality of goods and services. Moreover, a low ratio, as in the United Kingdom, can be interpreted as failure to meet needs as well as exceptional efficiency in meeting needs.

Despite all these caveats, however, the order of magnitude of the figures is such that, taken in conjunction with Britain's relatively good record in vital statistics, it is difficult not to conclude that the nation is getting a "bigger bang for the health care buck" than is the United States. Whether this degree of austerity can be pushed any further, without affecting the quality of care, is an open question.

After a decade and a half of severe financial restraints following World War II, the British embarked in the early 1960s on an ambitious program of capital expansion, centered around the prototype district general hospital, with strong emphasis on the expansion and better distribution of consultant (specialist) services. This was followed by expansion of the social services and renewed attention to the upgrading of general practice. By the early 1970s the rate of increase in the consolidated health and social services budget exceeded U.S. levels. For example, the increase in England, 1973 to 1974, was over 16 percent. Capital expenditures on hospital building were up 20 percent.

The prosperity was short-lived, however. By early 1975 the accelerating general inflation reached an annual rate of over 25 percent. This and other financial problems forced the government back to austerity budgets. Thus far, the reduction has been only in the planned rate of growth, not in actual expenditures. But most informed observers anticipate real reductions in health expenditures during the rest of the 1970s. The result has to be increased pressure, even on the favored geriatric services. On October 20, 1975, Prime Minister Harold Wilson announced the creation of a new Royal Commission to consider the many difficult problems now facing the NHS, most of which stem from the growing financial constraints.

Philosophy

The overriding philosophy animating all British geriatric care is that old people should be kept at home and as nearly independent as possible, except under extraordinary circumstances where constant medical and nursing services are needed. Irreversible terminal illness is not considered one of these extraordinary circumstances.

This philosophy, which differs so markedly from that in the United States, is a complex amalgam of public preference, traditional ways of practicing medicine, economic necessity, and advanced geriatric thinking. Dr. Michael Green, a leading geriatrician, probably speaks for the majority of health professionals in the United Kingdom as well as general public opinion when he says:

> Our aim should be to 'ensure attitudes and services that will allow old people to die at home, in comfort, and at an advanced age, having enjoyed their life up to the time of death.' This can only be achieved by providing effective and comprehensive services for practical and preventive health care.

The corollary of this philosophy is avoidance of heroics in keeping the dying alive through artificial procedures when there is no hope of recovery. The ethical case has been well put by Dr. M. Roth of the University of Newcastle upon Tyne:

> Civilization is concerned with values.... These same values should surely prevent active intervention to resuscitate or prolong a life which has become mindless, helpless, and painful. There is a distinction between actively terminating life (which doctors should never do) and not intervening when life in any real sense has passed. There is a grow-

ing tendency for medical means to be used, since they are there, without consideration of the value of what they achieve.³

Dr. Paul Beeson, then at Oxford, now at the University of Washington School of Medicine, has summarized this philosophy with particular cogency in a brief essay, "Quality of Survival:"

> There is another aspect of the quality of survival...that has to do with the troubling questions of prolonging life unnecessarily, with special emphasis on the increased technology available to maintain the function of the circulation and respiration, even when the brain is grossly damaged or when there is an irreparable disease process elsewhere....
>
> I would very much dislike to see the development of any legal policy of euthanasia....
>
> I have on the other hand no misgivings about the withholding of antibiotics and parenteral fluids in certain instances where beyond reasonable doubt the patient is hopelessly ill....
>
> Death deserves dignity. When the situation is irretrievable we should remove tubes from body orifices and needles from blood vessels....
>
> For my own guidance I have found Trudeau's dictum ('to comfort, always') immensely helpful. And comfort does not apply solely to the patient. The family must also be included. Most often comfort means compassion and 'staying with' the patient. Our most common sin is to desert dying people and find excuses for not coming in to see them....
>
> In conclusion it seems to me that policies relating to the general topic of quality of survival must be determined by different parties.... There are situations in which the doctor alone must determine policy based on the intimate nature of his relation with the patient, his family, and his life situation. There are others in which society acting through its representative government must make the decision. Increasingly ideal care becomes more and more expensive. It is going to be the task of government to decide on priorities in just the same way that it decides how many war planes, how many schools, or how many airports a country should have. We doctors will have to advise on some of these matters and if we are to give the best advice we must make our value judgments objectively, subordinating to the best of our ability our own special interests.

Sir George Godber, longtime Medical Director of the Department of Health and Social Security, has discussed the problems he faced in translating this philosophy into actual practice, especially with reference to patients with renal failure and babies with spina bifida.[4]

ACHIEVEMENTS AND PROBLEMS

The extent to which the British have succeeded in realizing these difficult objectives with respect to geriatric care is, of course, impossible to measure precisely. Certain facts are relevant, however. As of 1956, 43 percent of deaths in England and Wales took place in the hospital. By 1966 the figure was up to 54 percent. In America the trend was similar: in 1958, 61 percent died in hospitals or other institutions; in 1962-1965, 64 percent.

As already noted, the 1971-1973 life expectancy at birth in England and Wales was 69.0 for men, 75.2 for women. Compared with 1948-1950, this was a rise of 2.7 years for men, 4.2 years for women. During the comparable period in the United States, life expectancy for men rose by 2.4 years, to an average of 67.5; for women, by 4.5 years to 75.1. Thus, the improvement in the United Kingdom was slightly greater for men than in the United States; slightly less for women. At age 65, the 1971-1973 life expectancy in Britain was 12.2 for men, 16.1 for women; in America, it was 13.1 for men, 17.0 for women. There are even greater differences in the mortality rates for the elderly in the two countries.

How much of these distinctions can be accounted for by differences in health care—either a deliberate policy of not prolonging life unnecessarily or inadequate care—cannot be determined. Many of Britain's aged still bear the scars of two world wars and many decades of social and economic deprivation that preceded the National Health Service. Certainly, the British geriatric services do not lack for homegrown critics. A study of 200 elderly persons by three distinguished geriatricians in the early 1970s found that nearly 40 percent had needs not provided for.

Dr. Michael Green, a geriatrician, still complains about many of his fellow physicians, especially GPs. Their prognosis, he says, is wrong in nine-tenths of the patients transferred to a geriatric unit. The faulty prognosis usually errs on the side of pessimism, convinced that old people will never recover sufficient function after a stroke or that it is impossible for an old lady to live alone again. He also cites an estimate that "hospital treatment of pressure sores costs £60,000,000 annually in the United Kingdom." With the support of the DHSS, a working group was set up in 1974 by the British Geriatrics Society and the Royal College of Nursing to prepare guidelines to good hospital geriatric care.

To an American visitor, in 1975, it appears that the British are already making exceptional efforts along these lines. The author personally visited three long-stay institutions and an old people's home in the London and Oxford areas, accompanied a district nurse on her daily rounds, sat in on a patient assessment interview and a class for geriatric nurses, and talked with leading geriatricians and government officials at all levels from the DHSS down to the district health office and local authority social service office. One could not fail to be impressed by the universally compassionate and imaginative measures that were being undertaken, within the severe financial constraints, to permit the maximum proportion of old people to be sustained at home in reasonable comfort, even through serious illness or disability.

Most of the homes visited were old, shabby, and some not too clean. A few still lacked running water. Without exception, however, there was ample room, a kitchen with a stove and a teapot, numerous personal furnishings and mementos, usually growing plants, often a dog or bird. Also without exception, the old people—whose ages ranged from 71 to 100, whose ailments included diabetes, ulcerated varicose veins, arthritis, epilepsy, multiple sclerosis, and plain old age—were cheerful, hospitable, and obviously very fond of the district nurse.

The 100-year-old lady who still puts curlers in her hair every night, the totally helpless MS victim whose frail husband gets her up by means of an NHS pulley every afternoon, the woman with bleeding varicose ulcers who had just returned from a visit to Brighton arranged by the social services: these may not be typical of the entire NHS nor do they imply that to be old, infirm, and poor is a happy state of affairs in England—or anywhere else. But it does suggest that Dr. Green's objective is not too utopian to serve as a goal for a national geriatric program.

It would be grossly misleading, however, to conclude without emphasizing some of the serious geriatric problems and issues facing the British as they move into the second quarter century of their NHS. Several of these have already been suggested: the shortage of qualified health personnel trained in, and committed to, geriatric care, the waiting lists for most types of institutional accommodations, the still incomplete coordination of health and social services, and the increasing budgetary stringency handicapping both NHS and the social services. Most of these problems are relevant to the United States. [Discussion of only one is included here.]

ADEQUACY OF INSTITUTIONAL FACILITIES

The official norm for geriatric hospital beds, as noted, is 10 to 1,000 population 65 and over. With about 70,000 beds and a 65-plus population of 7.6 million, this goal has been nearly achieved on a national basis. There is, however, wide disagreement as to whether the norm is adequate.

In sharp contrast to the widespread public complaints and long waiting lists in some localities, most British health authorities agree that there is no overall shortage of beds—if all were in good buildings and in the right places. Among those expressing this view are Sir George Godber, Dr. Lionel Cosin, one of Britain's first and leading geriatricians, and John Owen, Director of St. Thomas' Hospital and the St. Thomas Health District, London.

Dr. Cosin believes there are already *more* beds than necessary; that what is needed is a greater professional commitment to home care and ambulatory care. To illustrate, he points to the success of his "floating bed" concept at Cowley Road Hospital in Oxford, a long-stay, chronic disease institution. These beds are routinely scheduled for two different geriatric patients each week—one for three days, one for four. The primary purpose is to enable severely disabled patients to be maintained at home by assuring them of periodic assessment stays in hospital, at the same time relieving their families or caretakers on a periodic basis.

An important byproduct, Dr. Cosin maintains, is higher morale and generally better care on the part of hospital professionals who remain more alert with the constant rotation of patients. In Dr. Cosin's philosophy, there is no such thing as a "bedfast" patient and—given the proper medical, nursing, rehabilitation, and support services—only 1 percent of those admitted to Cowley Road are expected to remain "chairfast," i.e., out of bed but unable to walk.

Regardless of opinion as to overall adequacy, however, there is no denying the widespread regional and other differences influencing individual access. In some southeastern resort communities, England's "Costa Geriatrica," where the proportion of the elderly reaches as high as 35 percent, the demand is very high and facilities overcrowded. In Scotland the proportion of old people is no greater, but the official bed ratio norm is 50 percent higher than for the rest of the country. Socioeconomic conditions also influence the need and demand for geriatric beds. The lower the income class, the higher the rate of admission. According to one study the demand in two hospital areas was 50 percent higher for the lowest economic class compared to the highest.

Interacting with the latter factor is the important influence of sex on need and demand. Not only do women live six years longer than men on average, but a much larger proportion are single, widowed, or divorced, and living alone. The proportions of the latter are rising rapidly. According to Dr. Ferguson Anderson, Professor of Geriatric Medicine, University of Glasgow, "In most large cities, there are four times as many older women living alone as there are men." As a result of their great age and lack of familial support, "women are occupying long-stay hospital beds for long periods before their deaths and this is perhaps the most important single problem in hospital geriatric practice today."

The question of adequacy of institutional facilities is thus highly complex, involving geographic, demographic, socioeconomic, cultural, and ethical values on the part of patients and the public at large as well as differences in medical practice. The British approach to geriatrics, with its heavy emphasis on rehabilitation, supportive social services, and the frugal management of both patients and facilities—what has been called a "social engineering" approach—has clearly paid off in terms of economical use of resources. Although differences in terminology prohibit precise comparisons between the United Kingdom and the United States, it is obvious that with less than one geriatric bed for every 100 elderly persons, and no "nursing homes" in the American sense of the term, they are making do with significantly fewer expensive inpatient facilities than we. [In 1973-1974, there were 5.5 nursing home beds per 100 persons 65 and over in the United States, see Table VII.]

Nevertheless, there would appear to be limits to which this approach can be pushed. In the words of one authority, "Although 95.5 percent of old people live at home, mostly by family help, the remaining 4.5 percent is putting serious pressure on the health and welfare services. Even an additional one percent would have a catastrophic effect."

CONCLUSION

Further improvements in the British geriatric services are certainly possible and, no doubt, will be undertaken, particularly with respect to the coordination of health and social services. But it is important to realize that there is no perfect solution to the manifold problems of health care delivery and financing in any country. What is involved, both in the question of optimum coordination and optimum provision of facilities, is no less than the patient's life style.

While health problems become increasingly dominant as we grow older and finally become the complete arbiter of ability to function, there is no way—even in a highly compassionate "cradle to grave" welfare society—that perfect coordination of all services related to health can be achieved without total abandonment of individual autonomy. In the end, some degree of overlap and noncoordination (otherwise known as pluralism) is the inevitable price that must be paid for democracy and individual freedom. The degree that any given society can and will tolerate varies in accordance with its population needs (age distribution plays an important role), resources, and historical traditions.

Clearly the British have made tremendous efforts to maximize efficiency in a high demand, comparatively low resource context. But there are limits to which professional dedication and patient manipulation can be pushed. With a 93 percent overall occupancy for geriatric beds and none at all available in some hospitals and many old people's homes, with the ever-rising number of elderly women without family support, and with the darkened financial picture, which will make it difficult even to keep up with the present bed/population ratios, it appears that some new policy directions—directed primarily at the reduction of demand on health services and personnel, by means other than the reimposition of financial barriers—may have to be explored. Among the first that come to mind:

1. more emphasis on prevention;
2. more emphasis on residential homes, sheltered housing, and other forms of congregate living, especially for single women;
3. increasing the retirement age for women from 60 to 65;
4. renewed emphasis on productive employment for both men and women, 65 to 70; and
5. employment of teenagers to provide certain social services to the elderly.

A few words about each of these is in order.

1. Much of the disease associated with current geriatric medicine can be traced to earlier years of poor nutrition, smoking, abuse of alcohol, and similar behavioral and social problems, as well as continuing environmental hazards. This fact is increasingly recognized by leading geriatricians, three of whom have declared that "the health and happiness of our aging citizens is largely dependent on the standards of preventive medical practice."

Dr. Thomas McKeown, University of Birmingham, has stated even more categorically:

> In developed countries, prevention of smoking, in particular, is the most powerful measure available, or likely to become available, for the protection of health. In terms of his expectation of life, a mature smoker would probably do better by giving up cigarettes and giving up doctors than by retaining both.

Dr. Green has called for the development of research and education in "preventive geriatrics" to investigate such questions as:

- the possible reduction of cardiovascular and bone diseases in postmenopausal women through estrogen therapy;
- lack of exercise as a factor in osteoporosis and heart disease;
- lack of calcium and vitamin D in osteoporosis and osteomalacia;
- effect of sensible diet and exercise on the aging process.

In general, he urges a combined geriatric-gerontological approach.

Despite such strong opinions on the part of leading physicians, preventive health services are as widely neglected in Britain as they are in most Western countries. The difficulties involved in changing individual habits and life styles are profound and, even if successful, many of the results would be evident only in the long run. However, some much more determined efforts will probably have to be made for the sake of the affected individuals and the health economy as a whole.

2. The shortfall in less expensive residential places and sheltered housing is even more acute than for inpatient beds, despite the rapid increase in both. The challenge to local governments, which have primary responsibility in these areas, is great and probably cannot be met in many areas without substantial assistance from the national government.

3. With a female retirement age of 60 and a life expectancy, at that point, of nearly 20 years, there were, in 1973, 6.4 million women of pensionable age. Only 12 percent were still economically active. The possibility of returning to productive work a substantial portion of the 1.7 million, 60 to 64, should be appealing in terms of both personal and national incomes and probably reduced demand on the geriatric services. But the opportunity must be limited in a society with over a million younger unemployed.

4. To some extent a similar argument could be made for both men and women, 65 to 70. However, the onset of illness and disability progresses more rapidly after 65, and optional retirement at 65 is probably essential at the present time. Far more attention could be given, however, to the provision of "phased retirement" and part-time or unpaid employment. If even a small portion of the personal social services for the over-75s could be provided by the over-65s there would be important advantages to all concerned: those rendering the service, those receiving the service, and the taxpayer.

5. Much the same argument could be made for the use of young people on a part-time basis—voluntary but with some strong incentives—to relieve the pressure on geriatric facilities and personnel. For example, school-age youngsters could work Saturdays or two afternoons a week as "home helps," delivering meals, providing transport, companionship, and performing numerous useful services to older people living at home, possibly also to those living in old people's homes....

NOTES

1. Official statistics are sometimes confined to England and Wales, sometimes to Great Britain (England, Wales, and Scotland), sometimes applied to the United Kingdom (Great Britain and Northern Ireland). Wherever available, data used in this selection are for the United Kingdom. The slight differences do not affect the broad trends and issues discussed here.

2. The term "nursing home" is applied, in Britain, to a group (185 in mid-1975) of independent (non-NHS) small hospitals that specialize in nonemergency surgery. With the projected phasing out of the remaining NHS pay-beds (DHSS Consultative Paper, Aug. 11, 1975), this group is planning to expand, partly with American and other foreign capital—a development that has aroused great controversy.

3. M. Roth, M.D., "The Implications of Present Practices in Geriatrics" in G. McLachlan, ed., *Patient, Doctor, Society* (Oxford: Oxford University Press, 1972), p. 120. Beeson's essay is in the same volume.

4. Sir George Godber, *Change in Medicine* (London: Nuffield Provincial Hospitals Trust, 1975), pp. 88-90 and *passim*.

Selection 51

Recharting National Health Priorities: A Canadian Perspective*

Everywhere the rising cost of health services continues, year by year, to outpace the growth of national economies. Should this trend continue, several countries would soon be spending a prohibitive 25 percent of their GNP on health. The problem would solve itself only if there were some limit, not too far removed from current levels, to the demand for health services. No such limit is in sight.

This assessment of the dilemma of health policy facing most of the economically developed nations today is based on a survey of 20 nations, including the United States, the U.S.S.R., and the major European countries made by a senior officer of the well-known management consulting firm, McKinsey & Co. In the effort to cope with this dilemma, the different nations are struggling with various efforts at reorganization, rationalization, and regulation of health services, improvement in financing mechanisms, manpower, power, and greater productivity, etc.

As governments begin to approach the acceptable limits of resources that can be allocated to health care, they are obviously faced with increasingly difficult choices. Basically, there seem to be three apparent possibilities: (1) reinstate traditional financial barriers, (2) impose monetary limits on prices and/or overall expenditures and ration the available services in one way or another, or (3) make a determined effort to reduce the demand through high priority attention to health promotion and health education.

The road that different nations will follow will depend, in good part, on their differing resources, values, and institutions. For a politically responsive democracy, the firm pursuit of any of these three routes, or even a more likely combination thereof, will be difficult. In this juncture, we in the United States, faced with one of the most complex sets of health care problems in the world, should welcome eagerly any tentative explorations bearing on the basic problems of redefining health priorities. In this respect we are particularly indebted to two leaders of the Canadian health "Establishment," Dr. John Evans, President, University of Toronto, and Marc Lalonde, Minister of National Health and Welfare.

Speaking to the Institute of Medicine, May 9, 1974, Evans identified four phases or "areas of emphasis" marking the "stages of evolution in health policy in Canada during the past two decades." Phase I, starting at the end of World

---

*Excerpt from A.R. Somers, Editorial, *New England Journal of Medicine* 291 (August 22, 1974): 415-416.

War II, concentrated on elimination of financial barriers. Phase II concentrated on development of health manpower. Phase III emphasized the organization and rationalization of health services. According to Dr. Evans,

> The most recent area of emphasis is on studies of the effect on health of external and environmental factors, personal habits and mode of living. It has become increasingly apparent that death and disability from trauma, lung cancer and coronary artery diseases will not be significantly lessened without fundamental changes in the attitude, behavior, and way of life of most members of society....

To illustrate the meaning of Phase IV, Dr. Evans held up a copy of a 1974 book by Lalonde, *A New Perspective on the Health of Canadians*. In this small volume, subtitled "A Working Document," Lalonde documents the need for "a new perspective" less in terms of cost than health status. He points out, for example:

1. Environmental factors and self-imposed risks are the principal or important contributing influences in the great majority of infant deaths and deaths at all ages up to 70.
2. Male mortality is particularly significant. In 1971, twice as many men as women died between the ages of 15 and 70.
3. Diseases of the cardiovascular system, injuries due to accidents, respiratory diseases, and mental illness are, in that order, the principal causes of hospitalization, accounting for some 45 percent of all hospital days. The role of the environment and self-imposed risks is evident.

The Minister's conclusion:

> The Government of Canada now intends to give to human biology [basic biomedical research], the environment, and lifestyle as much attention as it has to the financing of the health care organization [personal health services], so all four avenues to improved health are pursued with equal vigour.

As one who has advanced similar views for several years, I am delighted to find myself in the company of the chief health officer of Canada. However, the problems of implementing a "health promotion" as opposed to a "health care" strategy are so formidable, in our type of society, that many who may accept the Lalonde thesis philosophically may feel it is simply not worth the effort. As an antidote to unrealistic expectations as well as a basis for realistic action, it may be helpful to identify a few of the obstacles:

> 1. In a context of increasing financial constraints on the health field generally, it is extremely difficult to start any new program, no matter how modest in cost or how much it may theoretically be expected to contribute to greater cost-effectiveness for the field as a whole. This is true both at the na-

tional and community levels, the public and private sectors. Behind this is the knowledge that, "when push comes to shove," the forces supporting health care—including consumers as well as providers—can mobilize much more effectively than those supporting health promotion or health education.

2. The lack of agreement, in the scientific community as well as among health professionals, on the role of various risk factors in disease is notorious. Equally important is the widespread skepticism as to the possibility of significant modification of life style in our highly individualistic democratic society where so many value-producing forces, including television advertising, are lined up on the other side.

3. Even if effective behavior modification techniques could be developed and the opposition of all the vested interests overcome, some believe that the results would be worse than the current situation. Just as many decent citizens oppose the banning of pornography as a possible step toward general curtailment of free speech, so some who deplore the excesses of current life style fear that any serious effort at modification might lead to some sort of neo-Puritanism, thought control, or similar dangers.

None of these objections is frivolous. A great deal of money could be wasted on health promotion and health education in the absence of any demonstrably effective techniques. If effective techniques are developed, they could be seriously misused. There is no question that, if the programs are effective, some jobs—in the dairy, tobacco, and sugar industries, for example—could be affected.

But, as in so many areas of social policy, doing nothing is not the same as remaining neutral. We are now wasting a great deal of money on health care programs of dubious or marginal utility. Publicly-franchised airwaves are now being used to influence the behavior of millions of Americans, including impressionable children, in the direction of risk-taking and health-threatening behavior.

It is now clear that we no longer have the option of unlimited spending for personal health services. The choice now lies between increasingly stringent and probably arbitrary limits on supply, strenuous efforts to reduce demand, or a mixture of these interrelated factors. Since I do not believe that the American people will accept the reimposition of financial barriers as a legitimate way of controlling demand, this leaves the alternative of education and health maintenance. Fortunately, this is also the sensible course from the point of view of individual health.

Part IV

A Proposed Framework for Health and Health Care Policies

Part IV

A Proposed Framework for Health and Health Care Policies*

> Health cannot simply be given to the people; it demands their participation.
>
> René Sand, M.D. (1935)

During the mid-1970s, there was more talk about the need for a "national health policy" than in any preceding period—although the meaning of that term was not clearly defined. This was, of course, a sign of growing discontent with existing health policies and costs. The heightened concern was reflected in passage of the National Health Planning and Resources Development Act (P.L. 93-641), which in turn generated more interest. Among other provisions, it called upon the Secretary of Health, Education, and Welfare to develop a set of "guidelines concerning national health planning policy." But demands for reformulation of health policies were moving beyond the requirements of this law.

Two major 1976 conferences were devoted to this topic. The National Health Forum, conducted by the National Health Council, evidenced troubled skepticism about past policies and the directions in which we are moving.[1] The National Leadership Conference on America's Health Policy sponsored by two leading spokesmen on health issues in the House of Representatives—Paul Rogers, Chairman, Subcommittee on Health and Environment, Committee on Interstate and Foreign Commerce; and Dan Rostenkowski, Chairman, Health Subcommittee, Committee on Ways and Means—also severely questioned the efficacy of current activities and emphases.[2]

Former Congressman James Hastings, a major author of P.L. 93-641, set the tone of the latter conference by declaring in his keynote remarks that the nation appears to hold an implicit belief that more medical care means better health and that this

> socially acceptable attitude towards the consumption of medical services... is fueling the uncontrollable growth of our national health ex-

---

*Adapted from A.R. and H.M. Somers, "A Proposed Framework for Health and Health Care Policies," *Inquiry* XIV (June 1977): 115-170.

penditure at a rate that politically or economically cannot be sustained. It is these tenets that must be challenged before any commitment to a national program of health services financing paralyzes the force for constructive change.

Both gatherings produced widely divergent views as to what policies are desirable and possible. But agreement appeared to be emerging that the policies and politics of health care since World War II, with their almost exclusive concentration on enlarging "access to personal health services" were no longer adequate or appropriate. The various national health insurance proposals piling up in Congress appear to confirm this trend. While all are directed at broadening access, most also reveal a substantial concern with altering the delivery system, cost containment, or both.

This is not due to any illusion that the access problem has been solved, although there has been significant improvement, or that what remains to be done in this regard is not essential. On the contrary, there is probably increased sensitivity to the fact that millions of Americans still do not have satisfactory access, lacking either public or private health insurance, and many do not qualify even for welfare medicine—Medicaid—which is increasingly conceded to be unsatisfactory even for those who are eligible. This serious inequity can only be corrected through universal national health insurance.

However, the goal of universal access is now threatened by a variety of dissatisfactions and fears. Most of these derive from the painfully spectacular rise in health care prices and costs. Too much blame is generally assigned to the Medicare and Medicaid programs. Table XIV shows that the relative differential between increases in medical care prices and general prices was significantly greater in the years before Medicare than since.

For example, from 1960 to 1965, medical prices rose 108 percent more rapidly than all prices minus medical care. Between 1965 and 1970, the differential was 49 percent. Similarly, the price of medical services rose 72 percent faster than all services minus medical services, in the earlier period, but only 35 percent faster in the latter period. Obviously much of the difficulty is deeply rooted in the health care system. Nevertheless, there is little doubt that the government programs, by their sheer volume, magnified and exacerbated old practices and payment methods, and contributed to the problems.

More than anything else, it was the cost issue that led to the obvious questions: What are we getting for our $140 billion expenditure? How effectively is the money being spent? Do the annual 10 to 14 percent additional investments in health services pay off in commensurate improvements in health status? Have we passed the point of diminishing returns? Are the anomalies and waste in the organization and financing of health care delivery counteracting the gains from the additional expenditures? Are our priorities askew? There are obviously no ready answers; but neither are we completely in the dark.

HEALTH STATUS: COMPLEX CAUSES

In contrast to the disappointing decade of the 1960s, there has been real and gratifying improvement in national health status, 1970-1975, as measured by standard indices of death rates and life expectancy. The nation's crude death rate fell 6.3 percent, from 9.5 to 8.9 per 1,000 population (Table 1). The age-adjusted rate did even better, dropping from 7.1 per 1,000 to 6.4, almost 10 percent. Life expectancy increased from 70.9 to 72.4 years.

Unfortunately, neither these indices, nor any other available data, provide firm answers to the above questions. First, when examined in historical perspective, the 1970-1975 eperience is not as impressive as when viewed only in comparison with the preceding decade. Death rates have been dropping through most of this century. From 1900 to 1930, the crude rate declined about 1 percent a year. During the next 20 years, it fell at a rate of 0.7 percent a year. About 1950 the downward trend ceased and the rate was relatively static for two decades: 9.6 in 1950, 9.5 in 1960, and 9.5 again in 1970.

In that perspective the 1970-1975 drop of a little over 1 percent a year does not appear to represent any particular breakthrough. It is true that as the baseline becomes smaller and the population older, proportionate improvements become more difficult and represent greater achievement. But it must also be remembered that the 1970-1975 decline followed two decades of no progress; and, hence, part of the improvement can be regarded as catch-up. Altogether the average annual drop from 1950-1975 was about 0.3 percent.

The age-adjusted rates are considerably more favorable, but the basic message is similar. From 1900-1930 the average annual decrease was 0.9 percent. During the next 20 years the declines averaged 1.4 percent. But then the rate slowed down by half between 1950 and 1970. In the next five years the rate of decline returned to, and exceeded, the 1930-1950 averages. The average annual decline for the entire period before 1950 is remarkably similar to that from 1950 to 1975—0.85 and 0.80 percent, respectively.

Second, when examined in international perspective, it is clear that the United States does not enjoy the same relative position in terms of life expectancy as it does in terms of health care expenditures. In life expectancy as of the early 1970s, we were seventh from the top for women, 19th for men. In the latter case, particularly, we were surpassed by many countries with relatively modest resources and small per capita incomes. Clearly, neither financial nor scientific resources nor health care expenditures can be major factors in the differences. Inevitably one looks to differences in the environment, life style, and culture.[3]

Third, when one considers the major causes of mortality in the Untied States, it appears that numerous factors were involved in the recent overall improvement. In some cases, for example, heart disease and auto accidents, scientific knowledge, availability of good medical care, and environmental and behavioral influences all apparently combined to produce significant progress. With respect to cancer, on the other hand, scientific and technological progress have been more than cancelled out by increasing environmental and behavioral threats. Similarly with homicide and suicide, progress in emergency care and surgery has been unable to keep up with the growing risk factor of violence as a major health threat. In the case of infant mortality, where there has been impressive improvement, changing birth control policy and practice—an amalgam of technological, socioeconomic, and political considerations—undoubtedly played a major role.

In short, the data indicate that a large variety of socioeconomic, environmental, scientific, and health care delivery factors intermingle in indeterminate proportions to explain mortality rates and, inferentially, health status. It is interesting to note that the average annual improvement in death rates, whether measured in crude or age-adjusted terms, was as good before 1950—when technical medicine and the scientific revolution were far less advanced—as in the following quarter century. However, general standards of living and education were rising substantially, and the data may be primarily a reflection of that phenomenon.[4]

National health policy must include attention to all relevant factors. Any effort to concentrate resources on just one or two of these factors, to the exclusion of the others, can have only limited effect. This admonition applies both to those who maintain that "access to health care" is all that matters and to those who now say that health care is irrelevant. What is needed, now as in the past, is a balance of policies and resources involving all the relevant factors influencing individual and national health. In such a broad perspective, "health care" should be viewed as one essential element within the larger framework of a broad policy of "health promotion." Only in such a context can it achieve its maximum utility.

A NEW FOCUS: HEALTH PROMOTION

Any new design that will prove effective must, we believe, be based on two broad assumptions:

1. Responsibility for personal health rests primarily with the individual; not with government, not with physicians or hospitals, not with any third party financing program. Meaningful national health policies must be directed to increasing, rather than eroding, the individual's sense of responsibility for his own health and his ability to understand and cope with health problems.
2. If the individual's responsibility is to be effectively discharged, it must be supported by social policies designed to provide him with essential environmental protection, health information, and access to health care when needed.

In short, a policy of "individual responsibility" and a policy of "social responsibility" are complementary, not antithetical. Neither can be fully effective without the other. The term that seems best to suggest an approach that encompasses both assumptions is "health promotion." The overriding goal of such a national health policy may be stated as *the creation and maintenance of conditions under which individual Americans are most able and most likely to optimize their own health potential.*

This appears almost self-evident. Others may prefer different wording, but the objective itself can hardly arouse much dispute. Health is not a commodity that one individual can bestow on another. Health cannot be legislated or assured by regulation. In large measure, health has to be earned and maintained by the individual himself. However, it is equally true that the individual's conditions of life will either encourage or discourage his ability and motivation in this respect. These conditions have varied over time and at any given time. They vary from country to country and from community to community. They are, in large degree, the product of social and political choice, i.e., they represent decisions on the part of society.

The major conditions affecting individual and national health may be classified under several broad headings: genetic endowment, the environment, behavioral factors, access to good health services, and the scientific "state of the art" in all categories. For the purpose of this analysis focused on national policies, we omit genetics, except as it may be subsumed in those preventive procedures—screening and counseling—that are included in "personal health services."

For each of the other categories we have formulated a broad statement of objectives (hereafter referred to as "goals") with which we start each of the four following discussions. Although none may be fully attainable, this does not diminish their utility as guides for national policy. Other categorizations and different language are, of course, possible. But here again we believe that the essence of such a set of goals is virtually unassailable. Each of them, with its many problems and difficulties, must be dealt with in a comprehensive and balanced attack upon the overarching goal of maximizing the opportunities for better health for the populace. Health is multifaceted; policies must be developed accordingly.[5]

Our discussion of three of the goals, dealing with the environment, life style, and knowledge development, is brief, intended chiefly to stress their extreme importance to national health and to raise some of the major issues in relation to each. Fuller and more programmatically oriented discussion is reserved for personal health care.

NOTES

1. *A Declaration of Interdependence: Developing America's Health Policy, Proceedings of the 1976 National Health Forum* (New York: National Health Council, 1976).

2. The National Leadership Conference on America's Health Policy, April 1976, *Proceedings* (Washington, D.C.: National Journal, 1976).

3. For an excellent brief summary of the literature on the limited effectiveness of medical care on health status, see D.P. Rice and D. Wilson, "The American Medical Economy—

Problems and Perspectives," in T. Hu, ed., *International Health Costs and Expenditures* (Washington, D.C.: National Institutes of Health, 1976), HEW Publ. (NIH) 76-1067, pp. 41-43.

4. For a detailed historical review of this issue in the British context, see Thomas McKeown, M.D., *The Role of Medicine: Dream, Mirage, or Nemesis?* (London: Nuffield Provincial Hospitals Trust, 1976).

5. For closely related approaches, see Marc Lalonde, *A New Perspective on the Hof Canadians* (Ottawa: Ministry of National Health and Welfare, 1974); also R.J. Knobel and M.G. Holland, eds., *Georgia's New Health Outlook* (Atlanta: Georgia Department of Human Resources, 1976). See also *Daedalus* 106 (Winter 1977), entire issue, for discussions of the need for new health directions and policies.

Chapter Twelve

Knowledge Development

Goal 1: Development of basic and applied knowledge aimed at increasing our technical and economic capacities to attain the goals related to the environment (Goal 2), individual behavior (Goal 3), and health services (Goal 4), as well as in the biomedical sciences.

> Can there really be anyone left who still believes that science is separable from its political context? Such a suggestion, more in keeping with the gee whizzery of 15 years ago, could set science-policy thinking back at least as far.
>
> *New Scientist,* January 22, 1976

> How should priorities be set in a national biomedical and behavioral research program? Some say that there is no place for political concerns in setting research priorities.... In my opinion "politics" has an important and necessary function in the setting of priorities. The decision to have publicly supported activities demands political consideration. When programs are authorized, a priority has been set; when funds are appropriated another declaration of priority is made. Both of these occur in the context of our political system.
>
> Theodore Cooper, M.D. (1976)

There are, obviously, a host of impediments to substantial progress in respect to Goals 2, 3, and 4. Perhaps least appreciated is the paucity and uncertainty of essential knowledge of human health and the factors that enter into its protection. So impressed have we been with the "scientific and technological revolutions in medicine" that we often forget how new much of it is, how relatively restricted the discoveries compared to the needs, and how untested or unsure are many of the technologies we employ, even much of the underlying science.

The sparseness of knowledge relates to all the areas with which we are concerned—the biomedical science basis of personal health care as well as environmental and behavioral factors and methods of delivery. One of the nation's most distinguished physician-scientist-educators, Dr. Lewis Thomas, has recently warned of the

> misapprehension... that medicine has already developed into a full-fledged science. ... Instead, medicine is still the most immature and undeveloped, and, on balance, most unaccomplished of all the sciences.... We use the hybrid term "biomedical" science as shorthand to describe the whole inquiry that underlies modern

medicine.... There really isn't enough medical science yet to enable the term to stand alone....[1]

Other scientists and physicians may feel this is too harsh a criticism of the existing "state of the art," although most good physicians tend to agree that medicine is still more an "art" than a "science." But there are few, indeed, who would claim that existing knowledge respecting the causes and cures of cancer, heart disease, arthritis, diabetes, schizophrenia, and many other diseases is adequate. On the contrary, it is generally agreed that real progress in the capacity to deal with such diseases successfully—both treatment and prevention—depends largely upon advances in basic science.

We have also become increasingly aware that a great deal more epidemiological and/or clinical research is needed to test the efficacy of many commonly practiced medical and surgical procedures, which have been accepted largely on faith. Dr. A.L. Cochrane's now famous book, *Effectiveness and Efficiency*,[2] was one of the earliest to report that randomized clinical trials demonstrated that many widely accepted procedures produced generally negative results. The view is growing, even among physicians, that a great deal of current medical care is ineffective.[3] Much more clinical testing and measurement of "outcomes" will be essential before we can speak with confidence about "quality assurance" and the effectiveness of various devices for peer review. This too is an essential aspect of health-related research.

ENVIRONMENTAL, BEHAVIORAL, AND HEALTH SERVICES RESEARCH

The shortcomings in knowledge of human biology and medical practice are matched or exceeded by our ignorance of environmental and behavioral influences on health and factors relating to health services delivery. Starting in the 1950s, the federal government began to invest generously in the biomedical sciences, primarily through the National Institutes of Health. By 1975 such investment had increased to $2.9 billion (Table XII). Federal support has also increased for environmental, behavioral, and health services research. But such funds, especially in the field of behavior or life style, are still meager compared with those going to the biomedical sciences. A National Planning Association analysis of federally funded health-related research in 1976 resulted in the following breakdown:[4]

	Dollars (in millions)	Percent Distribution
Human biology	$1,044	38
Life style	105	4
Environment	844	30
Health services	786	28
Total	$2,779	100

In the case of the environment, serious concerns about the purity of water supplies, food, and milk, and research into the causes and control of contagious diseases go back over 100 years. However, the very success of the early public health and sanitation movements produced the illusion that environmental problems had been solved. Professional interest in, and public support for, such activities declined dramatically during the 1950s and 1960s with their overriding emphasis on biomedical research and personal health care. The new interest in the environment as a threat to health and even survival belatedly brought research funds to the Environmental Protection Agency, the Energy Research and Development Administration, National Aeronautical and Space Administration, the National Institute of Environmental Health Sciences, and the National Institute of Occupational Safety and Health, as well as a few older federal health agencies including the National Cancer Institute and the Center for Disease Control. However, investment in these areas is probably still inadequate in relation to the obvious needs.

We have, of course, developed a great many plausible theories and some definite knowledge about environmental and life style influences and the efficacy of health services, based on persuasive statistical and episodic evidence. These should be acted on even while we await positive scientific proof. But such "prudent" interventions are no substitute for the substantiating evidence we must seek.

Until we find out how to design and manage constructive interventions in the social and environmental factors influencing health, and how to inform, teach, and motivate people to take responsibility for their health, our expenditures for health care will probably continue to accelerate with declining effect on our health indices. The need for knowledge in these areas is no less urgent than in human biology.

MAJOR ISSUES IN RESEARCH POLICY

It is not difficult to achieve general agreement that we need to know more about matters we have been exploring intensively for a long time as well as about questions that have been relatively neglected. But this does not advance us very far, because the issues that remain after such basic agreement are complex and divisive, because we do not yet have adequate criteria for evaluating the relative effectiveness of what we are now doing, and because we do not know how best to translate convictions into public policy action—matters that themselves are in need of serious inquiry.

Following are some of the major issues in health research policy confronting the nation in the late 1970s.

How much of our national resources is it wise and productive to allocate to health and health care? This is a question that will elude scientific answer for the foreseeable future. Perhaps, in a free society, it can never be precisely answered. But it is important for all concerned to realize that the question is now being seriously raised in many quarters. The days of cornucopia in health expenditures appear to have passed, and the public mood is increasingly skeptical.

Even if it proves impossible, perhaps even undesirable, to come up with fixed percentages of gross national product (or other indices) that should be allocated to health, the very exercise of thinking in terms of relative contributions of full employment, education, housing, law enforcement, international relations, and other areas of national policy, as well as the four priorities identified as essential aspects of a rounded policy of health promotion, should be helpful to decision makers both in government and in the health professions. Research methodologies in this complex area will have to be as sophisticated as the issues are difficult and will inevitably involve many disciplines, including political science, economics, sociology, ethics, and law as well as those conventionally identified with health policy.

How much of the health allocation should be assigned to research? Is the current level of federal expenditure enough? According to HEW, the federal government already finances nearly 90 percent of the total health-related research effort. Private investment—most of this by drug companies—is obviously very limited. Is this a reasonable division of responsibility?

It is common to express some judgment on these questions by pointing out that research represents only a little over 2 percent of total health expenditures. But neither percentages nor gross amounts are instructive without answers about relative productivity of such expenditures. It does not automatically follow that more expenditures would bring bigger or better results. Some critics allege that available funds already exceed the qualified talent, resulting in a "trivialization" of research efforts. Some careful historical analyses of correlations, if any, between rising research expenditures and changing health status in this and other countries would be helpful.

Within whatever total is to be expended for health-related research, what is the most appropriate division among the four priority areas—environmental, behavioral, personal health care, and biomedical? Are present proportions satisfactory in relation to national needs? Should there be some transfer of resources from the biomedical field to the other three? Should the present biomedical investment be left relatively intact while substantially increasing the others?

Within each of the four areas, what should be the division between basic and applied research? According to the director of NIH, about 40 percent of its funds are spent for basic research on underlying mechanisms of disease, about 40 to 50 percent on clinical and evaluative programs, and the rest on technology and development.[5] Is this a reasonable division? If not, what would be?

The question of division of resources between basic and applied research—despite the large areas of ambiguity between the two—is as pertinent to the behavioral and environmental sciences as it is to the biomedical field, perhaps more so. The potential frontiers for primary investigations seem boundless and indefinable. It is not usually possible to foretell which explorations will prove fruitful, in what degree, and which will yield no return. But, in a world of limited resources, choices must be made.

PAYOFFS AND TRADEOFFS

In respect to all such questions, how are we to measure and evaluate payoffs? Within what time frame and by what criteria? A few examples indicate the difficulties.

1. The activities of the Occupational Safety and Health Administration (OSHA) have been criticized as lacking in cost-effectiveness. How are we to measure the relative value of one worker's life saved from occupational cancer versus higher product costs for millions of consumers?
2. The surprisingly low rate of compliance with therapeutic regimens among patients with hypertension and other chronic diseases—averaging only 50 percent for long term medications—has been carefully documented.[6] Is it worth the effort, in lives saved or lengthened, to add a major health education component to the usual treatment for these diseases?
3. Many of the newer developments in health care—Professional Standards Review Organizations (PSROs) and Health Maintenance Organizations (HMOs), for example—are intended to improve the quality of such care and to help control costs in the long run. But they may also increase costs in the short run. Is the payoff likely to be worth the extra investment?
4. Many scientists feel that the best hope for eventual conquest of cancer lies in the pursuit of basic biochemical knowledge with respect to mechanisms of cell control and the transmission of genetic information. Assuming they are correct, how do we measure the relative value of investment in such long range studies versus the need for immediate investment in controls with respect to known industrial and environmental carcinogens?

Many scientists, as well as practitioners in the various fields, resent such questions, feeling that attempts to appraise the value of their work on the basis of measurable results run counter to the spirit of science and could eventually congeal the inquiring energy, which is a fundamental source of progress—unpredictable as particular ventures may be and as erratic as the course of progress may be. There is, in the biomedical research community, a continuing faith in the inevitability of progress if we only continue along present directions. In the words of the prestigious President's Biomedical Research Panel:

> Biomedical science is more advanced, we have better tools with which to work than ever before, and the payoff is inevitable if we have the patience and perseverance to continue to build on the science base that exists today.[7]

But the public mood is no longer as uncritical as it once was. Even the Congress, which has frequently appropriated more to NIH than presidents have called for, has begun to ask questions respecting "payoffs" and "technology transfers" between the findings of basic research, medical care, and the national health. The Biomedical Research Panel was itself the product of such questioning on the part of the Senate Subcommittee on Health.

The panel's report was not particularly helpful on this issue. It not only reaffirmed uncritically the existing federal commitment to biomedical research but also urged NIH to hold fast to its "primary role," i.e., "conducting and supporting laboratory and clinical research attuned to the search for new knowledge." Distinctly in second place, it added, "and given adequate resources, of conducting and supporting clinical trials, selected demonstrations, and selected educational programs."

The panel was deeply concerned with two developments that it considered threats to the biomedical research effort:

1. growing competition for resources between the research mission of the NIH and the application and dissemination of knowledge, and
2. increasing and frequently changing public demands for allocation of resources according to public perceptions of important health goals, rather than on the basis of scientific opportunities. In response to these factors, there is public pressure for the Congress to play a strong role in setting program direction, emphasis, and budget levels.

During the Senate hearings, following publication of the panel report, some witnesses were strongly supportive, some critical. Among the latter, Dr. Lester Breslow, Dean of the School of Public Health, University of California at Los Angeles, attacked the report for (1) "the notion, common in the biomedical research community which the panel reflects, that essentially the only means of understanding how to prevent and otherwise control disease and to maintain health is through laboratory and clinical research," and (2) the "idea that the biomedical research community should ... bear no responsibility for the development of means for applying that knowledge and technology" and that "knowledge application and dissemination activities and clinical trials should be staffed and funded by resources dedicated solely to these purposes and should not compete with research budgets."[8] Dr. Breslow also criticized the panel's assumption that appropriate applications follow almost automatically the discovery of knowledge.

WHO SPEAKS FOR "THE PUBLIC"?

There is no intent here to claim that those interested in public health and epidemiology are any more public-spirited than the biomedical research community. It is not only understandable, but probably good, that each profession feels its work and its contribution are the most important. The point is that failure to accept the fact that public dollars carry with them an obligation to listen to public concerns, even if these are sometimes short-sighted or amateurish, can lead to further divergence between the public and scientific views, as well as divisions within the health field itself, with more extreme positions developing on each side, and eventual danger to the entire field.

A significant example of such differing views has arisen out of the research on recombinant DNA. In July 1976 the City Council of Cambridge, Massachusetts, requested Harvard University to halt temporarily construction of a new $500,000 laboratory for specialized genetic research. This unprecedented action grew out of the council's fears, based partly on the opinion of other scientists, that "the biologists who propose to tamper with the genetic apparatus of microorganisms, would create an Andromeda-like strain that might escape their control and spread an incurable disease to the population."[9] The Biomedical Research Panel sees the problem very differently:

> Genetic manipulations are undoubtedly the most exciting developments in this field [genetic chemistry]. By using the enzymic equipment of bacterial cells... genes from a wide variety of sources can be isolated and inserted into a heterologonous bacterial chromosome. When this chromosome is reproduced in a prokaryotic host, the foreign genes are replicated. Vast vistas are opened by these discoveries, since in principle this type of genetic manipulation could permit... the mass production of proteins (and other molecules) of medical and economic interest. If successful, this operation will open the door for minimum-risk substitution therapy with human enzymes, hormones, and antibodies produced in bacteria.[10]

The risks of scientific and technological progress have been present since the days of Prometheus. Fire, electricity, atomic energy, and genetic manipulation are all two-edged swords. Those who dare to penetrate these mysteries have repeatedly been accused of inviting the fate of the "Sorcerer's Apprentice." Thus, it is perhaps understandable that the recombinant DNA episode, although characterized by division within the scientific community, brought outcries that science was again threatened by constraints like those of "a new medieval church" and insistence that the "checks and balances" within the scientific community itself are sufficient.[11]

But science has become too important, too ubiquitous, in its effects, for such a position to be tenable in an open society. Activities of such far-reaching social consequences should not be left exclusively to professional scientists. Within the context of their training and discipline they tend to be dedicated to "knowledge for knowledge's sake." While this approach frequently does result in furthering the public interest, such is not always true. Even if true for the long run, the public's view of short run priorities cannot be ignored with impunity. Judgment on allocation of public resources in research, as in defense, involves not only expert specialized knowledge but also social values and differing levels of urgency and priority.

The scientist often sees the problem merely as a failure in communication: "The public must be made to understand." There is now a school of thought that maintains that "science questions" are too complex and too difficult to leave to Congress or public representatives to decide; that such issues should be referred to special "science courts" comprised of those who "really understand" the technical issues, i.e., other scientists.

Although there is much truth in the allegation that the average congressman cannot keep up with all the technical information he is asked to pass on today, the opposite view that public interest will be better served by turning such decisions over to those who have a professional, and perhaps even a financial, stake in the outcome is even less appealing. The constitutional view that war is too important to leave to the generals applies equally in the science field.

Decisions have to be based on a combination of scientific, ethical, political, and economic factors. The scientists have a monopoly on only one of these areas. Unless the long view of the scientist and the pragmatic needs felt by the public are put into balance and reconciled, we face not only a public perception of misdirected application of resources, but also the danger of a break in public tolerance of research, which could bring long term disaster.[12]

Probably the most promising way to avoid such a retrograde rebellion of public sentiment against basic science—in addition to more active public involvement in decision making—is by scientists collectively taking and demonstrating a holistic view of research and scientific purpose. Scientists must be concerned with the effectiveness of the linkages that tie the total enterprise together—from pure science, to clinical trials, to routine medical care, to improved national health status. Public appreciation of the continuum will depend in large measure on the scientific community itself evidencing its concern with the ultimate utilization and effects of the enterprise, irrespective of the particular segment on which the individual scientist specializes.

RESEARCH ON RESEARCH

Finally, it is essential to raise some questions with respect to the research enterprise itself, to undertake some "research on research." Elsewhere, we have examined the effect of federal research programs on medical schools and concluded that the results were not all positive (Selection 2). Here we question whether present federal procedures are most appropriate to the goals here stated and to the vitality of the research agencies themselves.

The National Institutes of Health, the National Institute of Mental Health, and the National Center for Health Services Research, as well as other research arms of the government, are accustomed to contracting out major portions, if not the bulk, of their research work. Considering that much of the country's research talents lie in our universities and research institutes, most of this is inescapable. But the process, as now pursued, has difficulties that bring it into conflict with the objectives enunciated above, and the process needs reexamination.

There is reason to believe that, in some instances, contracting out has had stultifying effects. Too often the responsible agency tends to become a mere conduit of monies, because it is several steps removed from the research itself. The agency administers the contract or the grant; it helps review applications, selects the contractor or grantee, decides on the amount of money to be spent, and checks that the funds are honestly used. No sweat or tears of the agency staff go into the study. There is a lack of emotional drive to get something done as a result of the study. The results of the research can be neglected or forgotten without any sense of loss or pain at the agency level.

If inhouse research becomes too small or insignificant, the agency may eventually lose its capacity to judge the quality of research. It can lose a sense of professional identity with the outside work. It can meet its formal obligations by simply recording that the grant was made in accordance with established procedures, expenditures were properly monitored, the product was (or was not) delivered, and, hopefully, it was published.[13]

Most academic investigators, to whom a large share of such contracts go, are not action-oriented or program-focused. They are interested in development of research methodologies, prestigious publication of research findings, and, not least, continued funding of their own research. They do not have much stake in the implementation of their findings.

Moreover, it is in reality the academic community that also makes most of the decisions on what research will be funded. Decisions are turned over to "peer" review committees composed mainly of academic consultants from outside the agency. Their loyalties and research interests are not necessarily the same as those of the agency, nor is their outlook primarily related to public policy.

It is a system which discourages, or at least obscures, accountability. It is also one in which purpose itself becomes shadowy. Hundreds of projects that have poured out of the machinery have never been integrated, compared, summarized or distilled to be useful as policy instruments to decision-making administrators, Congress, or even private influentials. A revised view of the social objectives of research will also demand new administrative procedures.

NOTES

1. *Conference on Future Directions in Health Care: The Dimensions of Medicine,* December 10-11, 1975, New York City, sponsored by Blue Cross Association, The Rockefeller Foundation. University of California Health Policy Program, pp. 94-95.

2. A.L. Cochrane, *Effectiveness and Efficiency* (London: Nuffield Provincial Hospitals Trust, 1972).

3. For example, Lewis Thomas, M.D., *The Lives of a Cell,* (New York: Bantam Books, 1974), pp. 36-37; Howard Hiatt, M.D., "Protecting the Medical Commons: Who Is Responsible?" *New England Journal of Medicine* 293 (July 31, 1975): 235-41.

4. M.S. Kaleda, C. Burke, and J.S. Williams, *The Federal Health Dollar: 1969-1976* (Washington, D.C.: National Planning Association, 1977), p. 69. The NPA definition of "environmental research" includes some programs conventionally assigned to other categories (p. 65).

5. Donald S. Frederickson, M.D., in *Conference on Future Directions, op. cit.,* p. 121.

6. D.L. Sackett, M.D. and R.B. Haynes, M.D., *Compliance with Therapeutic Regimens* (Baltimore: Johns Hopkins University Press, 1976).

7. Department of Health, Education, and Welfare, *Report of the President's Biomedical Research Panel,* Submitted to the President and the Congress of the U.S., April 30, 1976 (Washington, D.C.: U.S. Government Printing Office, 1976), p. 5.

8. Lester Breslow, M.D., "Testimony for U.S. Senate Subcommittee on Health on Basic Issues in Biomedical Research," June 17, 1976, (processed), p. 3.

9. Liebe F. Cavalieri, "New Strains of Life—or Death," *New York Times Magazine,* August 22, 1976, p. 8.

10. *Report of the President's Biomedical Research Panel, op. cit.,* Appendix A., pp. 25-26.

11. "Panel Expresses Fear of Curbs on Science's Freedom of Inquiry" (Report of meeting of American Association for Advancement of Science), *New York Times,* February 23, 1977.

12. At the instigation of Senators Jacob Javits and Edward Kennedy, who expressed concern about "a growing strain in the relationship between biomedical research and the general public" (Letter to Willard Gaylin, M.D., president, Institute of Society, Ethics, and the Life Sciences, Oct. 19, 1975), a conference was jointly sponsored by Case Western Reserve University Medical School and the Institute of Society, Ethics, and Life Sciences in April 1976 to enquire into the sources of tension and their bearing on future public policy. The Senators had written "... the public, which provides a considerable portion of all biomedical research funds, has an important role to play in allocation of these funds and in the formation of judgments on the potential benefits of research."

13. The Comptroller General of the United States, in a critical 1976 report, accused NIH of inadequate stewardship of both extramural and intramural research projects and recommended several important procedural reforms. *Better Controls Needed over Biomedical Research Supported by the National Institutes of Health,* Report to the Congress, July 1976.

Chapter Thirteen

The Environment

Goal 2: Protection of the natural environment essential to life and health and promotion of occupational, socioeconomic, and moral environments conducive to optimum physical and mental well-being.

> It isn't the pox that menaces us anymore, or the plague. It's strange new creatures of our own making, and they are all around us—in the air, our water and food, and in the things we touch.
> Russell Train (1976)

> We need a new philosophy of health—nothing less. It must be seen in the context of the totality of the person, in the context of a larger societal whole and the interactions between the person and the environment. Thus if a better basic income or better environment will produce a healthier individual or family, they should be part of the health strategy.
> Walter J. McNerney (1975)

THE NATURAL ENVIRONMENT

Man's obvious and fundamental dependence on the natural environment has been increasingly obscured during the past two centuries as progress in science and technology produced the illusion of mastery over nature. Industrialization, urbanization, the harnessing of nuclear as well as fossil fuel energy, improvements in transportation, communications, and climate control—all involving modification of the physical environment—have enabled us to support far larger populations at a far higher standard of living than could have been possible in the "natural" state. Pesticides and chemical treatment of water and land have been effectively used to increase food supply and to control disease. Biological vaccines have enabled us to immunize most Americans against most of the major infectious diseases.

In the celebration of such achievements, we have often lost sight of their price. Voices warning against the threats to life and health implicit in exponential population growth, too rapid consumption of irreplaceable resources, pollution of air and water by carcinogens and other toxic substances, violation of basic ecosystems, and similar transgressions against the natural environment have been raised with increasing intensity during recent decades. Natural scientists, social scientists, and statesmen joined in this effort.

With specific reference to disease, the National Institute of Occupational Safety and Health (NIOSH) lists some 12,500 chemicals with some toxic properties in commercial use today.[1] Epidemiological studies have demonstrated a close association between levels of air pollution and death rates from respiratory and heart diseases.[2] As to cancer—the second leading cause of death in the United States, which is expected to strike one in every four—an HEW Task Force reported:

> There is abundant evidence that the great majority of malignant neoplasms—probably over 90 percent—are induced, maintained, or promoted by specific environmental factors.... Carcinogenesis must therefore be regarded as one of the most significant potential consequences of environmental contamination.[3]

In other words, cancer appears to be, in large part, a manmade disease. The challenge is whether man has the wit and the will to protect himself from this new epidemic he has unloosed.

Spurred by such concerns and a growing bipartisan environmental/ecology movement, Congress adopted the National Environmental Protection Act of 1969, the Clean Air Act of 1970, and the Water Pollution Control Act of 1972. The federal Environmental Protection Agency (EPA) was established. A number of states enacted similar or stronger legislation. Antipollution standards were developed, and enforcement deadlines established. Real progress has been achieved, especially in major metropolitan areas. For example, according to the Illinois Environmental Protection Control Board, Chicago experienced a 21 percent drop in total mortality between 1970 and 1975, following enactment of a low sulfur fuel ordinance and a ban on leaf burning. Auto pollution has also decreased. There has been marked improvement in rivers, lakes, and shoreline areas as compared with the late 1960s. Federal support of family planning and the Supreme Court's 1973 abortion decision facilitated voluntary population control.

About 1973 however, the pendulum began to swing the other way. The unresolved energy crisis, the severe recession of 1974-1975, continuing international tensions, and the intense opposition of influential segments of organized labor and industry led to repeal, postponement, or nonenforcement of many pollution and conservation standards. Efforts to strengthen the Clean Air Act, including updated auto emission control standards, were defeated in the 94th Congress. Safety standards for the proliferating nuclear power plants are under severe pressures. The decision to accept the supersonic Concorde, at least temporarily, was made largely for foreign policy considerations. Opposition to abortion has been used to mount an attack on family planning generally.

On the other hand, 1976 saw passage of the long-debated Toxic Substances Control Act, permitting EPA to require testing of all chemicals in present use that might present an unreasonable risk of injury to health or the environment, and of new chemicals entering the environment. It specifically refers to polychlorinated biphenyls (PCBs) which can cause metabolic disorders, birth defects, and even cancer. The law is intended to phase out production of PCBs over the next two and half years.

Progress was also registered with respect to a national program of solid waste disposal. Despite considerable controversy over EPA's role in the regulation of pesticides, Congress extended the Federal Insecticide, Fungicide, and Rodenticide Act (FIFRA), thereby continuing authorization for the EPA pesticide programs.

It is not the purpose of this brief statement to discuss any of the vast range of policy issues subsumed under the heading of "natural environment." On many of the specifics there is wide disagreement among respected scientists, economists, and national leaders. Signs of progress with respect to population, toxic substances, disease control, and food and energy production appear to be about evenly balanced by increasing danger signals.[4]

It is our purpose to emphasize that protection of the natural environment is basic to national health, that national health policy must include this area as a major goal, and that such policy must be effectuated by a commensurate allocation of resources.

THE SOCIOECONOMIC ENVIRONMENT

The relationship between socioeconomic conditions and health has been abundantly documented. For example, a 1975 comparison between the per capita income of 105 nations and their life expectancy and infant mortality rates showed a predictably strong correlation among the three indices.[5] Countries with per capita incomes in the range of $2,000 to $5,600 enjoyed male life expectancy at birth of about 65 to 72 years; those with incomes estimated at $50 to $170 a year reported life expectancies as low as 26 years.

During the past few decades, improved socioeconomic conditions in the United States have played a major role in the generally improved health indices for most Americans. Nevertheless, as of 1973, there remained a discrepancy of 6.3 years in average life expectancy at birth of whites and blacks,[6] while infant mortality for nonwhites was 92 percent higher than for whites.[7] Socioeconomic factors clearly play an important role in this discrepancy.

It has now become clear that deteriorating socioeconomic conditions, especially in overcrowded urban slums, have become a breeding ground for health hazards that threaten the nation as a whole. Large scale unemployment has spawned its predictable share of health hazards. In 1975, Flint, Michigan, with a 20 percent unemployment rate, was reported to have the highest rate of alcoholism in the country.[8] Not only alcoholism and drug abuse, but also child abuse and crimes of violence have increased to alarming levels, almost cancelling out health improvements resulting from scientific advances in the practice of medicine and better access to care.

Corrective action will not come easily. Productive employment for all who are willing and able to work, including inner city youth, slum clearance, sheltered housing for the elderly, day care centers for working mothers, gun controls, more effective criminal justice: these and many other reforms needed to change the current health-threatening socioeconomic environment involve extremely difficult issues and some redistribution of national resources. However, these must now be recognized as health problems—health hazards for which traditional health care is an obviously insufficient answer.

OCCUPATIONAL SAFETY AND HEALTH

Occupational health has to be listed as an environmental problem as it is largely beyond the ability of the individual employee to control. Great progress has been made in the United States over the past half-century in this area. But there are no grounds for complacency. There were, in 1973, an estimated 14,200 work-related deaths and 2.5 million disabling injuries.[9] Worse, the injury rate was substantially higher in the early 1970s than it had been in the early 1960s. The rising incidence of occupational disease is not generally reflected in these figures. Although the precise amount of occupational disease probably never will be known, partly because of the multiple factors involved in the etiology of many conditions, HEW estimates 390,000 new cases each year and as many as 100,000 deaths.[10]

Passage of the Coal Mine Safety and Health Act of 1969 and the Occupational Safety and Health Act of 1970 were related both to pressure from organized labor and the environmental protection movement. Critics of the Occupational Safety and Health Administration (OSHA) contend that it has failed to establish its cost-benefit value. Each new mine disaster brings renewed criticism of the Department of Interior's stewardship of the coal mine program.

There clearly is need for reform in the divided jurisdictions (e.g., OSHA in the Department of Labor, NIOSH in HEW, and coal mine safety in Interior), structure, standard-setting, and enforcement. But this should not be used as an excuse for retreating from the goals of occupational safety and health. These are essential elements in the environmental protection of most American adults.

THE POLITICAL AND MORAL ENVIRONMENT

The relation of the moral tone of a society to individual health is far more important than is usually recognized. If health is a quality that has to be sustained by the individual himself, it follows that, on average, individuals who are motivated to want to live long and take care of their health will probably be the healthiest. This is not an argument for hypochondria or for making health an end in itself; it is an argument for a sense of purpose in life whose achievement can be furthered by means of a healthy body and mind. This purpose may be simply making a living for one's family or raising healthy, happy children. But, whatever it is, there must be a conviction that it is important and realistic enough to justify some self-denial of immediate health-threatening gratifications.

This, in part, anticipates the next goal: individual behavior. Here, we emphasize the role of external moral influences as conditioner of individual behavior and the responsibility of national leadership to help provide the people, especially youth, with a vision of community and individual challenges and goals that can be expected to stimulate a feeling of purpose in their lives.

Often in our national history, Americans have been animated by a sense of being part of a society with high purpose and moral values. In greater or lesser degree this was true in the early challenges of creating and governing a new nation with novel democratic aspirations, in the drive to conquer the wilderness and settle the west, in wars fought (ostensibly at least) for freedom or democracy, and in periodic broad movements for social and economic justice. Lack of such a shared sense of societal values often leads to widespread hedonism, alienation, lack of identification and self-esteem, and a slackness injurious to individual health. Some cynics insist that only war or other major disaster can now bind the nation together in purpose and morale. But other societies and, at times, this country, have demonstrated that this need not be so.

The Peace Corps, Vista, and similar undertakings sponsored by the American Friends Service Committee and other educational and religious groups all point in the right direction. The Rev. Jesse L. Jackson, a prominent civil rights leader, has called for a "self-development" crusade among Black Americans, especially in the inner cities.[11] Numerous commentators on the 1976 presidential primaries noted the growing popular appeal of traditional moral values. There is a crying need for strong national leadership, which could mobilize American youth for peaceful construction and reconstruction both at home and abroad such as, perhaps, some form of "Marshall Plan" for the cities. Such a crusade could help to establish a moral, as well as physical and socioeconomic, climate more conducive to the individual and national self-discipline essential to individual and national health (Selection 43).

One interesting vision of a new social ethic for society has been advanced by Glenn Seaborg, Nobel prize-winning chemist, discoverer of plutonium, and former Chairman of the Atomic Energy Commission. Unlike the many prophets of doom, Seaborg sees the world moving within the next generation toward a "steady-state" society, with the United States in the forefront:

> By the 1990s I suspect we will be a society almost 180 degrees different from what we are today.... I see us in 1994 as a highly disciplined society with behavior self-modified by social and physical conditions

> already being generated today. The permissiveness, violence, self-indulgence, and material extravagance which seem to be some of the earmarks of today will not be characteristic of our 1990 society....
>
> We ... will have a society that on the whole exercises a quiet, nonneurotic self-control, displays a highly cooperative public spirit, has an almost religious attitude toward environmental quality and resource conservation, exercises great care and ingenuity in managing its personal belongings, and shows an extraordinary degree of reliability in its work. Furthermore, I see such a society as being mentally and physically healthier and enjoying a greater degree of freedom, even though it will be living in a more crowded, complex environment.
>
> All this will not come about by making everyone subscribe and live up to the Boy Scout oath. I think it will come about as an outgrowth of a number of painful shocks—shocks of recognition, not future shocks—we will undergo over the coming years, one of which we are already getting in our current energy situation....
>
> The kind of general outlook that will prevail in 1994 will be a synthesis of today's low-technology communes and high-technology industries.... High technology, much better planned and managed, and important scientific advances will still be the basis for progress.
>
> But that progress will be guided by many of the new values being expressed by young people today. We will be more of a functional and less of a possessive society.... This will bring us a different kind of freedom, one more closely related to Hegel's definition when he said, "Freedom is the recognition of necessity."[12]

Whether the United States will, in fact, move in this direction or react to the anticipated series of "painful shocks" by reverting to violence, national and international, and increasingly authoritarian government, remains to be seen. The future of our society is at stake whether we do, or do not, take the necessary precautionary measures. But whether the issue is viewed starkly as a matter of survival, or more conservatively, as a question of preserving our health, our standard of living, and the freedoms we claim to cherish, the "moral environment" must also be viewed as an essential aspect of the total health environment.

In all of these areas, policies and strategies should be developed to emphasize health considerations whenever issues are raised in Washington, state capitals, or before influential, private sector bodies. Useful recommendations along this line are included in the reports of the 1975 National Conference on Preventive

Medicine sponsored by the NIH Fogarty International Center and the American College of Preventive Medicine.[13]

NOTES

1. Cited in Norton Nelson, M.D., Chairman, Task Force on Environmental Health, *Theory, Practice, and Application of Prevention in Environmental Health Services,* (New York: Prodist, 1976) pp. 3-4.

2. T. Hodgson, "Short-term Effects of Air Pollution on Mortality in New York City," *Environment, Science and Technology* 4 (July 1970); L.B. Lave and E.P. Seskin, "Air Pollution and Human Health," *Science* 169 (August 21, 1970): 723.

3. Cited in N.A. Ashford, *Crisis in the Workplace: Occupational Disease and Injury,* A Report to the Ford Foundation (Cambridge, Mass: MIT Press, 1976).

4. For an excellent worldwide summary of the positive and negative aspects of population control, see, L.R. Brown, "World Population Trends: Signs of Hope, Signs of Stress," *Population Reports,* George Washington University Medical Center, Department of Medical and Public Affairs, Washington, D.C., series J, no. 13, January 1977, pp. J-237-252.

5. "National Wealth and Its Effects," *New York Times,* September 28, 1975, p. E-3.

6. Department of Health, Education, and Welfare, National Center for Health Statistics, *Vital Statistics of the U.S. 1973 Life Tables,* Vol. 1, II-Sect. 5, pp. 5-12.

7. National Center for Health Statisitcs, *Monthly Vital Statistics Report: Final Mortality Statistics, 1974,* 24, no. 11, (February 3, 1976): 9-10.

8. Saul Friedman, "Falling Apart," *The Progressive,* February 1976, p. 38.

9. National Safety Council, *Accident Fact,* 1974 Edition, p. 25.

10. *The President's Report on Occupational Safety and Health,* May 1972, p. 111, cited in Ashford, *op. cit.*

11. Jesse L. Jackson, "Give the People a Vision," *New York Times Magazine,* April 18, 1976.

12. Glenn T. Seaborg, "The Recycle Society of Tomorrow," in L.C. Ruedisili and M.W. Firebaugh, eds., *Perspectives on Energy: Issues, Ideas, and Environmental Dilemmas* (New York: Oxford University Press, 1975), pp. 521-522.

13. *Preventive Medicine USA* (New York: Prodist, 1976).

Chapter Fourteen

Individual Behavior and Life Style

Goal 3: Universal access to a broad range of information with respect to health, illness, disability, and ways in which individuals can protect and improve their own health; and encouragement of public policies and social attitudes most likely to motivate people to translate such information into personal behavior and life style.

> It can be said unequivocally that a significant reduction in sedentary living and overnutrition, alcoholism, hypertension, and excessive cigarette smoking would save more lives in the age range 40 to 64 than the best current medical practice.
>
> Marvin M. Kristein, Charles B. Arnold, M.D.,
and Ernst L. Wynder, M.D. (1977)

During the last few years, assertions similar to the above have been increasing in volume and the range of sources. Documentation is accumulating regarding the direct connection between certain forms of behavior and specific disease consequences. For example, the Department of Health, Education, and Welfare has summed up the relation between smoking and health:

> The association between cigarette smoking and excess death rates has consistently been demonstrated in a large number of studies during the last 30 years.... The strength of the association has been firmly established by repeatedly showing that cigarette smokers have one and a half to two and a half times the overall death rates of non-smokers.... [S]ubstantial excess overall death rates occurred in populations grouped by age, sex, race, socioeconomic class, occupation, place of residence, and many other variables....
>
> The most important specific health consequence of cigarette smoking.... is the development of premature coronary heart disease (CHD).... A cigarette smoker is more likely to have a myocardial infarction and to die from CHD than a non-smoker....
>
> A second major health consequence.... the risk of developing lung cancer was found to be 10 times greater for cigarette smokers than for nonsmokers.... The risk of cancer of the larynx, pharynx, oral cavity, esophagus, and urinary bladder was also found to be significantly high....

> Cigarette smoking is the primary cause of chronic bronchitis and emphysema....[1]

Documentation for the connection between other specific behavior and health outcomes is, thus far, less definitive, but in many areas the evidence is sufficiently persuasive to cause almost universal acceptance, e.g., alcohol abuse and cirrhosis of the liver, alcohol abuse and auto accidents, drug addiction and hepatitis. In other areas, such as the influence of diet and a sedentary life style on coronary heart disease, or obesity on diabetes, professional opinion is not yet in total accord; but the consensus is now of such dimensions that the relationship can confidently be accepted as a guide to public policy.

For example, in 1972 the Inter-Society Commission for Heart Disease Resources, representing all major professional associations in this field, summarized the current state of knowledge on prevention of atherosclerotic diseases:

> Many studies [have been] conducted over the past 25 years.... Numerous risk factors for CHD have been identified, such as habitual diet high in saturated fat-cholesterol-calories, elevated blood lipids, hypertension, cigarette smoking, hyperglycemia (diabetes mellitus), obesity, sedentary living, psychosocial tensions, and a positive family history of premature atherosclerotic disease.... Certain risk factors can be avoided, controlled, or corrected by appropriate change in mode of life.[2]

Regarding obesity, the National Commission on Diabetes reported in 1975:

> Nutrition and eating patterns are important factors in both the etiology and treatment of diabetes.... Seventy percent of all adult-onset diabetic patients are overweight and the incidence of diabetes among individuals who accumulate excess weight between the ages of 25 and 44 is several times higher than normal.[3]

Detailed longitudinal studies generally corroborate the records of insurance companies and the observations of practicing health professionals on the positive relationship between appropriate living habits, better health, and longer life. For example, Dr. Lester Breslow and colleagues followed 7,000 adults for over five and a half years. The results of this now well-known study showed that seven simple habits—three meals a day at regular intervals, eating breakfast, moderate exercise, seven to eight hours sleep nightly, moderate weight, no smoking, and no alcohol or only in moderation—were associated with significantly longer life and better health.[4]

Such studies, of which the above are only random samples, confirm the growing appreciation of the critical, and undelegatable, role of personal responsibility in health. Willingness to testify publicly to this effect is now coming not only from scholars and longtime proponents of prevention but also from health insurance carriers, health practitioners, and spokesmen for organized medicine.

Five years ago, it would probably have surprised the medical world to read an editorial in the *Journal of the American Medical Association* stating:

> Many people mistakenly believe that health care is synonymous with medical care. Health is, to a large degree, a matter of personal responsibility that must be exercised within the limits of genetic endowment.... As a general rule... medical care has relatively little impact on health. Measurements that supposedly reflect health, such as morbidity, longevity, growth, and development are not measures of the quality of medical care being received.[5]

In 1977, not many health authorities would quarrel with that evaluation, even if surprised by the source. This change in attitude is also manifest by the growing number of legislative advances, most dramatically the rapid passage of the National Consumer Health Information and Health Promotion Act of 1976 (P.L. 94-317). This new law provides for a national program of "health information, health promotion, preventive health services, and education in the appropriate use of health care" and establishes an Office of Health Information and Health Promotion within the Office of the Assistant Secretary for Health, HEW.

CAN ANYTHING BE DONE ABOUT LIFE STYLE?

> One man's freedom in health is another man's shackle in taxes and insurance premiums. I believe the idea of a right to health should be replaced by the idea of an individual moral obligation to preserve one's own health—a public duty if you will. The individual then has the right to expect help with information, accessible services of good quality, and minimal financial barriers.
>
> John H. Knowles, M.D. (1977)

Given the near universality of informed opinion with respect to the role of life style and the Congressional mandate to establish a high level Office of Health Information and Health Promotion, the questioning now tends to focus on other issues. Since most individual behavior is culturally conditioned, is it possible to counteract the overpowering forces in American culture, such as commercial advertising and the prevailing hedonistic life style? What, specifically, can be done in a democracy about these deeply ingrained risk factors? What evidence is there to justify faith in, or support for, a new thrust in this direction? Have not previous efforts at public health information and health education been notoriously ineffective?

Some experience suggesting encouraging answers to these questions is available in the 1975 report of the NIH Fogarty International Center and American College of Preventive Medicine Task Force on Consumer Health Education,[6] and in the hearings[7] and report[8] of the Senate Subcommittee on Health, which led to passage of P.L. 94-317.

In evaluating such experience, it is important to distinguish among different types of health education programs. The Task Force classification system identified patient education, school health education, occupational health education, national, community, and media programs. Practitioners of each category can point to a few documented success stories that can be interpreted as having reasonably wide application to other similar programs.

The best documented examples involve those directed at individuals who already have some strong motivation: patients with a chronic illness or a disability, those facing an acute crisis such as surgery or childbirth, or employees whose livelihood may depend on overcoming alcoholism or some other job-threatening condition. This suggests that probably the quickest payoff will come in the area of patient education. For example, Blue Cross Association (BCA) reported in 1974,

> With respect to health care outcomes, studies have shown the quality-increasing effects.... At the University of Southern California Medical Center, the reorganization of the system of diabetic care and the initiation of a multi-faceted program of patient education was associated with a reduction of approximately two-thirds in the incidence of diabetic coma from 1968 to 1970. Similarly, in another study, a significantly higher percentage of congestive heart failure patients receiving educational support improved in their classification....

In regard to costs, BCA summarized:

> ... some studies do suggest large cost savings as a result of changes in the pattern of utilization. For example, the Tufts-New England Medical Center research, using a self-selected sample of male hemophiliac outpatients given post-period instruction and practice in self-infusion, yielded the following pre-post comparisons: Total inpatient days declined from 432 to 42, outpatient visits per patient decreased from 23.0 to 5.5, and total costs per patient went down 45 percent (from $5,780 to $3,209).

> At the USC Medical Center, a reorganization of the diabetic care system, incorporating a telephone "hotline" for information, medical advice, and the filling of prescriptions, counseling by physicians and nurses, and pamphlets and posters to promote the service, was associated with more than a 50 percent reduction in emergency room visits

per clinic patient and the avoidance of approximately 2,300 medication visits.[9]

Such results are in line with similar studies, leading Lawrence Green of Johns Hopkins University School of Hygiene and Public Health, who reviewed hundreds of such studies, to conclude, "the payoff is more than proportionate to the effort and costs."[10]

The effectiveness of programs directed to the general asymptomatic public or to school children is far more difficult to measure. But the modest gains registered in the past decade with respect to smoking and coronary disease in adults are encouraging. For example, the Surgeon General issued his historic report on cigarette smoking in 1964. Despite the continued rise in *total* cigarette consumption during the following decade, there has been a significant decline in the proportion of adult smokers. Male smokers over 21 dropped from 52.4 percent in 1965 to 39.3 percent in 1975; women smokers from 32.5 to 28.9.[11] In addition, there was a substantial decrease in the amount of tar and nicotine per cigarette. The recent decline in death rates from coronary heart disease has been in part attributed to this change in adult smoking habits.[12]

Probably the most successful study yet undertaken in this field is the Stanford Heart Disease Prevention Program sponsored by the National Heart and Lung Institute and directed by Dr. John Farquhar of the Stanford Medical School and Dr. Nathan Maccoby of the Stanford Institute for Communication Research.[13] The objectives of this five-year inquiry were to teach people between the ages of 35 and 69 about heart risk factors and to stimulate them to more healthful behavior. It compared risk factor reductions in three similar California communities exposed to different mixes of television spots, printed materials, and personal instruction. According to institute spokesmen:

> For the most part, the findings have been extremely encouraging. In general, Watsonville (the maximum-treatment town) has shown substantial change; Gilroy (the mass-media-only town) has changed a little; and Tracy (the control town) has changed negligibly or in the opposite direction. Moreover, within Watsonville, the intensively instructed respondents have changed more than have their randomized controls, who received our campaign messages only through the media and their mail boxes.

The particular data regarding triglycerides, cigarette smoking, cholestorol levels, etc., led the investigators to conclude that an educational campaign directed at an entire community can produce "striking increases in the level of knowledge of heart disease and risk factors and very worthwhile improvements in risk factor levels."

School health education is probably the least effective today, and probably the branch of health education least influenced by new developments in the field, including the entry of new types of professionals. Even in this area, however, there are a few encouraging examples which strongly suggest that a more determined effort could be expected to yield positive results.[14]

Such experiences are persuading increasing numbers of professionals and legislators at all levels that there is a potential for important gain from promotion of positive health behavior and that the variety of negative forces tending to undermine healthy behavior can be counteracted or significantly reduced. This suggests the value of a better balance between therapy and positive health promotion. When we consider that federal expenditures for life style activities accounted for about one-half of one percent of 1976 federal health expenditures,[15] it is clear that there is ample room for better balance.

The Stanford Program also indicates that if health promotion and behavior change programs are to be generally effective, especially for the asymptomatic, they must be accompanied by firmer professional guidance, supportive public policies, and mass communications designed to reinforce the message of health education. The need for such harmonization is illustrated by the current contradictions in such areas as cigarette smoking and tobacco subsidies, nutritional requirements of children, and school lunch and food stamp programs.

WHO SHOULD BE RESPONSIBLE?

Who should carry out this affirmative approach to health is a question that has taken on increased significance with passage of P.L. 94-317. What qualifications are required? The definition of "health education" adopted by the NIH-ACPM Task Force envisions a field going far beyond the traditional boundaries and training of the professional "health educator:"

> Consumer health education is a process that informs, motivates, and helps people to adopt and maintain healthy practices and lifestyles, advocates environmental changes as needed to facilitate this goal, and conducts professional training and research to the same end.

Under this definition, health education can, and should be, conducted by a variety of health, education, and communications personnel, in a variety of settings, starting with the physician in his office. Most health education leaders acknowledge this. P.L. 94-317 rejects the term "health education" in favor of "health information" and "health promotion." "Health education" would presumably continue more or less in its present role as one aspect of the broader field.

The role of the new Office of Consumer Health Information and Health Promotion (OHIHP) is yet to be determined. The mandate of the law is broad and challenging. But the authorized funds represent a miniscule fraction of what is being spent on health care; and, as of March 1977, no appropriations had been made. The major obstacles have a circular quality: Popular demand for such programs will not be large until the programs themselves are given adequate opportunity to demonstrate their value but, unlike medical care, they lack a constituency with job stakes in fund appropriations.

The significance of the legislation, however, goes far beyond the modest sums involved. For the first time, the federal government is, at least formally, on record as recognizing: (1) the crucial roles of individual information, responsibility, and behavior in determining personal and national health status, and (2) the responsibility of government to provide the necessary information and assistance to enable the individual to protect his health. This creates the potential for forging one of the major missing links in U.S. health policy.

NOTES

1. Department of Health, Education and Welfare, Center for Disease Control, National Clearinghouse for Smoking and Health, "The Health Consequences of Smoking," cited in *Congressional Record,* January 29, 1976, p. S.773.

2. "Primary Prevention of the Atherosclerotic Diseases," Report of Inter-Society Commission for Heart Disease Resources, *Circulation* 42 (December 1970, revised April 1972): 5, 18.

3. *Long-Range Plan to Combat Diabetes,* Report of the National Commission on Diabetes to the Congress of the U.S., summarized in American Diabetes Association, *Forecast,* December 1975, pp. 13-14.

4. L. Breslow, M.D., "A Quantitative Approach to the World Health Organization Definition of Health," *International Journal of Epidemiology* 1 (Winter 1972): 347-355; N.B. Belloc and L. Breslow, "Relationship of Physical Health Status and Health Practices," *Preventive Medicine* 1, (August 1972): 409-421; N.B. Belloc, "Relationship of Health Practices and Mortality," *Preventive Medicine* 2 (1973): pp. 67-81.

5. W.R. Barclay, M.D., "Hypertension: A Major Medical Care Challenge," *Journal of the American Medical Association* 235 (May 24, 1976): 2327.

6. A.R. Somers, ed., *Promoting Health: Consumer Education and National Policy* (Germantown, Md.: Aspen Systems Corp., 1976).

7. 94th Cong., 1st Sess., *Disease Control and Health Education and Promotion, 1975,* Hearings before the Senate Subcommittee on Health, May 1975 (Washington, D.C.: U.S. Government Printing Office, 1975).

8. 94th Cong., 1st Sess., *National Disease Control and Consumer Health Education and Promotion Act of 1975,* Report 94-330 to accompany S. 1466 (Washington, D.C.: U.S. Government Printing Office, 1975).

9. Blue Cross Association, *White Paper: Patient Health Education,* (Chicago: August 1974).

10. L.W. Green, Dr. P.H., "The Economics of Health Education: Does It Pay?" Paper presented to Blue Cross Association Press Seminar, November 16, 1974, New York City (processed).

11. HEW, Center for Disease Control and National Cancer Institute, *Adult Use of Tobacco—1975,* (Altanta, Ga.: 1976) Chart 1. For a comprehensive review of research in modification of cigarette smoking behavior, see D.A. Bernstein and A. McAlister, "The

Modification of Smoking Behavior: Progress and Problems," *Addictive Behavior* 1 (1976): 89-192.

12. W.J. Walker, M.D., "Government Subsidized Death and Disability," *Journal of American Medical Association* 230 (December 16, 1974): 1530. See also, J.B. Stamler, M.D., in J.E. Brody, "Drop Reported in Coronary Death Rate," *New York Times,* January 24, 1975.

13. Nathan Maccoby and John W. Farquhar, M.D., "Communication for Health: Unselling Heart Disease," *Journal of Communication* 25 (Summer 1975): 114-126; Stanford University, Institute for Communciation Research, *Annual Reports 1973-74* and *1974-75* (Stanford, Calif.); J.W. Farquhar and P.D. Wood, M.D., cited in "Heart Disease: The Message Gets Across," *Medical World News,* February 10, 1975, p. 8.

14. R.M. Hendrickson, "They're Learning to Be Healthy—And They Love It," *Prism* 3 (July-August 1975): 26-32; American Health Foundation, *Know Your Body: The Disease Prevention Program for School Children* (New York: 1976).

15. M.S. Kaleda, C. Burke, and J.S. Williams, *The Federal Health Dollar: 1969-1976* (Washington, D.C.: National Planning Association, 1977), p 69.

Chapter Fifteen

Personal Health Services

Goal 4: Universal access, as needed, to essential health services—preventive, diagnostic, therapeutic, rehabilitative, and longterm—with adequate personnel and facilities, quality protection, and controlled costs.

It is the body that is the hero, not science, not antibiotics—the task of the physician today is what it has always been, to help the body heal itself.

Ronald J. Glasser, M.D. (1976)

Despite the best efforts at prevention through knowledge development, control of environmental and behavioral threats to health, and the promotion of individual responsibility, millions of Americans will become ill each year. Millions will be disabled, and some two million will die. Access to individual services for the treatment of illness and the care of the sick and disabled will continue to be an essential element of health protection. This traditional response to health problems is the one on which government has concentrated its energies and enormous expenditures ever since World War II.

The results have been both positive and negative. Improvements in access, particularly for the poor and the elderly, better physical facilities, increased numbers of physicians and other health personnel, and higher technical quality have all played a part in the continuing improvement in life expectancy. But there is mounting criticism of the large remaining gaps in access, the degrading and low quality "welfare medicine," the unbridled cost inflation, the fragmentation of services, excessive indulgence in wasteful high technology "gadgeteering," and a breakdown in doctor-patient relationships.

Prescriptions for "reform" have been advanced with increasing frequency ever since the historic report of the Committee on the Costs of Medical Care in 1932. In recent years proposed panaceas and new programs, small and large, have proliferated at a feverish pace. But disappointments multiply at almost the same rate. This has led to increased pessimism—"everything has been tried and nothing works"—sometimes bordering on cynicism or even nihilism.[1]

The pessimism is understandable but not well-founded. In part, it derives from expecting too much of health care. It must be realized that such care is, for most people, a painful experience, often accompanied by fear and unwelcome results. The very need for it can be bruising to self-esteem. While there is vast room for improvement, health care will always retain some unpleasantness and frustration. Second, the capacities of medical science are limited. Not everything can be cured or even relieved. We remain mortal; Humpty Dumpty cannot always be put back together again. Too many physicians are reluctant to admit their limitations to patients; too many patients and families are unwilling to accept such realities.

Third, as already emphasized, medical care is but one important element in determining health status. If environmental and behavioral influences are neglected, health services alone can never prove fully satisfactory.

Fourth, it is not true that everything has been tried and nothing works. While numerous experiments and innovations have been attempted over the years, and some have been distinctly meritorious (e.g., the prepaid group practice plans of the Kaiser Foundation and at Puget Sound), in the main such undertakings have been drowned out by a veritable flood of public and private monies that have supported and encouraged the continuation of conventional practices, and subsidized their shortcomings on a massive, almost unrestricted, scale. Providers of care multiplied and prospered, and it looked as if it might go on forever. Except for the most idealistic and dedicated, there were no incentives to seek change or to practice self-restraint or frugality. In this atmosphere, it is not fair to condemn as failures all attempted experiments; it may be more accurate to say many never had a fair trial.

In short, it is our thesis that too much cannot realistically be expected of health services, that some of its shortcomings are inherent, but many are due to mistakes and abuses. Notwithstanding the frustrations of the past, health care will always be too important to reject or neglect. We cannot afford cynicism, nor is it justified. We can learn from past mistakes. We will not be able to correct all errors or solve all problems, but the improvements we can make are worth the effort. We here offer a number of suggestions for improvement; we do not offer panaceas.

FIVE BASIC PROPOSITIONS

Before moving to specific issues and proposals, we state several fundamental propositions that should be taken into account in the formulation of health care policies and which underlie our analyses.

Doctor-Hospital-Patient: Economic Relations

The health care economy is replete with many unusual and some unique economic relationships. One of the least understood involves the peculiar roles of producer or "provider," and purchaser or "consumer," in the typical doctor-patient relationship. In other parts of the economy, the seller tries to persuade potential buyers with various inducements of price, quality, and utility; but it is the buyer who makes the decision. Where circumstances permit the buyer no choice because there is effectively only one seller and the product is relatively essential, government usually asserts monopoly and places the industry under price and other regulations. Neither of these conditions prevails for most of health care.

Once an individual has chosen to see a physician—even then, there may be no real choice—thereafter the physician makes most significant purchasing decisions: whether the patient should return "next Wednesday," whether x rays are needed, whether drugs should be prescribed, whether hospitalization is required, etc. It is a rare and sophisticated patient who will challenge such professional decisions or raise advance questions about price, especially when the ailment is regarded as serious.

This is particularly significant in relation to hospital care. Nobody can be admitted to a hospital on his own say-so. The physician must certify to the need; he will determine what procedures will be performed, and when the patient may be discharged. The patient may be consulted, but in the main it is the doctor's judgments that are definitive.

Little wonder, then, that in the eyes of the hospital it is the physician who is the real "consumer." It is he who generates the hospital's revenues. It is the medical staff that represents the "power center" in hospital policy and decision making, not the administration.

Although usually there are, in this situation, four identifiable participants—the physician, the hospital, the patient, and the payer (generally an insurance carrier or government)—the physician makes the essential decisions for all of them. The hospital becomes an extension of the physician; the payer generally meets most of the bona fide bills generated by the physician/hospital; and for the most part the patient plays a passive role. In routine or minor illnesses, or just plain worries, the patient's options are, of course, much greater respecting use and price. But in illnesses that are of some significance, such choice tends to evaporate. And it is for those illnesses that the bulk of the health care dollar is spent. We estimate that about 75 to 80 percent of health care expenditures are determined by physicians, not patients. Thus, deterrent measures directed at patients or the general public are relatively ineffective, or undesirable (Selection 28, pp. 184-186).

Quality and Efficiency

It is frequently proclaimed—often as a defensive ploy—that quality and efficiency or economy are antithetical in health care. Common observation demonstrates that the contrary is more often true. Concern for efficiency and husbanding of resources bespeak an attitude of care and caution; indifference to these tends to slovenliness. Such attitudes are not compartmentalized; they spill over into quality of service. The mood becomes pervasive. For most people, a sense of responsibility is fostered by feeling at least partially "at risk" for the consequences of their actions.[2]

The cornucopia of easy money in recent years has contributed to financial irresponsibility that is evidenced in inappropriate or casual use of expensive facilities, equipment, and services. Assured open-ended reimbursement leads to insensitivity by all parties—patients, physicians, administrators, and carriers. This is as threatening to quality as to economy.

Limited Resources

The automatic "pass through" to government and insurance carriers of rapidly spiraling costs, set in a publicized environment of "the richest nation in the world," produced for a time a sense of unlimited resources. It developed a mood whereby every practitioner and institution could "do his own thing" without concern for the "Medical Commons"[3] or a heavy conscience. Economists who preached the inevitability of resource limitations were discounted as alarmists. Awareness of the realities has become more common. But the practices of the earlier period have become the accepted conventions, habit patterns that are very difficult to alter; they are the "natural" thing. This is one reason for the assumption that increased "intensity of care" is necessarily synonymous with "better care" and, therefore, justifies the additional cost.

There are many who say there is no choice but to wait for the inevitable citizens' tax revolt and/or industry rebellion against unabsorbable health insurance premiums which will bring an explosive reaction that will finally force reform. There are obvious dangers in this view. First, the explosion may be slow in coming, if at all, and there is needless waste and deprivation in the interim. Second, if such an explosion should come it will not produce an atmosphere appropriate to rational reform, but rather to intemperate reaction. We may then get more trauma than reform. We had better attempt our repairs while they may still be done in a climate of reason.

Overcapitalization

It is now widely recognized that the health care industry is overcapitalized. Many cities have hundreds of excess hospital beds; hospitals have proliferated a superabundance of high technology equipment; structural ostentations and luxury are the order of the day. Occupancy rates are low; in any given day, one-fourth of all community beds are vacant (Table VI). Expensive equipment is underused or, worse, used unnecessarily. "The imperatives governing the behavior of non-profit institutions produce, in the absence of sufficiently powerful countervailing pressures, strong tendencies to over-investment. Public policy in support of non-profits has exacerbated these tendencies. The wages of over-investment are financial peril."[4] The evils that flow from excess construction are multifold and very difficult to contain once the structures are in place.

Health Care in the Economy

In terms of employment and expenditures, health care is one of America's major industries—nearly 5 million workers (Table IV) and approaching 9 percent of gross national product (Table XI). It represents the livelihood of many more millions, an essential economic infrastructure for many communities, an expanding source of employment for unskilled and semiskilled labor, particularly among minorities, and has the added attraction of being relatively depression-proof. Small wonder that, when a new medical center is planned, the newspaper announcement will hail it for bringing "10,000 new jobs" into the community. It is now just as difficult to shut down a superfluous hospital (*vide* New York City), as it is to close obsolete military bases, and for similar reasons.

In short, the health industry has become a major prop for the general economy.[5] Increasingly, decisions on health care are founded more on considerations of general economic effects than upon health needs. Public policy cannot, and should not, be indifferent to jobs and community economic conditions, particularly in periods of persistent unemployment. But it is important that policy makers be informed and open about the basis of decisions—is it health or something else?

With these propositions as background, we now turn to a discussion of the principal issues involved in moving toward Goal 4. We concentrate on major shortcomings and some suggestions as to what might be done about them.

UNIVERSAL ACCESS

Access involves more than financial capability. Geographic and psychosocial factors are also important, but removal of financial barriers is the first indispensable element of access.

The predominant way of paying for personal health care is now through "third parties"—private or public health insurance and other public programs. According to Social Security Administration estimates, about 80 percent of the civilian population under 65 years of age had some degree of private health insurance in 1974 (Table VIII). Almost all persons over 65 were enrolled in Medicare. Nonetheless, some 38 million people were without either private or public insurance.

A large number of these were eligible for one or more other public programs such as Veterans Administration, CHAMPUS (for civilian dependents of military personnel), or workmen's compensation. About 13 million, other than the aged, were receiving welfare payments under categorical welfare programs and thus were presumably eligible for Medicaid coverage. Also an unknown, but relatively small, number of "medically indigent" qualified in a few states.

However, these numbers cannot be added to those covered by insurance. The overlaps are numerous and great. Many people covered by Medicare are also on "welfare;" their Medicare benefits have to be supplemented by Medicaid. Large numbers of those covered by relatively thin private insurance receive aid from public programs as well. The majority of those receiving health benefits from workmen's compensation also had coverage under private health insurance. Piecing together payments for medical services is common. Net figures are not known.

The Social Security Administration estimates conservatively that about 22 million, or 12 percent of the population, had no protection of any kind, from insurance or any public program, in 1974.[6] Moreover, for most of the insured such protection was only partial or temporary, with significant exclusions. Under varying conditions, within a normal range, we would venture that anywhere from 25 to 35 million Americans are now without means of financial access to needed medical services.

The Medicaid program, to which over 23 million people had to resort in fiscal year 1976, is almost universally condemned as highly unsatisfactory on many grounds. It is uncertain and degrading in its eligibility processes. It generally results in poorer quality care than is normally acceptable, and it is often replete with fraud and abuse. Experience with similar programs over many years, including pre-Medicaid times, suggests that much of this is inherent in a welfare system. "Reform" of Medicaid is not a promising avenue to pursue.

Private health insurance also has considerable instability. Most Americans have such insurance by virtue of their employment status. During severe recessions, layoffs can result in millions of persons, normally counted as covered, losing their eligibility. Needless to say, those without insurance are also those least likely to be able to pay their own bills. In 1974, 91 percent of white persons under 65 with incomes of $10,000 or more a year had hospital insurance, but only 28 percent of blacks with incomes under $5,000.[7] Less than 40 percent of the "working poor" are reported to have any kind of insurance.[8]

We appear to have arrived at a consensus in this country that this condition is inequitable and untenable. Virtually every significant interest group has endorsed some kind of national health insurance proposal, and all agree that government action is required to make access available to necessary health care for the entire population. It seems self-evident that universal coverage should be the primary criterion for acceptability of such a program. The proponents of almost all national health insurance (NHI) bills appear to agree, because they claim that their plans accomplish this. But, in fact, careful examination of the proposals shows that most fall far short of that accomplishment. For the most part this results from trying to patch together public programs with mandated private insurance—as in the Administration bills of 1972 and 1974. As in most such assembly jobs, the pieces do not fully mesh; large gaps remain. The resulting administrative difficulties are also prodigious. Moreover, such plans inevitably end up requiring means test eligibility for a considerable portion of the population who cannot qualify for any of the several insurance plans—which does not bring us very far from Medicaid and its deficiencies. Elsewhere we have detailed these shortcomings.[9] Here we confine ourselves to the conclusion that universal coverage without economic discrimination is achievable only through a single national uniform program financed primarily through taxation.

Such a plan can have serious hazards—of sheer size, administrative difficulties, inflationary potential, and excessive concentration of administrative and political power. We have spelled out such serious shortcomings of an earlier version of the Kennedy-Corman bill, for example. However, we believe that many of these dangers can be dealt with. There are various ways of constructing and operating a single national program without monolithic concentration, which could even incorporate some of the benefits of competition, as well as providing a powerful instrument for cost controls. We described one such possibility in 1972 (Selection 29). But there is no denying that risks remain under any plan.

Yet, we cannot have it both ways. We must decide whether the long-sought objective of universal and equitable access is worth the burdens and risks of a single public program. There is no other way. Moreover, the burdens and risks can and should be diminished by a phasing-in process. Our knowledge, administrative capabilities, and the political climate, are probably not ready to swallow so massive an undertaking all at once.

There are many possibilities for such gradual phasing-in. Former Commissioner of Social Security Robert Ball has proposed gradual extension of an improved Medicare program (liberalized benefits and better cost controls) to the entire resident population, starting with Supplemental Security Income recipients.[10] Another approach would cover specific age groups in sequence. For example, the Javits-Scheuer bills would cover children and pregnant women. Another approach would cover the entire population, but only for "catastrophic" illness, as in the Long-Ribicoff proposals. A fourth, more modest and gradual, is for prompt federalization of Medicaid—a suggestion very much welcomed by most states. It would have the obvious virtues of equalizing benefit and administrative standards and transfer a major portion of the financial burden to the federal government.

Gradualism is a wholesome American tradition. But it is important that with each step along the road we maintain a view of where we are going, and that the steps are, in fact, moving in the direction of perceived goals.

A BALANCE OF ESSENTIAL SERVICES

> The federal government, in deciding on the type and level of health insurance support, may ultimately have to make a choice. The basic options are either to spend money on preventive and maintenance-of-health services, which could significantly reduce the incidence of illness at a low per-person cost; or to underwrite high-cost treatment; but with the likely result of increasing sick persons' lifespans only marginally.
>
> Congressional Budget Office (1977)

In theory, there is widespread agreement that Americans should have access to "comprehensive care," i.e., preventive, diagnostic, therapeutic, rehabilitative, and long term services, as needed. The spectrum is sometimes defined more simply: primary, secondary, and tertiary care. Long term care is sometimes subsumed under primary care; sometimes added as a fourth element. The practice, however, is quite different from the theory. The different levels are often difficult to differentiate precisely. More important, the realities of health care financing and professional incentives tend to bias availability in the direction of the more specialized and expensive modalities.

Patterns of insurance strongly influence patterns of access, utilization, and costs. The imbalance is prejudicial to primary and long term care and health maintenance activities, compared to tertiary care. Although about 80 percent of the population under 65 had some hospital coverage under private health insurance in 1974, and almost the same number for surgery; only 62 percent had any coverage for physicians' office visits; 35 percent for nursing home care; 17 percent for dental care. Only 11 percent of the "working poor" had any coverage for out-of-hospital services.[11]

Moreover, these percentages understate the differences. Out-of-hospital benefits generally involve high deductibles, coinsurance, and other restrictions that erect financial and psychological barriers to use. When actual consumer expenditures are examined, we find that private insurance met 77 percent of hospital care expenditures, but only 51 percent for physicians' services (much of which was for services in hospitals), and 7 percent for all other care, including prescription drugs, dental care, nursing services, etc.[12]

A similar pattern is shown in Medicare expenditures. In fiscal year 1975, for example, the program paid for 72 percent of hospital expenditures for the elderly, 54 percent of physicians' fees (again, probably most of it for in-hospital services), 3 percent for skilled nurisng care, and 4 percent of all other.[13] Medicare also imposes higher cost-sharing and other limitations on nonhospital care. A strong imbalance is also found in Medicare's renal dialysis program. The law makes it substantially more expensive for the patient to do his own dialysis at home rather than at a hospital, although the cost of home dialysis is far less. The percentage of kidney patients using home dialysis has dropped sharply since kidney disease was brought under Medicare. One of the pioneers in development and use of the artificial kidney, Dr. Belding Scribner, has testified that in fiscal year 1977 "we will spend at least $150 million more on artificial kidney treatment than is really necessary."[14]

Such financing (as well as other kinds of government subsidy) encourages similar tendencies on the part of the providers, subsumed under the familiar maxims, "the technological imperative" and "the edifice complex." Today, most physicians are not in primary care. They are specialists or superspecialists, generally attuned to tertiary care (Table V). Most, sometimes all, of their clinical training takes place in hospitals. Prestige in the profession leans heavily to the accomplished diagnostician, who is greatly dependent on the imposing armamentarium of the tertiary institution. (The "battery of tests" syndrome has recently found a new rationalization in "defensive medicine.") Ample availability of funds encourages these tendencies.

Hospitals are driven by similar stimuli. Each wants to be bigger, to offer a broader range of services, to be the "best." Prestige comes from attracting prominent specialists to the staff, and this requires more and better technological equipment and plenty of beds—all of which leads to expanded capitalization, higher operating costs, and pressure to "fill the beds." If money to pay for all this appears virtually assured—some 92 percent of all hospitals costs were paid by third parties in fiscal year 1975[15]—there is not much to restrain these "natural" tendencies.

Such developments led the physician-in-chief, Massachusetts General Hospital, to observe, "We are doing too much for too few, at too great a cost, and with too little benefit."[16] In light of their training, it is often difficult to persuade physicians that postponement of death is not the sole purpose of health care. Matters such as pain, patient preference, medical expense, and social costs are competing considerations and, in some terminal contexts, may outweigh the prolongation of life. At the extreme, we have the appalling extent to which people in hopelessly vegetative or comatose states are kept indefinitely alive by a panoply of mechanical and chemical interventions, dramatized recently in the celebrated Karen Quinlan case.[17] It is doubtful that physicians would be quite so willing to continue such practices if government were not footing the bills.

There is still only meager scientific evidence as to what types of interventions render the most productive results and on what scale of measurement;[18] or, "where should we spend whose money to undertake the saving of lives with what probability?"[19] There is, however, growing evidence that the tendency to overspecialization and the justification of every new technological advance is a prime factor in the rising national health care expenditures and in our failure to develop a desirable balance of essential services.

In so sensitive an area of public policy there can be no definitive solutions, but there are measures that can be taken to improve the situation. First, and most obvious, is a proposal that has been advanced by several public bodies, but never acted upon: All health insurance, public and private, starting with Medicare and looking forward to national health insurance, should be required to provide a full range of benefits, balanced so as to remove any financial incentives in favor of one modality rather than another.

Specifically, these should include the full range of primary care services, long term institutional and home care for the aged and the chronically ilw,d essential preventive services at all ages. Efforts are already underway to define specific "packages" of preventive services, including appropriate screening, counseling, and behavior-change therapy, that would be health- and cost-effective at different ages and could be assimilated into current financing and organizational patterns without too great difficulty (Selection 46). Included among these are screening of newborn infants for certain genetic defects and parent counseling on this topic.[20]

It is not at all obvious that this would substantially increase premium costs, as some have argued. While conclusive data are not available, evidence from the Kaiser plans and some other prepaid group practice organizations indicates that the availability of adequate primary care facilities, including more preventive services than are available to the general population, has resulted in lower rather than higher costs. Experience in the United Kingdom, where home care, day hospitals, and other desirable forms of long term care are more readily available than in the United States, indicates that these, too, can be instruments for cost savings (Selection 50).

Second, methods of provider reimbursement by third parties, which are discussed in a later section, can be revised to constrain specialist and hospital ambitions in accordance with approved regionalization plans. The virtual guarantee that all costs will be met is an invitation to extravagance and, ultimately, to inappropriate care.

Third, every available means should be employed to strengthen and enlarge the role and acceptance of primary and long term care in the structure of medical services—through medical education, both undergraduate and graduate, residency selection procedures, health planning priorities, HMOs, family health centers, home care services, and financing mechanisms. The primary physician—if enough of them were to exist and if his training, available resources, and role recognition permitted—could contain the drive to hospitals and high technology care, even for the terminally ill, and help to assure a more balanced range of "essential services." As a widely experienced European authority put it, "The key to the proper use of hospital beds is not more and more regulation ... but a strong and organized system of primary care clearly coordinated into a wide range of related services."[21]

None of this is intended to suggest a prohibition of exotic, "elective," cosmetic care or anything else that some patient may desire for whatever reason. However, these should not be promoted by public policy or financed by public funds or by means, such as insurance, which place the burden on the wider community.

SUPPLY OF PHYSICIANS

By 1974 total employment in the health care industry had reached an estimated 4.7 million (Table IV), 5.5 percent of all employment. If related activities were added, e.g., the production of medical supplies and pharmaceuticals, the figures would show that more than 7 percent of the civilian labor force depends on the health care industry for its livelihood.[22] Because of space considerations, this discussion is confined to the physician. It is he, more than any other individual, who defines "essentiality" and determines the quality and cost of services.

The power of explicit public policy, when supported by generous funding and broad public approval, has rarely been so dramatically demonstrated as in the case of physician manpower. Throughout the 1940s and 1950s, while the federal government still assumed a "hands-off" posture, the physician-population ratio remained relatively constant. By the early 1960s there had developed a wide consensus that the supply of physicians was inadequate for the needs of a population growing in affluence, increasingly protected by health insurance, and making greater demands for medical care. Congress responded and, from 1963 onward, government has been heavily involved in financing the education of physicians, nurses, and other health personnel, conditioned upon the expansion of enrollments. Over 60 percent of the costs of all medical schools is now funded from government sources; two-thirds of that by the federal government.

The results have been prodigious. There were 88 medical schools in the United States in 1965; by 1975 there were 114 in operation, plus 11 more in various stages of planning or development.[23] And the capacity of the original schools had been substantially enlarged. In 1965 the schools graduated 7,409 physicians. In 1975 they graduated 12,714, a rise of 72 percent. The goal set by the Surgeon-General's Consultant Group in 1959,[24] which many regarded as utopian, was exceeded by 16 percent.

The momentum has not been halted. It is now anticipated that, by 1979, present medical schools will admit 15,946 first-year students, not including increases resulting from opening of new schools.[25] Thus, by 1983, graduate output should exceed 16,000, more than doubling the 1965 output. In addition, the 7 osteopathic schools are increasing their classes. They graduated about 500 in 1972. Simultaneously, there was a tremendous unanticipated increase of foreign medical graduates (FMGs) entering the country and remaining to practice. In 1963 only 11 percent of the nation's physicians were FMGs; by 1973 nearly 20 percent, over 71,000, were in this category—not including 6,000 Canadian graduates not classified as FMGs.[26] In 1973, 44 percent of all new licentiates were FMGs, as were 31 percent of all house staff in approved intern and residency programs, plus an unknown number in other programs. In each of the four years, 1970-1973, the number of FMGs entering the country exceeded the total number of new U.S. graduates. This development was greatly stimulated by preferential immigration and visa arrangements for foreign physicians and by the open-ended reimbursement for hospital house staff, which caused what many consider an excessive expansion of residencies, often in institutions ill-equipped to offer adequate training.

As a result of these two movements there has been a dramatic rise in the U.S. physician-population ratio, from 147 per 100,000 in 1965 to 176 in 1974 (Table V), a higher ratio than in most other industrial nations. However, a steadily declining proportion—only 91 percent of all active MDs in 1974—were engaged in patient care.[27]

On the other hand, the ratio of physicians to total health manpower is much lower in the United States than in most advanced nations. Health care in America is increasingly institution-based and heavily dependent on a wide array of allied health personnel. In addition to the multiplication of doctors, nurses, therapists, technicians, and other more or less traditional health occupations, we also embarked on a policy of supporting the development of a variety of new categories under the general heading of "physician extenders" (PEs), including physicians' assistants, Medex, nurse practitioners, Primex, and others. Dozens of new programs were established; and, by the end of 1975, some 6,200 PEs had been trained.[28] Support of such programs was specifically stressed in the National Health Planning Act of 1974 (P.L. 93-641) as one of the nation's top health care priorities. However, the cost-effectiveness of the new groups is still being debated and evaluation of this policy will have to be undertaken before long.

All this expansion has brought on some troubling questions. In accordance with classical economic theory, many economists had expected that an increase in supply of physicians would result in a lowering of prices. This did not occur. Physicians' fees continued to rise faster than the general cost of living, with sharp acceleration after Economic Stabilization Program controls were lifted (Table XIV).

Although cause and effect relationships are complex and largely speculative, this has led to considerable credence for the idea that physicians create their own demand. Moreover, a physician will, through his use of hospitals, referrals, prescriptions, etc., generate expenditures throughout the entire health care system. An Ontario study in 1974 concluded that every additional doctor in the province would add between $150,000 and $200,000 in health care costs. A small U.S. study of a group of seven internists practicing in a southern metropolitan area indicated that the average physician generated about $260,000 of total costs in 1972.[29] Some estimates are much higher.

Few are now thinking in terms of general shortages. On the contrary, the official mood has changed to a fear of surpluses, especially as projections indicate that by 1990 the country could have in the order of 600,000 doctors,[30] which would translate to a remarkable ratio of 236 doctors per 100,000 population, an increase of more than 50 percent over 1974.

Second, it was hoped that a substantial boost in physician supply would relieve the imbalance between "underserved" rural and inner-city areas compared to relative "surplus" areas. This did not occur either. If, indeed, doctors can generate their own demand, and payment is provided for, they will continue to practice in areas they prefer.

A third hope had been that a more favorable doctor-population ratio would help diminish a perceived maldistribution as between primary and highly specialized care. Some change has taken place in the last few years, under considerable pressure and financial assistance from both public and private sectors. The Association of American Medical Colleges (AAMC) estimates that about 44 percent of 1976-1977 residents in approved programs are in primary care, not including OB-GYN. Among graduates of U.S. medical schools, over 60 percent report choosing one of the primary care fields for first-year graduate training in 1976, up from 52 percent in 1975.[31] However, such data obscure the fact that increasingly pediatricians, as well as internists, are moving into particular subspecialties.

In any event, it is clear that Congress has become increasingly skeptical. For example, the Senate Labor and Public Welfare Committee stated in May 1976, "Like the geographical maldistribution problem, the specialty maldistribution problem has worsened over the past 20 years. In the United States too few physicians are in primary care fields while too many are in the surgical and other nonprimary care specialties."[32] Speaking of our reliance on foreign-trained doctors, the committee said it found the situation "unacceptable." It concluded,

"Over the past decade, while the federal government spent more than $3.5 billion for health manpower programs, these problems have grown worse."

P.L. 94-484

Consistent with these developments, Congress, after nearly three years of debate, altered its goals in the Health Professions Education Assistance Act of 1976 (P.L. 94-484). From the start of such legislation in 1963, the asserted goals had been: (1) to provide the nation with an adequate supply of trained medical manpower, and (2) to assist the medical schools to achieve fiscal stability. The latter goal still receives high priority through continuation of federal capitation grants, at the relatively generous authorization level of $2,000 to $2,100 per fulltime student,* conditional upon the school's fulfillment of certain requirements. However, Congress now says that the first goal has been met and the requirements no longer include expansion of enrollment. For the first time the legislation is conspicuously aimed at the two more complex problems of geographic and specialty maldistribution.

A third aim is the reduction in inflow of FMGs by removal of some of the special immigration and visa privileges and stricter requirements as to language and professional proficiency, although U.S.-born FMGs are treated differently. The conditions of medical school eligibility for capitation grants include the requirement that each school accept in its third-year class an "equitable number" of such U.S. FMGs. Although limited to two or three years, the schools have understandably been highly critical of this requirement—both as a threat to academic freedom and as conducive to inequitable admissions policies.

With respect to maldistribution, the law requires each school to reserve a specified percentage of first-year residency places for primary care (defined as family practice, general internal medicine, and general pediatrics): 35 percent for fiscal year 1978, 40 percent for 1979, and 50 percent for 1980. A new program of federally guaranteed, but interest-bearing, student loans, up to $10,000 a year, is established. Recipients may redeem up to 85 percent of such loans through service in designated "shortage" areas. In addition, National Health Service Corps scholarships are expanded. They cover tuition, all other reasonable expenses, and a $400 monthly stipend (automatically raised in accordance with federal salary increases) for living expenses. Each recipient must agree to one year of service in a "shortage" area for each year of scholarship received, with a minimum of two years. Failure to comply with this obligation is subject to heavy penalties.

Most of these Congressional actions are important moves in the right direction. However, it can be assumed that health manpower policy will continue to be highly volatile and politically sensitive, especially in relation to physicians. There will be need for continuous high level and objective monitoring and adjustment to changing circumstances. Among these "changing circumstances," we note especially the following five factors.

*Appropriations were smaller, ranging from $1,031 (1976) to $2,076 (1974).

First, one of the conditions for capitation grants is that the schools must maintain first-year enrollments no less than that in academic year 1976-1977 or 1977-1978, whichever is greater, leaving open the possibility of continued expansion both in existing and new schools. However, to expand beyond present physician-population ratios would commit the nation to substantial increases in future health care costs for which justification does not now exist.

Even the AAMC, originally a strong advocate of expansion, now agrees we have gone far enough. In an official communication to Congress, it said, "Whether or not further increases in physician production are in the nation's interest is highly debatable. The association recommends therefore no changes in first-year enrollments beyond those already scheduled, until further experience is gained in assessing the impact of recent rapid expansion." The association also described medical schools as "presently seriously overextended."[33] At some point, the federal government will have to conclude that tax subsidies can no longer be used to increase the physician-population ratio.

Second, in prescribing specified minimum percentages of residency positions for primary care physicians, Congress did not preclude absolute increases in residency posts in the other specialties. This does not go as far as the recommendations made by the National Academy of Sciences' Institute of Medicine (IOM) in a major 1976 study commissioned by Congress.[34] The IOM urged that, while training positions for primary care physicians be expanded, the number of all other post-MD graduate training slots available as of July 1, 1977 should be temporarily held at the level of residency positions filled as of July 1, 1975. The study specifically identified surgery as "oversupplied" and urged limiting the number entering surgical specialty training. It recommended that such actions remain in effect until a permanent commission, established by law to monitor specialty distribution, could determine the appropriate number of residencies for each specialty. The IOM recommendations appear more appropriate to the present circumstances.

Third, the Congressional actions to ease geographic imbalance create generous financial incentives which should prove very attractice. Even the steps taken merely to increase the overall supply of family practitioners should help this goal because such doctors display a greater than average disposition to locate away from population centers. The more equitable fee schedules we recommend later would also help.

But incentives directed exclusively to individual physicians cannot alone meet the need for good primary care. The importance of adequate physical, technical, and professional support services has been repeatedly demonstrated. Indeed, HEW has reported that the "opportunity to join a desirable partnership or group practice" is the single most important factor stated by primary care physicians as influencing location decisions.[35] The success of the Hunterdon (N.J.) Medical Center in attracting first-rate young family practitioners to a rural county is related primarily to their identification with a good community hospital and health care system.[36] Physician policies in this area will have to be constantly related to considerations of other types of health manpower, facilities, and regionalization.

In the longer run, one of the great difficulties in this redistribution objective will be the determination of "shortage" areas. There are probably less of these than it now appears, unless standards of supply are inflated. It is to be hoped that the program does not take on a life of its own and perpetuate itself beyond reasonable need.

Fourth, an end to overall expansion of medical schools should not preclude special financing to influence and augment training for family practice and other primary care specialties, including the fast-growing field of emergency medicine. The primary care issue is not just a matter of numbers or how the doctor is listed in the medical directories. It involves the physician's basic value system, his philosophy of patient care, and his personal professional priorities. The effective primary care physician must be prepared—not only technically, but philosophically and temperamentally—to assume continuing responsibility for the patient's overall health needs, including health maintenance. Medical school and residency training, and attitudes inculcated in those settings, must be reasonably consistent with the end-product that Congress and the public are demanding, or avoidable conflict and frustrations will continue to plague the profession and its educational institutions.

Fifth, the IOM also recommended that a major study be undertaken to reexamine the basis of physician fees and fee allowances in public and private health insurance programs. Such practices influence career choices and specialty as well as geographic distribution. The AAMC has pointed out that "Current fee schedules appear to place the greatest reward on short-term technical interventions in acute disease states. Comprehensive continuing care, which requires provision of less dramatic services by physicians and other members of the health care team, will not be achieved unless market forces provide the appropriate incentives."[37] We believe the evidence is sufficient to justify modification of Medicare and Medicaid reimbursement policies even before the results of the IOM-recommended study are available.

HOSPITALS AND RELATED FACILITIES

Many forces have combined to emphasize institutionalization of the ill and infirm in the United States. Immediately following World War II, in response to wide perception of a shortage of acute-care hospital beds, Congress acted to encourage and subsidize construction. The Hill-Burton legislation and related programs, plus the stimulus of private health insurance and growing governmental support of inpatient hospital costs, caused a rapid expansion. Between 1950 and 1975 community hospitals beds increased 88 percent, from 505,000 to 947,000, resulting in a rise from 3.35 to 4.5 per 1,000 population, or 34 percent (Table VI).

As in many such undertakings, the momentum continues long after objectives have been achieved. Before the end of the 1960s it was generally recognized that rural areas, to which Hill-Burton was primarily addressed, were over-bedded. In the early 1970s it became apparent that this was true of the nation as a whole. Elliot Richardson, then Secretary of HEW, and other Administration spokesmen began to point to the danger of a surplus as early as 1971. The case grows stronger every year. Despite the fact that hospital utilization continues to rise, the number of beds increased so much faster than the population that occupancy rates, relatively low for some time, have declined. The overall rate in 1975 was 74.8 percent, lower than in any year since 1961. The high point occurred in 1969 with 78.8 percent.

There are many serious consequences of low occupancy and overcapitalization. Financial waste—with construction costs running at around $75,000 to $100,000 per bed and the cost of maintaining an unoccupied bed estimated at up to three-fourths that of an occupied bed—is most conspicuous. The Kaiser Health Plan has demonstrated that adequate hospital care can be provided to its membership with 1.8 beds per 1,000.[38] Even allowing for differences in the Kaiser population and that of the nation, the discrepancy in the two ratios is striking.

In addition to the obvious waste implicit in low occupancies, they create pressure for unnecessary hospitalization and unnecessary use of ancillary services. Utilization review procedures appear to have provided some check on the former but have done little to restrain the rapid proliferation of highly sophisticated and expensive diagnostic tests and devices that are the hallmark of modern inpatient care. The 23 percent rise in nonpayroll expenses of community hospitals between 1974 and 1975, most of which is for new equipment for such procedures, contrasts dramatically with the rise of less than 2 percent in average daily census (Table VI). A considerable proportion of the continued rise in the personnel-patient ratio and in payroll expenses is also due to this factor.

A significant part of the problem is imbalance as between: (1) acute care beds and equipment versus long term facilities, and (2) institutional versus ambulatory care. While community hospitals were expanding steadily for three decades, all other hospital categories were declining; not only proportionately but in absolute numbers. Moreover, only a small fraction of the increase in short term beds can be attributed to substitution. Tuberculosis hospitals have been almost eliminated, quite properly. Nonfederal psychiatric beds have been reduced by more than half since their peak in 1960—to 330,000 in 1975.[39] The justification here is less clear. Some mental patients are now better treated in short-term institutions. Others have been returned to the community, usually on medication, but frequently neither they nor the community is adequately prepared. Still others have simply been transferred from state-supported mental hospitals to private but publicly reimbursed nursing homes. In such cases the net cost to the taxpayer is greater, while the quality of care may or may not be improved. The decline in all other nonfederal long term beds, including those for chronic diseases—from 0.5 to 0.3 per 1,000 population—appears inconsistent with the aging of the population and is also probably best explained in terms of changing methods of financing and the tremendous boom in the nursing home industry.

In part because of the increase in the elderly, but in much larger part due to the coming of Medicaid and, to a lesser extent, Medicare, the middle 1960s witnessed a great expansion of private investment in nursing homes. Between 1954 and 1973 nonhospital long term beds of all types increased by 134 percent to an estimated 1,328,000. The large majority of these are in nursing homes, and all the increase was in this category. The remainder represent residential homes for the aged or infirm and "personal care homes."

In 1964, a year before passage of Medicare and Medicaid, we had 576,000 nursing home beds. By 1973-1974, we had 1,188,000, a 106 percent increase, resulting in a striking ratio of over 55 beds per 1,000 persons 65 years old and over (Table VII). Only about 12,000 of the 16,000 facilities had either Medicare or Medicaid certification, and about two-thirds of these, with half the beds, had only Medicaid certification.[40] Expenditures for nursing homes in 1974 were about $7.5 billion, over 40 times greater than in 1950. During the 1950s expenditures increased about 10 percent a year on average. In the early 1960s, when Medical Assistance for the Aged (MAA) was implemented, spending rose at an average rate of more than 20 percent per year; with the advent of Medicare and Medicaid, it accelerated even faster.[41]

Even so, there are still widespread allegations of a "shortage" of nursing home beds. But, we must ask: Shortage in relation to what? If we think in terms of "warehousing" most of our elderly and infirm in institutions, the shortage is indeed great and can never be fully corrected. That the current demand for beds exceeds the supply is also true. But the proper question is: What alternatives are we offering and what options do our present financing arrangements make available? Very little. In short, public policy appears to be pushing the infirm aged into institutions and then claiming a "shortage." Alternatives—probably cheaper and, for many patients, more satisfactory—can be developed.[42]

The heavy financial burden of over-institutionalization has led to many attempts to develop ambulatory facilities, including community mental health centers, neighborhood health centers, migrant labor health centers, home care and day care for the elderly, etc. Support for such activities has, however, been relatively meager. Health maintenance organizations (HMOs) have received the most attention as a means of deemphasizing hospitalization. For a time, HEW declared the HMO to be the "centerpiece" of its health policies. The objective was admirable, but the outcome has been disappointing (Selection 34). The proportion of the population covered by such plans has remained very small, about 3 percent, and stable.

In the effort to further discourage the trend to institutionalization, Hill-Burton funds have been officially discontinued, although some residual monies were still being used in 1976 for loan-guarantee programs. Section 1122 of the Social Security Act and certificate-of-need laws in about half the states were intended to discourage unnecessary beds and services. The experience with such devices is still too recent and scattered to offer firm conclusions about their effectiveness, although fragmentary evidence suggests that the countervailing forces towards expansion are still stronger. A few areas have already demonstrated the savings possible through reduction of beds.[43]

Many hospitals, bowing to the new mood, have shifted their attention from more beds to replacement and modernization, more space per bed, more technical equipment, and greater provision of physical amenities for both patients and staffs, frequently with little or no discernible relationship to the quality of patient care. In the view of many authorities, overindulgence in expensive equipment and technical procedures, many of unproved therapeutic value, is now one of the biggest obstacles to the rationalization of health services and cost containment.[44]

The time has almost certainly come for a moratorium on additional beds and expensive new equipment, with exceptions for the latter only after controlled clinical trials have demonstrated greater cost-effectiveness than existing equipment and procedures. The counter-arguments are not persuasive. In relation to beds, some argue that the lowest occupancy rates are in small rural hospitals. True, occupancy rates tend to rise in relation to hospital size. But this is a relative matter. The average rate, at none of the sizes, is impressively high. It is also pointed out that the lowest rates are in pediatric and maternity services, where beds are not easily adapted to the more crowded medical-surgical services. True again, but it is surely cheaper and more sensible to convert unneeded special beds than to build additional ones.

It is also sometimes argued that U.S. bed-population ratios are much lower than in some other nations. This is partly a matter of noncomparable categories, partly of differing patterns of hospital care. For example, there are virtually no nursing homes in the American sense of that term in Britain; most general hospitals consequently have large geriatric wards. Such differences are reflected in utilization statistics; for example, our admission rates are among the highest in the world while our average length of stay is among the lowest.

The increase in the number of medical schools has been accompanied by construction and expansion of university teaching hospitals, often irrespective of community needs. The argument is made that good medical education requires that each school operate its own "tertiary care" hospital. Yet, there are numerous examples to show that medical education can be conducted as well and, in the case of primary care, probably even better in existing community institutions. Nor is it necessary that the instruction, that takes place in the most highly specialized hospitals, be on the same campus, or even in the same city as the school.

In the debate pro and con new equipment, the CT (computerized tomography) brain and body scanners have become a symbol as well as the most expensive recent example. The original cost of a single CT varies from $300,000 to $600,000 and operating costs average about $370,000 a year.[45] While some physicians claim that the scanner represents the most revolutionary advance in medical diagnosis since discovery of the x ray, others say that the technology is still in the developmental stage, and that there is no justification for the current widescale proliferation, not only in hospitals but also in private physicians' offices.[46]

Granting the scanner's positive potential, the logical first step was not proliferation but controlled clinical trials to determine cost-effectiveness and, insofar as possible, objective technological assessment of the probable social impact. It may now be too late in this case but the lesson should not be lost to public policy. While millions of Americans suffer from neglect in underfinanced and understaffed long term facilities and others are told there is no money to support such universally essential services as home care and health education, the nation cannot afford to indulge every new technolgoical advance, even though it may prove beneficial to a small number of patients.

The Institute of Medicine underlined the seriousness of the bed situation in 1976 by declaring that:

> the evidence clearly indicates that significant surpluses of short-term general hospital beds exist or are developing in many areas of the United States and that these are contributing significantly to rising hospital care costs....

It recommended:

> that a national planning goal be established... to achieve an overall reduction of at least 10 percent in the ratio of short-term general hospital beds to the population within the next five years and further significant reductions thereafter. This would mean a reduction from the current national averages of approximately 4.4... beds per 1,000 population to... approximately 4.0 in five years and well below that in the years to follow....[47]

Without passing judgment on the precise validity of any specific bed-population ratio as a planning goal, we agree with the IOM as to the desirability of a gradual reduction in existing ratios. It seems doubtful, however, that this can be achieved without at least a temporary moratorium on new construction. Thereafter, the entire policy should be reexamined in approximatley three years.

Robert Ball has suggested a fairly drastic approach to a long range policy in this area, as part of his NHI proposal: Federal control would be established over hospital plant investment through annual national capital expenditure allocations. State and local planning groups would make the allocations within their areas. Depreciation would *not* be included in reimbursement to individual institutions. Instead, such amounts, based on replacement costs, would be deposited in state or local funds, along with the federal allocations. Institutions seeking replacement and/or new capital would be required to submit justification to the appropriate authority. Facilities would be precluded from the acquisition of capital from other sources except gifts.[48]

To achieve their long term aims, and to remain viable, any such restrictions on new construction and technological expansion must be accompanied by a serious drive to make more rational and effective use of existing facilities and equipment and to relate different levels of institutions to one another, both geographically and professionally. For some years ample legislative lip service has been paid to such objectives.

The Comprehensive Health Planning Act of 1966 and its state counterparts, the Regional Medical Program, and the National Health Planning and Resources Development Act of 1974, among others, represented strong proclamations of the virtues of health care planning and "regionalization." But they were little more than proclamations; and, despite the efforts of a few good planning agencies, not much progress has been made toward these broad goals. The proclamations were not fortified by clear definition of goals, forthright development of strategies or techniques, or adequate fixing of responsibility and accountability. Most important, no significant incentives were established to motivate hospitals to forego their own institutional ambitions. On the contrary, reimbursment policies continue to encourage and support autonomous behavior. The new planning instrumentalities—typically large, cumbersome, committees composed of interest group representation and ill-defined "consumers"—have not been such as to inspire confidence in either the providers of care or the public (Selection 38). The understandable professional and institutional resistance is reinforced by the conspicuous public irresolution.

A containment policy for acute care beds and equipment should be accompanied by a diversion of resources to ambulatory care and to more suitable chronic care facilities, whether under the umbrella of regionalization or not. For the time being, we cannot afford to restrict skilled nursing home beds in the absence of adequate alternatives. They will undoubtedly need to expand at a modest rate for a number of years. But governmental planning and resources should not be directed at promoting growth, but rather toward the development of more satisfactory and less expensive alternatives in the various forms of noninstitutional care.

QUALITY PROTECTION

Of obvious critical importance, quality is perhaps the most elusive problem in health care (Selections 5, 6, 39-41). If the nature of treatment depends upon the accident of who happens to see the patient first and there is confusion as to where to obtain primary care, quality is likely to be impaired. If there is a surplus of surgeons, it naturally creates a strong impetus for unnecessary and sometimes dangerous surgery. If there is an inadequate supply of health workers concerned with health education and prevention, resulting in avoidable self-abuse or neglect by patients, the quality of health care will be affected. If there are more obstetrical units than needed in a community, the low patient volume will affect quality adversely.

Clearly, quality is in part a product of the availability and organization of services. Here we deal only with a relatively few aspects, relating mainly to the qualifications and competence of physicians and hospitals. It is useful to be reminded, however, that important as these considerations are, quality will not be assured no matter how well they alone are handled.

Traditionally, government has relied almost exclusively on professional licensure to assure public protection against poor quality care. For physicians, this meant a one-time, lifetime license, encompassing the entire range of medical practice, generally revokable only for gross moral turpitude. In most states, hospitals have been licensed only since World War II; nursing homes for an even shorter period.

These minimal state controls were gradually augmented by voluntary standards imposed by professional organizations: certification of medical specialists by "boards" made up of their peers, and accreditation of hospitals by the Joint Commission on Accreditation of Hospitals (JCAH). As a result of JCAH pressure, as well as legal responsibililty technically delegated by the governing boards, the medical staffs of many of the better hospitals have long maintained a system of peer review, operating through a network of specialized committees. Also, the more advanced hospitals limit the practice of specialized procedures to physicians who are "board certified" in that field. Osteopaths, nurses, nursing homes, home care organizations, and other groups have also established voluntary standard-setting bodies, with varying degrees of effectiveness.

During most of this period there was a common faith that the competence and performance of doctors and hospitals could safely be left to the self-policing and self-discipline of the profession itself. In the late 1960s and 197(ne feeling increased that this was not enough. A variety of proposals emerged for reform of professional "credentialing" procedures, including compulsory "continuing education," periodic relicensing and recertification, substitution of "institutional" for individual licensure for some of the health professions, federalization or national standards for licensing, and even a basic rethinking of the entire evaluation and examination process for physicians.[49]

As a result of such pressures and developments, there has been substantial progress. As of mid-1976, 11 states had statutory provisions for relicensure linked to continuing education. The American Board of Medical Specialties (ABMS) and its 22-member boards have endorsed the principle of periodic recertification. Two specialty boards—Family Practice and Internal Medicine (mandatory for the former)—have held recertification examinations. Three others are in the process of developing such exams.[50] A major problem has been the formulation of tests that would be useful measures of actual medical practice, not simply academic knowledge. The National Board of Medical Examiners and related organizations are investing serious effort in this area.

Historically, the federal government's principal effort at quality control was through the Food and Drug Administration (FDA). The enormous technical and political difficulties facing this agency, as it attempts to monitor the great and growing number of new and reconstituted drug products proposed for the market each year, are being compounded by the increased chemical complexity and variety of new formulations, by the long lead time frequently required for adverse side effects to become evident, and the impatience on the part of all parties—manufacturers, doctors, and patients—to try the latest "wonder drug." The definition and extent of required clinical trials, and who should do them, remain controversial issues.

In 1976, after years of debate, FDA authority was extended to medical devices (P.L. 94-295). In addition to the general requirement for the registration of all devices, and establishment of safety standards, certain life-saving items such as pacemakers and dialysis machines will now require premarketing clearance.

In 1965, the federal government started to intervene more directly in the quality of health care services, as a concomitant of its greatly increased expenditures in that field. The Medicare *Conditions of Participation* established criteria—in varying degrees of detail—which hospitals, nursing homes, home health agencies, and independent laboratories have to meet to participate in the program. The original statute accepted JCAH accreditation as sufficient for hospital certification except for the addition of mandatory utilization review. JCAH subsequently added this requirement to its own standards. Despite the fact that JCAH has since tightened many of its procedures and standards, questions about the adequacy of its accreditation have been increasing.[51]

The 1972 Social Security Amendments (P.L. 92-603) increased federal institutional quality controls: (1) The *Conditions of Participation* for nursing homes (skilled nursing facilities and intermediate care facilities) were consolidated and made applicable to both Medicare and Medicaid (this had been achieved earlier for hospitals); and (2) the law introduced the concept of Professional Standards Review Organizations (PSROs). Building on the experience of a few county medical societies, medical foundations, and federally supported Experimental Medical Care Review Organizations (EMCROs), PSRO combined the concept of professional "peer review" of medical practice with statutorily defined "public accountability."

Implementation of PSRO has proved difficult, expensive, and slow. The first few years after passage were mainly devoted to reducing the resistance of some elements of the profession and to debates over structure, standards, and methodology.

In this atmosphere of uncertainty, it is not surprising that progress was slow. As of February 1977, four years after passage of the law, the nation has been divided into approximately 200 PSRO areas. One hundred and four "conditional" PSROs are performing review; 55 more are in the "planning" stage. HEW anticipates that 120 will be "conditional" by the end of fiscal year 1977 and most of the remainder into "planning."[52]

The law itself has significant limitations. PSRO jurisdiction is currently confined to institutional care, but it is clear that what happens in the hospital is in part predetermined by the kind of care received before admission, and the degree and character of recovery are dependent on the quality of posthospital care. Failure to provide for public representation, at either the local or federal levels, creates a problem of credibility. But on the positive side, the technical methodology of standard setting and peer review, like that of proficiency examinations, has received a great deal of attention and support from several specialty organizations as well as independent investigators.[53] Under leadership of the American Society of Internal Medicine, an effort is being made to extend professional quality controls to ambulatory as well as hospital care.[54]

The role and utility of PSROs remain unclear. An indepth study of 18 of the nation's "better" quality-assessment programs (including several PSROs), sponsored by the Institute of Medicine, found a widespread "lack of demonstrated effectiveness." This was because the program goals were not well specified, there was little agreement on the definition of "quality," and even when deficiencies were identified, the programs had difficulty in accomplishing improvements.[55] Despite the continuing ambiguities and uncertainties, which we have emphasized from the outset, it now appears much wiser to emphasize the positive aspects of PSRO, correcting the deficiencies wherever possible, rather than scrapping the whole effort for some hypothetical alternative.

However, it is now clear that "quality" issues are too complex and too pervasive for control by mechanisms such as JCAH and PSRO alone. Several recent developments have highlighted the need for broader action: (1) the growing malpractice furor, (2) the revelation of widespread abuse in the Medicaid programs, involving both cost and quality factors; and (3) increasing public concern for the "appropriateness" of certain aspects of health care.

1. The malpractice controversy is discussed in detail in Selections 10 and 41. As there indicated there have been some salutary results. Of the many dilemmas created by the spiraling of malpractice costs, one that appears to have escaped due attention should be mentioned. These costs have underlined, for hospital governing boards, the doctrine enunciated in the classic *Darling* case[56]—the hospital's duty to assure competent medical staff and to admit to membership only those physicians that the staff, after investigation, holds to be capable and qualified to exercise privileges.

While court decisions on this issue have been inconsistent, the leading cases now appear to buttress the hospital board's responsibility for, and authority over, the quality of care provided within the institution.[57] This move to join responsibility and liability with commensurate authority appears proper, but it also raises some problems which have not yet been effectively confronted by either the profession or the courts. For example, what happens to physicians refused hospital privileges? The doctor rejected for lack of qualifications will, as a result, be facing probable further professional deterioration. But he will continue in practice.

2. The miserable care rendered to Medicaid patients in "Medicaid mills" and nursing homes in several states has been a matter of record since the early 1970s. More recently it has been spotlighted for public view. The litany of abuses revealed by the Senate Special Committee on Aging, the New York State

Temporary Commission on Living Costs and the Economy (Stein Commission), the New York State Moreland Act Commission, and others, has attracted repeated first-page stories, indignant editorials, and strong political criticism.

A few states have attempted some corrective action, directed primarily at financial abuses rather than at quality. HEW has acknowledged its inability to monitor adequately this vast program across 50 states, blaming Congress for failure to finance the necessary personnel and the states for poor administration. Congress has reacted by legislating stronger measures against fraud, including establishment of a new Office of Inspector-General in HEW. This should help to control some of the more egregious abuses. However, we now have ample evidence that welfare-type medical programs inherently encourage low quality and produce an environment conducive to corruption.

3. Advances in technology and the heightened complexity of procedures inevitably elevate risks, as well as potential benefits. They have increased the urgency of the old issue of "appropriateness." Beyond the question of whether a particular procedure is well performed is the prior question of whether the procedure should be performed at all. Dr. Francis Moore has sharply pointed out:

> Modern intensive care in surgery has become a most elaborate matrix of interactions, electronic devices, and operative procedures... the opportunities for error have been multiplied a thousand-fold. Every patient that emerges from intensive care does so despite many misadventures.[58]

The debates over estrogen therapy for postmenopausal women, mammography for women under 50, coronary bypass surgery, some diagnostic and therapeutic procedures for elderly patients with minimal life expectancy, and life-preserving measures for the terminally ill, all demonstrate the importance of appropriateness as a quality issue. All raise questions that involve not quality alone, or cost alone, but subtle cost-benefit relationships and ethical considerations that vary with the age of the patient, life expectancy, underlying physical and mental condition, the "state of the art" for various diagnoses, etc.

Thus far, we have usually left all such decisions, both medical and nonmedical aspects, in the hands of physicians alone. To continue to do so becomes increasingly unsatisfactory. By training and by temperament, doctors are peculiarly prone to the "technological imperative"—to do "everything possible" for the patient regardless of the odds against a favorable outcome; if the technology is available it should be used. But many doctors feel it is unfair that they should have to "play God" and believe that society should help to make these difficult decisions.

In October 1976 California became the first state to grant terminally ill persons the right to authorize withdrawal of life-sustaining procedures when death is believed imminent.[59] In January 1977 New Jersey became the first state with professional guidelines for withdrawal of life-support systems from patients, such as Karen Quinlan, who are in a comatose state and for whom there is no hope of recovery.[60] The guidelines, established by the Medical Society of New Jersey, the Association of Osteopathic Physicians and Surgeons, and the New Jersey Hospital Association, with endorsement of the New Jersey Department of Health, the state Attorney General, and the state Board of Medical Examiners, provide for establishment of a "prognosis committee" at each hospital. The committee could, under carefully specified conditions, authorize the patient's physician to "proceed with the appropriate course of action," with immunity to any criminal or civil liability.

Absolute answers to the issue of appropriatness will never be available. The risk of undertaking certain procedures will always have to be weighed against the risk of not undertaking them. The patient and/or his family will increasingly be expected to share responsibility. The legal requirement of "informed consent" will not prove adequate. The relationship between intelligent and responsible decision making by the patient and responsible patient education by the doctor is clear. It would be difficult to overemphasize the importance of patient education as a characteristic of good patient care.

Quality is inevitably a moving target that can only be copied with by an attitude of public accountability and incessant vigilance by the health professions, especially physicians, public authorities, educators, health administrators, and individual patients. But there are a number of specific steps that seem justified and feasible on present evidence:

1. The Administration should promptly develop plans for, and the Congress urged to adopt, legislation to replace Medicaid with a program that does not distinguish the "poor" from other people. Meanwhile, the Administration should call on organized medicine to join with it in devising ways of strengthening PSROs and other devices to correct the gross qualitative abuses in Medicaid and other programs aimed primarily at low income groups. Sophisticated professional methodologies for distinguishing the "A-" doctor from his "B+" colleague are no substitute or excuse for professional failure to take action against the small number of "D-" offenders, who probably should not be practicing at all.

2. Special efforts should be made to incorporate the various modalities of long term care into the mainstream of health care. The existing attitudinal "iron curtain" between acute and chronic care, with the latter starved for professional concern and quality controls as well as funds, must be replaced by recognition of the continuum of comprehensive care. As suggested earlier, such a qualitative improvement, if properly integrated, need not represent additional costs.

3. Periodic specialty recertification and, for all physicians not board-certified, periodic relicensure should both be mandatory within a few years. It appears desirable, for many reasons, to retain state licensing authority but this should probably be coupled with some form of national standard-setting and monitoring to exert moral pressure on any laggard jurisdictions and to assist with the technical aspects of relicensure.

4. PSRO review should be extended to all hospital patients and to ambulatory and long term care. Knowledgeable public members should be added to PSRO policy bodies at the local and federal levels.

5. Procedures and requirements for state licensure of hospitals, nursing homes, and other health care facilities should be strengthened. Greater emphasis should be placed on their health care responsibilities and competence, including more explicit bylaw requirements with respect to physician privileges, defined inservice training programs for all staff, and revocation of license for insufficient utilization of specific services as well as poor care of individual patients. Particular attention needs to be paid to independent clinical laboratories whose work has, in some localities, become something of a scandal.

6. Machinery should be set in motion to develop an effective and ethically acceptable methodology for clinical trials for new, and some old, surgical, diagnostic, and other significant procedures.

7. The ethical, legal, and medical aspects of "the right to die" should be fully studied at the highest level of public and professional competence. If feasible, national guidelines—acceptable both professionally and socially—should be formulated and disseminated.

Effective implementation of all the above will call for creative and cooperative working relations between the responsible public agencies and the relevant professional organizations. Neither can do the job alone.

CONTROLLED COSTS

Health care spending in the United States reached $139.3 billion in fiscal 1976.... In the two years since price controls expired, health care expenditures have risen $33 billion or 31 percent. At the same time, the economy in general has been rising at a relatively slower pace. As a result, health expenditures as a portion of GNP have grown from 7.8 percent in 1974 to ... 8.6 percent in 1976.

U.S. Department of Health, Education,
and Welfare, *HEW News* (1976)

Failure to move forward incrementally towards greater cost effectiveness of health care can only, by default, precipitate far cruder measures, such as across-the-board hospital rate freezes and cuts in health insurance benefits. Such solutions to the complicated problems of containing costs of the multi-billion dollar hospital industry would, of course, single out the ill and disabled citizens in our society to bear the consequences....

Katharine G. Bauer (1976)

Prodigious inflation of health care costs has persisted for three decades, and there are no signs of abatement. On the contrary, since the demise of the Economic Stabilization Program (ESP) it has accelerated (Tables XI, XII, XIV). Concern has understandably deepened.

The causes have been subjected to repeated investigations, private and public, at all levels of government. They have been discussed in this volume, as early as 1961 (Selection 16), and frequently since then. They are multiple and complex, but no longer obscure—although hardly devoid of controversy. But understanding causes is not the same as identifying, or obtaining agreement on, remedies.

The phenomenon of rising costs and prices prevails, in greater or lesser degree, in most advanced countries, regardless of varying methods of paying for health services—which underscores the great difficulty of establishing effective controls, particularly in democratic societies. However, appreciation of the difficulties should not reduce us to a sense of hopelessness. We are not prisoners of some ironic fate. Nothing will be done if we wait for perfect or all-embracing solutions or only those whose effectiveness can be proved in advance. Nor will anything significant be undertaken if we seek only remedies that will not meet political resistance nor impinge on any group's present privileged position. The problem is urgent enough to require and justify some risk-taking.

It is well to be reminded that the "reasonable costs" formula for institutional care and "reasonable charges" for practitioners, to which we have become so accustomed in the past decade, were not the usual methods of government payment before Medicare. Workmen's compensation and vendor programs for welfare patients usually remunerated physicians on the basis of fixed-fee schedules. The inflationary blank checks created by open-ended "reasonable costs"—unilaterally determined by the institutions themselves—and "reasonable charges"—effectively determined by the practitioners themselves—were mandated by government in a law that organized medicine opposed. The results could easily have been foreseen. Within the first year of Medicare we wrote:

> ... there will be increasing recognition of the basic deficiencies in the principle of individual hospital cost reimbursement—inherently inflationary, inefficient, and inequitable. There will be mounting criticism, but the critics will be unable to agree upon an alternative.... [61]

About physician reimbursement, we said, "The inescapable question is being raised as to whether it is feasible for the government to guarantee to any group or profession payment at any level the group may unilaterally elect."[62]

It may be argued that such provisions were a necessary compromise if any Medicare law was to be passed; adjustments could be made later. In any case, the evidence is now in: the payment system is untenable over the long pull. Yet, after a decade of constant jaw-boning, mutual recriminations, limiting amendments, and regulatory tinkering, the initial reimbursement principles remain essentially intact.

The major effort to contain prices came in 1971 as part of the Economic Stabilization Program, the first peacetime imposition of general wage and price controls in American history. During the first two phases of ESP, August 1971-December 1972, the health industry was treated like the rest of the economy. In Phase III, health care, along with construction, food, and oil, remained under controls while other industries were gradually decontrolled. In the final stages of Phase IV, starting in early 1974, plans were developed for continuing controls on health care, including use as well as price. Hospitals, nursing homes, and physicians declared war on ESP and initiated a series of legal battles. Before the new regulations could go into effect, the battle had been won by the providers. ESP died in April 1974. The lesson may be that any attempt to impose price controls on the health industry alone is probably politically, and perhaps constitutionally, unfeasible. A different approach—utilizing the Medicare/Medicaid reimbursement provisions—was written into the Social Security Amendments of 1972 (P.L. 92-603). In addition to PSRO, this included mandatory requirements with respect to hospital planning, and efforts to set some boundaries to "reasonable costs" and "reasonable charges." Regulations to implement the new provisions began to appear in 1974 and 1975, resulting in more court suits and further bitterness between providers and government. In 1975-76, the last year for which data are available, hospital charges rose more than twice, and physician's fees almost twice, as much as general prices (Table XIV).

The new drive for national health insurance (NHI), which started around 1970-1971, was in part motivated by a belief that it could be used to contain costs. Paradoxically, the continued increases contributed to a decline of enthusiasm. With costs apparently out of control, could the nation embark on so large an enterprise? "Costs too much" became the most common argument against NHI. But, if costs continue their upward spiral, that may become the trigger for bringing it on, inevitably accompanied by stringent controls. In any case it is clear that the alleged imminence of national health insurance should no longer be used as an excuse for delaying action on costs. The need is urgent now. If and when NHI does arrive, we should already have developed some knowledge and experience with control policies and strategies.

The time for a positive containment policy is politically propitious. Supporters and opponents of NHI, conservatives and liberals, organized labor and management, even most of the health care industry, agree that some kind of fiscal restraints are needed. But what kind? Ideally, the simplest and the most palatable answer lies in the regulatory discipline of a free and competitive market. But, as indicated in Propostion 1 (p. 412), economically effective competition does not exist, and is impractical, for most of the industry. We must, therefore, turn primarily to the more cumbersome and complex instruments of public regulation. In political terms, this decision has already been made and is undoubtedly irreversible.

Many cost control proposals have been offered. Several have already been discussed, including the importance of avoiding a surplus of physicians. Here, we limit ourselves to a brief examination of seven areas.

Capital Facilities and Equipment

Institutional capital expenditures are obviously a major factor in annual expenses, not only because of their own great cost but because they are significant determinants of operating costs and utilization. Once built, a hospital bed will be costly to maintain whether used or not. It is estimated that operating cost for every new piece of equipment will equal the original cost in a period of about two years. For the CT scanner, the first year's operating cost may equal or exceed the purchase cost. Although the data undoubtedly reflect some accounting idiosyncracies, it is interesting to note that, in 1975, community hospitals reported that operating expenses exceeded total land, plant, and equipment assets by 24 percent and came to 83 percent of total assets, including endowment and other cash funds.[63]

In recognition of these relationships and the growing evidence that hospitals were expanding unnecessarily, over half the states have passed some form of certificate-of-need (C/N) program for review and approval of capital expenditures for construction or substantial expansion of health care facilities. The Medicare/Medicaid programs now require such reviews under Sec. 1122 of the Social Security Act (Sec. 221 of P.L. 92-603), and almost all states have agreements with HEW for this purpose. Under P.L. 93-641, state capital approval programs will be mandatory after 1979, as a condition of continued federal funding of health care programs within the state. Nationwide networks of health systems agencies (HSAs) and state health planning and development agencies are being set up as successors to the former Comprehensive Health Planning bodies. As of February 1977, 205 HSAs had been designated, with an anticipated total of 212.[64]

Most of the C/N laws are less than five years old and it is difficult to appraise their effectiveness (Selections 36 to 38).[65] P.L. 93-641 has thus far survived numerous political and legal attacks, including a major challenge by the Association of American Medical Colleges on behalf of teaching hospitals. Even in the case of New York, which has had a mandatory C/N program for a decade, it is impossible to be sure whether the amount and distribution of resources are significantly different today from what they would have been without the program. However, it is acknowledged that the programs have been operating under severe handicaps.[66]

The C/N programs are inherently at odds with the present reimbursement system. As long as the institutions can demonstrate that they are able to pay for the proposed new facility or equipment, because of assured third party reimbursement, it is politically extremely difficult to prohibit construction or purchase. Conversely, unless unnecessary and expensive additions are prevented in advance, it is almost impossible to deny reimbursement. If either type of control is to prove effective, both will have to be strengthened and coordinated.

To this end we have earlier suggested a temporary moratorium on acute hospital beds and, with certain exceptions, on expensive equipment, to be accompanied by a complementary restriction on additional residencies. In the next section we recommend changes in institutional reimbursement consistent with this policy. Some authorities also advocate annual fixed "caps" for capital expenditures within a state or region as well as the nation.

With or without such "caps," the C/N apparatus will have to improve its performance. The first stage of C/N review takes place in the HSAs. There has been criticism, especially from state officials, that these bodies are not accountable to any public authority. However, the HSAs are not empowered to make final C/N decisions. They furnish recommendations and evidence to the state. Their effectiveness will depend on the degree of technical competence they can muster and the reputation they achieve for ability to withstand the intense local pressures that normally accompany the highly charged issues of health facilities. In large degree, this can also be said of the state agency. That is why the organizational structure of these bodies is so important. On the basis of the available evidence on C/N administration, thus far, we recommend:

1. The advisory councils at both the HSA and state levels must be bolstered to provide a strong and knowledgeable constituency with some stake in cost containment. The present requirement of 51 percent "consumer" representation does not do that, because the definition of "consumer" is so restrictive as to disqualify some of the strongest and best informed people with an interest in control, e.g., health insurance officials and public trustees of Blue Cross plans, HMOs, or other community health organizations. Such individuals, together with representatives of union and management purchasers of care, offer the base for a potential balancing of constituency interests. To date, consumer representation has generally been weak or uninformed, which has contributed to provider domination of most of these bodies.

2. Important as is the role of advisory councils, they should not have final decision-making power, in appearance or in fact. This belongs in a visible and accountable public authority, either an independent commission, department of health, or similar body.

3. The councils should be small enough to instill a sense of responsibility in each member, and members should not be selected to represent particular interest groups. The prevalence of bodies with large numbers—sometimes 50 or more—has not only produced inefficiency but has further contributed to provider domination. Interest-representing bodies invite suspicion of conflict of interest and diminish political credibiltiy.

4. C/N agencies need authority to decertify. For example, an agency may be faced with a request for approval of a fine modern hospital in an area that has all the beds it needs in a poor obsolete institution close by. The agency's position becomes untenable: either electing for obsolescence or a surplus of beds.

(Experience indicates that competition alone will not drive the original hospital out of business, as logic might suggest.) Decertification authority would, of course, be politically difficult to exercise, but it is an important weapon to have in the closet. In the case indicated, it might serve as an instrument to persuade the old hospital to modernize, alter its functions, or to merge with the proposed institution.

Institutional Rates

> The current reimbursement system gives the manager of the system neither the carrot nor the stick he could use with the constituencies within his system.
>
> Lawrence M. Klainer, M.D. (1976)

There is now increasing, albeit reluctant, agreement on the necessity for some kind of institutional rate, or price, controls, especially for hospitals to which this discussion is confined. Hospitals consume the largest portion of the health care dollar, are the fastest growing sector, and for many years have experienced far higher price increases than any other segment of the industry. The American Hospital Association has been on record for years favoring state rate regulation—at least partly to avoid federal regulation.[67]

The Economic Stabilization Program (ESP) episode demonstrated the enormous difficulty of establishing federal price controls for a single industry. More enduring have been the efforts embodied in P.L. 92-603 to modify and limit the concept of "reasonable costs" under Medicare and Medicaid. Under Section 223, HEW established a hospital classification system based primarily on size and geographic location. For each class, reimbursement ceilings were set for "routine" services (excluding special care units and ancillary services) at a given percentile of the "reasonable costs" of all hospitals in the same class. Originally the 90th, this was reduced to the 80th, plus 10 percent of the median for each class. Institutions were permitted to seek exemptions and/or, under certain circumstances, charge the patient any difference between actual costs and the Medicare rate. The regulation became effective in July 1974.

According to the AHA, the rates in several hundred hospitals were affected by the limits. But since the ceilings apply only to "routine" costs of Medicare and Medicaid patients, it is legally permissable to transfer such costs to ancillary services and to non-Medicare/Medicaid patients. There is no statistical evidence of any effect on overall rates; in fact, as already noted, the 1974-1975 hospital per diem rise was the greatest of any single year during the past decade.

Largely in recognition of the inherent shortcomings of the concept of retroactive cost reimbursement, interest has shifted to various forms of "prospective" or predetermined rates.[68] One of the first tentative efforts in this direction was the much publicized Medicare "incentive" reimbursement experiment program. First authorized under the Social Security Amendments of 1967, and expanded under Sec. 222 of P.L. 92-603 and Sec. 1526 of P.L. 93-641, it has not been very productive thus far.[69] The program is voluntary, and few hospitals saw much point to participation if there was to be a risk and no certainty of gain. Most were doing well enough without such "incentives." Moreover, it made the common erroneous assumption that the nonprofit hospital is subject to the same incentives as ordinary business.

In 1976, and again in early 1977, the Ford Administration proposed a ceiling of 7 percent on hospital reimbursement increases under Medicare and Medicaid, based on the anticipated consumer price index rise for the year. This would have required a change in the basic Medicare law, and passage was successfully opposed by the hospital industry.

Early in 1977, the Carter Administration announced its intention to seek legislation to limit the annual percentage increase in hospital revenues from all sources as well as to set national and state ceilings on new capital expenditures.

Meanwhile, Congressional initiative was led by Senator Herman Talmadge, Chairman of the Senate Finance Committee's Subcommittee on Health. His 1976 Medicare-Medicaid reform bill (S. 3205) included a new "performance based" hospital reimbursement plan. It recreated the "target-rate" incentive approach of Sec. 222 (reward the efficient and penalize the inefficient) but made it mandatory, and combined that with the methodology of Sec. 223 (classification of hospitals for valid comparisons). Despite some adjustment, this approach suffered from the demonstrated shortcomings of each of the previous ones. The rate setting was limited to "routine" costs. The omitted items, said to be unpredictable or not directly subject to the hospital's own control—such as malpractice insurance, utility costs, and capital expenses—were estimated at 60 to 65 percent of total costs. Thus only a minor portion of costs were subject to the target rates. The prospect for effective cost containment on this basis is dim.

State Rate Review

Some form of hospital rate setting or rate review activity, either statutory or voluntary, was in process in over half the states as of January 1977, a rapidly expanding development that started in New York in the late 1960s.[70] The few common elements include: (1) review of proposed budget and/or rate schedule by some body external to the institution; and (2) the principle that payment will be made on the basis of "prospective," as opposed to "retrospective," rates.

Otherwise, the programs vary widely—in objectives, authority, jurisdiction, and methods of operation. Some emphasize controls on facility and program expansion; some stress better hospital management; others seek to equalize rates to all payers; still others simply try to narrow the spread between the rise in hospital rates and other prices.

Due to differences of interpretation, there is disagreement as to the exact number of states with statutory programs, either ten or 12. Some limit their jurisdictions to Medicaid and/or Blue Cross reimbursement. Others include all payers except Medicare. Maryland, Rhode Island, and Washington include, or plan to include, Medicare under experimental agreements with HEW.

In states with nonstatutory programs, the activities are purely voluntary, without legal status. In most, this simply means that Blue Cross uses prospective, rather than retrospective, rates as the basis for reimbursement, often with allowance for later adjustments for unanticipated events. In three states, the review is performed by the state hospital association. Several states follow the "Indiana model," wherein Blue Cross-determined rates are applied to all patients other than Medicare. There are other variations.

In general, there appear to be four broad categories: (1) *rate setting:* unilateral imposition of rates or maximum per diem payment limits, by a government agency—New York and New Jersey have such authority; (2) *rate review for approval:* hospitals are required to submit advance annual rate schedules for approval or adjustment; (3) *budget review for approval:* hospitals are required to submit revenue and expenditure budgets and projected service volume to justify a proposed rate schedule—Maryland and Washington have mandatory programs of this type, Indiana a voluntary one; (4) *rate review for comment:* submission and public disclosure of hospital budgets and proposed rates; outside body may comment or criticize but has no further authority—California, Montana, and Arizona employ variations of this pattern. Only one state—Rhode Island—sets rates within the limits of an overall cost ceiling (maxi-cap) on permissible increases in total hospital expenditures.

Operating procedures vary widely—from formula-based rate promulgations to "education," public disclosure, and jaw-boning. Units of payment to be reviewed and/or approved may be "charges," per diem costs, per case costs, or case-mix categories (diagnosis related groups). Budget preparation, criteria for evaluation, and standards for "exceptions" differ. Means for resolving conflicts may include negotiation, arbitration, formal hearings, or court action. Several states, desperately trying to contend with ever-growing Medicaid costs, are groping and shifting from one formula to another, while confronting equally frustrated hospitals facing operating deficits.

The results of all this experimentation are uncertain. C. R. Gaus, Director, Health Insurance Studies, Social Security Administration, summarized the findings of an extensive two-year evaluation study of prospective rate setting in Pennsylvania, New York, New Jersey, and Rhode Island, commissioned by SSA:

> The programs under study were moderately successful in lessening the pace of hospital cost inflation....[But] in many cases the results did not pass the rigorous statistical tests of significance and therefore must be interpreted with caution. Another sobering factor is that, even with highly significant statistics, the magnitude of savings (1-3 percent) per year that could be attributed to the system would not even approach bringing hospital cost increases into line with inflation in other sectors of the economy.... Prospective reimbursement is no panacea. On the

other hand, several percentage point savings per year compounded over 10 years would be large savings to us taxpayers.[71]

Katharine Bauer, an authority in this field, has concluded, more pessimistically:

> Rate setting, per se, is just a highly complicated tinkering operation, plugging up leaks in one small section of a rudderless ship that is cracking at the seams.... In the absence of a broader policy of health regulation, expectations of cost containment through most of the types of rate setting programs currently in operation should be kept modest, commensurate with the modesty of their own operational objectives, i.e. to blunt the spiral of hospital inflation by discouraging duplicative expansions and overbedding, and *by encouraging types of potential cost savings in areas of hospital functioning not affected by physician decisions.*" (Italics supplied.)[72]

A New/Old Proposal: Negotiated Rates

Obviously, the problem of controlling the runaway costs in the health care industry is much too broad to be solved by any one device. Institutional rate controls constitute only one of many areas in need of close, and probably simultaneous, attention. They are probably of lesser urgency than controls over capital facilities and equipment and the number of physicians. Moreover, in a context of ever-increasing federal funding, state controls are inherently of limited efficacy.

It does not follow, however, that "modest" objectives are unimportant. On the contrary, one of the major obstacles to effective health care cost containment has been the unrealistic quest for a single panacea. Prospective reimbursement is such an obvious reform that it can hardly fail to be adopted in the near future. The irony is that, far from a revolutionary new control, it merely reestablishes normal business pricing practices. In the words of one well-informed hospital administrator:

> The health care industry erroneously believes that prospective reimbursement is unique to the industry. Actually, almost all businesses operate on a prospective basis. They have established prices before the consumers use their services or purchase their products, and the prices are not subject to adjustment. Moreover, before the existence of cost reimbursers, hospital rates were prospective. Room rates and charges for ancillary services were established, and patients were billed. Hospital financial management was much simpler then, and it can be much simpler in the future if we eliminate retroactive determination of reimbursement rates, particularly because the payers do the determining.[73]

While not universally accepted, this realistic view is shared by a substantial number of industry leaders. Moreover, as Katharine Bauer points out in her excellent study, the methodology of rate setting is gradually improving as is the essential data base.[74] What is principally lacking today, we believe, is not a specific methodology or magic all-purpose formula but a political and structural framework that will permit the industry and government to work together toward solution of the problem, taking into account two circumstances that have changed dramatically since 1965: (1) the gradual universalization of third party payments, and (2) the gradual acknowledgment of limited resources.

Under these circumstances, rate setting inevitably becomes essentially a political process. The rest of this discussion is framed about three essentially political questions: (1) How can rates be set most equitably and acceptably, and by whom? (2) Can prospective rates be made to stick? If not, is the exercise worth the effort? (3) Should there be preestablished national and state ceilings ("caps") on operating expenditures?

1. The search for "correct" rates does not lend itself to a "scientific" answer. Detailed data and analysis are, of course, essential. They set a context and framework for decisions but cannot furnish definitive answers regarding what should be done. They will not tell us whether a hospital should emphasize expensive technologies or primary care, whether it should have a salaried emergency room staff as opposed to reliance on "attending"physicians or whether members of the medical staff should sit on the board of directors. Such questions ultimately come down to values and judgment.

Who then can best be depended on for fair judgments most acceptable in a democratic society? The conventional answer of "government" is inadequate, because it begs the essential question, "With what instrumentalities and how?" Whether done in the name of government or not, this is a task in which all affected parties have a responsibility and must participate. We know from experience with regulatory agencies in other fields that no matter how much legal authority is vested in them, the majority of important decisions, if they are to prove viable, emerge from negotiations among the parties.

For such reasons, "negotiated" rates have long been advocated by some of the most public-spirited hospital leaders. They were recommended in the excellent report of the Secretary's (HEW) Advisory Committee on Hospital Effectiveness in 1968.[75] The rationale is that no single regulator is more likely to arrive at balanced and equitable decisions than the product of hard bargaining by buyers and sellers. Nor is any other type of decision making likely to appear more reasonable and be more acceptable to the public. Such decisions can work because both parties accept responsibility for the agreed rates, while arbitrary "caps" have a way of being systematically penetrated until they break down.

In an analytical study of government controls in the Canadian health care system, Lewin and Associates stated as one of their conclusions:

> Perhaps the major lesson for the United States in the Canadian experience is that a negotiated approach to resolving issues relating to

medical insurance activities is feasible. Good negotiations are marked by a number of characteristics—arm's length bargaining, competent analysis, controlled conflict.[76]

Our proposal, therefore, is that the Social Security Act be amended either to repeal "reasonable costs" as a basis of reimbursement or to define "reasonable costs" as the rate levels that emerge from the following process: There should be required, periodic, nationwide, bilateral negotiations between spokesmen for the hospitals (presumably the American Hospital Association, various state associations, and other appropriate representational organizations) and representatives of the major purchasers of services, governmental and private (presumably HEW, Blue Cross Association, and perhaps state insurance commissioners). State officials, however, should not be assigned primary negotiating responsibility. Once Medicaid has been federalized or absorbed into NHI, the states will inevitably lack the necessary incentive to the hard, arm's length bargaining required to make the negotiating process work.

The mission of the negotiators should be to arrive at a firm prospective all-inclusive national rate schedule, providing for appropriate geographic and type-of-hospital variations, that is binding on both parties for a specified period, for example, two years. A condition for effectiveness would be a formal or informal understanding by the hospitals and state commissioners that the agreed rates would apply to all other purchasers of care, to assure equity.

The results of the bargaining process should be subject to approval by an independent National Board of Review, which would have three major functions: (a) establishment and periodic review of the national guidelines, (b) review of the current rate schedules to determine that no relevant law, public policy, or due process has been circumvented, and (c) in the event that the bargaining parties are unable to arrive at agreement, to arbitrate the difference.

2. We start with the premise that prospective rate setting should mean what it says: a fixed price for a defined product for a fixed period of time. Conceivably, the negotiators may decide that the "product" or "unit" for which the rate is set, may differ for different institutions with different case mixes. They could be paid on the basis of itemized charges, per diem costs, the number of patients served, or patient stay by diagnosis. In some cases, the "rate" could include both inpatient and outpatient care, or even total health care on a capitation basis for the entire service area, thus approximating the HMO concept. The law and the guidelines should encourage flexibility in this respect.

In two respects, however, the guidelines should be clear and firm: (a) rates should not vary according to the source of payment, and (b) rates should be all-inclusive, not limited to "routine" costs or those easier for hospital management to control.

The rate must also put both parties at risk if it is to be fair and if the process is to contain sufficient incentives for serious bargaining on both sides. The buyer takes the risk that actual costs may fall below the bargained rate. The providers assume the risk that costs may be higher. While it is a premise of this entire process that, with proper budgeting and resolute administrative management, costs for a period of two years fall within the boundaries of reasonable predictability (in fact, it can be presumed that the necessity for prediction will serve as a spur to firmer management), yet it must be foreseen that some hospitals, for good or bad reasons, may exceed anticipated costs.

What happens if a number of hospitals, no longer able to shift costs from the prospectively rated services to others not covered, protest "We're going bankrupt; we will have to shut down if we don't get an upward adjustment?" In the American political climate, will government and the other purchasers be able to stand firm, and should they? The danger is that, if adjustments are made, except under the most extraordinary and rare contingencies, the system will break down. The providers need not then take the original negotiation too seriously. The theoretical case for the buyers standing firm is great, even if it means that the defaulting hospitals have to be placed under new management. Perhaps that would be a long run gain for the hospital economy—an empirical method for getting rid of weak management.

Part of the answer will depend on the respect achieved by the National Board of Review and by the negotiating process itself; part on the stake that the negotiators perceive that they have in the success of the system. There is some reason for optimism on the latter point, because the obvious alternative is likely to be some form of government fiat.

Yet, we must acknowledge the possibility that the political circumstances might force an untoward number of "adjustments." We would maintain that the process remains worthwhile. The process of prospective rates through negotiation does oblige hospitals to expose their plans and budgets for review and justification in advance of expenditure. This in itself is a sobering influence. It also promotes good managerial practice. If overruns occur, they will be publicly exposed and must be publicly reviewed and adjudicated. And this, too, has inherent containment incentives.

3. The final question overlaps with the first in that it relates to the context and boundaries of the negotiations. Should the negotiations on "rates" be contained within a preestablished national, regional, or state expenditure ceiling—expressed in dollars or in terms of a maximum allowable annual percentage increase—or should the ceilings emerge as a result of the rate negotiations? Opponents of "caps"—public spokesmen as well as providers—fear, with some reason, that such a policy may lead to undue restraints on scientific and technological innovation, freezing of existing structures and programs, and excessive politicalization of allocation decisions. Proponents acknowledge the risks but insist that "caps" provide the only way to contain unacceptable escalation of hospital costs. If that view prevails, as current trends appear to suggest, the negotiation process we propose should start at the first stage. To minimize the risks and to place rate negotiations in a balanced context, the regulated must be in on the "take-off," that is, the expenditure ceilings themselves must be the product of fair negotiation.[77]

No rate determination policy yet invented is without some vulnerable points. And none will work perfectly or exactly as anticipated. But we know we have done poorly in the past, and traditional methods offer little prospect for improvement. This proposal has at least promise for effectiveness. As a minimum, its new demands and new hopes may break through the paralyzing cynicism that this problem and its depressing experience have imposed on the hospital economy.

Physician Reimbursement

Physicians' fees are the second largest segment in national health care expenditures—about 19 percent in 1976, representing over $26 billion (exclusive of salaries of physicians on hospital payrolls or serving in the Armed Forces). The amount is itself large enough to warrant high priority attention. But since physicians play the primary role in determining most other health care costs, the way in which they are paid takes on much greater significance insofar as it may affect their attitudes and behavior.

Since the end of ESP, HEW has tried to control physicians' fees in Medicare by setting an upper limit to increases in the "prevailing rates" component of "reasonable charges," determined by an "economic index" in accordance with Sec. 224 of P.L. 92-603. The index attempts to reflect changes in operating expenses of physicians in private practice and in the earnings levels in the economy as a whole; it is annually revised. The complexity of the formula is beyond the comprehension of anyone other than an accomplished statistician and has been a growing source of bewildered resentment. More important there are no signs that it has had any effect commensurate with its trouble.

The Ford Administration gave tacit acknowledgment to this failure in 1976 when it proposed a flat ceiling of 4 percent annual increases in fees. It was not acted upon; most people feeling that it was unlikely to be effective. Physicians have too many available devices for circumventing such arbitrary ceilings, such as subdividing units of treatment and charging separately for each. And, as long as physicians are permitted to charge patients more than the approved Medicare level, they will continue to do so.

Essentially, the same conclusion must be drawn regarding "reasonable charges" for physicians as for the "reasonable costs" of hospitals: a decade of frustrating multiple manipulations has demonstrated they just do not work. This does not prove that some other method will work better, but it does demand that some basic departure from the failed method be tried.

The change should follow along the same lines proposed for determining hospital reimbursement. The "reasonable charges" provisions of the Social Security Act should be amended so fees can be fixed in advance on the basis of rates negotiated nationally and regionally between the third party buyers and appropriate medical societies, very much in the same manner as proposed for the hospitals. The fees should reflect geographic differences, specialty levels, differential diagnoses and procedures, and other significant variants. The agreed rates should probably be fixed for a period of two years.

Predetermined rate schedules have some history and precedents in physicians' fees that offer reasonable encouragement regarding their feasibility. As mentioned earlier, some government programs have long operated with fixed fees. Some insurance companies have done the same in experimental programs. Several state medical societies developed "relative value schedules" as early as the 1950s. While these do not set fees in monetary terms, they do establish accepted relationships among such fees by procedures. Some of the specialty societies have also developed relative value scales over a number of years.

While the Federal Trade Commission has recently challenged the legality of such schedules, with the well-intentioned belief that they inhibiit competition, it is doubtful that the notion that there can be effective price competition among doctors in the medical marketplace will stand up. In any case, that is a matter that Congress can decide. The point here is that doctors are not strangers to predetermined schedules and fees; the technical problems are manageable.

If agreed-on rates are arrived at, it would no longer be necessary to make distinctions between "assignments" and reimbursements to the patients, a Medicare albatross long admitted to be a source of inflation and discrimination. Both parties would agree on what should be the "full payment" in all cases (except for the 20 percent coinsurance). For the first time, there might be some predictability in the price of physicians' services over at least two years. If NHI comes along, a workable model would be available for setting universal fees.

Negotiated rates do not remove the possibilities for evasion available to physicians. But they can produce a working climate that is likely to diminish them. As in the case of hospitals, it can be reasonably anticipated that having agreed to a "fair" level of reimbursement, the antagonisms and self-justification that lead to evasion will be minimized. In addition, the medical societies, having been direct parties in the negotiations, may be expected to assume greater responsibility for compliance.

There are increasing signs that medical societies might prefer such an arrangement to their present profitable but increasingly vulnerable and exasperating situation. The societies in a few states, notably South Carolina and Georgia, are reported to be considering moving to negotiated fee schedules with HEW, even in the absence of any statutory requirement. It is certainly credible to anticipate that most societies might welcome negotiated rates if only to escape continuation of the present unilaterally imposed and incomprehensible Medicare formula and the unknown demons that may lie ahead.

Competition

There are some substantial segments of health care where competition can be significant and should be further promoted. While hospitals are not usually in price competition with one another, the vast array of nonpayroll items they purchase could be highly competitive. These include drugs, appliances, equipment, consultant services, contracted housekeeping services, etc.

But for such competition to be fully operative, the buyer must have strong incentives to "shop around," to bargain, or even to refrain completely from too high priced a purchase. That is one of the objectives of the proposed prospective fixed rates. If the hospitals were placed at risk by having to live within predetermined rates, there would be reason for them to assume the more demanding role of a frugal buyer. Prepaid group practice plans may already have such motivation.

More price competition could also be encouraged in consumer purchases of prescription drugs and appliances. Studies have shown that large numbers of doctors do not know the comparative prices among different items they prescribe. It should not be difficult to devise a method to keep doctors currently informed, and this could have a moderating effect on their prescribing patterns, including the number of pills in a single prescription. Encouragement of generic prescribing would also help. In addition, price posting by retailers would enable consumers to do comparative shopping or at least to know in advance the price that will be charged. The 1974 Maximum Allowable Cost (MAC) Medicare regulation—which limits reimbursement to pharmacists to acquisition cost plus a dispensing fee and, in the case of chemically identical drugs, to the lowest priced of those generally available—is a step in the right direction.

For a time, shortly after Medicare went into effect, it was presumed that the fast growth of for-profit or investor-owned hospitals would introduce a strong element of competition into the hospital field. For a variety of reasons—among them, the extraordinary rise in construction and investment costs—the boom in proprietary hospitals lasted only a short time. By 1975 they represented 13 percent of all community hospitals, but only 8 percent of the beds.[78] Mainly they are located in smaller communities and frequently are not in direct competition with other hospitals. Whether they have had a price-moderating influence is not clear. A 1976 study prepared for Blue Cross found that investor-owned hospitals had higher per diem costs and higher charges for comparable diagnoses than the nonprofits.[79] Although this finding was challenged in two studies commissioned by the American Federation of Hospitals, chief spokesman for the investor-owned institutions,[80] the net evidence was such as to "test the conventional wisdom" in this area. Despite their considerable contribution to hospital management concepts and practices (a substantial number of voluntary hospitals have contracted with for-profit hospital corporations for ongoing management services), and the probability of some continued growth, it does not seem likely that the proprietary institutions will play a major role in overall hospital financing for the foreseeable future.

The most actively advocated device for large scale competition by those who still maintain a belief in the possibility of a free market in health care is the HMO. Some of its proponents believe that we must not only make such organizations available throughout the country as an active competitor with traditional fee-for-service medicine, but there must be enough HMOs or other capitation-type organizations to compete with one another.[81]

We enthusiastically endorse HMOs as an alternative delivery system (Selections 19, 20, 32, and 34). We believe that they have real potential for conserving costs—mainly through greater emphasis on ambulatory care and concomitant reductions in hospital utilization. (There is, of course, the opposite danger of underutilization.) But HMOs have a long history that does not justify reliance on the prospect of rapid increase as an important aggregate influence on costs.

In the 30 or more years of their existence, growth has been disappointly slow; they have hardly kept up with the expanding medical economy. Even official encouragement and subsidies by government have had small effect. While one can find many flaws in the governmental action—administrative neglect that belies the enthusiastic rhetoric, and the excessive requirements imposed by the HMO Act of 1973 for qualification—it is clear that the HMO formula has limited appeal. In 1976 only about 3 percent of total U.S. population was enrolled, although the percentage was, of course, higher in areas where HMOs exist.

The Congress amended the HMO Act in 1976 to remove many of the restrictions. It had earlier legislated "dual choice," that is, each employer with a health insurance plan must offer an option to employees to select HMO coverage, where one exists. The dual choice device was originated by the Kaiser Foundation Health Plan and is an option primarily of preference, not price. These and other encouragements to HMO development are desirable, and are likely to lead to some expansion. But it must be acknowledged that a real proliferation of HMOs is a long term and evolutionary possibility at best. The government can encourage and support, but it should not mandate.

Utilization

By conventional and relatively crude measures, the role of utilization has been a relatively minor factor in rising costs, both in Medicare and the population as a whole. The proportion of Medicare Part B enrollees using covered services changed only slightly between 1968 and 1974, moving from 79 percent to 81 percent.[82] The proportion of elderly admitted to short term hospitals did increase, but the decline in length of stay resulted in a net decrease in the number of days of care, from 3,575 per 1,000 enrollees in 1967 to 3,556 in 1973. In the population as a whole, the number of ambulatory physician contacts per person has been remarkably stable since 1971, averaging about five per person.[83] The pattern is similar in respect to use of community hospitals.

Such raw data are, however, not very instructive. They do not tell us whether utilization is too high, too low, or about right. As most averages, they may conceal that there is as much underutilization as overutilization, although it is now known that the poor are using as much or more services than middle and upper income classes. The crude data represent only contact units or number of hospital days. They do not tell us the character of such encounters. Great changes could be taking place without altering such data. That obscures the important issue in utilization—as in quality—the changing patterns or "intensity" of care. Has a significant elaboration of procedures been compressed into about the same number of so-called "contacts" or hospital days? Has fragmentation of services caused additional contacts for the same amount of care?

For example, physicians now generally concede that they order an unnecessary number of laboratory and radiological tests. They call it "defensive medicine," and recently they have placed the blame on fear of malpractice suits (and earlier on private health insurance). Whatever the cause, this is excess utilization. Similarly, the medical literature reflects the general view that too much surgery is being practiced. In short, the costs of utilization are determined less by the number of contacts than by what is done, or not done, during such interaction. Thus, in economic terms, as well as quality terms, primary attention must be directed to the latter.

It is conventional to say that "what will be done" is determined by the "state of the art." That is only partly true. There are numerous other factors that will determine how, when, and what part of "the art" will be employed, such as:

1. The relative availability and accessibility of appropriate acute and long term care facilities. Many hospitals have large case loads of the chronically ill who would be better served by nonhospital long term programs if only they were available.

2. The relative availability of expensive equipment and procedures. If every hospital aspires to become a tertiary care institution and equips itself accordingly, there will be an inevitable tendency, if not pressure, to use such procedures more than would otherwise be the case. In medical care, as in other fields, choices are frequently available to the decision maker. The environment in which the physician operates is an important conditioner of the option he selects.

3. The character and coverage cf health insurance or other third party coverage. It has long been known that the unbalanced protection of most health insurance creates pressures on both doctors and patients for unnecessary use of hospitals. Similarly, as we noted earlier, there is a well-known differential in use of hospitals and elective surgery between members of prepaid group practice plans and patients with other types of insurance.

4. Physician motivation. In large part this is related to the above three items, plus the physician's educational experiences, especially the nature of his residency. These factors help determine the physician's attitude with respect to economy and costs, collegial status, and the patient. His own monetary incentives and the monetary needs of his hospital play a role. So does his self-image as specialist or family practitioner.

Since utilization problems overlap many other considerations, most of these factors, and what might be done about them, have been discussed earlier. Here we reiterate only two points. First, if PSRO provisions for utilization review are broadened as recommended, and responsibly implemented and supported, any additional bureaucratic layer would be redundant and purposeless. It is in the medical care financing and delivery system culture that the more important changes need to be made.

One addition does seem called for. The recent experiments by some Blue Cross plans with a "second opinion" in cases of recommended surgery is worth consideration for Medicare and Medicaid. The early evidence not only indicates the probability of substantial cost saving, if done on a selective basis, but it also introduces an element of consumer choice and judgment that is otherwise largely absent from medical care decisions.

Second, the many factors affecting utilization again emphasize that the primary decision maker is the physician, not the patient. Proposals to use deterrent cost sharing as a utilization monitor aim at the wrong target. Far more important and potentially effective would be incentives aimed at the physician. That is admittedly more complicated.

Hospital Organization

The language and therefore the assumptions, underlying much of the economic discussion of hospitals, are frequently inconsistent with realities of hospital organization. We speak of "incentives for the hospital," "place the hospital at risk," and "hospital management." The words encourage an illusion that there exists a unified institution with an identifiable and responsible decision-making center with internal control. This is not the reality.

The typical hospital is a tripartite arrangement of trustees, administration, and medical staff with the formal lines of authority often in conflict with the practice. By historical accident, a central feature of the American hospital has been its use as a place for the private practitioner to bring his private patients for treatment, but where he had no administrative or financial responsibilities. In return, the doctor was expected to donate care for the indigent, who once constituted the majority of hospital patients. That structure long ago became an anachronism.

Ultimate responsibility for policy has always rested with lay trustees. They can have control over the administrator, if they wish to exercise it, but neither they nor he has effective control of the medical staff which, individually or collectively, dominate most significant decisions. In the eyes of physicians, the administrator is in charge only of nonmedical aspects of the hospital's operations. Thus, in the hospital business, it is customary to speak of "dual control." The two lines often overlap and are blurred. While physicians have no financial or budgetary accountability, they do control most of the hospital's activities which determine both revenues and expenditures. In effect, dual control often means no control.

Obviously, this situation enormously complicates the problem of effectuating the proposals made to influence hospital behavior. In their present state of disjunction, it is difficult to say who, if anybody, can control the behavior of "the hospital." Awareness of this serious limitation on authority may be the reason that attempted reforms, dealing with hospitals, are often watered down to the point of ineffectuality, as in the case of the 1976 Talmadge bill's numerous exceptions to the application of prospective rates.

That problem is also harrassing the Canadian system. A recent report states:

> The current incentives in the Canadian hospital insurance program place only the administrator at risk. While difficult to achieve, it is important that incentives in such programs be structured so there is a community of interests within the institution to restrain expenses and utilization.[84]

Our proposals for stronger controls over capital development and for negotiated prospective rates should help increase motivation to bridge the structural duality. The existence of firm and all-inclusive predetermined rates, designed to contain individual and collective professional ambitions, should be conducive to more integrated decision making and coordinated behavior. This may, over the long run, set the stage for more basic structural reform. In addition, the demands of public negotiation and public justifications should motivate, if not require, more responsible involvement of the medical staffs.

Beyond such devices, the integration of the hospital will require highly professionalized and respected management. Fortunately, the trends are in that direction. But cultures do not change quickly. The image of the hospital as "the doctor's workshop" bemuses trustees and administrators just as it does the general public. Only slowly are we coming to think of the hospital as an institution that primarily serves patients, rather than physicians. The implications for that distinction are greater than often recognized.

In the interim, we should consider what can be done now to strengthen hospital management vis-à-vis the numerous centrifugal forces within the institution. Hospital administrators complain of the necessity of hiring more allied health personnel than they need to meet the required certification and accredition procedures, requirements which they blame, in turn, on the numerous "guilds."[85] This is a problem that has been with us for years but has become more obvious with rising hospital wage levels and the constant proliferation of specialized technologies. Institutional, rather than individual, licensure has been suggested as one remedy.

Whether this is the answer or not, it is clear that ways must be found to strengthen managerial capability and at the same time to increase employee sense of identification with the institution, its goals, decisions, and financial status. Relevant experience such as the Quebec experiment with employee representation on hospital boards and the "codetermination" or *"mitbestimmung"* movement in Western Europe should be watched for possible guidance.

Fraud

Only a brief word need be said here about the mounting publicity on medical fraud, particularly in Medicaid, which the Senate Subcommittee on Long-Term Care of the Special Committee on Aging estimated had mulcted taxpayers of $1.5 billion in fiscal year 1975, probably an underestimate, since fraud by its nature is not always detectable. There has been universal revulsion. Congress has increased the federal penalties for such fraud and mandated an Office of Inspector-General in HEW to help uncover it. These should be promptly implemented. While fraud directly involves only a very small portion of the industry, its persistence has a corrosive effect on the whole. Three aditional observations may be worth noting:

1. The revelations indicate that HEW must take a much more active role in monitoring Medicaid. Many of the states, which have the most immediate responsibility, have neither the resources nor the skills to deal with the subtle instruments of modern fraud.
2. However active the government is, it will never fully succeed in mastering the situation unless the professional societies take on a full measure of earnest self-policing and cooperation with the authorities. The medical societies have protested that they do not have the power to suspend a physician, as the bar associations can disbar a lawyer. True, but the power of the profession to influence licensing authorities and to discipline recalcitrant members and to establish the ethical climate of the profession is prodigious.
3. It is insufficiently appreciated that welfare medicine has always contained a larger self-corrupting component. Means tests, the identification of pauperism, and discriminatory designations of selected populations not only seem to dictate a two-level quality of care but also have always generated a set of attitudes in both providers and patients that raises the tolerance level for corruption. It is significant that there is far less fraud in Medicare than in Medicaid. A properly designed national health insurance program, which abjures means tests, would probably not be characterized by "Medicaid mills" or by patients so intimidated by the pauper designation as to acquiesce readily to being accessories to exploitation.

* * *

This extended discussion on controlling costs should not be misleading. We do not believe there is anything inherently right or wrong about spending 8 or 9 percent of the gross national product, or even more, for health care. The question is whether we are spending these vast amounts wisely or effectively. While we must be concerned with whether Americans are being taxed or charged for more than they are receiving and, ultimately, with the question of how much of the nation's resources can we sensibly allocate to health care, our immediate concern here is with the relation of health care payment policies and practices to the maintenance of individual health. To the extent that such policies and practices do appear to be contributing commensurately to health, we would not quarrel with costs. But, to the extent that the practices have acquired a life and momentum of their own, not significantly related to considerations of health, they must be challenged and corrected.

Not only is there substantial question as to whether the costly increments in spending each year are contributing to health, there is the even more disturbing question of whether "easy money" and indifference to economy and efficiency do not establish a climate wherein quality of care is negatively affected. A point can be reached in the levels and manner of expenditure that is not merely wasteful, but is actually harmful. As we have said, economy is not the enemy of quality. More often the two are likely to be complementary and mutually advantageous disciplines.

NOTES

1. For example, Ivan Illich, *Medical Nemesis: The Expropriation of Health* (New York: Pantheon Books, 1976); Rick Carlson, *The End of Medicine* (New York: John Wiley & Sons, 1975).

2. A small but carefully controlled study of short term, voluntary, nonteaching hospitals in Massachusetts found that "higher costs per case were significantly associated with a higher, not lower, medical-surgical death rate even after case mix severity is taken into account." The authors conclude that there is "no incompatibility between the goals of efficiency and quality of care." The primary managerial variables of interest were identified as "visibility of consequences, participation in decision-making, and the ratio of scheduled group meetings to unscheduled meetings." S.M. Shortell, S.W. Becker, and D. Neuhauser, "The Effects of Management Practices on Hospital Efficiency and Quality of Care," in Shortell and Brown, eds., *Organizational Research in Hospitals* (Chicago: Blue Cross Association, An *Inquiry* Book, 1976), pp. 100-04.

3. Howard Hiatt, M.D., "Protecting the Medical Commons: Who Is Responsible?" *New England Journal of Medicine* 293 (July 31, 1975): 235-241; A.R. Somers, *The Philadelphia Medical Commons* (Philadelphia: Blue Cross and Blue Shield, 1976.)

4. Bruce C. Vladeck, "Why Non-Profits Go Broke," *The Public Interest,* (Winter 1976): 87.

5. See, e.g., National Commission for Manpower Policy, *Employment Impacts of Health Policy Developments,* Special Report 11 (Washington, D.C.: October 1976).

6. M.S. Mueller and P.A. Piro, "Private Health Insurance in 1974," *Social Security Bulletin* 39 (March 1976), p. 4. The article uses the term "insurance protection" but the authors inform us that the interpretation used here is correct. Telephone interview with M.S. Mueller, September 3, 1976.

7. Department of Health, Education, and Welfare, National Center for Health Statistics, *Hospital and Surgical Insurance Coverage Among Persons Under 65 in the U.S., 1974,* 25, no. 2 (May 19, 1976): 4.

8. Karen Davis, "The Case for National Health Insurance," *Trustee,* March 1976, p. 21.

9. H.M. and A.R. Somers, "Major Issues in National Health Insurance," *Milbank Memorial Fund Quarterly* 50 (April 1972): Part 1, pp. 177-210.

10. R.M. Ball, "A Self-Supporting Comprehensive National Health Insurance Plan," National Academy of Sciences, Institute of Medicine, February 4, 1977, manuscript.

11. Davis, *op. cit.*, p. 21.

12. M.J. Mueller and P.A. Piro, "Private Health Insurance in 1974," *Social Security Bulletin* 39 (March 1976): 18.

13. Marion Gornick, "Ten Years of Medicare: Impact on the Covered Population," *Social Security Bulletin* 39 (July 1976): 17.

14. H.M. Schmeck, Jr., "Law on Kidney Aids is Termed Unfair," *New York Times*, August 29, 1976.

15. M.S. Mueller and R.M. Gibson, "National Health Expenditures, FY 1975," *Social Security Bulletin* 39 (February 1976): 14.

16. Alexander Leaf, M.D., at Duke University Medical Center Board of Visitors Meeting, April 3, 1976.

17. *Matter of Quinlan*, 70 N.J. 10 (1976).

18. A.L. Cochrane, *Effectiveness and Efficiency* (London: Nuffield Provincial Hospitals Trust, 1972).

19. R. Zeckhauser and D. Shepard, "Where Now for Saving Lives?" Discussion Paper Series No. 42 D, J.F. Kennedy School of Government, Harvard University, May 1976, and bibliography.

20. *Genetic Screening* (Washington, D.C.: National Academy of Sciences, 1975).

21. Brian Abel-Smith, "Value for Money in Health Services," *Social Security Bulletin* 37 (July 1974): 25.

22. U.E. Reinhardt, "Health Manpower Policy in the United States," paper presented to University of Pennsylvania Bicentennial Conference on Health Policy, November 11-12, 1976 (in press).

23. American Medical Association, "Medical Education in the United States, 1974-75," *Journal of the American Medical Association* 234, no. 13 (December 1975): 1333.

24. *Physicians for a Growing America* (Washington, D.C.: U.S. Department of Health, Education, and Welfare, Public Health Service, 1959), p. v.

25. American Medical Association, *op. cit.*, pp. 1337-1338.

26. *Health U.S. 1975* (Washington, D.C.: U.S. Department of Health, Education, and Welfare, National Center for Health Statistics, 1975), p. 117.

27. American Medical Association, Center for Health Services Research and Development, *Physician Distribution and Medical Licensure in the U.S. 1974* (Chicago: The Association, 1975), p. 12.

28. *Forward Plan for Health, FY 1978-82* (Washington, D.C.: U.S. Department of Health, Education, and Welfare, Public Health Service, August 1976), p. 55.

29. Reinhardt, *op. cit.*, pp. 40-42.

30. HEW, Bureau of Health Resources Development, *The Supply of Health Manpower: 1970 Profiles and Projections for 1990* (Washington, D.C.: 1974), pp. 48, 53, 54.

31. *The Position of the AAMC on the House and Senate-Passed Bills on Health Manpower (H.R. 5546)* (Washington, D.C.: Association of American Medical Colleges, Aug. 18, 1976), p. 8; Attachment II, Table 1.

32. "Senate Bill Puts Controls on Doctor Training," *Congressional Quarterly Weekly Report*, June 5, 1976, p. 1433.

33. Letter to Senator Edward M. Kennedy from John F. Sherman, Vice President, Association of American Medical Colleges, August 20, 1976, p. 2.
34. Institute of Medicine, *Medicare-Medicaid Reimbursement Policies* (Washington, D.C.: National Academy of Sciences, March 1976).
35. *Forward Plan for Health, FY 1978-82, op. cit.,* p. 54.
36. H.B. Curry *et al., Twenty Years of Community Medicine* (Frenchtown, N.J.: Columbia Publishing Co., 1974).
37. Association of American Medical Colleges, "Comments on Institute of Medicine Social Security Studies," June 1976, p. 18.
38. J.J. Boardman, Jr., "Utilization Data and the Planning Process," in A.R. Somers, ed., *The Kaiser-Permanente Medical Care Program: A Symposium* (New York: The Commonwealth Fund, 1971), p. 65.
39. *Hospital Statistics, 1976 Edition,* (Chicago: American Hospital Association), Table 1, pp. 3-4.
40. *Medical Care Expenditures, Prices, and Costs: Background Book* (Washington, D.C.: HEW, Social Security Administration, 1975), p. 82.
41. *Ibid.,* p. 80.
42. For example, A.R. Somers and F.M. Moore, "Homemaker Services: An Essential Option for the Elderly," *Public Health Reports* 91, (July-August, 1976): 354-359; Congressional Budget Office, *Long-Term Care for the Elderly and Disabled* (Washington, D.C.: U.S. Government Printing Office, February 1977).
43. The Community Service Society of New York reported that Medicaid and Blue Cross were able to avoid spending $6.5 million in 1974 and 1975 because of penalties for excess bed capacity in New York State. The State Health Department said 4,365 beds had been closed during the two years under a state law setting penalties and decertification of beds when occupancy falls below minimum levels. "Medicaid and Blue Cross Saving Millions on Excess-Bed Penalties," *New York Times,* October 17, 1976.
44. For discussion of this issue, see M.E. DeBakey, M.D., and H.H. Hiatt, M.D., "Medical Technology: How Much is Enough?" in National Leadership Conference on America's Health Policy, *Proceedings* (Washington, D.C.: National Journal, 1976).
45. U.S. Congress, Office of Technology Assessment, *The Computed Tomography (CT or CAT) Scanner and Its Implications for Health Policy,* prepared at request of U.S. Senate Committee on Labor and Public Welfare and Committee on Finance (Washington, D.C.: U.S. Government Printing Office, September 1976, draft), p. 57.
46. See, for example, Hiatt, *op. cit.,* note 44; S.H. Shapiro and S.M. Wyman, "CAT Fever," *New England Journal of Medicine* 294 (April 22, 1976): 954-956; D.F. Phillips and K. Lille, "Putting the Leash on CAT," *Hospitals* 50 (July 1, 1976): 45-49. For general discussion of the need for, and problems of, assessing the social impact of new medical technologies, including nine specific case histories, see U.S. Congress, Office of Technology Assessment, *Development of Medical Technology: Opportunities for Assessment* (Washington, D.C.: U.S. Government Printing Office, August 1976).
47. Institute of Medicine, *Controlling the Supply of Hospital Beds* (Washington, D.C.: National Academy of Sciences, October 1976), pp. vii, ix. A later HEW-commissioned report, prepared by InterStudy, stated that hospital capacity could be reduced 5 to 10 percent over the next five years by retiring idle capacity, and another 10 percent by eliminating "unnecessarily utilized capacity." American Hospital Association, *Washington Developments* 6 (April 27, 1977): 1.

48. Ball, *op. cit.*, pp. 1-2, 9-10.

49. For example, *Health Professions Educational Assistance Act of 1974* (S.3585) and *Hearings* related thereto; National Board of Medical Examiners, Committee on Goals and Priorities, *Evaluation in the Continuum of Medical Education* (Philadelphia: National Board of Medical Examiners, 1973); H.S. Cohen and L. Miike, *Developments in Health Manpower Licensure,* HEW Publ. (HRA) 74-3101, Washington, D.C., 1973.

50. American Board of Medical Specialites, *Annual Report 1975-1976* (Evanston, Ill: 1976), and unpublished data, September 1976.

51. For example, J.S. Lublin, "Outfit That Accredits Hospitals Helps Set Quality of Patient Care.... Are Surveys a 'Whitewash'?" *Wall Street Journal,* January 13, 1975.

52. Jean Hochheimer, Bureau of Quality Assurance HEW, telephone communication, February 24, 1977. Among the numerous controversies over area designations, Texas was reduced from nine to one in 1976 at the insistence of state medical society.

53. For example, R.H. Brook, A.D. Avery *et al., Quality of Medical Care Assessment Using Outcome Measures,* 3 vols. (Santa Monica, Calif.: Rand Corporation, 1976).

54. American Society of Internal Medicine, Conference on Assessing Physician Performance on Ambulatory Care, June 1976, *Proceedings* (San Francisco: The Society, 1976).

55. R.J. Haggerty, M.D., Chairman, *Assessing Quality in Health Care: An Evaluation* (Washington, D.C.: National Academy of Sciences, Institute of Medicine, 1976). See also, R.H. Brook and K.H. Williams, *Evaluation of the New Mexico Peer Review System 1971-1973* (Santa Monica, Calif: Rand Corporation, 1977); W.J. McNerney, "The Quandry of Quality Assessment," *New England Journal of Medicine* 295 (December 30, 1976): 1511-1515.

56. *Darling v. Charleston Community Memorial Hospital,* 33 Ill. 2d 236, 211 N.E. 2d 253 (1965).

57. Stephen M. Blaes, "The Legal Perspective," *Trustee* (May 1976): 9-11.

58. F.D. Moore, M.D., "Surgical Biology and Applied Sociology: Cannon and Codman Fifty Years Later," *Harvard Medical Alumni Bulletin* 49, no. 3 (1975):12-21.

59. L. Ledbetter, "California Grants Terminally Ill Right to Put an End to Treatment," *New York Times,* October 2, 1976. For comparison of "right-to-die" bills introduced into the various state legislatures, as of 1976, see Society for the Right-to-Die, Inc., *Death with Dignity: Legislative Manual,* 1976 Ed. (New York: The Society, 1977).

60. A.A. Narvaez, "New Jersey Adopts Plan on Patients in Coma," *New York Times,* January 26, 1977.

61. H.M. and A.R. Somers, *Medicare and the Hospitals* (Washington, D.C.: The Brookings Institution, 1967), p. 259.

62. *Ibid.,* p. 261.

63. *Hospital Statistics, op. cit.,* pp. xix, xxii, 4.

64. R. Hutchings, HEW, Health Resources Administration, telephone communication, March 24, 1977.

65. See, for example, D.S. Salkever and T.W. Bice, *Impact of State Certificate-of-Need Laws on Health Care Costs and Utilization,* National Center for Health Services Research, HEW Publ. (HRA 77-3163), 1977.

66. B.C. Vladeck, "Interest-Group Representation and the HSAs: Health Planning and Political Theory," *American Journal of Public Health,* 67 (January 1977): 23-29.

67. For example, AHA, "Guidelines for Review and Approval of Rates for Health Care Institutions and Services by a State Commission," (Chicago: 1972).

68. F.L. Sattler, ed., *Hospital Prospective Payment: Issues and Experiences* (Minneapolis: InterStudy, June 1976).

69. For a summary of studies and demonstrations under way as of mid-1976, see, T.W. Galblum, *Research in Health Care Reimbursement,* U.S. Department of Health, Education, and Welfare, HEW Publ. (SSA) 77-11901.

70. Katharine Bauer, "Hospital Rate Setting—This Way to Salvation?" in M. Zubkoff and I.E. Raskin, eds., *Hospital Cost Control* (New York: Milbank Memorial Fund, in press); AHA, "Report on Rate Regulatory Programs," January 1977 (processed); F.L. Sattler and D. Burns, *Abstracts of State Rate Review and Prospective Payment Legislation* (Minneapolis: InterStudy, May 1976); H.A. Cohen and R.J. Davidson, "The Maryland Health Services Cost Review Commission: The Perspective of the Regulator and the Regulated," Health Insurance Association of America, *HIAA Viewpoint,* January 1977; B.M. Kinzer, *Experience with the Health Regulatory System in the Commonwealth of Massachusetts* (Chicago: Teachum Inc., 1977, in press).

71. C.R. Gaus and F.J. Hellinger, "Results of Hospital Prospective Reimbursement in the U.S.," paper presented to NIH Fogarty International Center, International Conference on Policies for the Containment of Health Care Costs, June 3, 1976, Bethesda, Md. (processed), pp. 16-17. See, also, references in note 70.

72. Bauer, *op. cit.*

73. H.G. Barth, "Prospective Reimbursement Holds Promise, Poses Problems," *Hospitals* 50 (October 1, 1976): 81.

74. For a useful survey and analysis of the range of data and data-collecting procedures now employed by the federal and state governments and Blue Cross for rate-setting or rate-review purposes and recommendations for improvements, see, K.G. Bauer, Principal Investigator, *Improving the Information for Hospital Rate Setting* (Cambridge, Mass: Harvard University Center for Community Health and Medical Care, 1976).

75. HEW, Secretary's Advisory Committee on Hospital Effectiveness, *Report,* (Washington, D.C.: U.S. Government Printing Office, 1968), p. 28.

76. Lewin and Associates, *Government Controls on the Health Care System: The Canadian Experience, Summary* (Washington, D.C.: Lewin and Associates, 1976), p. 10.

77. In a novel experiment all 23 hospitals in the Rochester, New York, area are participating in a two-year experiment whereby their reimbursement is set by a regional panel representing the hospitals, two Blue Cross plans, consumer groups, and state and federal governments. Payments are related to an overall community health plan that could entail closing of underused or duplicate services. *Medical World News,* January 10, 1977, p. 11.

78. *Hospital Statistics, 1976 Edition, op. cit.,* p. 4.

79. *Investor-Owned Hospitals: An Examination of Performance,* a study by Lewin and Associates for Blue Cross Association (Chicago: Health Services Foundation, 1976), pp. 176-177.

80. *Ibid.,* pp. 126-173, 180.

81. C.C. Havighurst, "Regulation of Health Facilities and Services by Certificate-of-Need," *Virginia Law Review* 59 (October 1973): 1143-1229; Paul Ellwood, Jr., M.D., "Alternatives to Regulation: Improving the Market," in Institute of Medicine, *Controls on Health Care* (Washington, D.C.: National Academy of Sciences, 1976), pp. 49-72.

82. Gornick, *op. cit.*, p. 7.

83. HEW, Health Resources Administration, *Baselines for Setting Health Goals and Standards*, HEW Publ. (HRA) 76-640, p. 60.

84. *Government Controls on the Health Care System: The Canadian Experience, op. cit.*, p. 6.

85. For example, L.W. Cronkhite, Jr., M.D., in National Leaderhsip Conference on America's Health Policy, *op. cit.*, p. 40.

Epilogue

Health Care, Technology, and the Political System: The Sorcerer's Apprentice Revisited

Epilogue

Health Care, Technology, and the Political System: The Sorcerer's Apprentice Revisited*

The specter of the automated robot or unloosed genie that starts out as the obedient, hard-working servant of man and ends up as his potential master has haunted poets and philosophers throughout the ages. Goethe's sorcerer's apprentice, Aladdin's genie, and the Jewish legend of the Golem are all variations on this theme. In *R.U.R.*, Karel Capek's successful play of the early 1920s, the universal robots revolt successfully against their human masters, kill all of them, and are only saved from extinction themselves when one robot couple learns the secret of humanity—the capacity for love and suffering.

An equally terrifying vision of an imminent future in which Western society has become a hypertechnologized, hypersexed, and violence-prone slum is portrayed in a number of recent films such as Stanley Kubrick's widely acclaimed *Clockwork Orange*. According to this view, rather than being conquered by the robots, man's own personailty is debased and vulgarized almost beyond recognition.

In the beginning, modern industrial technology was greeted with fear and hostility. The Luddites, breaking up the new mechanical looms in the English textile mills at the beginning of the Industrial Revolution, have become symbols of this fear. During the hundred years of almost continuous technological progress, from the mid-19th to the mid-20th centuries, their fears and those of the artists were generally dismissed as irrational.

Classical economists were confident that the marketplace was an effective self-regulating mechanism, with both supply and demand governed by man's basic rationality. Marxists rejected the market as regulator but were confident that government, acting on behalf of the masses, could control technology and turn it to constructive ends. Those whose economic and political philosophy fell somewhere between these extremes—European democratic socialists, Keynesian liberals, American pragmatists, and others—looked to various combina-

---

*Excerpt from A.R. Somers, "Health Care and the Political System: The Sorcerer's Apprentice Revisited," presented to the National Center for Health Services Research and Development, Conference on Technology and Health Care Systems in the 1980s, January 1972, San Francisco, and to the Association of University Professors of Opthalmology, January 1972, Key Biscayne, Florida; published in *American Journal of Ophthalmology*, 73 (April 1972): 600-609, and in U.S. Department of Health, Education, and Welfare, National Center for Health Services Research and Development, *Technology and Health Care Systems in the 1980s: Proceedings of a Conference*, Morris F. Collen, Chairman, HEW Publ. 73-3016, pp. 37-45.

tions of competitive and regulatory disciplines. Fearing overconcentration of power in government as well as uncontrolled private enterprise, the liberals and pragmatists agreed that the political process was not only a reliable brake on the excesses of capitalism but an effective device for spreading the benefits of technology to the population at large.

In the past few years, however, there has been a rapid increase in the ranks of those who fear that technology, like the apprentice's robot, may now be out of control; that the economic philosophy of continuous growth, with which it is associated, may be doing more harm than good; and that government, far from being an effective regulator of technological excess, may have already been captured by it.

The physical scientists and ecologists were the first to warn of danger. For example, in January 1972, 33 leading British scientists, including the distinguished biologist Sir Julian Huxley and other environmentalists, endorsed a report, "Blueprint for Survival," that is the one of the starkest doom warnings yet. They warned that the world is heading for an inevitable social and enviromental breakdown—"within the lifetime of someone born today"—unless man fundamentally alters his long-imbedded drive for growth and industrialization. Here is part of their reasoning:

> Continued exponential growth of consumption of materials and energy is impossible. Present reserves of all but a few metals will be exhausted within 50 years, if consumption rates continue to grow as they are. Obviously, there will be new discoveries and advances in mining technology, but these are likely to provide us with only a limited stay of execution.
>
> At the same time, we are sowing the seeds of massive unemployment by increasing the ratio of capital to labor so that the provision of each becomes ever more expensive. In a world of fast diminishing resourses, we shall quickly come to the point when very great numbers of people will be thrown out of work, when the material compensations of urban life are either no longer available or prohibitively expensive, and consequently when whole sections of society will find good cause to express their discontent in ways likely to be anything but pleasant for their fellows.

More recently, social scientists are beginning to agree. Odin Anderson points out that the automobile has become "an independent variable determining the shape of our living patterns." John Kenneth Galbraith saw the origins of corporate giantism, "the new industrial state," and the military-industrial complex in the imperatives of advanced technology. Jay Forrester of the Massachusetts Institute of Technology says, "Our greatest challenge now is how to handle the transition from growth into equilibrium."

"The Luddites were *not* all wrong!" according to the British economist, Ezra Mishan, whose "Mishanic Message" of antitechnology and antigrowth is attracting scholary attention. Senators and Congressmen, trying to cope with miliary technology, and its victims of smog in many of our major industrial comnunities undoubtedly agree.

Whether the Luddites were, in fact, right or wrong; whether man, the clever pprentice, by stealing the secrets of his master—God or Nature or the Cosnos—has unloosed forces which he can no longer control is a question that only he future can answer. There is no question, however, that the comfortable opimism of the late 19th and early 20th centuries has been shattered and that the fficacy of all three major supports of this optimism—technology, economic rowth, and government as the ultimate regulator of both—is now widely quesioned.

We in the health field have, in one sense, less reason for concern than some of our brethren in the physical sciences. Despite advances of recent years, technology still plays a relatively minor role. And despite the rapid recent increase in government financing, health care is still predominantly a private sector activity. Nevertheless, the general trends are clearly present: more and more technology, ever rising costs, more and more billions of dollars being spent, more and more government involvement.

How and why has this happened? What is the nature of the interaction between technology and the political process? What have been the major benefits? The principal dangers? The net results? Should the process be reversed? Can it? It not, what then?

A WORKING HYPOTHESIS

There is no easy or graceful approach to this outsize topic. I will start with a working hypothesis, a broad general construct which may throw some light on the crucial interaction between technology and the political process. It consists of four related propositions:

1. There is a dynamic expansionist force inherent in modern technology that leads to economic growth, higher costs, and increasingly centralized financing and administrative control, ending, almost inevitably, with government.

2. The primary results of this growing financial and administrative centralization, combined with ever larger markets or service areas, are likely to be positive, with direct benefits in the form of more goods and services for more people. At this point, the driving force of technology appears fully compatible with the democratic goal of maximizing benefits for the maxium number of people.

3. However, there are a number of serious negative results, including overpopulation, overcrowding, pollution of our living environment, the vastly increased power—for evil as well as for good—of the bureaucracies in control of

technology; the alienation of millions of young people, blacks, country folk, and others who feel themselves redundant in this highly structured, technocratic society, and the general overemphasis on material goods and values.

4. Whatever the net balance of positive and negative effects, the growth of techonology is probably irreversible—at least until far more of the world's population has experienced more of its benefits. The challenge, therefore, is to bring this formidable force under social control and to develop political and other institutions adequate to this task.

Each of these four propositions will be discussed briefly with special reference to medical technology and the increasing "politicization" of medicine in the United States.

The Expansionist Force of Modern Medical Technology

There is a dynamic expansionist force inherent in modern technology that leads to economic growth, higher costs and increasingly centralized financing and administrative control, ending, almost inevitably, with government.

Among the many paradoxes associated with the triumphs of modern medical technology none is more striking than this: The more advanced and more effective the technology, the greater the overall costs of health care. There are many reasons: the capital investment in the new equipment, the often high cost of maintenance, the need for specialized personnel to operate it, the need for an institutional setting in which it can be operated (which usually means additional overhead costs), the longer life expectancy of the population (which means more health care over the lifetime of the individual and over the year for the nation as a whole), the ever rising, albeit often unrealistic, expectations on the part of the consumer-patients, leading to an elasticity of demand that is almost total.

In many industries the more effective the technology, the lower the unit cost of production. This is possible as a result of the efficiency of mass production. There *are* examples of efficient mass production in the health services industry, including the manufacture of drugs, the automation of laboratory tests, and computerized business services. Diagnostic screening could be handled on a mass basis from the production point of view.

But health care, by and large, does not lend itself to the mass production approach. There seems little hope that the rising costs of medical care can ever be balanced by the same sort of productivity increases that we have witnessed in industry in general.

Some authorities disagree on this point. Some see the progress of technology permitting replacement of the physician and other very expensive personnel with lower cost, highly specialized, technicians. According to this view, even if total costs rise and unit costs cannot be cut, still we will be able to provide more services to more people. Presumably this would be a net gain.

I see little evidence, however, that things will work out this neatly. First, this view minimizes the effectiveness of health professionals in resisting technological replacement. For example, the introduction of unit dosage into hospital pharmacy might be expected to reduce hospital costs by eliminating the necessity of a resident pharmacist. This is not likely to happen, however. On the contrary, the pharmacist is seeking, understandably, to upgrade his role and salary to that of a "clinical pharmacist."

More important, the technologists generally underestimate the continuing importance of interpersonal relations in health care. Much nonsense has been uttered in the recent past with respect to the doctor-patient relationship and TLC ("tender loving care"). Many now make the opposite mistake and tend to overlook the often crucial role of subjective factors in illness, the importance of treating the "whole man," and the essentiality of the professional's role as educator, as well as technician, in helping the patient to prevent or cope with his illness.

Moreover, heavy emphasis on technological economies and productivity may lead to overemphasis on those health services which can most easily be mass-produced—drugs, laboratory tests, x-ray studies, even some types of surgery. But these are precisely the areas where there is already danger of too much, rather than too little, consumption. I will return to this point later.

This is not to say that many more effective cost controls cannot be devised. They can and should. But, if past experience is any guide, futher improvements in medical technology will, almost inevitably, lead to futher increases in the cost of care and futher pressures to spread or socialize those costs, over larger and larger population bases, as well as to bring in outside controls in the effort to moderate the rise.

In most of the world, the cost of health care, like the cost of education, is already paid for almost entirely by government—because this is the only social entity with the necessary financial resources. We would undoubtedly have gone the same route long before now except that our wealth and the special circumstances of collective bargaining in U.S. industry enabled us to absorb the rising costs of health care through the price of other goods and services. Every bikini, every tin can, incorporates in its price the cost of health care for the garment worker and her family, for the steel worker and his family. The major theme of medical economics for the first two decades after World War II was the "great cost pass-through" to the general consumer.

After 1965 the story began to change. The private sector proved unable to absorb the total costs, especially for high risk groups such as the aged. For the first time, the federal government was brought into the picture as a major factor in health care financing. Within four years, the public share of total U.S. health expenditures increased from less than 26 percent, a figure never before exceeded except in war, to 38 percent. Costs are now passed through to the taxpayer as well as the consumer.

But this does not mean that a viable equilibrium has been achieved. On the contrary, the pressures are even greater in 1972 than in 1965. Describing the successful 1971 drive for a major federally funded campaign against cancer, *Medical World News* editorializes, "The politicization of cancer suggests a possible politicization of the entire biomedical enterprise."

Along with the rise in the government share of expenditures has come a phenomenal increase in the total expenditure figure itself. Consumer dissatisfaction with rising prices forced even a reluctant Administration to inflation control measures for the economy in general and the health care industry in particular. Both state and federal governments are trying to put the lid on rising health insurance premiums.

A taxpayer revolt at state and local levels is forcing even conservative politicians to call for national health insurance. Adoption of some sort of universal health insurance system seems inevitable. Despite our wealth, despite our preference for nongovernmental financing, despite the ingenuity and efforts of private insurance carriers, despite the fears of many providers and consumers, there seems to be no other way that we can cope with the ever rising costs of modern medical technology.

The Honeymoon of Technology and Government

The early results of this growing centralization of control, combined with ever larger market or service areas, are likely to be positive, with direct benefits in the form of more goods and services for more people. At this point, the driving force of technology appears fully compatible with the democratic goal of maximizing benefits for the maximum number of people.

Due to a number of fortunate circumstances in the United States—particularly in size and natural resources and our constitutional and other traditions—science and technology, on the one hand, and politics and government, on the the other, have generally coexisted in a state of creative or dynamic tension. In general, government has done that which the people were unable to do for themselves—and not much more.

In the medical field the atmosphere has sometimes been acrimonious, but never fatally so. The expansion of government health care programs has, thus far, been generally limited to categories of persons who could not provide their own care and for whom no adequate source of support existed in the private sector. The unit costs of health services have generally not been lowered. This is not only because of the limits of mass production in health care but because provider organizations tend to be stronger than consumer organizations, and once a program becomes "politicized" it becomes especially vulnerable to such pressures.

Thus far, however, the tax base has proven flexible enough to absorb the rising costs, chiefly by involving broader governmental units and larger population bases. So, thanks to "politicization," millions of Americans—including Indians, disabled veterans, the indigent, and nearly all over 65—who would otherwise be denied the fruits of the new technology have access to some health services. At the same time, the incomes of most providers have improved substantially.

Medical research, professional education, and construction of facilities have been liberally supported, both by public and private funds. Belatedly, but now quite generously, government is supporting research into new methods of organizing and financing health care, with strong emphasis on new technology.

Further triumphs of such technology, such as telemedicine, which may give new meaning and potential to the individual doctor-patient relationship, and computerized medical records, which could make possible lifetime continuity and true comprehensiveness of care, are just over the horizon. The honeymoon of government and politics has obviously been productive of many social goods.

The Faustian Dilemma: Is The Price Too High?

However, there are a number of serious negative results, including overpopulation, overcrowding, pollution of our living environment, the vastly increased power—for evil as well as for good—of the bureaucracies in control of technology, the alienation of millions of young people, blacks, country folk, and others who feel themselves redundant in this highly structured, technocratic society, and the general overemphasis on material goods and values.

War, violence, crime, the arrogance of power, and the exploitation or alienation of the weak: None of these evils is peculiar to the age of technology. They have been with us since the dawn of history. But just as the hydrogen bomb is infinitely more lethal than the bow and arrow or the gun, so the destructive possibilities inherent in modern production, transportation, communications, space, biochemical, and other technologies give pause to even the congenital optimist. Some students see in this train of events the eventual self-destruction of the human race.

Thus far, the fear that sophisticated medical technology—experimental surgery, computer medicine, telemedicine, mind and mood control drugs, biological engineering, etc.—perverted in the hands of some native Hitler seems unfounded. But this does not mean there have been no negative effects. Among those who feel that many patients have suffered unnecessarily, either as a result of experimentation or incompetence, is Dr. Bernard Towers. He states:

> When I consider the sheer power, for both good and harm, that resides in such a simple technical procedure as setting up an intravenous saline drip, I am frightened for the safety of the patient.

Advanced medical technology has helped to exacerbate two preexisting evils—inflation and fragmentation. In both cases, this results from acceptance of the advantages of technology and politicization without willingness—either on the part of the industry or government—to apply the voluntary restraints or public controls necessary to provide relative price stability and coordination of services.

The term "bureaucratic" is so frequently and indiscriminately applied as an epithet to condemn government in general that one hesitates to use the term.

Certainly, the characteristic is not peculiar to government—either in its technical or pejorative sense. Bureaucracy is primarily an attribute of large scale operations, regardless of public or private status. To many a ghetto patient, the worst "bureaucrats" are not in Washington but in the nearest medical school or teaching hospital.

The fact remains, however, since governments tend to be larger than private enterprises, the danger of bureaucracy in government is increased. Moreover, once a government program is established and aquires a constituency of its own, it is harder to discontinue it, regardless of social utility, than a similar program in the private sector, which usually has to depend on a direct relationship between user satisfaction and willingness to pay the price.

Within government, the further removed the agency is from actual operating responsibilities, the greater the difficulty of evaluating its preformance and of maintaining accountability to Congress and to the people, and the greater the danger of self-perpetuating, unresponsive offices and personnel. In short, the cliché is not without substance.

Sometimes one wonders if all the goings and comings in Washington and throughout the industry, all the conferences, the projects, the rising expenditures, and the protocols have any appreciable effects on the nation's health. . . .

The clue to many, if not most of our health problems, not only among the young but the middle aged, appears to be life style. This, in turn, is at least partly related to morale. The symptoms of alienation, boredom, apathy, and irresponsibility with respect to health are all about us. Odin Anderson calls it "the short-range hedonistic model" and hopes that it will be replaced by "the long-range moderate and balanced pleasure model." It seems that the more effective the technology, the less responsibility many consumers exercise with respect to their own health. This phenomenon has been widely noted in the case of venereal disease, where the easy reliance on contraception and penicillin has led to widespread disregard of elementary hygiene. When we have heartburn, rather than cut down on eating we take *Alka-Seltzer*. Emotional problems? Rather than face up to the cause, we take a tranquilizer. Tired? A pep pill. And so on.

A related issue involves the effect of technology in inducing an artificial rise in use, whether or not medically indicated. For example, a recent Temple University publication points out:

> The fact that typical equipment designs [of clinical chemistry laboratories] can handle more than the usual daily needs of even a large hospital may lead the administration to adopt standing orders for a battery of screening tests for each admission.

The drug industry is that portion of the health care industry most clearly in line with general technological trends and the economies of mass production. Its achievements have been tremendous. Chemotherapy is today one of the most powerful arms of modern medicine. But overused and abused it becomes a powerful pollutant. Its effluence is the current drug culture and its Frankenstein offspring, the heroin epidemic. Here, indeed, the sorcerer's apprentice has lost control.

The Challenge Before Us

Whatever the net balance of positive and negative effects, the growth of technology is probably irreversible—at least until far more of the world's population has experienced more of its benefits. The challenge, therefore, is to bring this formidable force under social control and to develop political and other institutions adequate to this task.

It is possible that the Congressional vote on the supersonic transport plane and the reduced appropriations for space exploration may have marked the end of the honeymoon between American technology and the American government.

In the health field, the antitechnology sentiment is passive among doctors and patients alike. "Everyone" laments the loss of the traditional doctor-patient relationship—even those who never had it. "Everyone" deplores the increasing depersonalization of care—even those who never knew good personal care. Senator William Fulbright's accusations aganist the "military-industrial complex" for its "arrogance of power" are echoed in a hundred journalistic diatribes against overspecialism, the hospital (which Walter McNerney calls a "technological emporium") and the nascent "medical-industrial complex." After a year of frenetic activity, the epidemic of heart transplants seems to have come to an end—at least for the time being. One Houston cardiologist, who was involved in a number of the operations, calls the whole experiment "dehumanization by technology."

But how many Americans would be willing to pay the price of a clampdown on science and technology? How many really agree with Professor Mishan that for the average man life was better a half century ago and the whole world would be better off now if we had stopped technological and economic growth around 1919? At that time U.S. steel workers were still working a 12-hour day, child labor was the rule, southern blacks still lived in a state of serfdom little different from their previous slavery, and medicine had just passed the point that Dr. Lawrence Henderson of Harvard identified as that when "for the first time in human history, a random patient with a random disease consulting a doctor chosen at random stood better than a 50-50 chance of benefiting from the encounter."

If 1919 is not the right date, how about 1950? Or 1972? Who is to decide on the magic hour when the human race is supposed to have achieved the optimum balance between the good and bad results of technology? We in this comfortable hotel room? Or the unemployed steelworker and his family? Or the hundreds of millions still living in preindustrial dark ages? In Gary, Indiana, where massive layoffs in the steel industry have produced a community-wide depression, a shopkeeper was asked to suggest a solution. His prescription: "Make those smoke stacks blow their beautiful dirty smoke again!"

Even if we in the affluent West do become frightened enough of pollution, disappearing natural resources, and the drug epidemic to impose effective restraints on our own technological and economic growth, we obviously lack the power to enforce any such decision on the whole world. We represent only about 6 percent of the 3.5 billions who inhabit this planet and the technological abundance that is becoming superfluity or worse to us is still a vision of hope to the vast majority.

What will probably happen is that the present striking imbalance between U.S. consumption of world resources and that of the rest of mankind will not continue indefinitely. Either we will share voluntarily, or involuntarily, or we will spend more and more of our gross national product on armaments to try to defend our privileged position—another way of reducing domestic consumption.

In any case, the politics of growth—how to cut up an everexpanding economic pie based on a continually expanding landmass, population, technology, and GNP—may now be superseded by the politics of equilibrium. The result could be futher exacerbation of domestic intergroup and political tensions. Control over technology, especially communications, could become a major source of conflict. Small groups, enjoying privileged positions—known to some as islands of excellence, to others as ivory towers of élitism—will be hard put to defend their privileges. Basic scientific research could be threatened.

Still, it seems unrealistic to anticipate any immediate dramatic change in national policy. The multitude of conflicting pressures coming to bear on government in a democracy tend to maintain a relatively constant and centrist position. To talk of stopping technology or reversing the trend to government involvement seems romantic nonsense, a copout on the issues that we may—just possibly—be able to do something about. Tough, practical, inescapable problems, such as the following:

- How to assure that technology is kept under accountable human control?

- How to restrain technological innovation to a rate that is socially assimilable—from the point of view of employment, consumption, and our value systems—without impairing the creative drive that has contributed so much to our past progress?

- How to broaden, strengthen, and futher democratize governmental and other decision-making institutions?

- How to decentralize government to the point that people can, once again, feel some sense of meaningful participation and, at the same time, adjust boundaries to conform more nearly to expanding market and service areas?

- How to maintain—if necessary even build in—effective counterweights to government at all levels so as to minimize the danger of repression while avoiding the opposite dangers of anarchy or stalemate?

- How to share our technological and other resourses with other nations, peacefully, and to our mutual advantage?
- How to improve the decision-making process at all levels so that good intentions can be matched by clear understanding of probable consequences?

In the health care field, the acid test of our ability to cope with these problems will probably come with our eventual decisions on national health insurance. But these decisions, in turn, will be greatly influenced by what we do, or do not do, today and tomorrow, with respect to a multitude of subsidiary or related issues, including medical education, professional licensing, hospital franchising, regulation of the private health insurance industry, HMOs, Medicaid, drug abuse, day care centers, consumer health education, etc.

Vitally important, of course, is the question as to who will control the health care technology of the future: The health professions and consumers through their elected representatives? Or the technologists themselves, both in and out of government? If the latter happens, I believe it will be primarily due not to greed on their part but to default by those who have the greatest stake in accountable democratic controls.

Finally, our ability to cope with the basic issues listed above will depend on the nature and effectiveness of our national research effort—with respect both to the pursuit of biomedical knowledge and its application. Significantly, Dr. Towers with all his fears of new "iatromechanical" and "iatrochemical" techniques, concludes with a plea for greater use of the computer:

> It seems to me that intelligent use of the computer could give medicine the most powerful, and yet most *in-nocent* (in the literal meaning of the word) technique ever discovered. All knowledge, all understanding, involves four stages, all of them requiring the handling of information. They are, in order, information accumulation, filtering (selection), storage, and retrieval. The last stage involves not simply the regurgitation of data previously "memorized" but the juxtaposition and synthesis (in both space and time) of data culled from various sources, and at various times. This is the essential element in scientific discovery, in "insight" in the exercise of clinical "diagnostic flair." This is the process that the good clinician uses continually, a process of analysis and synthesis, with many feedback loops, both positive and negative. Cyberneticians refer to the process as "systems analysis;" and this concept marks a radical break with the linear, cause-effect paradigm of "good" natural science which was at the basis of what Bernard called "l'iatromécanique" and "l'iatrochimie." ... I see the computer as a tool to help us to a much deeper understanding of man, of man seen in "biological space-time."

In other words, some forms of technology, appropriately applied, could be our salvation. But with or without the insights of the computer, with or without the advantages to medicine, Dennis Gabor, the physicist, has the last word:

> The insane quantitative growth must stop; but innovation must not stop—it must take an entirely new direction. Instead of working blindly toward things bigger and better, it must work toward improving the quality of life rather than increasing its quantity. Innovation must work toward a new harmony, a new equilibrium; otherwise it will only lead to explosion.

The ultimate challenge to man, the clever, competitive, conceited apprentice, is whether he can learn to use his new-found knowledge with the wisdom, self-discipline, and humility necessary for survival. In the words of that great philosopher, Pogo, "We have met the enemy—and it is us."

Appendix:
Tables and Figure

TABLE I U.S. Death Rates: Crude; Age-Adjusted, By Sex and Race; and By Age. Selected Years, 1920-1975 (per 1,000 population)

	1920	1930	1940	1950	1960	1970	1975
Total, crude	13.0	11.3	10.8	9.6	9.5	9.5	8.9
Total age-adjusted	14.2	12.5	10.8	8.4	7.6	7.1	6.4
Male	14.7	13.5	12.1	10.0	9.5	9.3	8.5
Female	13.8	11.3	9.4	6.9	5.9	5.3	5.0
White	13.7	11.7	10.2	8.0	7.3	6.8	6.1
Male	14.2	12.8	11.6	9.6	9.2	8.9	8.1
Female	13.1	10.6	8.8	6.5	5.6	5.0	4.5
All other	20.6	20.1	16.3	12.3	10.5	9.8	8.5
Male	20.4	21.0	17.6	13.6	12.1	12.3	11.0
Female	21.0	19.2	15.0	10.9	8.9	7.7	6.5
Male, by age:							
Under 1 year	103.6	77.0	61.9	37.3	30.6	24.1	18.3
1-4 years	10.3	6.0	3.1	1.5	1.2	0.9	0.8
5-14	2.8	1.9	1.2	0.7	0.6	0.5	0.4
15-24	4.8	3.5	2.3	1.7	1.5	1.9	1.8
25-34	6.4	4.9	3.4	2.2	1.9	2.2	2.0
35-44	8.2	7.5	5.9	4.3	3.7	4.0	3.5
45-54	12.6	13.6	12.5	10.7	9.9	9.6	8.6
55-64	24.6	26.6	26.1	24.0	23.1	22.8	20.3
65-74	54.5	55.8	54.6	49.3	49.1	48.7	44.1
75-84	122.1	119.1	121.3	104.3	101.8	100.1	95.2
85 and over	253.0	236.7	246.4	216.4	211.9	178.2	175.7
Female, by age:							
Under 1 year	80.7	60.7	47.7	28.5	23.2	18.6	14.4
1-4	9.5	5.2	2.7	1.3	1.0	0.8	0.6
5-14	2.5	1.5	0.9	0.5	0.4	0.3	0.3
15-24	5.0	3.2	1.8	0.9	0.6	0.7	0.6
25-34	7.1	4.4	2.7	1.4	1.1	1.0	0.9
35-44	8.0	6.1	4.5	2.9	2.3	2.3	1.9
45-54	11.7	10.6	8.6	6.4	5.3	5.2	4.6
55-64	22.4	21.2	18.0	14.0	12.0	11.0	10.1
65-74	50.5	46.8	42.2	33.3	28.7	25.8	22.5
75-84	115.9	106.6	103.7	84.0	76.3	66.8	60.3
85 and over	224.7	221.4	227.6	191.9	190.1	155.2	140.3

Sources: U.S. Bureau of the Census, *Historical Statistics of the U.S., Colonial Times to 1970*, pp. 61-62; U.S. Department of Health, Education, and Welfare, National Center for Health Statistics, *Health U.S. 1975*, HEW Publ. (HRA) 76-1232, p. 231; National Center for Health Statistics, *Monthly Vital Statistics Report, Final Mortality Statistics, 1975*, (HRA) 77-1120, Vol. 25, No. 11 Supplement (February 11, 1977): 11, 22. See these sources for technical footnotes.

TABLE II Life Expectancy at Birth: Selected Countries, Latest Available Period

Country	Data Period	Males Life Expectancy	Males Rank Order	Females Life Expectancy	Females Rank Order
Sweden	1972	71.97	1	77.41	1
Norway	1966-70	71.09	2	76.83	2
Netherlands	1972	70.8	3	76.8	3
Demark	1970-71	70.7	4	75.9	6
Japan	1972	70.49	5	75.92	5
Israel	1972	70.14	6	72.83	23
Switzerland	1960-70	69.21	7	75.03	9
Germany, Democratic Republic of	1969-70	68.85	8	74.19	10
Bulgaria	1965-67	68.81	9	72.67	24
Canada	1965-67	68.75	10	75.18	8
Ireland	1965-67	68.58	11	72.85	22
France	1971	68.5	12	76.1	4
New Zealand	1960-62	68.44	13	73.75	16
Australia	1960-62	67.92	14	74.18	11
Italy	1964-67	67.87	15	73.36	20
United Kingdom	1968-70	67.81	16	73.81	14
Belgium	1959-63	67.75	17	73.51	18
Greece	1960-62	67.46	18	70.70	30
United States	1972	67.4	19	75.2	7
Spain	1960	67.32	20	71.90	26
Germany, Federal Republic of	1968-70	67.24	21	73.44	19
Poland	1970-72	66.83	22	73.76	15
Austria	1972	66.8	23	74.1	12
Hungary	1970	66.28	24	72.05	25
Romania	1970-72	66.27	25	70.85	29
Czechoslovakia	1970	66.23	26	72.94	21
Finland	1966-70	65.88	27	73.57	17
Uruguay	1963-64	65.51	28	71.56	27
Portugal	1970	65.30	29	71.02	28
Yugoslavia	1970-71	65.30	29	70.14	32
Singapore	1970	65.1	31	70.0	33
U.S.S.R.	1970-71	65	32	74	13
Albania	1965-66	64.9	33	67.0	34
Sri Lanka	1967	64.8	34	66.9	35
Argentina	1965-70	64.06	35	70.22	31

Source: Adapted from U.S. Department of Health, Education, and Welfare, National Center for Health Statistics, *Health: United States 1975*, HEW Publication (HRA)76-1232, pp. 221,223.

TABLE III U.S. Death Rates: Crude, Selected Causes, and Years, 1950-1975

	Deaths per 100,000 Population			
	1950	1960	1970	1975[a]
All causes	963.8	954.7	945.3	896.1
Major cardiovascular diseases	494.4	515.1	496.0	459.4
Diseases of the heart	356.8	369.0	362.0	339.0
Cerebrovascular diseases	104.0	108.0	101.9	91.8
Arteriosclerosis	20.4	20.0	15.6	13.7
Hypertension	8.3	7.1	4.1	3.0
Other	4.9	11.0	12.5	11.9
Malignancies	139.8	149.2	162.8	174.4
Neoplasms of digestive organs and peritoneum	—	—	46.6	47.8
Neoplasms of respiratory system	—	—	34.2	41.5
Neoplasms of genital organs	—	—	20.3	20.2
Neoplasms of breast	—	—	14.7	15.3
Leukemia	—	—	7.1	7.0
Other neoplasms	—	—	39.9	42.6
Pneumonia	26.9[b]	32.9[b]	29.0	24.7
Influenza	4.4	4.4	1.8	2.2
Diabetes mellitus	16.2	16.7	18.9	16.8
Cirrhosis of liver	9.2	11.3	15.5	15.1
Bronchitis, emphysema and asthma	—	—	15.2	11.9
Certain diseases of early infancy	40.5	37.4	21.3	12.8
Tuberculosis, all forms	22.5	6.1	2.6	1.5
Hyperplasia of prostate	4.2	2.5	1.1	0.6
Syphilis and its sequelae	5.0	1.6	0.2	0.2
Ill-defined symptoms and conditions	14.9	11.4	12.7	15.3
Accidents	60.6	52.3	56.4	47.6
Motor vehicle	23.1	21.3	26.9	20.9
All other	37.5	31.0	29.5	26.7
Suicide	11.4	10.6	11.6	12.6
Homicide	5.3	4.7	8.3	10.2

[a]Provisional, based on 10 percent sample of deaths.
[b]Excludes pneumonia of newborn.
— not available

Sources: U.S. Bureau of Census, *Statistical Abstract of U.S., 1975*, p. 64; U.S. Department of Health, Education, and Welfare, National Center for Health Statistics, *Monthly Vital Statistics Report, Annual Summary for the U.S., 1975*, Vol. 24, No. 13, p. 26.

TABLE IV Health Manpower: Selected Occupations, Estimates, 1974

Health Field Occupation	Persons Active		
Total [a]	4,672,850	to	4,707,650
Administration of health services			48,200
Ambulance attendant			260,000
Basic sciences in health field			60,000
Biomedical engineering			12,000
Chiropractic			16,600
Clinical laboratory services			172,500
Dentists			107,300
Dental hygienist, assistant, and lab technician			172,500
Dietetic and nutritional services			72,700
EKG, EEG, and operating room technicians			25,500
Environmental sanitation			20,000
Food and drug protective services			47,900
Funeral directors and embalmers			50,000
Health education	22,500	to	23,000
Health information and communication	7,400	to	10,500
Medical assistant			16,000
Medical records			60,000
Midwifery			4,000
Nursing and related services			2,319,000
Registered nurse			857,000
Practical nurse			492,000
Nursing aide, orderly, attendant			936,000
Home health aide			34,000
Occupational therapy	13,500	to	14,500
Optometry and opticianry	37,100	to	37,300
Ophthalmic assistant			20,000
Orthotic and prosthetic technology	2,800	to	3,800
Pharmacy			132,900
Physical therapy			26,100
Physician (M.D.)			350,600
Physician (D.O.)			12,100
Physician's assistant			2,000
Podiatry			7,100
Psychology			35,000
Radiologic technology			100,000
Rehabilitation: counseling, speech, audiology, etc.	56,995	to	57,950
Respiratory therapy technician	18,000	to	19,000
Secretarial and office services in health field	275,000	to	300,000
Social work			38,600
Veterinary medicine			33,500
Other	4,000	to	19,200

[a] Each occupation is counted only once. For example, all physicians are in medicine and osteopathy.

Source: National Center for Health Statistics, HEW, unpublished data.

TABLE V Doctors of Medicine: Total, Total Active, Primary Care Potential, and Ratios to Population, Selected Years 1949-1975

Specialty	1949	1955	1960	1965	1970	1974	1975
				Number[a]			
Total physicians[b]	202,683	219,852	245,313	292,088	334,028	379,748	393,742
Total active physicians	192,951	208,181	232,624	277,575	310,845	330,266	340,280
Primary care potential[c]	112,958	110,036	112,226	125,949	118,639	127,394	131,618
Internal medicine	11,588	16,321	27,154	38,690	41,872	51,572	54,331
Pediatrics[d]	4,315	6,567	11,609	15,893	18,819	21,645	22,730
Family and general practice	97,055	87,148	73,463	71,366	57,948	53,997	54,557
Obstetrics-gynecology	5,074	7,198	14,656	16,833	18,876	20,987	21,731
			Percentage of Total Active Physicians[a]				
Primary care potential[c]	58.5	52.9	48.2	45.4	38.2	38.6	38.7
Internal medicine	6.0	7.8	11.7	13.9	13.5	15.7	16.0
Pediatrics[d]	2.2	3.2	5.0	5.7	6.1	6.6	6.7
Family and general practice	50.3	41.9	31.6	25.7	18.6	16.3	16.0
Obstetrics-gynecology	2.6	3.5	6.3	6.1	6.1	6.4	6.4
			Physicians per 100,000 Total Resident Population[a]				
Total physicians[b]	132.9	130.2	133.5	146.6	159.5	175.6	180.8
Total active physicians	126.5	123.2	126.6	139.3	148.4	152.7	156.2
Primary care potential[c]	74.1	65.1	61.1	63.2	56.6	58.9	60.4
Internal medicine	7.6	9.7	14.8	19.4	20.0	23.9	24.9
Pediatrics[d]	2.8	3.9	6.3	8.0	9.0	10.0	10.4
Family and general practice	63.7	51.6	40.0	35.8	27.7	25.0	25.0
Obstetrics-Gynecology	3.3	4.3	8.0	8.4	9.0	9.7	10.0

Appendix 497

a For 1949-1960, data are for midyear; for 1965-1975, data are for year end.
b Includes physicians who are inactive, not classified, and whose addresses are unknown, but excludes those with temporary foreign addresses.
c For 1949-1955, includes only physicians in private practice; for 1960-1975, includes all active federal and nonfederal phycians (excludes inactive, not classified, and address unknown).
d Includes pediatric allergy and pediatric cardiology.

Notes: Large increases and decreases among specialties between 1965 and 1970 occurred as a result of the Reclassification of Physicians Project conducted by the American Medical Association. Classification by specialty was based on the most hours reported on the Physicians' Professional Activities questionnaire rather than on an arbitrary selection by the physician. For a detailed explanation, see *Reclassification of Physicians, 1968*, Center for Health Services Research and Development, American Medical Association.

Because of different data collection procedures, physician data before and after 1963 are not fully comparable. Both published and unpublished data prior to 1963 are for midyear and usually do not include the U.S. medical school graduates for the respective years nor the foreign medical school graduates engaged in medical training programs in the United States. Data since 1963 are for the year end and include both of these categories.

Sources: Physicians for 1949-1973: American Medical Association, *Distribution of Physicians in the U.S*, annual editions and unpublished reports. Physicians for 1974-1975: American Medical Association, *Physician Distribution and Medical Licensure in the U.S*, annual editions. Population: U.S. Bureau of the Census, *Current Population Reports*, Population Estimates Series P-25, Nos. 361, 417, 462, 478, 516, 600, 634, 336, 392, 436, and earlier reports. Totals include population in outlying areas (Puerto Rico, Virgin Islands, etc.) to correspond with physician data.

TABLE VI Community (Nonfederal Short Term) Hospitals, Selected Data and Years, 1950-1975[a]

						Average Annual Percentage Increase			
	1950	1965	1970	1974	1975	1950-1965	1965-1970	1970-1975	1974-1975
Total civilian population (in thousands)	150,790	191,605	201,722	209,676	211,355	1.6	1.0	0.9	0.8
Number of hospitals	5,031	5,736	5,859	5,977	5,979	0.9	0.4	.5	0.03
Number of beds (in thousands)	505	741	848	931	947	2.6	2.7	2.3	1.72
Beds per 1,000 population	3.4	3.9	4.2	4.4	4.5	1.0	1.7	1.4	0.9
Admissions (in thousands)	16,663	26,463	29,252	32,943	33,519	3.1	2.0	2.8	1.75
Admissions per 1,000 population	110.5	138.1	145.0	157	159	1.5	1.0	1.9	1.27
Average daily census adjusted (in thousands)[b]	372	620	727	793	806	3.4	3.2	2.1	1.64
Patient days per 1,000 population, adjusted[b]	900	1,181	1,315	1,379	1,391	1.8	2.2	1.1	0.87
Occupancy (percent)	73.7	76.0	78.0	75.3	74.8	0.2	0.5	-0.8	-0.66
Average length of stay (days)	8.1	7.8	8.2	7.8	7.7	-0.2	1.0	-1.2	-1.28
Outpatient visits (in thousands)	—	92,631	133,545	194,838	196,311	—	7.6	8.0	0.76
Total expenses (in millions)	$2,120	$9,147	$19,560	$32,751	$39,110	10.2	16.4	14.9	19.42
Expenses per inpatient day, adjusted[b]	$15.62	$40.56	$73.73	$113.21	$133.08	3.3	12.7	12.5	17.55
Nonpayroll expenses (in millions)	$917	$3,503	$8,139	$14,890	$18,361	9.4	18.4	17.7	23.31
Personnel, full-time (in thousands)[c]	662	1,386	1,929	2,289	2,399	5.1	6.8	4.5	4.8
Personnel, full-time, per 100 census, adjusted[b,c]	178	224	265	289	298	1.5	3.4	2.4	3.1
Payroll expense per employee	$1,817	$4,072	$5,921	$8,057	$8,649	5.5	7.8	8.3	9.3
Payroll expenses as percent of total expense	56.7	61.7	58.4	54.5	53.1	0.6	-1.0	-1.8	-2.5

[a] These data include all nonfederal, short term hospitals for all years. The AHA definition of "community" hospitals was revised in 1972 to exclude about 100 small institutions whose services are not open to the general public, i.e., college and prison infirmaries. This change does not significantly affect the data.
[b] Except in 1950, weighted equivalents of outpatient visits are added to inpatient days.
[c] Includes part-time equivalents.

Sources: American Hospital Association, *Hospital Statistics, 1976 Edition*, Table 1, p. 4; population: 1950-74: *Statistical Abstract of the U.S., 1975*, p. 5; 1975: *Current Population Reports*, Series p-25, no. 634 (July 1976).

TABLE VII Nursing Homes: Selected Characteristics 1964, 1969, and 1973-1974

ITEM	1964	1969	1973-1974	ITEM	1964	1969	1973-1974
NURSING HOMES[a]				RESIDENTS IN NURSING AND PERSONAL CARE HOMES—Cont.			
Estimated number (thousands)	14.6	15.0	16.1	Male (thousands)	194	252	318
Beds, total (thousands)	576	879	1,188	Female (thousands)	360	563	757
Average per home	39	59	74	Under 65 years old (thousands)	66	93	114
Per 1,000 persons 65 years old and over	32.2	45.2	55.2	65 years old and over (thousands)	488	722	960
Employed in homes[b] (thousands)	246	495	722	Percent of total residents	88.0	88.6	89.4
Per 100 residents	47.4	63.5	65.7	Male:			
Average monthly resident charge (dollars)	185	335	478	Under 65 years old (thousands)	36	45	52
Primary source of payment:				65 years old and over (thousands)	158	207	266
Medicare (percent)		3.4	4.1	Percent of total male:	81.3	82.2	83.5
Medicaid (percent)		13.3	49.9	65-69 (thousands)	40	23	29
Public assistance (percent)	46.0	36.5	46.0	70-74 (thousands)		29	37
Other (percent)	54.0	46.9		75-79 (thousands)	74	39	47
				80-84 (thousands)		52	55
Residents, total (thousands)	519	778	1,099	85 and over (thousands)	43	64	98
RESIDENTS IN NURSING AND PERSONAL CARE HOMES				Female:			
				Under 65 years old (thousands)	30	48	62
				65 years old and over (thousands)	330	515	695
Total (thousands)	554	815	1,075	Percent of total female:	91.6	91.5	91.8
				65-69 (thousands)	64	30	36
White (thousands)		779	1,009	70-74 (thousands)		56	62
Negro and other (thousands)		37	65	75-79 (thousands)		95	115
				80-84 (thousands)	157	137	167
				85 and over (thousands)	109	198	315

[a] Excludes those providing personal care, domiciliary care, or room and board only (an additional 5,600 homes in 1973-1974).
[b] Full-time equivalent.

Source: Department of Health, Education, and Welfare, National Center for Health Statistics, *Vital and Health Statistics*, Ser. 12, Nos. 5, 9, 21, and 23. Count based on periodic surveys.

TABLE VIII Private Health Insurance: Estimated Percent of Population Covered, by Age and Specified Type of Care, Selected Years 1962-1974

	Hospital Care	Physicians' Services				Dental Care	Prescribed Drugs (out-of-hospital)	Visiting Nurse Service	Nursing Home Care
		Surgical Services	In-hospital Visits	X-Ray and Laboratory Examinations	Office and Home Visits				
All Ages									
1962	70.0	65.0	—	35.0	—	0.5	26.0	23.0	3.0
1967	73.9	72.2	—	47.0	—	2.4	36.2	41.6	9.2
1970	75.9	73.9	71.7	70.2	—	6.0	49.7	52.6	16.0
1973	75.8	75.1	73.4	73.1	—	10.4	59.8	58.7	33.1
1974	77.6	75.7	73.6	72.7	59.4	15.8	67.3	64.9	33.2
Under 65									
1962	—	—	—	—	—	—	—	—	—
1967	77.0	75.2	65.6	50.0	—	2.6	39.0	44.6	8.9
1970	78.6	76.9	75.1	73.8	—	6.6	53.5	56.4	15.4
1973	78.0	77.6	77.2	76.9	—	11.4	64.6	62.9	33.4
1974	79.9	78.3	77.5	77.5	62.3	17.4	73.2	70.1	35.2
65 and Over									
1962	—	—	—	—	—	—	—	—	—
1967	45.0	44.1	31.1	18.7	—	0.4	9.7	13.0	15.2
1970	51.4	46.7	41.1	37.4	—	.6	15.9	18.8	24.7
1973	57.4	53.6	41.1	40.8	—	1.1	18.5	22.3	30.3
1974	57.9	54.0	40.3	31.7	35.5	1.9	16.9	21.0	15.8

— not available.

Source: *Social Security Bulletin*, annual article on private health insurance, February 1975 and March 1976.

Appendix 503

Table IX follows on page 504

TABLE IX Private Health Insurance: Financial Experience, by Type of Carrier, 1965 and 1974 (amounts in millions)

Type of Plan	Total Income	Subscription or Premium Income	Claims Expense Amount	Claims Expense Percent of Premium Income	Operating Expense Amount	Operating Expense Percent of Premium Income	Net Gain from Underwriting Amount	Net Gain from Underwriting Percent of Premium Income	Net Income Amount	Net Income Percent of Total Income
				1965						
Total....................	—	$10,001.3	$8,728.9	87.3	$1,417.7	14.2	$−145.3	−1.5	—	—
Blue Cross-Blue Shield plans...	$4,229.8	4,169.0	3,912.9	93.9	238.9	5.7	17.2	.4	$78.0	1.8
Blue Cross..............	3,036.5	2,993.7	2,853.4	95.3	132.3	4.4	8.5	.3	51.3	1.7
Blue Shield.............	1,193.3	1,175.3	1,058.5	90.1	106.6	9.1	8.6	.7	26.7	2.2
Insurance Companies.........	—	5,224.0	4,265.0	81.6	1,140.0	21.8	−181.0	−3.5	—	—
Group..................	—	3,665.0	3,413.0	93.1	454.0	12.4	−202.0	−5.5	—	—
Individual..............	—	1,559.0	852.0	54.7	686.0	44.0	21.0	1.3	—	—
Independent plans...........	608.3	608.3	551.0	90.6	38.8	6.4	18.5	3.0	18.5	3.0
Community..............	216.2	216.2	198.6	91.8	16.3	7.6	1.3	.6	1.3	.6
Employer-employee union....	366.3	366.3	329.0	89.8	20.5	5.6	16.8	4.6	16.8	4.6
Medical society..........	.7	.7	.5	72.5	.1	9.5	.1	18.0	.1	18.0
Private group clinic.......	12.1	12.1	10.8	89.5	1.1	8.9	.2	1.6	.2	1.6
Dental society...........	13.0	13.0	12.1	93.3	.8	6.2	.1	.6	.1	.6

TABLE IX (Continued)

Type of Plan	Total Income	Subscription or Premium Income	Claims Expense		Operating Expense		Net Gain from Underwriting		Net Income	
			Amount	Percent of Premium Income	Amount	Percent of Premium Income	Amount	Percent of Premium Income	Amount	Percent of Total Income
1974										
Total............................	—	$28,399.9	$24,766.8	87.2	$3,992.8	14.1	$-359.7	-1.3	—	—
Blue Cross-Blue Shield	12,611.8	12,367.0	11,639.5	94.1	911.0	7.4	-183.5	-1.5	$61.3	0.5
Blue Cross......................	8,757.7	8,647.6	8,311.1	96.1	470.2	5.4	-133.7	-1.3	-23.6	-.3
Blue Shield.....................	3,854.1	3,719.4	3,328.4	89.5	440.8	11.8	-49.8	-1.3	84.9	2.2
Insurance Companies............	—	13,867.0	11,109.3	80.1	2,916.9	21.0	-159.2	-1.1	—	—
Group policies	—	10,590.0	9,392.2	90.6	1,376.7	13.0	-378.9	-3.6	—	—
Individual policies	—	3,277.0	1,517.1	46.3	1,340.2	47.0	219.7	6.7	—	—
Independent plans...............	2,221.0	2,165.9	2,018.0	93.2	164.9	7.6	-17.0	-.8	38.1	1.7
Community.....................	855.4	847.5	798.1	94.2	57.2	6.7	-7.8	-.9	.1	
Employer-employee union.......	938.0	897.0	853.4	95.1	62.7	7.0	-19.1	-2.1	21.9	2.3
Private group clinic.............	34.8	33.4	26.5	79.3	5.0	15.0	1.9	5.7	3.3	9.5
Dental service corporation ...	392.8	388.0	340.0	87.6	40.0	10.3	8.0	2.1	12.8	3.3

— means data not available.

Source: *Social Security Bulletin*, annual article on private health insurance, 1966 and 1976.

TABLE X Personal Health Expenditures[a]: Amount and Percentage Distribution, by Source of Funds, Selected Fiscal Years, 1929-1975

Fiscal Year	Total	Private				Public		
		Total	Direct Payments	Insurance Benefits	Other	Total	Federal	State and Local
			Aggregate Amount (in millions)					
1929	$ 3,165	$ 2,882	$ 2,800[b]	—	$ 83	$ 282	$ 85	$ 197
1940	3,414	2,891	2,799[b]	—	92	523	133	389
1950	10,400	8,298	7,107	$ 879	312	2,102	979	1,124
1960	22,729	17,779	12,576	4,698	525	4,930	2,102	2,828
1965	33,498	26,540	17,577	8,280	683	6,958	2,840	4,118
1970	60,113	39,568	24,272	14,406	890	20,545	13,403	7,142
1975	105,745	63,779	35,553	26,894	1,331	41,966	28,866	13,100
1976[c]	120,431	72,013	39,099	31,359	1,556	48,418	33,683	14,735
			Percentage Distribution					
1929	100.0	91.1	88.5[b]	—	2.6	8.9	2.7	6.2
1940	100.0	84.7	82.0[b]	—	2.7	15.3	3.9	11.4
1950	100.0	79.8	68.3	8.5	3.0	20.2	9.4	10.8
1960	100.0	78.3	55.3	20.7	2.3	21.7	9.2	12.4
1965	100.0	79.2	52.5	24.7	2.0	20.8	8.5	12.3
1970	100.0	65.8	40.4	24.0	1.5	34.2	22.3	11.9
1975	100.0	60.3	33.6	25.4	1.3	39.7	27.3	12.4
1976[c]	100.0	59.8	32.5	26.0	1.3	40.2	28.0	12.2

[a] Includes all national health expenditures (Table XII) except: expenses for prepayment and administration, government public health activities, and research and medical facilities construction.
[b] Includes any insurance benefits and expenses for prepayment (insurance premiums less insurance benefits).
[c] Preliminary estimates.

Source: M.S. Mueller and R.M. Gibson, "National Health Expenditures, FY 1975," *Social Security Bulletin*, February 1976, p.17; "National Health Expenditures, FY 1976," *Social Security Bulletin* April 1977), pp.5, 9.

TABLE XI National Health Expenditures: Aggregate and Per Capita Amounts and Percent of Gross National Product, Selected Fiscal Years 1929-1976

Fiscal Year	GNP (in billions)	Amount (in millions)	Per Capita	Percent of GNP
1929	$ 101.3	$ 3,589	$ 29.16	3.5
1940	95.4	3,883	28.98	4.1
1950	264.8	12,027	78.35	4.5
1960	498.3	25,856	141.63	5.2
1965	658.0	38,892	197.75	5.9
1970	960.2	69,201	333.57	7.2
1974	1,361.2	106,321	495.01	7.8
1975	1,452.3	122,231	564.35	8.4
1976[a]	1,611.8	139,312	637.97	8.6

[a] Preliminary

Source: R. M. Gibson and M. S. Mueller, "National Health Expenditures, FY 1976," *Social Security Bulletin,* April 1977, p.4.

TABLE XII   National Health Expenditures: Aggregate Amount and Percentage Distribution, by Type of Expenditure, Selected FYs 1929-1976

Type of expenditure	Aggregate amount (in millions)									
	1929	1935	1940	1950	1955	1960	1965	1970	1975	1976[a]
Total...............................	$3,559	$2,846	$3,883	$12,027	$17,330	$25,856	$38,892	$69,201	$122,231	$139,312
Health services and supplies.........	3,382	2,788	3,729	11,181	16,392	24,162	35,664	64,065	114,652	131,022
Personal health care expense.........	3,165	2,585	3,414	10,400	15,231	22,729	33,498	60,113	105,745	120,431
Hospital care	651	731	969	3,698	5,689	8,499	13,152	25,879	48,224	55,400
Physicians' services[b]	994	744	946	2,689	3,632	5,580	8,405	13,443	22,925	26,350
Dentists' services..................	476	298	402	940	1,457	1,944	2,728	4,473	7,810	8,600
Other professional services.........	248	150	173	384	552	848	989	1,385	2,190	2,400
Drugs and drug sundries[c]...........	601	471	621	1,642	2,282	3,591	4,647	7,114	10,269	11,168
Eyeglasses and appliances...........	131	128	180	475	605	750	1,151	1,776	1,785	1,980
Nursing-home care..................	—	—	28	178	291	480	1,271	3,818	9,100	10,600
Other health services...............	64	63	95	394	770	1,037	1,155	2,225	3,442	3,933
Expense for prepayment and administration......................	128	91	160	430	730	1,012	1,495	2,515	5,954	7,336
Government public health activities..	89	112	155	351	384	401	671	1,495	2,953	3,255
Research and medical facilities construction	207	58	134	847	938	1,694	3,228	5,137	7,579	8,290
Research[d]	—	—	3	110	194	592	1,391	1,846	2,942	3,327
Construction.......................	207	58	131	737	744	1,102	1,837	3,291	4,637	4,963

TABLE XII (Continued)

Percentage Distribution

Type of expenditure	1929	1940	1950	1960	1965	1970	1975	1976[a]
Total	100	100	100	100	100	100	100	100
Health services and supplies	94.2	96.0	93.0	93.4	91.7	92.6	93.8	94.0
Personal health care expense	88.2	87.9	86.5	87.9	86.1	86.9	86.5	86.4
Hospital care	18.1	25.0	30.7	32.9	33.8	37.4	39.5	39.8
Physicians' services[b]	27.7	24.4	22.4	21.6	21.6	19.4	18.8	18.9
Dentists' services	13.3	10.4	7.8	7.5	7.0	6.5	6.4	6.2
Other professional services	6.9	4.5	3.2	3.3	2.5	2.0	1.8	1.7
Drugs and drug sundries[c]	16.7	16.0	14.7	13.9	11.9	10.3	8.4	8.0
Eyeglasses and appliances	5.1	4.6	3.9	2.9	3.0	2.6	1.5	1.4
Nursing-home care	—	0.7	1.5	1.9	3.3	5.5	7.4	7.6
Other health services	1.8	2.4	3.3	4.0	3.0	3.2	2.8	2.8
Expense for prepayment and administration	3.6	4.1	3.6	3.9	3.8	3.6	4.9	5.3
Government public health activities	2.5	4.0	2.9	1.6	1.7	2.2	2.4	2.3
Research and medical facilities construction	5.8	3.5	7.0	6.6	8.3	7.4	6.2	6.0
Research[d]	—	0.1	0.9	2.3	3.6	2.7	2.4	2.4
Construction	5.8	3.4	6.1	4.3	4.7	4.7	3.8	3.6

[a] Preliminary
[b] Services of salaried physicians in hospitals are included in hospital care; but self-employed physicians' services in hospitals are included in this line. Anesthesia and x-ray services are sometimes classified as hospital care expenditures and sometimes as expenditures for physicians' services, depending on billing practices.
[c] Costs of drugs used in hospitals are included with hospital care.
[d] Research expenditures of drug companies are in "Drugs and Drug Sundries."

Source: R.M. Gibson and M.S. Mueller, "National Health Expenditures, FY 1976," *Social Security Bulletin*, April 1977, p. 15.

TABLE XIII Public Programs: Expenditures for Health Services and Supplies, by Program, Type of Expenditure, and Source of Funds

Fiscal Years 1965 and 1976

(in millions)

FY 1965

Program and source of funds	Total	Hospital care	Physicians' services	Dentists' services	Other professional services	Drugs and drug sundries	Eyeglasses and appliances	Nursing-home care	Government public health activities	Other health services	Administration
Total	$7,636.3	$4,778.0	$527.1	$33.3	$31.8	$133.3	$28.4	$449.7	$688.1	$961.4	$25.0
Temporary disability insurance (medical benefits)	50.9	38.3	11.3	—	.6	.4	.4	—	—	—	—
Workers' compensation (medical benefits)	580.0	203.0	336.4	—	17.4	11.6	11.6	—	—	—	—
Public assistance (vendor medical payments)	1,367.1	582.4	113.5	28.7	8.2	116.2	—	448.4	—	69.7	—
General hospital and medical care	2,514.7	2,499.8	2.5	.4	—	.4	.4	—	—	11.2	—
Defense Department hospital and medical care (including military dependents)	936.8	436.4	29.2	—	—	—	—	—	—	469.8	1.4
Maternal and child health services	224.1	39.4	10.5	3.1	5.6	1.6	4.7	—	—	157.7	1.3
School health	132.0	—	—	—	—	—	—	—	—	132.0	—
Other public health activities	669.9	—	—	—	—	—	—	—	668.1	—	1.8
Veterans' hospital and medical care	1,120.9	963.2	9.7	1.1	—	3.1	6.6	1.3	—	115.4	20.5

Appendix 511

Medical vocational rehabilitation............	34.2	15.5	14.0	—	—	—	4.7	—	—	—	5.6—
Office of Economic Opportunity..............	5.6	—	—	—	—	—	—	—	—	—	—
Federal	3,080.7	1,789.2	105.3	14.9	5.4	51.9	12.2	183.3	221.1	672.2	25.0
Workers' compensation (medical benefits)........	11.3	7.3	2.8	—	.7	.2	.3	—	—	—	—
Public assistance (vendor medical benefits).......	555.0	236.4	46.1	11.7	3.3	47.2	—	182.0	—	28.3	—
General hospital and medical care................	137.9	123.0	2.5	.4	—	.4	.4	—	—	11.2	—
Defense Department hospital and medical care (including military dependents).....	936.8	436.4	29.2	—	—	—	—	—	—	469.8	1.4
Maternal and child health services.................	69.1	13.3	6.3	1.7	1.4	1.0	2.0	—	—	41.9	1.3
Other public health activities	222.9	—	—	—	—	—	—	—	221.1	—	1.8
Veterans' hospital and medical care.................	1,120.9	963.2	9.7	1.1	—	3.1	6.6	1.3	—	115.4	20.5
Medical vocational rehabilitation.............	21.2	9.6	8.7	—	—	—	2.9	—	—	—	—
Office of Economic Opportunity...............	5.6	—	—	—	—	—	—	—	—	5.6	—
State and Local........	4,555.5	2,988.8	421.8	18.5	26.4	81.4	16.2	266.4	447.0	280.2	—
Temporary disability insurance (medical benefits).	50.9	38.3	11.3	—	.6	.4	.4	—	—	—	—
Workers' compensation (medical benefits)........	568.7	195.7	333.6	—	16.7	11.4	11.3	—	—	—	—
Public assistance (vendor medical payments).......	812.1	346.0	67.4	17.1	4.9	69.0	—	266.4	—	41.4	—

TABLE XIII (Continued)

Fiscal Years 1965 and 1976
(in millions)

Program and source of funds	Total	Hospital care	Physicians' services	Dentists' services	Other professional services	Drugs and drug sundries	Eyeglasses and appliances	Nursing-home care	Government public health activities	Other health services	Administration
General hospital and medical care	2,376.8	2,376.8	—	—	—	—	—	—	—	—	—
Maternal and child health services	155.0	26.1	4.2	1.4	4.2	.6	2.7	—	—	115.8	—
School health	132.0	—	—	—	—	—	—	—	—	132.0	—
Other public health activities	447.0	—	—	—	—	—	—	—	447.0	—	—
Medical vocational rehabilitation	13.0	5.9	5.3	—	—	—	1.8	—	—	—	—
Total	$53,300	$30,396	$6,632	$469	$793	$1,023	$114	$5,856	$3,255	$1,627	$3,133

FY 1976[1]

Program and source of funds	Total	Hospital care	Physicians' services	Dentists' services	Other professional services	Drugs and drug sundries	Eyeglasses and appliances	Nursing-home care	Government public health activities	Other health services	Administration
Medicare (health care insurance for the aged and disabled)	17,777	12,809	3,548	—	284	—	—	302	—	835	—
Temporary disability insurance (medical benefits)	74	53	18	—	1	1	1	—	—	—	—
Workers' compensation (medical benefits)	2,125	1,072	902	—	66	43	43	—	—	—	—
Medicaid (public assistance vendor medical payments)	15,320	4,888	1,774	390	397	944	—	5,365	—	728	835

Appendix 513

General hospital and medical care	6,902	6,786	19	4	—	2	—	—	—	—	91
Defense Department hospital and medical care	3,232	2,050	161	6	—	11	—	—	—	25	977
Maternal and child health services	593	90	57	14	46	13	18	—	—	5	350
Government public health activities	3,255	—	—	—	—	—	—	3,255	—	—	—
Veterans' hospital and medical care	3,793	2,555	39	55	—	9	31	189	—	34	881
Medical vocational rehabilitation	229	93	114	—	—	22	—	—	—	—	—
School health[2]	—	—	—	—	—	—	—	—	—	—	—
Federal	36,247	21,394	4,884	288	540	550	61	3,417	1,243	1,322	2,548
Medicare (health insurance for the aged and disabled)	17,777	12,809	3,548	—	284	—	—	302	—	835	—
Workers' compensation (medical benefits)	66	43	17	—	4	1	1	—	—	—	—
Medicaid (public assistance vendor medical payments)	8,381	2,666	968	213	216	515	—	2,926	—	422	455
General hospital and medical care	1,265	1,149	19	4	—	2	—	—	—	—	91
Defense Department hospital and medical care	3,232	2,050	161	6	—	11	—	—	—	25	977
Maternal and child health services	306	47	42	10	36	11	11	—	—	5	144
Government public health activities	1,243	—	—	—	—	—	—	—	1,243	—	—
Veterans' hospital and medical care	3,793	2,555	39	55	—	9	31	189	—	34	881

514 HEALTH AND HEALTH CARE

TABLE XIII (Continued)

Fiscal Years 1965 and 1976
(in millions)

Program and source of funds	Total	Hospital care	Physicians' services	Dentists' services	Other professional services	Drugs and drug sundries	Eyeglasses and appliances	Nursing-home care	Government public health activities	Other health services	Administration
Medical vocational rehabilitation	183	74	92	—	—	—	17	—	—	—	—
State and local	17,053	9,002	1,748	181	254	474	53	2,439	2,012	306	585
Temporary disability insurance (medical benefits)	74	53	18	—	1	1	1	—	—	—	—
Workers' compensation (medical benefits)	2,059	1,029	885	—	62	41	41	—	—	—	—
Medicaid (public assistance vendor medical payments)	6,939	2,222	806	177	180	429	—	2,439	—	306	379
General hospital and medical care	5,636	5,636	—	—	—	—	—	—	—	—	—
Maternal and child health services	287	43	15	4	10	3	6	—	—	—	205
Government public health activities	2,012	—	—	—	—	—	—	—	2,012	—	—
Medical vocational rehabilitation	46	19	23	—	—	1	4	—	—	—	—
School health[2]	—	—	—	—	—	—	—	—	—	—	—

[1] Preliminary
[2] Data no longer available

Sources: B. Cooper, "Public and Private Expenditures for Health, FYs 1965-68 and Calendar Years 1965-67," Social Security Administration, *Research and Statistics Note* 22 (November 11, 1968); Table 4; R.M. Gibson and M.S. Mueller, "National Health Expenditures, FY 1976," *Social Security Bulletin*, April 1977, p. 11. For technical footnotes, see these sources.

TABLE XIV Consumer Prices and Medical Care Components, Average Annual Percentage Change, Selected Periods, 1950-1976, and Total Percentage Increases, 1965-1976

	1950-1960	1960-1965	1965-1970	1970-1975[a]	1975-1976	Total Percentage Increase 1965-1976
CPI, all items	2.1	1.3	4.2	6.8	5.8	80.4
Less medical care	—	1.2	4.1	6.7	5.5	78.8
CPI, all services	3.6	2.0	5.7	6.5	8.3	95.7
Less medical care	—	1.8	5.4	6.3	7.9	90.7
Medical care, total	3.9	2.5	6.1	6.9	9.6	106.4
Medical care services	4.2	3.1	7.3	7.6	10.1	125.8
Hospital service charges[b]	—	—	—	—	12.4	—
Semiprivate room	6.6	5.8	13.9	10.2	13.8	253.9
Operating room charges	—	—	11.4	11.0	14.8	231.5
X-ray diagnostic services	—	—	5.1	6.1	11.8	92.1
Physicians' fees	3.4	2.8	6.6	6.9	11.3	113.5
Dentists' fees	2.5	2.4	5.3	6.3	6.4	86.8
Routine laboratory tests	—	—	3.3	6.3	6.0	69.3
Drugs and prescriptions	1.7	-.8	.7	1.6	6.1	25.8

[a] The Economic Stabilization Program was in effect for more than half this period, August 1971-April 1974.
[b] This index was not introduced until January 1972.
— not available.

Source: Derived from *Consumer Price Index*, U.S. Bureau of Labor Statistics.

FIGURE I   Proportion of Gross National Product Spent on Health Services, International Comparisons, 1960, 1969, and 1973

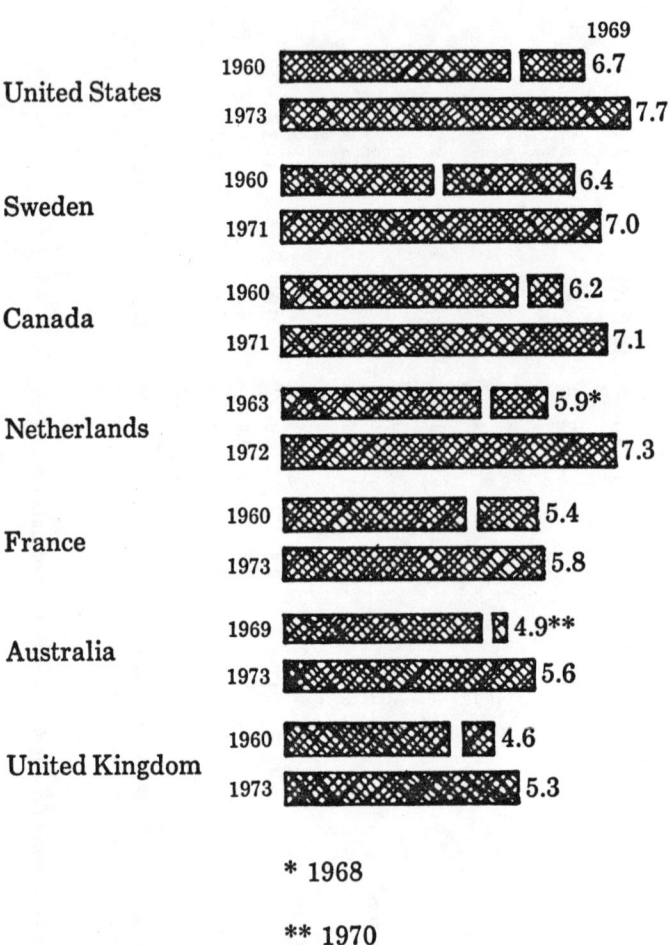

* 1968

** 1970

Source: Robert Maxwell, Principal, Health Economics Office, McKinsey & Co., Inc., London, "International Health Costs and Expenditures: An Hors d'Oeuvre," in T. Hu, ed., *International Health Costs and Expenditures*, U.S. Department of Health, Education, and Welfare, HEW Publ. (NIH) 76-1067, 1976, p. 7.

Index

A

Abbeyfield Society, 381
Academic Medicine. *See* Medical schools
Access
  financial factors, 431-433, 452-472
  hospital facilities, 441-446
  manpower supply, 436-439
  quality of care, 446-452
  type of care, 433-436
Accidents. *See* Occupational health
Accreditation, 25, 447, 448
Acion, Jan, 257
Advisory Committee on Hospital Effectiveness, 136, 240, 461
Advisory Council on Social Security, 159
Aetna Life and Casualty, 134
AFL-CIO, 98, 110, 181
Age Concern, 381
Amalgamated Clothing Workers of America, 119
Ambulatory care, 46, 67, 85-86, 87, 94, 185, 226, 228, 252, 366 443, 449, 467
  geriatric day hospitals, 380
  public accountability, 283-284
  quality protection, 285-288
American Academy of Family Practice, 286
American Academy of General Practice, 59
American Arbitration Association, 300
American Bar Association, 295
American Board of Family Practice, 286, 447
American Board of Internal Medicine, 286, 447
American Board of Medical Specialties, (ABMS), 447
American Cancer Society, 312
American College of Hospital Administrators, 299
American College of Physicians, 34, 37, 278, 286
American College of Preventive Medicine, 308, 417, 422, 424
American College of Surgeons, 34, 35, 37, 157, 283, 287, 299

American Federation of Labor (AFL) Medical Service Plan of Philadelphia, 119
American Geriatric Society, 379
American Hospital Association (AHA), 34, 97, 128, 131, 159, 165, 181, 208, 228, 230, 236, 283, 294, 313, 457
American Medical Association (AMA), 28, 34, 35, 68, 121, 149, 160, 161, 162, 165, 171-172, 179-180, 181, 183, 222, 277, 279, 294, 295, 354
American Nurses Association, 165
American Pediatric Society, 353
American Psychiatric Association, 34
American Society of Internal Medicine, 278, 286, 288, 449
American Surgical Association, 299
Anderson, Ferguson, 387
Annenberg Institute of Communications, 347
Argonaut Insurance Company, 290, 291
Associated Hospital Service of New York, 133
Association of American Medical Colleges (AAMC), 43, 438, 440, 441, 455
Association of Osteopathic Physicians and Surgeons, 451
Atchley, Dana W., 73

B

Babcock, Kenneth, 37
Ball, Robert, 433, 445-446
Bandura, Albert, 350
Barnett, Arnold, 352
Barr Committee. *See* Advisory Committee on Hospital Effectiveness
"Basic Principles for Rehabilitation of the Injured Worker," 157-158
Bauer, Katharine, 452, 460, 461
Baylor College of Medicine, 346
Beeson, Paul, 384
Bell, W. G., 355
Biggs, Herman, 143
Biomedical research, 7-15, 40, 316, 402, 403, 406
Biomedical Research Panel, Presidents, 405, 406, 407

517

Blue Cross (BC), 94-95, 110, 111, 112, 113, 114, 119, 120, 121, 123, 125, 128-131, 133, 159, 164, 165, 175, 181, 243, 236, 248, 249, 283, 359, 458, 459, 466, 469
Blue Cross Association (BCA), 133, 168, 344, 422-423
Blue Cross-Blue Shield Plans, 134, 138
Blue Shield (BS), 94, 111, 112, 113, 123, 130, 136-141, 244, 283, 344
Brecher, Edward, 57
Breslow, Lester, 406, 420
British Geriatric Society, 379, 385
British National Health Service (NHS), 186, 190, 364, 366, 367-368, 369, 372-375
  financing, 378, 382-383
  geriatric care, 377-390
  home health aides, 355
  research grant system, 10
British United Provident Association (BUPA), 367
Brookings Institution, xvii
Brotherston, John, 375
Bureau of Health Education, 308
Busse, Ewald, 379
Byrnes, John W., 160, 161

C

California Medical Association, 69
California Physicians Service (CPS), 112-113
Canada, 150, 391-392, 461-462, 470
Carnegie Report, 43-44
Carter, Tim Lee, 189
Casualty Actuarial Society, 148
Cater, Douglass, 351
Catholic Hospital Association, 208
Center for Disease Control, 308, 403
Certificate-of-need (C/N), 188, 239, 241, 242, 251, 260-261, 382, 443, 455-457
  impact of regionalization, 262-267
  market regulation versus, 255-260
  problems, 268-274
Certification
  admissions, 244
  hospital, 447
  physician, 286, 298, 447
CHAMPUS, 146, 431

Cherkasky, Martin, 91
Chicago Union Health Service, 119
Child Abuse Prevention and Treatment Act of 1974, 347
Children
  abuse, 347
  impact of television on, 348-349
Church, Frank, 358
Civil Service Commission, U.S., 134
Clean Air Act of 1970, 412
Coal Mine Safety and Health Act of 1969, 414
College of Medicine and Dentistry of New Jersey-Rutgers Medical School, xvii, 226, 326
Commission on Medical Malpractice, 290, 292, 293
Committee for National Health Insurance, 181
Committee on Economic Security, 180
Committee on the Costs of Medical Care, 104, 259, 427
Committee on the Nation's Health, 180
Commonwealth Fund, 43
Community Health Association of Detroit (CHA), 120
Community Nursing Services of Philadelphia, 248
Communiversity, 46, 49
Comprehensive care, 43, 206-208
  insurance plans, 118-125, 126-128, 132-133, 135
  models, 208-229
Comprehensive Health Planning (CHP), 239, 240, 241, 252, 270
Comprehensive Health Planning Act of 1966 (P.L. 89-749), 309, 446
Comprehensive Training and Employment Act of 1973 (CETA), 356
Comptroller General of the United States, 357-358, 359
Congress, U.S., 134, 168, 170, 180, 231, 232, 240, 241, 252, 412, 439, 441, 450
  See also specific committees and subcommittees
Consumer health education, 189, 307-308, 421-424, 451
  definition, 424
  hospital-based, 319-320, 322-331

need for, 310-319
  recommendations, 320-322
Consumer-patients
  expenditures, 103-104, 504-507
  health care utilization, 76-84
  health insurance preferences, 123-125
  health responsiblity, 79, 309, 419-25
  hospital attitudes, 92-93
  media influence, 347-349
  medical records access, 298
  participation, 41-42, 67-68, 71, 311
  Patient's Bill of Rights, 283
  representation, 270-271, 283, 311
  right to die, 450-451, 452
  suit-prone, 69
  See also Consumer health education; Doctor-patient relationship; Malpractice
Continuing education, 26, 286, 298, 447
Cooper Hospital, New Jersey, 272
Cooper, Theodore, 401
Cornell Medical Index, 71
Cosin, Lionel, 386-387
Cost controls, 452-455, 471-472
  capital expenditures, 255-275, 455-457
  competition, 465-469
  fraud, 471
  hospital organization, 469-470
  hospital rates, 243-244, 267-268, 457-464
  physician reimbursement, 464-465
Council of Europe, 364, 364-365
Council on Medical Education and Hospitals, 34
Cowley Road Hospital, Oxford, England, 387
Crichton, Michael, 310-311
Cronkhite, Leonard, 219, 220
Crowe, Beryl, 245
Cushing, Harvey, 64

D

Danderyd Hospital, Stockholm, Sweden, 371
Darley Ward, 43, 67, 70, 213-215
Darling case, 301, 449
Dawson, Marshal, 151
Dearborn, Ned, H., 53

Death rates, 237, 315, 346, 397, 412, 414, 423, 492, 493
  infant mortality, 371, 413
  occupational, 51, 53, 414
Defensive medicine, 302, 469
Delaware Valley Hospital Council, 258
Delivery systems, 195-196, 229-233
  European, 364-376
  franchised hospitals, 99-100, 216-217
  Garfield system, 218-219
  group practice, 221-223
  hospital-based model, 206-217, 225-229
  Kaiser model, 223-225
  neighborhood health centers, 219-221
  price competition, 465-467
Denmark, 368
Denver General Hospital, Denver, Colorado, 43
Derbyshire, Robert, 298
Directors of medical education (DME), 47
Disability insurance, 94
Doctor-patient relationship, 56, 60, 82-83, 286-287, 345
  changes, 65-68
  dependency, 62-63
  deterioration of, 68-70
  educational, 71-74
  medical school setting, 39-42
  traditional, 61-62, 63-65
Dodd, Walter, 147
Downey, E. H., 52-54, 156
Drug therapy, 72
Dubois, René, 317, 320
Duke University, 59-60
Dunbar, Flanders, 70

E

Ebert, Robert, 46, 47
Economic Stabilization Program (ESP), 236, 240, 241, 246, 454, 457
Edwards, Charles, 233
Egeberg, Roger, 292
Eisenhower, Dwight, 181
Eldercare program, 160, 161, 179
Elderly, 333-334, 354-355, 443, 500
  geriatric care, 377-390

520 HEALTH AND HEALTH CARE

health insurance, 160, 161, 162, 169, 181, 502
home services, 355-362
hospital utilization, 95, 96, 467
population growth, 377-378
See also Medicare; Nursing homes
End-stage renal disease (ESRD) program, 265-267
Energy Research and Development Administration, 403
Engel, Arthur, 364, 370
Environment
 protection, 411-417
 research, 402-403
Environmental Protection Agency (EPA), 403, 412, 413
Essex County Medical Society, 119-120
Evans, John, 48, 391, 392
Ewing, Oscar, 180
Experimental Medical Care Review Organizations (EMCROs), 448

F

Family practice, 38, 56, 59, 226
Farquhar, John, 423
Federal Employees Health Benefits Program (FEP), 113, 133-135, 138, 200, 203, 222
Federal government
 health expenditures, 236-237
 quality controls, 447-449
 rehabilitation program, 153-158
 research grants system, 7-15
Federal Insecticide, Fungicide, and Rodenticide Act (FIFRA), 413
Federal Trade Commission (FTC), 465
Federation of American Hospitals, 466
Finance Committee, Senate, 161, 168, 172, 240
Fishbein, Morris, 169
Flexner, Abraham, 43, 48
Flexner Report, 27, 43
Fogarty International Center, 308, 417, 422
Food and Drug Administration (FDA), 313, 447-448
Foreign medical graduates (FMGs), 288, 437, 438, 439

Forgotson, E. H., 27, 31
Franchised hospitals, 99-100, 216-217
Franks Commission, 10
Fraud, 471

G

Gabor, Dennis, 490
Garfield, Sidney R., 218
Garfield system, 218-219
Gaus, C. R., 459-460
General Accounting Office (GAO), 232
General Motors Corp., 237
Genetic research, 407
Geriatric care, 377, 379-390
 See also Elderly; Home health care; Homemaker-home health aids; Nursing homes
Gibbon, John H., Jr., 128
Gilpin, Robert, 12
Glasser, Ronald J., 427
Godber, Sir George, 385, 386
Goldwater, Barry, 159
Great Britain
 See British National Health Service
Greater Delaware Valley Regional Medical Program, 248
Green, Michael, 383, 385, 389
Greenberg, Selig, 147, 152
Gregg, Alan, 36
Group Health Insurance (GHI), 94-95, 119, 120, 124, 132-133, 134
Group practice, 77
 growth, 221-223
 health insurance plans, 114, 120, 122, 123, 132, 133
 negative characteristics, 36
 quality control, 36-37, 123, 127, 128, 133
 See also Health Maintenance Organizations
Gunderson, Gunnar, 35

H

Halifax Medical Center, Daytona Beach, Florida, 301
Hamilton, Alice, 54
Hamilton Hospital, New Jersey, 272

Index 521

Hanse, Horace, 28-29
Hardin, Garrett, 244-245, 246
Harvard University, 407
Hastings, James, 395, 396
Haverford College, xvii
Havinghurst, Clark, 257, 258
Hawaii Medical Service Association (HMSA), 138, 344
Hawley, Paul R., 35
Health
  definition, 317-318
Health and Hospitals Corporation of New York, 217
Health care
  costs, 100-105, 125-126, 235, 248, 316, 333-335, 368-369, 396, 443, 464, 479-481, 504-516, 517-518
  utilization, 76-84, 236, 258
  See also Delivery systems; Health care regulation; Quality of care
Health Care Administration Board (HCAB), 263, 265, 268, 269, 270, 273
Health care cororations (HCC), 228, 230
Health care facilities
  definition, 268
  See also Hospitals; Neighborhood health centers; Nursing homes
Health care personnel, 87, 436-439, 493
  credentials, 31-33, 447
  shortage, 60
  unionism, 97-98
  utilization, 77
  See also Medex; Nurse practitioners; Physician extenders; Physicians; Physicians assistants; Primex
Health care regulation
  capital expenditures, 255-275, 455-457
  planning, 239-242, 250-254, 262
  rates, 243-244, 267-268, 457-464
  See also Certificate-of-need
Health departments, 248, 264, 266
Health education
  See Consumer health education
Health, Education, and Welfare, Department of (DHEW), 136, 168, 220, 231, 232, 233, 240, 241, 265, 266-267, 276, 292, 329, 347, 404, 412, 414, 419, 421, 440, 442, 443, 448, 450, 455, 457, 459, 461, 464, 465, 471

Health Information Foundation-National Opinion Research Center (HIF-NORC), 103, 104, 120
Health insurance, 431
  comprehensive prepayment plans, 118-125, 126-128, 132,-133, 135
  cost regulation, 125-130
  coverage, 94, 120, 134, 137, 359, 431, 434, 502
  development, 109-111, 130-135, 236-237
  financial structure, 504-505
  participation, 431-432, 434, 502
  pricing policies, 113-114, 120-121, 127, 128, 134, 135
  problems, 114-118, 121-125, 136-138
  public programs, 143-179, 512-516
  recommendations, 135-136, 138-141
  types, 112-115
  utilization, 94, 124, 135
  See also National health insurance
Health Insurance Association of America, 181
Health Insurance Benefits Advisory Council (HIBAC), 168, 358, 359
Health Insurance Plan of Greater New York (HIP), 45, 94-95, 114, 119, 120, 121, 123, 126-127, 131, 134, 175
Health Maintenance Organization Act of 1973, 111, 231-232, 467
Health Maintenance Organizations (HMOs), 44, 138, 221, 223, 231-232, 255, 258-259, 443, 466-467
Health Manpower Training Act of 1971, 40
Health of Regionville, 76-77, 83
Health Professions Educational Assistance Act of 1963, 15
Health Professions Educational Assistance Act of 1976 (P.L. 94-484), 439-441
Health Security Program, 181
Health Services and Public Health Act of 1968, 381
Health Subcommittee, House, 395
Health Systems Agencies (HSAs), 240, 251, 252, 455, 457
Hershey, Nathan, 32
Hiatt, Howard, 246

Hill-Burton program, 34, 172, 222, 239, 240, 241, 251, 252, 441, 442, 443
Hollingshead, A. B., 77-78, 82-83
Holmes, Oliver Wendell, 68
Home health agencies, 167, 355, 356, 357, 358
Home health aides. *See* Homemaker-home health aides
Home health care, 248, 355
  financing, 357-359
  Great Britain, 381-382
  recommendations, 361-362
  services, 356
Homemaker-home health aides, 60, 355-356, 359-360
Hospital Association of New York, 97
Hospital Association of Risk Managers, 301
Hospital associations, 97, 290-291, 294, 451, 459
Hospital Plan for England and Wales, 372
Hospitals, 248, 249, 250, 429, 430-431
  accreditation, 35, 447, 448
  ambulatory care, 46, 67, 85-86, 87, 226, 228, 366, 380
  community, 35, 40, 41, 44-49, 86, 213-215, 228, 236, 440, 442, 466, 467, 498
  consumer education, 313-314, 319-331
  cororate liability, 90, 301, 449
  development, 85, 86-87
  European, 365, 366, 367, 368, 369, 370-375, 380-381
  expenditures, 236, 442, 455-456
  franchise system, 99-100, 216-217
  geriatric care, 380-381, 386-388
  licensure, 297, 497
  malpractice, 288, 289, 290, 291, 294, 299, 300
  market competition, 465-467
  organization, 89-91, 469, 470
  personnel, 31-33, 97-98
  preventive programs, 301
  prices, 87, 102-103, 236
  prognosis committee, 451
  proprietary, 88-89, 173, 230-231, 257, 466

  regionalization, 86, 91, 206-217, 225-233, 446
  regulation, 34-35, 243-244, 255-275, 447
  reimbursement, 128-129, 171-176, 457-464
  risk control programs, 301
  supply, 441-446
  teaching, 40, 45, 46, 48, 59, 65, 67, 86, 87, 226, 365
  types, 87-91
  utilization, 86-87, 92-96, 121, 135, 138, 226, 258, 368, 387, 442, 467-469, 498
  voluntary, 88-92, 98, 173, 466
  See also Nursing homes; Professional Standards Review Organization
Hospital Survey Committee, Philadelphia, 248, 249, 250
Hunterdon Medical Center, Flemington, New Jersey, 225-227, 440

I

Industrial Medicine, 150
  See also Occupational Health
Institute of Medicine (IOM), 296, 391, 440, 441, 445, 449
Insurance Services Office (ISO), 289, 293
Interior, Department of, 414
International Association of Industrial Accident Boards and Commissions (IAIABC), 146, 149-150, 152, 154
International Ladies Garment Workers Union, 119
Inter-Society Commission for Heart Disease Resources, 420

J

Jackson, Jesse L., 415
Jacobi, Abraham, 353
Javits, Jacob, 188, 433
Johns Hopkins Hospital, Baltimore, Maryland, 78-79, 81, 227
Johnson, Lyndon B., 107-159, 161
Joint Commission on Accreditation of Hospitals, 34, 283, 287, 447, 448
Joint Underwriters Association, 290

Index 523

K

Kaiser Foundation Health Plan, 114, 119, 120, 121, 123-124, 132, 134, 138, 186, 198-199, 203, 232, 440, 467
Kaiser-Permanente Medical Care Program, 223-225, 344
Karolinska Hospital, Sweden, 371
Keene, Clifford, 203
Kennedy, Edward, 181, 200
Kerr-Mills program, 160, 161, 162, 177, 178, 181
Kessler, Henry H., 150-151
Kidd, Charles V., 14
King-Anderson bill, 159, 161
Kittredge, John, 343, 344
Koch, Edward, 358
Koos, E. E., 76

L

Labor, Department of, 153
Labor and Public Welfare Committee, Senate, 438-439
Labor Health Institute of St. Louis, 119
Lalonde, Marc, 391, 392
Lambertville Family Health Center, New Jersey, 226
Lankenau Hospital, Philadelphia, 313
Larson Commission, 121, 123, 222
Lee, Roger, 35
Liberty Mutual Center, 154
Liberty Mutual Insurance Company, 155
Licensure
 continuing education, 298
 criticisms, 27-31
 disciplinary action, 28-31, 297
 health care facilities, 260, 261, 265, 447
 hospitals, 297, 447
 physicians, 27-33, 297-298, 447
 purpose, 27
 relicensure, 298, 447
 task delegation, 31-33
Liebert, Robert, 346
Life expectancy, 333, 377, 385, 397, 413, 493
Lifetime Health Monitoring Program (LHMP), 336-343, 345

Lippmann, Walter, 351
Local Authority Social Services Act of 1970, 381
Logan, Robert, 374-375
Long-Ribicoff bill, 186, 187, 433

M

Maccoby, Nathan, 423
Magnuson Report, 180
Malinowski, Bronislaw, 62
Malpractice, 449
 delegation of authority, 32
 insurance, 237, 288-291
 legal reforms, 293-296
 professional response to, 298-299
 suits, 68-70, 232, 290, 292-293, 300
Manpower, *See* Health care personnel
Maternal and Child Health and Crippled Children's Program of 1935, 188, 232, 241, 260, 277
Maud Commission, 373
McCarran Act, 198
McGee, Lemuel C., 72
McKeown, Thomas, 389
McNerney, Walter, 258, 344
Meals-on-wheels, 356, 382
Medex, 437
Medicaid, 101, 177-179, 181, 188, 232, 239, 240, 241, 244, 260, 273, 277, 334, 359, 396, 432, 443, 448, 449-450, 454, 457, 458, 471
Medical Assistance for the Aged (MAA), 160, 181
Medical care. *See* Health care
Medical care foundations, 277
Medical licensing boards, 26, 29
Medical practice acts, 297
Medical procedures
 appropriateness of, 302, 450-451, 469
Medical records, 230
 patient access, 298
Medical schools, 27, 37
 academic freedom, 13-14
 community hospital affiliation, 40, 41, 44-49
 federal grant support, 7-15, 439
 growth, 436-437
 health care delivery role, 42-44

patient relationship, 39, 41-42
  problems, 38-41
Medical societies, 28, 37-38, 69, 119-120, 123, 127, 128, 148, 149, 176, 217, 222, 232, 277, 286, 290, 294, 297, 298, 300, 448, 451, 465, 471
Medical Society for Care of the Elderly, 379
Medical technology
  development, 3-6, 479-481, 482-485
  political process and, 481-490
Medicare, 101, 184, 188, 205, 232, 237, 239, 240, 243, 260, 265, 267, 277, 334, 358, 359, 431, 433, 434, 443, 448, 454, 457, 459, 464, 466, 467, 471
  deductibles and coinsurance, 164-165
  formulation of, 158-163, 203
  implementation, 166-169
  reimbursement, 170-177
  structure, 163-164
Medicare-Medicaid reform bill (S. 3205), 458, 470
Medicredit, 181
Menninger, Karl, 71-72
Mentally ill
  attitudes toward, 77-78
  hospital facilities, 442
  psychiatric care, 71-72, 78, 82-83, 93, 369
Mercy Community Hospital model, 209-211, 212
Metropolitan Life Insurance Company, 313
Metropolitan University Hospital model, 211-212
Metzger, Norman, 97-98
Michigan State University, 45
Mills, Wilbur, 160
Monmouth Medical Center, New Jersey, Health Education Program, 322-327
  financing, 328-329
  teaching methods, 328
  VD hotline, 326, 327-328
Montefiore Medical Group, 131
Morgenstern, Joseph, 349
Moss, Frank, 358
Mount Sinai School of Medicine, 45
Mt. Zion Hospital, San Francisco, 227
Myrdal, Gunnar, 370

N

National Academy of Sciences, 295-296, 440
  See also Institute of Medicine
National Advisory Commission on Health Manpower, 222
National Aeronautical and Space Administration, 403
National Assistance Act of 1948, 380, 381
National Association of Insurance Commissioners (NAIC), 292-293
National Board of Medical Examiners, 447
National Board of Review
  proposed, 462
National Cancer Institute, 403
National Healthcare Act, 181
National Center for Health Services Research, 408
National Center for Health Statistics, 315, 347
National Commission on Community Health Services, 209
National Commission on Diabetes, 420
National Conference on Preventive Medicine, 308, 337, 338, 416-417
National Conference on Private Health Insurance, 136
National Consumer Information and Health Promotion Act of 1976 (P.L. 94-317), 308, 421, 422, 424
National Council for Homemaker-Home Health Aide Services, 356, 357, 358
National Council of Senior Citizens, 159
National Council on Health Education
  proposed, 314
National Council on Health Planning and Development, 252
National Environmental Protection Act of 1969, 412
National Governors' Conference, 181
National Health Council, 395
National Health Forum, 395
National health insurance (NHI), 432, 445-446, 454
  catastrophic insurance issue, 186-188
  cost, 196, 197
  cost control issue, 188

cost-sharing issue, 184-186
criteria for, 192-195
financing mechanism, 182-184
impact of, 195-196
legislative history, 179-181
long term care issue, 189
preventive care issue, 189
problems, 197-200
proposal, 200-203
National Health Planning and Resources Development Act of 1974 (P.L. 93-641), 188, 233, 240, 241, 250-254, 261, 270, 395, 437-438, 446, 455, 458
National health policy guidelines, 397-399
environmental protection, 411-417
health-related research, 401-409
life style modification, 419-425
universal access, 427-472
National Health Service. *See* British National Health Service
National Health Service Corps, 439
National Heart and Lung Institute, 423
National Institute of Enviromental Health Sciences, 403
National Institute of Mental Health, 408
National Institute of Occupational Safety and Health (NIOSH), 403, 412, 414
National Institutes of Health (NIH), 8, 10, 15, 251, 308, 402, 404, 406, 408, 417, 420, 424
National Labor Relations Act (NLRA), 97, 98, 251
National Leadership Conference on America's Health Policy, 395
National Planning Association, 402
National Professional Standards Review Council, 277
National Service Act, 381
National Service Corps
proposed, 320-322
Neighborhood health centers, 60, 220, 231, 311
Netherlands, 355, 369
Newhouse, Joseph, 258
New Jersey Health Care Facilities Planning Act (NJSA 26:2Hl, et seq.), 261-267

New Jersey Hospital Association, 274-275, 435
New Jersey Medical Society, 451
New York State Moreland Act Commission, 450
New York State Temporary Commission on Living Costs and the Economy, 450
New Zealand, 368
Nilsson, Goth, 369
Nixon, Richard, 221, 321
Nork case, 301
Norway, 355, 368
Nurse practitioners, 59, 437
Nursing homes, 355, 357, 398, 443, 447, 448, 449, 500
See also Elderly

O

Occupational health, 414
casualties, 51-55, 414
rehabilitation programs, 153-158
workmen's compensation, 145-152, 153, 431
Occupational Safety and Health Act of 1970, 414
Office of Economic Opportunity (OEO), 60, 220, 231
Office of Health Information and Health Promotion (OHIHP), 421, 424-425
Office of Inspector-General, 450, 471
Office of Vocational Rehabilitation (OVR), 153, 155
Organized labor, 110, 116, 119, 159, 223
Osler, William, 63-64, 70
Our Lady of Lourdes Hospital, Camden, New Jersey, 267
Outpatient departments. *See* Ambulatory care

P

Paramedicals. *See* Medex; Nurse practitioners; Physician extenders; Physicians assistants; Primex
Parsons, Talcott, 64-65
Passaic Valley Health Facilities Council, 264
Patients. *See* Consumer-patients

Patient's Bill of Rights, 283
Pellegrino, Edmund, 286-288
Pennsylvania Hospital, 247
Pennsylvania State University, 45, 59
Perloff Committee, 181, 228
Perth Amboy Hospital, New Jersey, 260-262, 271
Philadelphia Blue Cross, 128-129
Philadelphia College of Physicians, 247, 248
Philadelphia County Medical Society, 128
Philadelphia General Hospital (PGH), 248
Philadelphia Health Management Corporation (PHMC), 257, 258
Physician extenders (PEs), 437
Physicians, 247, 428-429
 certification, 286, 298, 447
 choice of, 146-150
 distribution, 439-441
 European system, 366, 367-368, 374, 388-389
 geriatric specialists, 379
 health educator role, 71-74, 303, 424, 451
 hospital role, 86, 90-91, 469
 income, 237
 licensure, 26-33, 297-298, 447
 malpractice, 288-289, 290, 291, 294, 298-299, 300
 peer review, 127, 128, 232, 277, 287, 297, 447, 448
 prepayment plan opposition, 122-123
 professional changes, 21-26
 quality controls, 35-38
 reimbursement, 176, 453, 464-465
 strikes, 96, 237, 238
 suit-prone, 69
 supply, 436-437, 439-440, 496
 utilization, 77, 79, 368
 See also Doctor-patient relationship; Foreign medical graduates; Medical schools; Professional Standards Review Organization
Physicians assistants, 32, 59-60, 437
Popper, E. M., 80
President's Commission on the Health Needs of the Nation, 180

President's Committee on Health Education, 308
Preventive care, 83, 189, 333, 335-336, 343-344, 389
 life style factors, 419-425
 Lifetime Health Monitoring Program, 336-343
Primary care, 388, 439, 440, 441, 496
Primex, 437
Problem-Oriented Medical Information System, 230
Professional Standards Review Organization (PSRO), 188, 232, 244, 277-280, 283, 448-449, 454
Prudential Life Insurance Company, 346
Psychiatric care, 71-72, 78, 82-83, 93, 379
Psychogeriatrics, 379
Public accountability, 281-283
 ambulatory care, 283-285
Public Health Service, 11, 36-37, 163
Public Health Service Act, 251

Q

Quality of care, 33-35, 36-38, 123, 127, 128, 133, 147, 285-288, 296-299, 447-452
Quinlan, Karen, 264, 435, 450

R

Ravdin, I. S., 37, 128
Redlich, F. C., 77-78, 82-83
Regional Comprehensive- Health Planning Council, 248
Regional Medical Program (RMP), 209, 239, 240, 252, 264, 266, 446
Rehabilitation, 72, 153-158
Renal Disease Program, 265-267, 434
Reston, James, 321
Rhode Island Medical Society, 148
Rice, Dorothy, 258
Richardson, Elliot, 452
Right to die, 450-451, 452
Robert Wood Johnson Foundation, The xvii
Rochester, New York, Home Care Association, 358
Rockefeller, Nelson, 181

Roemer, Milton, 80, 93, 94
Rogers, Paul, 395
Roosevelt, Franklin, 180
Roosevelt, Theodore, 179
Ross-Loos, 114, 121
Rostenkowski, Dan, 395
Roth, M., 383-384
Rothenburg, Michael, 350
Royal College of Nursing, 385
Royal College of Physicians, 379
Royal Commission on Local Government in England, 373
Rush-Presbyterian-St. Luke's Hospital, Chicago, 227
Rusk, Howard, 72
Rutgers University, 137, 226, 326

S

Sand, René, 83
San Joaquin County Foundation for Medical Care, 122, 127, 133, 134
San Joaquin Medical Society, 127, 232, 277
Sargent, Francis W., 219
Saskatchewan Swift Current Program, 127
Scheuer, James, 188, 433
Scott, H. William, Jr., 309
Seaborg, Glenn, 415-416
Seebohm Committee, 381
Select Committee on Government Research, House, 15
Shain, Max, 93, 94
Smoking, 79, 419, 423
Social Class and Mental Illness, 77-78, 82-83
Socialized medicine. *See* British National Health Service; National health insurance; Sweden
Social Security Act, 180, 358
 Amendments of 1965. *See* Title XVIII, Title XIX (below)
 Amendments of 1967, 457
 Amendments of 1972 (P.L. 92-603), 188, 240, 241, 251, 260, 265, 277, 359, 443, 448, 454, 455, 457-458, 464
 Title V, 188, 232, 241, 242, 260, 277
 Title VI, 34, 172, 222, 239, 240, 241, 251, 252, 451, 452, 453
 Title XVI, 251
 Title XVIII, 161, 162-177, 355, 358
 See also Medicare
 Title XIX, 161, 177-179, 358
 See also Medicaid
 See also Hill-Burton program; Maternal and Child Health and Crippled Children's program; Medicaid; Medicare
Social Security Administration (SSA), 160-161, 166, 168, 172, 173, 256, 356, 431, 459-460
Society of Patient Representatives, 283
Solo practice, 37-38, 77, 119, 120, 122, 123, 127-128, 132
Special Committee on Aging, Senate, 459
 See also Subcommittee on Long Term Care
Specialities, 57, 379, 434, 438
Specialty societies, 277, 278, 286, 299, 447, 449, 465
Stanford Heart Disease Prevention Program, 423
State Health Planning Councils (SHPCs), 262, 264, 266, 269-270, 273
States
 certificate-of-need programs, 188, 239, 241, 242, 251, 260-275 382, 443, 455-457
 cost containment, 133, 188, 243-244, 458-460
 franchised hospital system, 99-100
 public health insurance, 179-181
 regulatory role, 240-243, 251
 rehabilitation programs, 153-158
 workmen's compensation, 145-152
St. Barnabas Hospital, New Jersey, 272
Stein Commission, 450
St. Joseph's Hospital and Medical Center, New Jersey, 254-265, 271, 272
Straus, Donald, 121
Strickland, Stephen, 351
Subcommittee on Health, Senate, 406, 422, 458
Subcommittee on Health and Environment, House, 395
Subcommittee on Long Term Care, Senate, 354-355, 358, 359, 360, 471

Supreme Court, U. S., 412
Sweden
  national health system, 186, 190, 355, 365-367, 368, 369, 370-372

T

Talmadge, Herman, 458, 460
Task Force on Consumer Health Education, 308, 350, 422, 424
Task Force on Medicaid and Related Programs, 136, 181
Television
  impact of, 313, 347-351
Tennessee Medical Society, 37
Terry, Luther, 57
Thomas, Lewis, 401
Town-gown conflict, 7-15
Toxic Substances Control Act, 413
Truman, Harry, 162, 180

U

Ullman, Al, 181
Unionism, 97-98, 249, 298
United Mine Workers (UAW), Welfare and Retirement Fund, 95, 119, 120, 126, 132
University of Colorado, 43
University of Indiana, 45, 46, 47
Utilization review (UR), 246, 442, 458

V

Van Steenwyk, E. A., 121
Veneral disease, 79-80, 316
  hotline program, 326, 327-328
Vocational Rehabilitation Council, 154
Violence
  epidemiological approach to, 351-354
  increase of, 346-347
  media role, 347-351
Violence Profile, 347

W

Wagner-Murray-Dingell bill, 180
Water Pollution Control Act of 1972, 412
Ways and Means Committee, House, 159-161, 162, 168, 189, 240, 258
Wesley, John, 65
White, Mary, 323
Wienerman, E., 34
Wiggins, Walter S., 35
Wilson, Harold, 383
Windsor Medical Services (WMS), Windsor, Ontario, 119-120, 122, 127
Workmen's compensation, 145-146, 431
  disability determination, 150-152
  physician selection, 146-150
  rehabilitation, 153-158
World Health Organization (WHO)
  health definition, 317

Y

Youth Horizons, 327

ABOUT THE AUTHORS

Anne and Herman Somers, both nationally recognized authorities on health care, are prolific contributors to the literature of health care. Their writings have appeared in the leading health care journals and books for over 25 years. They have long experience as consultants and advisors to private and public organizations.

Herman M. Somers is Professor of Politics and Public Affairs, Princeton University, and is a noted health care economist.

Anne R. Somers is Professor of Community Medicine and Family Medicine, College of Medicine and Dentistry of New Jersey—Rutgers Medical School, and editor of *Promoting Health: Consumer Education and National Policy* (Aspen Publications, 1976).